DATE DUE

DEMCO 38-296

TRAUMA ANESTHESIA
AND
CRITICAL CARE
OF
NEUROLOGICAL INJURY

Edited by
Kenneth J. Abrams, MD
Assistant Professor of Anesthesiology and Surgery
Mount Sinai School of Medicine
New York, New York;
Director of Anesthesiology
Elmhurst Hospital Center
Elmhurst, New York

Christopher M. Grande, MD, MPH
Executive Director, ITACCS
Baltimore, Maryland

Senior Consulting Editors
Elizabeth A.M. Frost, MD   **Donald S. Prough, MD**

TraumaCare Series
Series Editor
Christopher M. Grande, MD, MPH
Executive Director, (ITACCS)
Baltimore, Maryland

Futura Publishing
Company, Inc.
Armonk, NY

ıblication Data

Trauma anesthesia and   ⸱eurological injury / edited by
  critical care of   ande.

.... and Critical Care Society."
Includes bibliographical references and index.
ISBN 0-87993-625-8
    1. Neurological intensive care.   2. Anesthesia in traumatology.
3. Nervous system—Wounds and injuries.   I. Abrams, Kenneth J.
II. International Trauma Anesthesia and Critical Care Society.
III. Series.
    [DNLM: 1. Central Nervous System—injuries.   2. Anesthesia—
methods.   3. Critical Care—methods.   4. Emergencies.   WL 354
T7773   1997]
RC350.N49T73   1997
617.4′8044—dc21
DNLM/DLC
for Library of Congress   97-14865
                                                                 CIP

Dedication

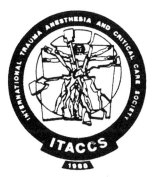

This volume is dedicated to the head-injured and those who care for them.

*This book is dedicated to my children:
Harris and Gayle Abrams,
my most precious legacy*

KJA

*To my lovely wife,
Dr. Lesley Wong, with love
and gratitude for all the years
of understanding and support.*

CMG

Acknowledgments

Trauma Anesthesia and Critical Care of Neurological Injury is the product of the hard work of extraordinarily talented contributors who have generously and tirelessly given their time and expertise. We thank them for their patience and support of our project. This text appears under our names and, thus, we accept full responsibility for its contents. In the development, we ourselves learned a great deal from these distinguished scientists and physicians. We thank our publisher, Steven Korn, for helping this dream become reality.

Kenneth J. Abrams, MD - Special thanks and appreciation to my secretarial staff Rolanda Taylor-Brown and Rosalie O'Hara, and to my Administrative Assistant, Marilynn Finz, who worked diligently without complaint. Tremendous gratitude to my faculty and colleagues for allowing me the time to devote to this project. A special note of recognition to my mentors, Dr. Joel A Kaplan and Dr. Paul L. Goldiner, for their guidance and support. My most sincere gratitude and thanks to Dr. Philip Podrid, whose never-ending support and encouragement has inspired my career. Most of all I thank Dr. Merceditas M. Lagmay for her love and understanding.

Christopher M. Grande, MD, MPH - I recognize that for an author/editor of any book, one of the most important benefits of participating in a book project is what one learns, not only about the technical subject matter being presented, but also about one's self and one's colleagues. This book project has been very satisfying in that regard. Indeed, I have much to be grateful for, given my past 10-year affiliation with the ITACCS organization, which has afforded me many opportunities for personal and professional growth and experience. On a personal level, it is also important to recognize those who supported me over the past decade, and whose loyalty and faith in me have enabled me to go "one step beyond." The space here does not allow me to thank each and every one of these wonderful people to whom I owe great debts of gratitude. However, most importantly has been my lovely wife, Dr. Lesley K. Wong, for going that one step beyond with me.

Finally, we thank our patients who inspire us to learn more about the injuries that afflict them.

Senior Consulting Editors

Elizabeth A.M. Frost, MD
Professor and Chair, Department of Anesthesiology, New York
Medical College, Valhalla, New York

Donald S. Prough, MD
Rebecca Terry White Distinguished Chair, Professor and Chair,
Department of Anesthesiology, The University of Texas Medical
Branch, Galveston, Texas

Contributors

Kenneth J. Abrams, MD
Assistant Professor of Anesthesiology and Surgery, Mount
Sinai School of Medicine, New York, New York; Director of
Anesthesiology, Elmhurst Hospital Center, Elmhurst, New
York

Neal Bodner, MD
Memorial Same Day Surgical Center, Hollywood, Florida

Anne F. Boudreaux, MD
Fellow in Critical Care Medicine, University of Florida,
Gainsville, Florida

Tor Buxrud, MD
Consultant Anesthesiologist, Department of Anesthesiology
and Intensive Care, Akershus Central Hospital, Oslo; Flight
Anesthesiologist; Norwegian Air Ambulance, Aal and
Dombaas, Norway

Pierre A. Carli, MD
Professor of Anesthesiology, SAMU de Paris, Department of
Anesthesiology and Surgical Intensive Care, Hospital Necker,
Paris, France

Joseph Darby, MD
Director, Trauma/Neurosurgical ICU; Assistant Professor, Department of Anesthesia and Critical Care Medicine, University of Pittsburgh, Pittsburgh, Pennsylvania

George Desjardins, MD, FRCPC
Assistant Professor of Anesthesiology, University of Miami School of Medicine, Division of Trauma Anesthesia and Critical Care, Ryder Trauma Center, University of Miami/ Jackson Memorial Medical Center, Miami, Florida

Douglas S. DeWitt, PhD
Associate Professor, Department of Anesthesiology, The University of Texas Medical Branch, Galveston, Texas

Elizabeth A.M. Frost, MD
Professor and Chair, Department of Anesthesiology, New York Medical College, Valhalla, New York

T. James Gallagher, MD, FCCM
Professor of Anesthesiology and Surgery, Chief, Critical Care Medicine, University of Florida, Gainsville, Florida

Joseph P. Giffin, MD
Professor of Anesthesiology, SUNY Health Science Center at Brooklyn, Chairman, Department of Anesthesiology, Long Island College Hospital, Brooklyn, New York

Christopher M. Grande, MD, MPH
Executive Director, ITACCS, Baltimore, Maryland

Eiichi Inada, MD
Professor of Anesthesiology, Department of Anesthesiology, University of Teikyo Medical School, Tokyo, Japan

Ronald A. Kahn, MD
Assistant Professor of Anesthesiology, Divisional Director, Vascular Anesthesia, Mount Sinai School of Medicine, Division of Cardiothoracic Anesthesia, Mount Sinai Medical Center, New York, New York

Yoo Goo Kang, MD
Director, Liver Transplantation Anesthesia Department, University of Pittsburgh, Pittsburgh, Pennsylvania

Susan G. Kaplan, MD
Assistant Professor of Anesthesiology, Temple University School of Medicine, Attending Anesthesiologist, Albert Einstein Healthcare Network, Philadelphia, Pennsylvania

Thomas E. Knuth, MD
Chief, Trauma and Surgical Critical Care, Eisenhower Army Medical Center, Fort Gordon, Georgia

W. Andrew Kofke, MD
Professor and Vice Chairman, Department of Anesthesia, West Virginia University, Morgantown, West Virginia

Andrew B. Leibowitz, MD
Assistant Professor of Anesthesiology and Surgery, Mount Sinai School of Medicine; Associate Director, Surgical Intensive Care Unit, Director, Surgical Nutrition Service, Mount Sinai Medical Center, New York, New York

Kazuo Okada, MD
Professor of Anesthesiology, University of Teikyo Medical School, Tokyo, Japan

Gilles A. Orliaguet, MD
Assistant Professor of Anesthesiology, SAMU de Paris, Department of Anesthesiology and Surgical Intensive Care, Hospital Necker, Paris, France

John M. Oropollo, MD
Assistant Professor of Surgery and Medicine, Mount Sinai School of Medicine, Associate Director, Surgical Intensive Care Unit, Co-Director, Neurosurgical Intensive Care Unit, Mount Sinai Medical Center, New York, New York

Irene P. Osborn, MD
Assistant Professor of Anesthesiology, Department of Anesthesiology, New York University School of Medicine, New York, New York

David Powner, MD
Professor of Anesthesia and Critical Care, University of Pittsburgh School of Medicine, Pittsburgh, Pennsylvania

Donald S. Prough, MD
Rebecca Terry White Distinguished Chair, Professor and Chair, Department of Anesthesiology, The University of Texas Medical Branch, Galveston, Texas

Anthony P. Randazzo, III, MD
Assistant Professor of Anesthesiology, Mount Sinai Medical Center, Division of Trauma Anesthesia, Elmhurst Hospital Center, New York, New York

Vance Shearer, MD
Assistant Professor of Anesthesiology, Southwestern Medical Center, Dallas, Texas

Sharyn Tarricone, MD
Instructor in Anesthesiology, Albert Einstein College of
Medicine, Bronx, New York

Steven J. Tryfus, MD
Assistant Professor of Anesthesiology, Mount Sinai Medical
Center, Division of Trauma Anesthesia, Elmhurst Hospital
Center, New York, New York

Albert J. Varon, MD
Professor of Anesthesiology, University of Miami School of
Medicine; Director, Division of Trauma Anesthesia and
Critical Care, Ryder Trauma Center, University of Miami/
Jackson Memorial Medical Center, Miami, Florida

Charles B. Watson, MD, FCCM, FCCP(AN)
Chair, Department of Anesthesiology and Critical Care
Medicine, Bridgeport Hospital, Bridgeport, Connecticut

Torben Wisborg, MD, DEAA
Consultant Anesthesiologist and Chairman, Department of
Anesthesiology and Intensive Care, Hammerfest Hospital,
Hammerfest; Flight Anesthesiologist, Norwegian Air
Ambulance, Bergen, Norway

Mark H. Zornow, MD
Professor, Department of Anesthesiology, The University of
Texas Medical Branch, Galveston, Texas

Foreword

One cannot overemphasize the importance of neurological trauma as a source of morbidity and mortality. In our society at large, statistics are changing but as of this writing, trauma is still the leading cause of death in the first four decades of life and the third leading cause of death overall. Approximately half of these deaths result from traumatic brain injury, which is also a major cause of post injury morbidity.

Many patients with neurological injuries will be managed at general hospitals rather than trauma centers for a variety of complicated reasons. Anesthesiologists may be requested to provide care for patients with overt or hidden neurological injury. For example, a patient scheduled for open reduction of fractured ankle may be progressively developing cerebral edema from a closed head injury. For these reasons, a new book on anesthesia for neurological injury is timely and appropriate.

Because of the international group of experts that Drs. Abrams and Grande have gathered as authors, the scope of this book reaches far beyond the intraoperative management of the patient with head injury. This book also covers the very important facets of prehospital care that occupy anesthesiologists and emergency physicians in many parts of the world. The book also provides extensive coverage of spinal cord injury, another very important facet of neurological injury. Further evidence of the holistic approach of this book are the chapters on critical care of the neurologically injured patient, diagnostic evaluation, nutritional support following neurotrauma, rehabilitation of neurological injuries, and finally, brain death and organ procurement. We predict that this text will become a valuable reference on the shelf of any anesthesiologist who commonly or occasionally manages traumatized patients with neurological injury.

Adolph H. Giesecke, MD
Jenkins Professor of Anesthesiology
Former Chairman of Anesthesiology University of Texas
Southwestern Medical School Dallas, TX

John K. Stene, MD, PhD
Associate Professor of Anesthesia
Penn State College of Medicine
Hershey, PA

Series Editor's Foreword

On behalf of the International Trauma Anesthesia and Critical Care Society (ITACCS), we are pleased and honored to present this volume.

In 1993, after completing the extensive *Textbook of Trauma Anesthesia and Critical Care* (Mosby-Yearbook, St. Louis, 1993), the conclusion was reached that, despite a work of that size, several areas required an in-depth examination at a higher level of magnification. Since that time, ITACCS has focussed on exploring several key issues in trauma anesthesia and critical care individualy and more thoroughly in a series of smaller books, constituting the ITACCS Library. One of those areas pertain to the perioperative management of central nervous system injuries. In keeping with its commitment to the improvement of trauma care, and the support of educational and scientific programs dedicated to that process, ITACCS is proud of its role in bringing this volume to press.

ITACCS is deeply indebted to Dr. Kenneth J. Abrams for doing the lions' share of this book project by melding the superb work of the contributing authors into a timely, well-referenced, multidisciplinary approach to head and spinal cord trauma. They have endeavored to present the reader with a comprehensive treatment of the subject, following the patient from the time of injury, at the scene, during transport, through the emergency room, the operating room, and the intensive care unit. The description of current medical and surgical practice found in this volume reflects contemporary thoughts, and is unique as it is presented within the context of a historical prespective. We are also deeply appreciative of the efforts of the consulting editors, Dr. Elizabeth A. M. Frost and Dr. Donald S. Prough, and especially of Dr. John K. Stene and Dr. Adolph H. Gieseke for having undertaken a critical editorial review of the work assembled by Dr. Abrams and myself before the volume was released to the publisher.

It is not the past or the present of neurological traumatology that deserves the most attention, but rather the future. In order to make a quantum leap that is necessary in truly improving the care of the head and spinal cord injured, three important things must occur:

1) Heightened awareness of the subspecialty of traumatology.
2) Heightened awareness and commitment from the lay communities including the public-at-large, and governmental bureaucracies.
3) A dramatically improved commitment to increased research, education, and clinical support of head and spinal cord injuries, once they have occurred.

ITACCS is poud to present this textbook as one important piece of the future of traumatology.

Christopher M. Grande, MD, MPH

Preface

Although trauma has just recently been surpassed by AIDS as the most common cause of death in the 25–40 year age group, in the United States, it remains a significant cause of mortality and perhaps more importantly, morbidity.

While the herculean efforts to combat HIV have mitigated against much of the severity of this dreaded illness and improved longevity and quality of life, relatively small advances have been made in the treatment of trauma, particularly neurotrauma.

Significant injury, with its residual disability, has a profound impact on patients, their families, and society. Nowhere is the devastating effects of trauma more evident than in neurological trauma. Approximately 50% of all trauma patients suffer neurological injury following blunt trauma; the vast majority of these manifest as head injury. These injuries tax our struggling health care system in all aspects: prehospital resuscitation, intrahospital care, and post-injury rehabilitation. Financially, the impact is profound and often long-lasting, with many years of potential productive life lost to injury. We, as health care providers and physicians, must take a proactive role in formulating the appropriate systems and means to properly care for these victims in order to restore their health and productivity.

It is with this broad view in the forefront that we embarked on *Trauma Anesthesia and Critical Care of Neurological Injury.* We have attempted to approach the effects of neurological trauma along a continuum of care. The primary focus of this book is to stress the importance of understanding the continuing dynamics associated with central nervous system injuries, and to emphasize the essential role of the trauma anesthesiologist in prevention of secondary injury and promotion of optimal outcome.

Trauma Anesthesia and Critical Care of Neurological Injury starts from the scene of the accident and addresses the importance of the "initial responder" in prehospital care and transport of the critically injured. Chapters 3 through 9 discuss the problems inherent in the early stages of intrahospital evaluation and care. Specific sections include discussions on the priorities of resuscitation, immediate intrahospital considerations, airway management, cerebral protection, fluid management, diagnostic evaluations, and anesthetic management in the neuroradiology suite. The next five chapters concentrate on the practical issues of intraoperative and intensive care of patients with head and spinal cord injuries. The subsequent two chapters discuss new pharmacological therapies, and diagnostic and monitoring modalities on the horizon, and their potential impact on the care rendered following neurological injury. Finally, the book concludes with the final outcome, either rehabilitation of the recovering patient and in the case of unfortunate outcomes, the importance of organ procurement and transplantation. Most of the chapters stress a common theme of multispecialty cooperation, communication, and teamwork in order to accomplish the laudable goals of reduced mortality and improved functional morbidity.

Since, by design, *Trauma Anesthesia and Critical Care of Neurological Injury* crosses multiple disciplines, its usefulness goes beyond that of the anesthesiologist. It is intended to serve as a comprehensive reference and a practical textbook to traumatologists, anesthesiologists, neurologists, neurosurgeons, intensivists, emergency medicine physicians, and the many other trauma specialists required for the successful recovery of neurologically injured patients.

Kenneth J. Abrams, MD
Christopher M. Grande, MD, MPH

Contents

Contributors iv

Foreword: Dr. Adolph Giesecke, Dr. John Stene ix

Series Editor's Foreword: Christopher M. Grande xi

Preface: Dr. Kenneth J. Abrams,
          Dr. Christopher M. Grande xiii

1 **Prehospital Anesthetic Management of
   Neurological Trauma**
   Torben Wisborg
   Tor Buxrud 1

2 **Interhospital Transport of Neurotrauma Patients**
   Gilles A. Orliaguet
   Pierre A. Carli 47

3 **Priorities in Initial Resuscitation and
   Perioperative Management: Multitrauma Patients
   with Head, Chest, and Other Major Injuries**
   Thomas E. Knuth
   Charles B. Watson 69

4 **Initial Intrahospital Resuscitation of the Patient
   with Head Trauma**
   George Desjardins
   Albert J. Varon 95

5 **Airway Management in Neurological Injuries**
   Steven J. Tryfus
   Kenneth J. Abrams
   Christopher M. Grande 121

6 **Neuronal Cell Pathophysiology and Modalities of
   Brain Protection**
   Ronald A. Kahn
   Neal Bodner 153

7 **Fluid Management and Resuscitation in Neurological Trauma**
Donald S. Prough
Douglas S. DeWitt
Mark H. Zornow 189

8 **Diagnostic Imaging in Neurotrauma**
Susan G. Kaplan   227

9 **Anesthesia for Neurodiagnostic Evaluation**
Irene Osborn
Sharyn Tarricone 269

10 **Intraoperative Anesthetic Management of Closed Head Injuries**
Elizabeth A.M. Frost 291

11 **Intraoperative Management of Spinal Cord Injury**
Joseph P. Giffin
Vance Shearer 307

12 **Critical Care Management of Closed Head Injury**
T. James Gallagher
Ann F. Boudreaux 341

13 **Critical Care Management of Spinal Cord Injury**
Ann F. Boudreaux
T. James Gallagher 365

14 **Nutritional Care following Neurotrauma**
Andrew B. Leibowitz
John M. Oropello 383

15 **Therapeutic Advances in Neurotrauma**
Gilles A. Orliaguet
Pierre A. Carli 405

16 **Recent Advances in Central Nervous System Monitoring**
Eiichi Inada
Kazuo Okada 435

17 The Role of the Anesthesiologist in Rehabilitation
Anthony P. Randazzo, III 457

18 Brain Death and Organ Procurement
W. Andrew Kofke
Joseph Darby
David Powner
Yoo Goo Kang 499

Index 539

$$\boxed{1}$$

Prehospital Anesthetic Management of Neurological Trauma

Torben Wisborg, MD, DEAA, Tor Buxrud, MD

"The brain is my second favorite organ."
—Woody Allen

Prehospital Strategies in Neurological Injuries

Primary Versus Secondary Injury

Head injury patients have for long been known to "talk and die."[1] Although sustaining an injury that definitely did not initially destroy nervous tissue enough to hinder the expression of meaningful words, these patients develop a series of reactions leading to death from cerebral herniation. This constitutes the basis of "secondary brain injury." At the cellular level, a combination of hypoxia and cerebral hypoperfusion leads to an intracellular oxygen deficit that in turn results in energy failure with intracellular swelling, release of neuro-

From *Trauma Anesthesia and Critical Care of Neurological Injury,* edited by K. J. Abrams and C. M. Grande. © 1997, Futura Publishing Co., Armonk, NY.

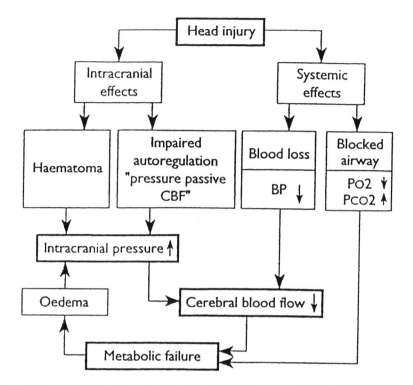

Figure 1. Interaction of systemic and intracranial adverse effects (referred to as "avoidable factors"). From ref. 78 with permission of the author and publisher.

transmitters, and neuronal excitation increasing the already failing energy consumption. At the visceral level, hematoma, edema, and an impaired autoregulation of blood flow combined (Fig. 1) with disruption of the blood-brain barrier increases intracranial pressure. Cerebral blood flow is reduced to ischemic areas, leading to a vicious cycle and increasing the area of neuronal death. Similar changes seem to occur in the spinal cord.[2]

Some of this secondary brain injury is preventable. Among the factors aggravating the secondary brain injury, hypoxia, hypercapnia, and hypotension, combined with a delay in surgical evacuation of intracranial hematomas, are best documented (Table 1). A number of clinical studies have shown that taking away the impact of these "avoidable factors" in patients with serious head injury reduces mortality and morbidity.[1,3–6] One large series found that the incidence

Table 1
Avoidable Factors Aggravating the Initial Brain Injury by Constituting
the Basis for a "Secondary Brain Injury"

- Hypoxia
- Hypercapnia
- Hypovolemia
- Hypotension
- Unrecognized extracranial injuries
- Delayed surgical evacuation of intracranial hematoma

of hypoxia on arrival in the neurosurgical unit decreased from 22% to 8% while the frequency of endotracheal intubation increased from 11% to 82%. Overall mortality was reduced from 45% to 32%.[3]

Some injuries carry an inherent risk of aggravation, not only from secondary brain injury, but also from extension of the primary injury. The unstable fracture of the spine, especially of the cervical spine, is a nightmare for all personnel dealing with neurological trauma.

Most head-injured patients do not require surgery. Only 20–40% have surgically removable mass lesions or extrameningeal hematomas.[7,8] Data suggest that, in patients without other extracranial/extraspinal lesions endangering the circulation, no urgency exists to rush the patient to the hospital. On the contrary, careful immobilization and thorough resuscitation at the scene reduces the degree of secondary brain injury.[1,3–5] With injury-to-hospital times below 1 hour, a twofold increase in transportation time had no adverse effect on outcome, provided this time was spent in preventing "avoidable factors."[4]

Prehospital Treatment: Aims and Means

Advanced prehospital treatment of neurological injuries aims at reducing the consequences of the primary nervous tissue injury, while minimizing the risk of further damage. This is achieved by: (1) precluding the occurrence of "avoidable factors" by proper airway management and ventilatory and circulatory support; (2) prompt recognition and treatment of associated injuries; (3) protecting the spinal cord from damage by unstable fractures when treating/transporting the patient; and (4) careful transportation by a combination of anesthesiologists, other physicians, and nonphysician emergency medical technicians, paramedics, ambulance personnel, and nurses/

nurse anesthetists. As a rule these professionals are limited in number at the scene. The amount of equipment is also reduced. Assuming the prehospital service is delivered by an anesthesiologist, there will seldom be any on-line medical direction and the physician has to make decisions alone. In addition, helpers such as ambulance personnel, paramedics, and nurses are few and may well be occupied with other casualties. One has therefore to become more or less self-contained, not only concerning equipment, but also in decision-making. The realization of this point is one of the most important hurdles an anesthesiologist has to overcome when moving from the "safe" hospital environment to the prehospital service. Another important hurdle is the realization that one has to act as part of a small team, where each team member may be responsible for the security of the team. In airborne missions, the physician may have to act as a navigator for the pilot, while the third crew member is performing a rescue mission below the helicopter (Fig. 2).

Most advanced prehospital units carry equipment comparable to that of an intensive care unit including monitors, infusion pumps, drugs, and airway/circulation support equipment. In emergency medical services employing anesthesiologists, anesthetic drugs and a ventilator are part of the armamentarium. In addition, a limited number of tools for extrication, and collars, splints, and stretchers for immobilization, are a natural part of the equipment (Fig. 3).

Thus, the advanced prehospital trauma anesthesia management of neurological injuries includes all available in-hospital procedures, with the exception of diagnostic imaging and surgery. There is no evidence to support prehospital trepanation or other surgical procedures.

Limitations to the prehospital phase are mainly related to environment and time. At the scene of a crime or in other dangerous environments (e.g., traffic, temperature, avalanches, etc.) the prehospital team must await clearance from the police/rescue personnel before entering, and may have to leave the scene before more than the most necessary tasks have been done. The objective of the treatment has to be borne in mind: to avoid further damage and reduce the secondary brain/spinal injury, which includes surgical evacuation of removable hematomas without *undue* delay.

When to Suspect Neurological Injury

In most trauma patients, the injury is obvious. Any facial or head injury should raise the suspicion of an underlying intracranial

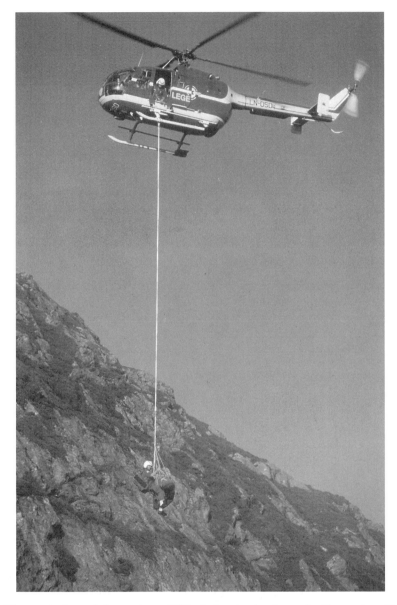

Figure 2. One of the authors (TW) sitting in the door of a Norwegian Air Ambulance operated Eurocopter BO 105 ambulance helicopter guiding the pilot during a underhanging rescue operation. Photo: T. Hillestad, Norwegian Air Ambulance.

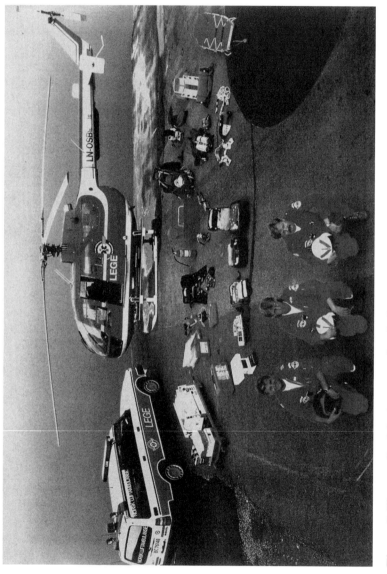

Figure 3. The anesthesiologist-manned ambulance service with emergency car, helicopter and medical equipment in addition to diving, mountain rescue and extrication devices. The crew consists of a pilot, a rescuer and an anesthesiologist. Photo: T. Hillestad, Norwegian Air Ambulance.

injury. Even without such injury any alterations in consciousness *must* raise suspicion of neurological damage. Nevertheless, initial treatment follows ordinary rules to eliminate hypoxia and hypoperfusion as causes of altered mental status. With intracranial lesions the level of consciousness is the cornerstone of diagnosis. Frequent examinations using a uniform approach minimizes inter- and intraobserver variability, and is the best means to detect changes indicative of deterioration (see Neurological Assessment and Scoring below). It is important to remember that a number of patients eventually dying from head injury may have had a period of time after their head injury when they were talking and were described as being completely lucid. In one series, this proportion, of all patients succumbing after head injury, was found to be around 10%.[1] Likewise, it may be underlined that even without a skull fracture, and with completely normal consciousness, but the risk exists of an intracranial hematoma.[9] A skull fracture, even with full consciousness, increases this risk considerably. In both respects, children have a reduced risk, compared to adults.[9]

An injured cervical spine, especially in patients with altered consciousness, evokes great fear among prehospital care providers. Cervical spine injury seems to occur in 2–4% of all major trauma cases, and in contrast to earlier views, there seems to be no difference in incidence between patients with or without head injury.[10,11] Spinal cord injury occurs in 30–70% of patients with cervical spine injury.[11,12] Motor vehicle accidents remain the major cause of cervical spine injury, being responsible for some 50–70%, mainly among men between 15 and 35 years old.[11,12] (see chapter on Epidemiology of Neurological Trauma). Other situations in which one has to be clinically suspicious are falls, especially head-first falls, ejection from automobiles, shallow water diving, other sudden decelerations (e.g., airplane crashes), high-impact contact sports and other major trauma in general. A thorough review of the literature[13] concluded that the only trauma patient in which one can exclude spinal injury is the *fully* alert patient without any pain or tenderness in the neck. For the prehospital treatment, this implies cervical spine precautions for all patients.

Initial Assessment

Primary Survey

The primary survey is a prioritized series of observations aimed at simultaneously identifying and treating life-threatening conditions. By the time this survey has been completed, any necessary resuscitation has already started. When the patient is stable, a thorough secondary survey may be undertaken. It is assumed that the patient is in a safe environment, i.e., no danger of fire, further traffic accidents, firearms, or assault. In general, the patient is not moved unnecessarily. If necessary, the cervical spine is immobilized following the procedure described in the American College of Surgeons Manual of Advanced Trauma Life Support (ATLS™)[14] (discussed in detail below).

The patient is examined where he is found. The primary survey follows the steps "A-B-C-D-E" for mnemotechnical reasons, although most of the survey is carried out simultaneously while obtaining the history. If the patient is unable to report about the accident, detailed accounts of the incident *must* be obtained from bystanders or rescue personnel. Important details include: time of the accident, directions of falling/ejection from automobile, speed of vehicles, and if possible, any past medical history, allergies, and time of last oral ingestion.

Airway and cervical spine: Is the patient able to maintain a patent airway? Is the airway blocked by the tongue, or foreign materials? Chin lift or jaw thrust, combined with suctioning or manual removal of foreign debris is the initial maneuver. *The cervical spine is assumed to be unstable until proven otherwise*, which implies that the head is kept in a neutral position and no movements are allowed before immobilization is applied, and that enough personnel are present to maintain the cervical spine in neutral axis.

Breathing: A patent airway does not guarantee adequate ventilation. The chest has to be exposed for evaluation of breathing. Signs of ventilatory impairment are: asymmetrical chest movements, a respiratory rate <10 or >30 breaths per minute, abnormal respiratory efforts and signs of chest injury. Tension pneumothorax, open pneumothorax, and flail chest with pulmonary contusion are the major injuries compromising ventilation in trauma patients. The initial management is bag-valve ventilation via a face mask. (Prehospital endotracheal intubation is discussed below.) Oxygen should be given to all trauma patients as soon as possible, i.e., during the primary survey.

Circulation: The loss of erythrocytes and intravascular volume is disastrous and yet often easily correctable when identified. Hypotension is assumed to be due to hypovolemia until proven otherwise. During the primary survey, i.e., when the patient examination is done with eyes and fingers, level of consciousness, skin color, and pulse should be evaluated. In head-injured patients, altered consciousness may obviously be caused by the head injury, but this assumption is made when the depressed mental status is present *in spite of* an adequate circulating blood volume. A conscious patient has at least enough blood volume to maintain cerebral perfusion. Pale, white, cold extremities, and especially paleness of the face are signs of hypoperfusion, although a cold outdoor environment may reduce peripheral circulation. Pulses are palpated at the carotid or femoral artery for pulse rate and quality, with rates above 100 and a "fine" thready pulse, suggesting a compromised circulation.

External bleeding should be controlled by direct pressure during the initial survey. Internal bleeding is impossible to diagnose or exclude in the prehospital setting. Isolated head injury bleeding is seldom a problem, and intracranial bleeding is *never* sufficient in adults to explain general circulatory compromise, except for the late and ominous sign of Cushing's reflex caused by intracranial hypertension. On rare occasions, one may experience profuse bleeding from the galeal arteries. Such bleeding is difficult to control by compression, and may be one of the few indications for the prehospital use of surgical clamps. Underneath a galeal tear may be a cranial fracture, and possibly, no bony protection of the meninges, which mandates that clamping be performed with great care.

Disability: The initial survey for disability is a brief neurological assessment that only involves determining the level of consciousness on a four-level scale (AVPU) and pupillary size and reactivity. It is an integral part of the survey already when approaching the patient. The conscious levels are: **A**—Alert, **V**—responds to *V*ocal stimuli, **P**—responds to *P*ainful stimuli, and **U**—*U*nresponsive. Although at this time one may unintentionally observe motor function in the extremities, that sign is part of the secondary survey.

The eyes are briefly examined for pupillary size and reaction.[15] The finding of bilaterally fixed and unreactive pupils is a poor prognostic sign indicating severe hypoxia or intracranial hypertension. A unilateral fixed and unresponsive pupil may herald tentorial herniation due to a large hematoma or intracranial hypertension.[16]

Exposure: The fifth part of the initial survey in the ATLS concept is the total undressing of the patient to facilitate thorough examination. In the prehospital setting this is often unsuitable, as decreased light and temperature extremes do not allow extended examinations.

Resuscitation Phase

Simultaneously with the initial survey the resuscitation phase is started. It is begun while surveying the patient. For the spontaneously breathing patient with an uncompromised airway, oxygen is supplied. Nasal cannulae are inefficient to raise the FiO_2 (an FiO_2 >0.85 is the aim), and a disposable face mask with an oxygen reservoir is preferable. Even better is the use of a face mask, bag and valve (bag-valve-mask apparatus [BVM]) synchronized with the patient's own respiratory movements. If breathing is insufficient, initial ventilation is with a bag-valve with a face mask. However, the endotracheal tube is the only device currently approved in the trauma setting that allows an FiO_2 close to 1.0 and offers protection against aspiration of gastric contents.

Independent of the result of the initial evaluation of the circulation, intravenous access is established. Two separate large-bore cannulae are desirable. The need for rapid infusion may be evaluated, but infusions should be prepared and mounted. Urinary output is a good indicator of renal perfusion, and thus, of circulating volume. Due to the danger of urinary tract infection and the limited time spent on-scene and during transportation, the prehospital placement of a urinary catheter is seldom advocated.

Airway management and circulatory resuscitation are discussed in greater detail below.

At this time, it is assumed that the prehospital trauma anesthesia team has secured vital functions and will immobilize the patient before extrication or transfer to a stretcher. The patient may now be brought to an ambulance or helicopter, and monitoring may be established simultaneously as the patient is thoroughly assessed neurologically.

Neurological Assessment and Scoring

In assessing the neurological function of an injured patient one physician has to report a largely qualitative observation to another, allowing for later reassessments that are comparable to the initial survey. To overcome this problem the Glasgow Coma Scale (GCS) was introduced in 1974.[17] This scale is the most widely used scoring system for neurological injury, and is also used for nontraumatic neurological conditions. It has a favorably low interobserver variability, which allows a longitudinal assessment of the patient by differ-

Table 2
The Glasgow Coma Scale (GCS)

Behavior	Response	Score
Eye opening	Spontaneous	E4
	To speech	3
	To pain	2
	Nil	1
Best motor response	Obeys	M6
	Localizes pain	5
	Flexion withdrawal	4
	Abnormal flexion	3
	Abnormal extension	2
	Nil	1
Verbal response	Oriented to time, place and person	V5
	Confused conversation	4
	Inappropriate words	3
	Incomprehensible sounds	2
	Nil	1

Best score = 16.
Lowest score = 3.

ent observers.[18] The patient (Table 2) is scored according to three different reactions: A score is calculated by addition of the points gained in each aspect. Motor function score from the best extremity is recorded. GCS has been shown to correlate to mortality.[16] A GCS of 8 or less is considered a severe head injury, 9–12 a moderate head injury, and GCS 13–15 a mild head injury. However, one single figure is difficult to interpret. If a patient is examined *shortly* after the injury, he or she may have a GCS below 13 and thus be classified as having a moderate head injury, although the patient may have a GCS of 15 a short while later. Head injury is a dynamic process, and the initial response is largely identical. Repeated examinations starting in the prehospital phase and extending into the hospital may illustrate the changing scores provided these examinations are performed in a structured fashion.

The GCS does not precisely reflect general hemodynamic alterations, as in hemorrhagic shock. Though the brain may be lightly injured, its function may be described as deteriorating by the GCS in a bleeding patient.[19] For this purpose, the GCS has been combined with a physiological score using the respiratory rate and mode, systolic blood pressure and capillary refill as physiological parameters

Table 3
The Trauma Score

Variable	Measurement	Score
Respiratory rate (breaths per minute)	10–24	4
	25–35	3
	>35	2
	<10	1
	0	0
Respiratory effort	Shallow	1
	Retractive	0
Systolic blood pressure (mm Hg)	>90	4
	70–90	3
	50–69	2
	<50	1
	Unmeasurable	0
Capillary refill	Normal	2
	Delayed	1
	Absent	0
Glasgow Coma Scale (GCS)	14–15	5
	11–13	4
	8–10	3
	5–7	2
	3–4	1

Best score = 16.
Lowest score = 1.

to form the Trauma Score (TS) (Table 3). This easy-to-use scoring tool allows good correlation between TS and mortality[21] and high inter-rater reliability in prehospital care.[22] The TS has been further revised to adjust for underestimation of the severity of some head injuries, and to eliminate the need for difficult and unreliable evaluations of respiratory mode and capillary refill. The Revised Trauma Score (RTS) is based on only GCS, systolic blood pressure, and respiratory rate.[23] The RTS has demonstrated substantially improved reliability in outcome predictions compared to the TS.[23]

The scores are very efficient as quality assurance tools, where patient information from one institution may be compared to large pools of information, as in the Major Trauma Outcome Study.[24] They are equally well suited to give an objective indication of the case load on a prehospital emergency medical service (EMS). They also give a good indication of the severity of trauma when calculated prehospitally, and thus the need for referral to trauma centers. However, their value as accurate predictors for single patients have been questioned.[25] A recent, comprehensive review covers the issue of trauma patient scoring.[26]

Neurological scoring in children and infants may be difficult for a number of reasons. A special Coma Scale has been advocated for neurological testing in children.[27]

Progressing along the trauma patient care process, the patient is now in the ambulance or helicopter, monitoring is established (as discussed below), a neurological assessment has been performed and the appropriate therapeutic interventions are complete. It is time for reporting to the base or dispatching hospital for physician-manned services without on-line medical control. The patient is assigned to the appropriate institution and transportation may begin.

Prehospital Performance of Specific Procedures

Airway Management

All head-injured patients should be ventilated to optimize oxygenation and reduce hypercapnia. Aims for the ventilation are $PaO_2 > 15$ kPa (110 mm Hg), and $PaCO_2$ 4.0–4.5 kPa (30–35 mm Hg). Head injury reduces ventilation and produces hypercapnia, recently underlined by a series of prehospital blood-gas analyses, where a very close correlation was found between GCS and level of hypercapnia.[28] Hyperventilation by the bag-valve-mask (BVM) is difficult, even in the hands of experienced personnel.[29] Prehospital care providers are placed in a dilemma between the risk of a possible aggravation of a cervical spine injury versus the need for airway intervention.

Several studies have failed to document anecdotal reports of quadriplegia resulting from intubation in patients with unstable cervical spine fractures.[13,30] Recently, it was even suggested that ventilation with the BVM is the technique producing most cervical spine displacement in patients with cervical spine fractures.[29]

Endotracheal intubation permits the best possible ventilation, high FiO_2, and protection of the patient against aspiration of gastric contents. It is our opinion that endotracheal intubation is the method of choice in the prehospital treatment of head-injured patients. Prehospital endotracheal intubation may be achieved in several ways: blind nasal, nasal with laryngoscopy, oral, or through a cricothyrotomy. No method has been scientifically proven safer than others, and in our opinion, the prehospital anesthesiologist has to use the technique with which he or she is most familiar. This view has recently been supported by a review of methods used by a large number of trauma anesthesiologists.[31] Nasal intubation in patients with suspected basal skull fractures carries the risk of intracranial placement of the endotracheal tube. This is also the reason for the reluctance to place nasogastric tubes. If a cuffed endotracheal tube is in place aspiration is unlikely, and if the flight level during air evacuation is limited to <8,000 feet above sea level, or the cabin pressure is kept at sea level, gastric distention by gas is unlikely.

Indications for prehospital endotracheal intubation are listed in Table 4. We consider the administration of general anesthesia with the use of muscle relaxants before intubation compulsory except in the patient who is unlikely to strain or cough on intubation, and/or unable to produce any significant increase in blood pressure after stimulation by laryngoscopy, i.e., the dying or arresting patient. The use of general anesthesia permits intubation in patients with higher GCS than if only nonreacting patients are intubated without pharmacological support, and thus improves airway protection and permits appropriate ventilation in a larger patient population.[32] The anesthetic technique is discussed in detail below. During the intuba-

Table 4
Indications for Prehospital Endotracheal Intubation and Induction of Anesthesia after Head Injury

Neurological
  Glasgow Coma Scale (GCS) ≤ 8
  Focal symptoms, asymmetrical pupils
  Significantly deteriorating level of consciousness or GCS
  Convulsions
  Bilaterally dilated pupils
  Spontaneous hyperventilation
Airway-related
  Obstructed airway due to injuries/bleeding in face/mandible/oral cavity
  Loss of protective pharyngeal/laryngeal reflexes
  Suspected aspiration of gastric content
  Clinically insufficient ventilation
Others
  As part of pain relief for other injuries
  Before lengthy or complicated extrication

tion procedure one person is assigned to provide stabilization of the head and cervical spine. Neck flexion should be avoided and the cervical spine maintained in a neutral position by a gentle manual in-line axial stabilization. A thorough discussion is found in the chapter on Airway Management in Central Nervous System Injuries, and elsewhere.[13]

In services without the ability to induce general anesthesia in the field, indications for intubation have to be restricted. The use of an oropharyngeal airway may be an adjunct to the BVM ventilation, making it easier to maintain a patent airway. Especially in head-injured patients, it is easy to induce nausea and vomiting by the insertion of the airway, and this maneuver has to be done with great care and attention.

It is wise to remember the neurological assessment before inducing anesthesia and relaxation. The in-hospital neurological examination may be greatly disturbed by deliberate muscle relaxation that nevertheless may be necessary to provide a secure airway and adequate ventilation.

Circulatory Resuscitation

The choice of intravenous fluids for circulatory resuscitation, the estimation of the severity of hemorrhagic shock, strategies for resuscitation, and special considerations for the neurologically injured patient are detailed in the chapter on Fluid Management and Resuscitation in Neurological Trauma. Only techniques suitable for prehospital infusion, technical difficulties, and primary goals are discussed in this section.

Intravenous access is best achieved in visible, peripheral veins using catheter-over-needle intravenous cannulae. As large a cannula as possible is chosen. It is often possible to place 14 G/2.0 mm O.D. cannulae (allowing a flow of 270 mL/min) in forearm veins. Starting as peripherally as possible, it allows for later attempts more centrally. It is wise to use the right upper extremity initially, as the left arm is most easily accessible during transportation in ambulances and in some helicopters. If no visible peripheral veins are found, it is often possible to access the greater saphenous vein which lies anterior to the medial malleolus, even without seeing it. It is *always* there. When a vein has been successfully punctured, the cannula must be secured to the skin to prevent dislodgement in patients who are wet, cold, and dirty. Specifically, it is recommended that the cannula to be taped in a circular fashion around the extremity, allowing the tape to adhere to itself.

If no peripheral veins are found, the external jugular may be punctured. Before applying the cervical collar, the vein is digitally compressed just above the clavicle. In-line manual stabilization of the cervical spine is maintained. Though theoretically inappropriate, it may be helpful to raise the foot-end of the stretcher a few degrees immediately before and during puncture. When the cannula is in place and secured, the cervical collar may be applied.

The third approach is the femoral vein. It lies just medially to the femoral artery, and may be punctured with an intravenous cannula of ordinary length in slim adults, although a longer cannula is preferable. Venipuncture is easiest if a saline-filled syringe is mounted on the needle before puncture to allow constant aspiration while searching for the vein, and to identify the correct placement of the catheter more easily. The femoral vein accepts cannulae of great dimensions, but infusions below the diaphragm are less desirable when suspicion of intra-abdominal injury exists.

If these attempts are unsuccessful, further approaches rely on the experience of the anesthesiologist or professional in charge. In adults, the experienced anesthesiologist would probably prefer to try to catheterize the subclavian vein. Cannulation is possible without compromising the cervical spine protection (in contrast to the internal jugular vein approach), and with a large-bore catheter-over-needle the procedure does not take long. As with the external jugular puncture it may be helpful to *briefly* elevate the foot-end of the stretcher. Alternatively, venous surgical access may be performed. This is traditionally performed at the greater saphenous vein, but has the disadvantage of being below the diaphragm in case of abdominal or pelvic injury. Both approaches carry a certain risk of infection, which has to be accepted as the price for obtaining venous acces. In children, and increasingly in adults, the intraosseous route may be chosen after failed attempts at peripheral cannulation. Through this approach all relevant medications may be given, and large volumes of fluid may be infused.[33-35] Our suggested approach to prehospital vascular access is illustrated in Figure 4.

The infusion rate of fluid from plastic bags through a venous cannula is governed by gravity, viscosity, temperature, diameter of the cannula, and intravenous pressure/resistance. It is often necessary to apply pressure around the infusion bag, especially in vehicles where height above the patient is reduced. Traditionally, this has

Peripherally in arms *(use right first)*

↓

Peripherally in feet

↓

External jugular *(remember cervical spine stabilization)*

↓

Femoral vein

ADULTS   CHILDREN

↙   ↘

Subclavian   Intraosseous

↓   ↓

Cut-down/intraosseous   Cut-down/subclavian

Figure 4. Suggested approach to prehospital vascular access.

been done with pneumatic devices manually inflated around the bag. Thus pressure decreases as the fluid leaves the bag. The pneumatic infusion device manufactured by Alton Dean Medical, Inc. (Utah, USA) overcomes this problem by using any source of pressurized gas, maintaining a constant infusion pressure, adjustable between 0 and 300 mm Hg. It can be used in vehicles as well, provided there is access to pressurized gas.

The diameter of the cannula chosen should be as large as possible. The vein will often accommodate a larger catheter than is possible to introduce by the cannula-over-needle technique, if a vein dilator and guidewire are used. However, this procedure takes time, and should be done only if a low flow in the primary cannula may be improved by a larger catheter.

Even when using infusion fluids heated to 37°C in the ambulance or helicopter, the fluid will often be cold when entering the circulation, especially in frigid and outdoor prehospital settings. Several devices have been invented to overcome this problem, but few have been of any practical benefit. The Norwegian Army invented the Heatpac™ personnel and infusion heater (Norwegian Defense Research Establishment, NATO no. 8465–25–128–3804), which is able to heat 0°C fluid to 12°C with a flow rate of 25 mL/min at an ambient temperature of ÷ 20°C, and 16°C fluid to 25°C under identical conditions.[36,37]

Recent research in animal models indicates that rapid infusions in uncontrolled hemorrhage may in fact increase mortality and morbidity rates.[38–41] The significance of these studies to the prehospital treatment protocols remains to be evaluated. In our opinion, the head-injured patient with hypotension needs rapid restoration of circulating volume to avoid the risk of secondary brain injury. The possible risk of infection or induced hypothermia are secondary considerations.

Immobilization and the Extrication Phase

Immobilization and extrication are procedures carried out mainly by ambulance or rescue personnel, according to the local organization. These procedures are unfamiliar to the anesthesiologist or other physician not trained in prehospital emergency medicine. Extrication is the phase of rescue where the patient is released from a situation in a vehicle that hinders the free transfer to a stretcher. The extrication phase carries danger to the patient and challenges to the anesthesiologist in the field and will be considered in detail. Extrication should be a coordinated process in which the prehospital anesthesiologist and ambulance personnel secure the patient, while rescue or fire personnel remove obstacles from the patient. Merely lifting the patient out of a damaged vehicle involves the risk of aggravating injuries. These procedures should always be planned and discussed among identified individuals responsible for the medical team and for the rescue team, before commencing. In more complicated situations, the use of advanced tools may carry danger to the personnel as well as to the patient, which further underlines the need for this coordination.

Before extrication is begun, the primary survey and resuscitation should be completed as quickly and as far as possible, and during the extrication the prehospital anesthesiologist and ambulance personnel should continuously support the cervical spine and survey vital functions. In lengthy extrications, it may be necessary to establish intravenous access and perform other procedures before the patient is released, in addition to administration of oxygen. Small portable monitors (discussed below) may be applied to the patient before extrication.

Thorough immobilization includes securing the patient's head and total spinal column in the neutral midline position before moving the patient. Immobilization devices are tools to *reduce* the danger of secondary spinal injury, although they *will not* be able to completely preclude it. Immobilization starts with gentle, manual in-line stabilization of the head during the airway assessment in the primary survey. The head is brought to and kept in the neutral position, unless this procedure results in increased pain, muscular defense (i.e., spasm), neurological symptoms, or a compromise of the airway.

After life-threatening conditions have been excluded, a rigid cervical collar is applied, which reduces the possibility of compression of the cervical spine but does not preclude movement of the neck.[42] It is of paramount importance that the collar is chosen according to the size of the patient because a collar that is too high may cause traction of the cervical spine, and one that is too short may merely compress soft tissue. With the collar in place, the patient is secured to some kind of backboard. Ideally, the whole spine should be immobilized, i.e., from the sacrum to the head, but in sitting patients, as in cars, short boards extending from the lumbar spine to the head are applied. Because many adult patients have a distance of several centimeters from the posterior margin of the occiput to the posterior margin of the scapulae in the neutral, supine position, padding below the head may be necessary. In children the opposite is true, and padding below the scapulae may be required to prevent the large occiput from causing cervical flexion during immobilization on a backboard. After the patient is safely positioned and tightly strapped to the backboard he or she may be moved.

Many services use the log-roll maneuver to place lying patients on the board. In this maneuver, the patient is rolled with the arms beside the body as a unit (Fig. 5).[43] This method of rolling seems to

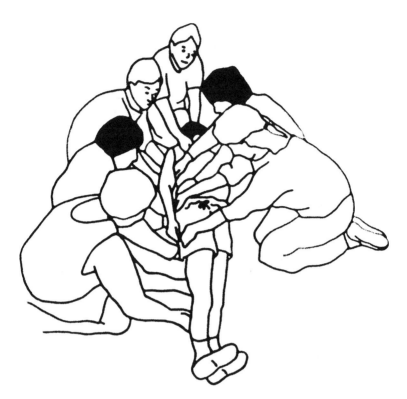

Figure 5. The log-roll maneuver.

be able to give a high degree of movement in the spine with unstable fractures,[44] whereas the scoop stretcher offers better protection. The scoop stretcher consists of two separate parts that interlock when applied (Fig. 6). It may be slid under the patient virtually without movement and offers the possibility for carrying or transfer to an ordinary stretcher while maintaining the spine immobile. Another recent invention is the vacuum mattress, which consists of thousands of tiny isopore balls within a plastic mattress. When air is evacuated from the mattress (by a simple hand- or foot-operated suctioning device), it becomes rigid, and may be carried in almost all positions. It is particularly suitable for patients trapped in difficult positions, where the soft, air-filled mattress may be molded to slide under and fit to the body. Thereafter, it may be emptied by vacuum and used as a stretcher in extrication and transportation (Fig. 7).

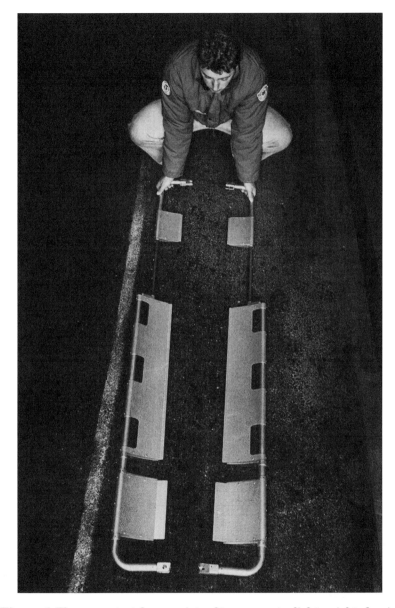

Figure 6. The scoop stretcher consists of two separate, light weight aluminium parts. When slid under the patient they will lock together to form a rigid stretcher, adjustable in length. Photo: T. Hillestad, Norwegian Air Ambulance.

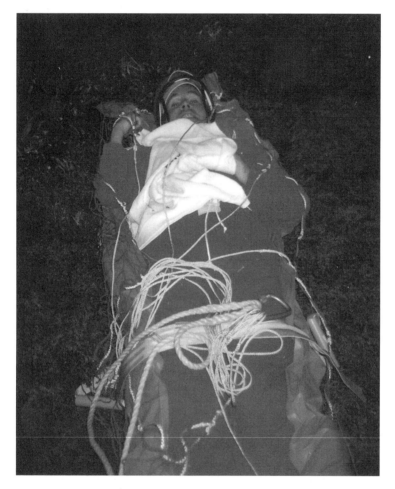

Figure 7. The vacuum mattress shown with a patient wrapped into the deflated, and thus rigid, mattress. When emptying the mattress for air, by applying vacuum, it becomes rigid and useable as an ordinary stretcher. During the evacuation of air it may be molded as to suit the patient. Photo: L. Fossedal, Norwegian Air Ambulance.

Exposure and Helmet Removal

Exposure of the patient at the scene is recommended only to the degree necessary for the initial survey for external bleeding, to observe penetrating foreign bodies and to be able to choose the right level of treatment for the patient. The risk of hypothermia should delay a thorough exposure and secondary survey until reaching the hospital, or at least the ambulance or helicopter. If necessary, the exposure is done by cutting the clothes in the midline of all extremities, unwrapping the body, and leaving the cloth underneath the patient initially.

Motorcyclists and others wearing protective helmets present a special problem to the rescuers. These patients have a high risk of cervical spine injury, and often a depressed level of consciousness. The helmet must be removed to allow airway assessment and procedures, to be able to treat the patient in case of vomiting, and to allow placement of the head with the cervical spine in neutral midline position. The procedure is illustrated in Figure 8a-d. One person is assigned to maintain manual in-line cervical stabilization. This rescuer sits beside the patient's body and supports the head by holding the mandible with one hand, and the occiput with the other. A second rescuer releases the chinstrap and applies outward traction on both sides of the helmet while the helmet is lifted. To avoid the nose with the chinpiece of the helmet, it may be necessary to roll the helmet slightly backwards. The rescuer controlling the head is in command, and is responsible for avoiding neck movement. When the helmet is removed, the rescuer at the head-end of the patient takes over the manual in-line stabilization, while the other applies the cervical collar.

Specific Treatment of Spinal Cord Injury

Spinal cord injury may be obvious at the scene, e.g., in patients manifesting neurological deficit in the extremities. Although catastrophic to the patient, there is potential for recovery. Mortality for this group is low,[45,46] although a number of very high-level spinal cord-injured patients die at the scene. The economic implications for society are equally dramatic.[45] Any treatment that could improve outcome would be of immense importance.

Pathophysiological changes in the spinal cord are comparable to those in secondary brain injury.[2] Therefore, it must be assumed

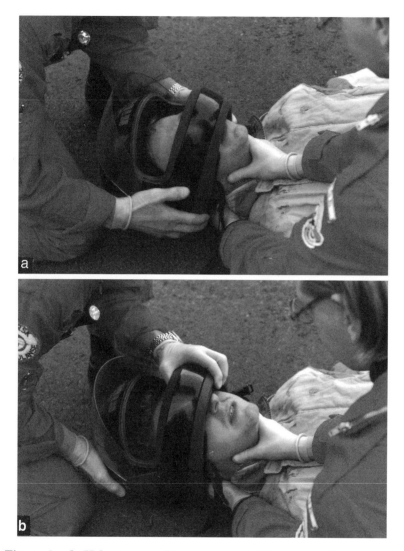

Figure 8 a, b. Helmet removal in sequences. **(a)** One person is assigned to maintain manual in-line cervical stabilization. This will be the rescuer sitting beside the patient's body. He will support the head by holding the mandible with one hand, and the occiput with the other. A second rescuer releases the chinstrap and applies outward traction on both sides of the helmet while the helmet is lifted up. **(b)** To avoid the nose with the chin-piece of the helmet it may be necessary to roll the helmet slightly backwards. The rescuer controlling the head is in command, and is responsible for avoiding movement of the neck.

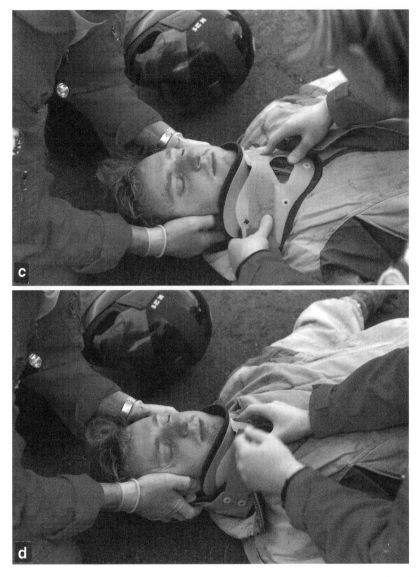

Figure 8 c, d. (c) When the helmet is removed, the rescuer at the head end of the patient takes over the manual in-line stabilization. **(d)** The other rescuer applies the cervical collar. Photos: T. Hillestad, Norwegian Air Ambulance.

that meticulous attention to "avoidable factors" will give equally good results in spinal cord injury. In addition, several pharmacological trials have been performed. One that has proved valuable is the early administration of high-dose steroids.[46,47] However, this therapy results in statistically significant improvements only when started within the first 8 hours after injury. As 8 hours were used as the cut-off point, one may assume that earlier administration would be more beneficial, which is why this therapy should start prehospitally. In the study, 30 mg/kg body weight of methylprednisolone was given as an intravenous bolus over 15 minutes, followed after 45 minutes by a 23-hour infusion of 5.4 mg/kg/hour of methylprednisolone. This therapy did not result in dramatically improved results, but even minor neurological improvement may have major functional importance.

Spinal cord injury may result in loss of sympathetic tone in the lower body, and even in loss of the cardioaccelerator nerve supply to the heart. Hypotension in the trauma patient should nevertheless be considered a result of hemorrhage until proven otherwise. Initial treatment is fluid loading, not vasopressors. Bradycardia should be treated symptomatically. A high level of preparedness should be taken to prevent pulmonary edema, which may result from the fluid load and decreased cardiac reserve due to loss of sympathetic stimulation.

Specific Treatment of Intracranial Hypertension: Mannitol

Control of intracranial hypertension is achieved primarily by securing adequate ventilation by induction of anesthesia and relaxation, followed by tracheal intubation. Other "avoidable factors" should be eliminated. Proper positioning, i.e., elevation of the upper body approximately 30° and avoidance of rotation in the cervical spine, is another element in treatment.

The use of mannitol to control raised intracranial pressure (ICP) is controversial, especially in later phases of trauma treatment. A number of studies have given contradictory results concerning the efficacy. Part of the discrepancy may be different experimental models. Most neuroanesthesiologists today recommend the use of mannitol in the early phase after a head injury with poorly controlled intracranial hypertension. This applies to both prehospital and in-hospital treatment.[48] However, many head-injured patients are hy-

Table 5
Indications for Prehospital Administration of Mannitol

In the prehospital setting mannitol is recommended for:
- treatment of severe focal symptoms (paresis, asymmetrical pupils)
- signs of severe intracranial hypertension (bilaterally dilated, fixed pupils in spite of adequate oxygenation, ventilation and circulation)
- GCS ≤ 7
- rapid neurological deterioration as evidenced by falling GCS

povolemic, and the diuretic effect of mannitol may increase existing hypovolemia and thus aggravate the head injury. Recent interest has therefore focused on treating multitraumatized patients with hypertonic saline. Hypertonic saline seems to have the same effect as mannitol on intracranial hypertension, in addition to a pronounced volume-expanding effect.[49] Hypertonic saline might therefore be preferable to mannitol, but more experimental work, especially clinical studies, has to be undertaken before it is recommended as a routine.

Indications for prehospital administration of mannitol are listed in Table 5. The aim of prehospital mannitol treatment is to save time. The infusion of mannitol increases urine production within 15–30 minutes. If a hospital cannot be reached within 30 minutes, we recommend the insertion of a urethral catheter. Mannitol is infused, rather than injected, during 10–20 minutes, to avoid sudden changes in blood pressure and thus possible changes in cerebral blood flow and intracranial pressure.[50] Dosage is 0.5–1 g/kg initially, supplemented by 0.2–0.5 g/kg every 4 hours.

Prehospital Induction of Anesthesia in the Neurologically Injured Patient

The induction of anesthesia and muscular relaxation places the anesthesiologist in control of the airway, ventilation, and to a certain degree, cerebral metabolic rate. The semiconscious patient thrashing around on a stretcher with an unprotected cervical spine, unable to protect himself from aspiration and with insufficient ventilation is in immediate danger and aggravates the secondary brain injury. Early intervention in this category of patients is of proven value.[3,28,51] On the other hand, induction of anesthesia in these circumstances is difficult and may be dangerous to the patient.[7] Except in the patient without any reflexes, in an arrest or pre-arrest situation, the performance of intubation without prior administration of general anesthesia is inappropriate, especially in head-injured patients.[52]

For simplicity and safety, the prehospital approach to induction of anesthesia has to be rather uniform with respect to drugs, equipment, and technique. In prehospital practice the use of inhalational agents including nitrous oxide is difficult and unnecessary. (Some services are using Entonox, a 50% N_2O/O_2 mixture for analgesia. We have no experience with this in prehospital use.) All intravenous agents are theoretically possible to use. For a detailed discussion the reader is referred to the chapters on Anesthesia for Neurodiagnostic Evaluation and Intraoperative Management of Closed Head Injuries. We suggest using a barbiturate (we use thiopental), a benzodiazepine (we use midazolam), an analgesic (we use morphine and fentanyl), and two neuromuscular blocking agents (we use succinylcholine and vecuronium). Equipment includes a laryngoscope with two blades, Magill's forceps, various endotracheal tubes, and tape or gauze for fixation, a failed intubation kit with cricothyrotomy equipment, self-inflating ventilation bag, oxygen, a hand/foot-operated suctioning device with large capacity, and, in the helicopter, a pressure-driven ventilator. When indicated, anesthesia is induced primarily where the patient is found, although it is preferable to place him on a stretcher. The equipment listed above must be present. Adverse environmental factors may dictate the transferral of the patient to an ambulance or a helicopter prior to induction, although space in vehicles often hampers optimal cervical spine stabilization.

All patients are considered as having an unstable cervical spine. They are also assumed to have a full stomach, placing them at risk of gastric aspiration, as well as raised ICP. Many of the patients, in addition to head injury, have other injuries, and may thus be hypovolemic. The anesthetic technique should therefore reduce the risk of cervical movement during intubation, prevent gastric aspiration, prevent increases in ICP, and maintain cardiovascular stability. If possible, the anesthetic may well reduce the ICP.

Monitoring during induction in the prehospital phase reflects these concerns. Monitoring should *at least* include ECG, noninvasive automatic blood pressure measuring, and pulse oximetry. Capnography is highly desirable. A complete discussion of prehospital monitoring follows.

As in the hospital, an anesthetic plan is made prior to induction. Our "ideal" anesthetic technique includes the use of three persons, one of whom may be a professional not from the helicopter team, e.g., an ambulance technician. It is of great importance that all personnel involved are well aware of the plan. After the primary survey and resuscitation are completed the patient is ventilated with 100% O_2 via bag and mask. Fluids are being infused, and monitoring is as previously described, with the monitors visible to the anesthesiologist. Drugs are prepared in syringes and the paramedic takes responsibility for the manual in-line stabilization of the cervical spine. Now the front portion of the cervical collar may be removed to allow the assistant to apply cricoid pressure and, if necessary, remove any obstruction to emergency cricothyroidotomy. The anesthesiologist ventilates and administers the drugs intravenously. Intubation is done in a rapid-sequence procedure with administration of hypnotic and muscular relaxants almost simultaneously. We prefer direct orotracheal intubation, and are reluctant to pass nasogastric tubes before the cranial base has been x-rayed. Confirmation of tube position is done by auscultation with a stethoscope and, if available, capnography. The patient is initially ventilated manually, and eventually by the ventilator, and the cervical collar replaced. The endotracheal tube is *secured well* (we recommend adhesive tape in a circular fashion around the neck, allowing the tape to adhere to itself, but avoiding compression of the jugular veins), and the patient is strapped to the backboard again.

After intubation, vital signs are rechecked, bearing in mind that a simple asymptomatic pneumothorax may develop into a tension pneumothorax after positive pressure ventilation, and that circulation may be disturbed by the altered intrathoracic pressures as well as the anesthetic drug effects.

Prehospital Monitoring

The use of monitors prehospitally is intended as a supplement to what is visible and audible without any equipment. A monitor constructed for prehospital use should ideally be light, easy to carry and apply, visible from different angles and under different lighting conditions, and battery-operated with a battery capacity of several hours which allows recharging with 12 or 24/28 V in vehicles. The software should allow for configuration by the user to give only significant information. Alarms should be both audible and visual, and of an intensity to attract attention in environments with a high level of noise and poor lighting. Alarms should be configurable to react only to variables considered significant for the situation.

The monitor should be understandable to nonphysicians, and

reveal only information from connected equipment (i.e., if no ECG leads are attached, it should not show a flatline ECG). Trend recording is desirable. Interface to computers may be desirable, as may be the possibility for radio transmission of signals to a medical control. Built-in printers should be unnecessary, as paper copies may be obtained via an interface to a printer. Also, they occupy space and consume electrical power.

For practical reasons it is desirable to assemble as many functions as possible in one monitor; however, the EMS is then much more vulnerable in case of equipment failure. A backup unit should always be available.

Parameters that are included in a prehospital monitoring system are as follows:

ECG has been an established natural component of all patient monitoring schemes, mainly to detect arrhythmias and cardiac ischemia. Although arrhythmias are frequent after head injury, this population does not have a high prevalence of ischemic heart disease. ECG monitoring is highly susceptible to electrical noise and motion, and may thus be misinterpreted and cause confusion. However, the ECG comes along with most monitors, but should not be the first variable monitored.

Blood pressure is of great importance in trauma patients, and it is desirable to have a reliable, automatic oscillometric blood pressure cuff as part of the monitor. The equipment gives systolic, mean, and diastolic blood pressure through direct measurement of oscillations in the cuff. It is the most power-consuming part of most monitors, and the measurement interval has to be easily adjustable. Invasive blood pressure is relevant for secondary transports, but seldom is relevant in the primary prehospital setting.

Pulse oximetry provides an instant picture of the oxygenation of arterial blood and, if combined with a graphic display of the plethysmographic wave, may give qualitative information comparable to that of an arterial wave [53,54]. Some monitors have, however, a self-adjusting scale, in which a decreasing plethysmographic amplitude suddenly may be "inappropriately" enlarged by scale adjustment, leading to false impressions. Other pitfalls in pulse oximetry include the inability of the pulse oximeter to react to methemoglobin and carboxyhemoglobin. The pulse oximeter reports only the difference between oxy- and deoxyhemoglobin. It is necessary to emphasize that a high oxygen saturation shown by pulse oximetry does not indicate adequacy of ventilation, which is indicated only by the carbon dioxide level in the arterial blood.

End-tidal CO_2 (ETCO$_2$) gives an indication of the arterial level of carbon dioxide. It confirms endotracheal tube position, and gives early warnings about greater changes in circulation. Because the arterial CO_2-level is of paramount importance for cerebral circulation, the recent invention of portable capnographs is one of the great advances in prehospital monitoring. In mainstream measurements, the analyzer is attached directly to the endotracheal tube and analyzes virtually without delay. Although placed directly at the endotracheal tube, it is small and light, and is troublesome only in small children and infants. At present, we are not aware of battery-operated side-stream ETCO$_2$-analyzers. Their advantage is the absence of the analyzer at the endotracheal tube connection; their disadvantage is a short delay in measurement depending on sample tube volume and sampling flow rate. The use of ETCO$_2$ analyzers in moving vehicles has not yet been scientifically evaluated. The disposable, colorimetric ETCO$_2$ analyzers have been evaluated as adjuncts to confirming correct endotracheal tube position,[55] but precision seems lacking for continuous determinations of ETCO$_2$.

It is useful to measure temperature in cases with suspected hypothermia. It assumes low priority in the prehospital phase of neurological injury, because there are few possibilities to actively heat the patient, and protection against thermal loss should be performed irrespective of patient temperature.

Neuromuscular blocking monitors are also of little relevance in the prehospital phase. Intubated patients must be relaxed, and a relative overdosage has minor consequences.

An example of a portable monitor suitable for prehospital use is shown in Figure 9.

When in the helicopter or ambulance little or nothing is heard of audible alarms. It is therefore important that visible alarms are sufficient to attract attention. In some aircraft, there are no curtains between the cockpit and cabin, which is inappropriate from a flight safety and a medical point of view. If the monitor has to be used in such an environment it is advantageous to be able to dim the light emitted from the monitor screen for night and instrument flight conditions.

Patient Transportation

Three concerns are addressed in this section: (1) *who* is to treat and transport the patient; (2) *in which vehicle*; and (3) *to what institution*—if one is in the position to choose. It is important to under-

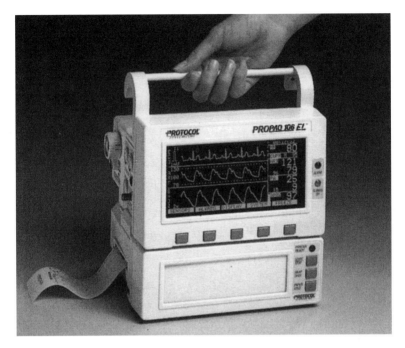

Figure 9. An example of a portable monitor suitable for prehospital use with the following parameters: ECG, automated blood pressure, invasive pressure, temperature, pulse oximeter and capnograph (Protocol, Beaverton, OR, USA). Courtesy Jean Mette Medical A/S.

stand that every prehospital caregiver is presumed to be treating patients to the best of his abilities, and that the recommendation of a certain staffing model or configuration of a fleet of vehicles does not indicate any underrating of existing services. This discussion addresses the optimal standards of care, and should, in fact, underline the need for improved services when less than optimal in the interest of patient care.

Prehospital Personnel: Anesthesiologists in the Field

Staffing of prehospital services varies throughout the world. The prevailing question is whether or not physician staffing is beneficial. Several investigators have tried to evaluate this problem with varying conclusions.[4,56–59] In some studies, physicians were able to perform procedures that other professionals were not trained or certified to perform,[4,58] whereas in others, medical judgment has been the most substantial contribution from physicians.[56] A recent paper attempted to determine whether the physician should be an anesthesiologist or a general practitioner.[59] Fifty percent of the life-saving missions were considered to be dependent on the use of anesthesiologists. This suggests that the use of anesthesiologists prehospitally improves patient care.[59] Cost of physicians in contrast to paramedics was estimated to be 7% of the total program cost in another study,[56] with "benefits far outweighing costs."

The working environment in a prehospital service is quite different from in-hospital work. Through proper training, personnel can be prepared for difficulties and changes, and thus maintain appropriate judgment and performance under unusual conditions. However, experience seems to be very important to ensure proper performance.[60]

There is probably no single optimal staffing model for prehospital EMS. In services with a high load of relatively homogenous patients, full-time nurses or paramedics probably perform as well as physicians in "routine" patients, especially with on-line medical control. However, in services employing part-time professionals, with heterogenous patients or without on-line control, physicians have the best capability to perform judgment and exercise skills. According to local organization these physicians should be thoroughly trained in airway management, venous access, induction of anesthesia and emergency medicine/intensive care procedures, all of which are capabilities of the anesthesiologist.[59]

Vehicles

Most of the scientific differences between land ambulances and airborne units are due to differences in staffing, equipment, and treatment protocols. Rapid transportation per se is seldom of importance, except in situations of uncontrolled hemorrhage and in long travel distances. However, working conditions and treatment possibilities on board vehicles differ greatly.

Some helicopters are small and allow access to the upper part of the patient only, while Figure 10 others offer excellent conditions. Most helicopters have satisfactory lighting and heating, while the noise level and vibration varies considerably. Size of the cabin seems to have some influence on time consumption to perform specific Ad-

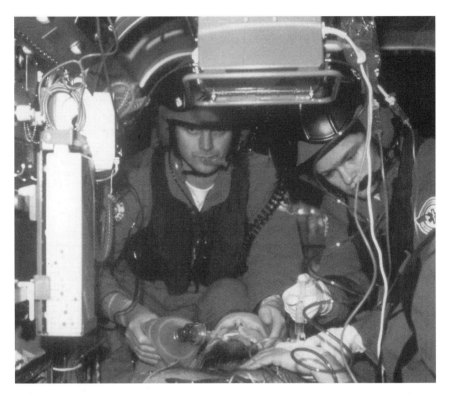

Figure 10. The interior as seen from behind in a Norwegian Air Ambulance Eurocopter BK 117, a medium-sized ambulance helicopter, which offers moderate good conditions as regarding space. Photo: T. Hillestad, Norwegian Air Ambulance.

vanced Life Support (ALS) interventions,[61] although working conditions in the helicopter in general requires most procedures be performed before takeoff. The ride in a helicopter eliminates acceleration and deceleration of any importance although airspeed may exceed 100 mph. Norwegian Air Ambulance uses twin engine small and medium-sized helicopters for air ambulance missions (Eurocopter BO 105 and BK 117), while the Royal Norwegian Rescue Helicopter Service operated by the Royal Norwegian Air Force uses large-size off-shore helicopters for rescue operations (Westland Sea-King).

Land ambulances may differ considerably in size, interior, and quality of ride.[62] They are, for obvious reasons, confined to roads, and are thus susceptible to traffic jams. The ride consists of accelerations and decelerations, especially with eager and tense drivers, and treatment while driving is almost impossible. Patients are loaded uniformly with the head first in the direction of driving, and rapid decelerations produce a flow of blood toward the brain and a concomitant increase in ICP. Drivers should be instructed in slow, gradual stops if possible. If the patient suddenly deteriorates during transport in a land ambulance, the vehicle should be stopped and the patient evaluated unless uncontrolled bleeding is obviously the reason.

Fixed-wing aircraft are used mainly for secondary transports and in rural areas for primary transports. Airborne working conditions are generally excellent, although the noise level may dictate the use of headsets as in helicopters. Airspeed is higher than that of helicopters. Patients are uniformly positioned parallel to the axis of the aircraft, and thus acceleration and deceleration become important determinants for intravascular volume displacements and ICP. Speed and incline angle is greatest during takeoff, while a long descent track and slow braking during landing may reduce decelerative forces. A patient with raised ICP should thus be placed with the head forward, while the hypovolemic patient theoretically should benefit from the opposite placement. If intracranial air is suspected (cranial fractures, penetrating injuries) the cabin pressure should be kept at sea level (1 atmosphere) if possible, and the patient should breathe or be ventilated with 100% O_2.

Motion sickness may be a problem for both patient and personnel. Good ventilation, a slightly reduced cabin temperature (15–20°C), intermittent visual ground contact and, if possible, a moment's relief from patient treatment are helpful tricks. In some patients, intravenous treatment and prophylaxis with metoclopramide, for example, may be indicated, while prophylactic medication of personnel should be discussed with the flight safety officer and company physician in advance. Noise may be stressful to even unconscious patients, and prophylactic application of a headset or ear protection should be a natural part of the preflight checklist.

Triage/Assignment

Triage is the process of awarding treatment and transportation priority according to patient needs. Considering isolated head and spinal cord injury only, patients with deteriorating neurological function *in spite of* proper airway, breathing/ventilation and circulation should receive high priority on the suspicion of a rapidly expanding, evacuable intracranial hematoma. On the other hand, the multiply-injured patient with a possible suspected uncontrolled hemorrhage needs urgent surgery as erythrocytes are lost every moment. This patient receives the highest priority for transportation.

Assignment to special institutions may be relevant, provided control of correctable factors is achieved at the scene. If the patient has an unprotected airway or is hypovolemic, the most appropriate institution is the nearest hospital with an in-house anesthesiologist and surgeon for immediate attention to injuries. If, on the other hand, these factors are controllable by the personnel present, time may be better spent at the scene inducing anesthesia, stabilizing the circulation, and assessing the patient. Thus proper assignment *and* warning of the institution chosen to allow preparation of CT scanner, radiologist, surgeons, and operating suite before arrival are possible. Assignment should ideally be part of the written procedures, after thorough discussion with hospitals, neurosurgeons, EMS, and prehospital anesthesiologists in question. As an aid for assignment the recently revised Prehospital Trauma Triage Algorithm by the American College of Emergency Physicians may be helpful with appropriate local modifications (Fig. 11).[63]

Documentation and Quality Assurance

Proper documentation of all findings, observations and treatment is of great importance not only to the patient, but also to the prehospital unit. Documentation should be written during treatment on self-copying forms, providing one copy to the receiving institution and one to the EMS. The graphical design of the form may vary according to local needs, but it is essential that the data elements are well defined and easily (and unequivocally) understood by different observers. After the mission, forms should be collected and stored at the EMS base. To allow for medical supervision and all kinds of quality assurance and improvement activities, it is desirable to have the records contain the full name and date of birth of the patient. Special demands with respect to confidentiality in terms of access and storing of the records arise. It is likewise desirable to obtain discharge reports from hospitals and add morbidity/mortality data to the prehospital EMS records. Legislation concerning this issue

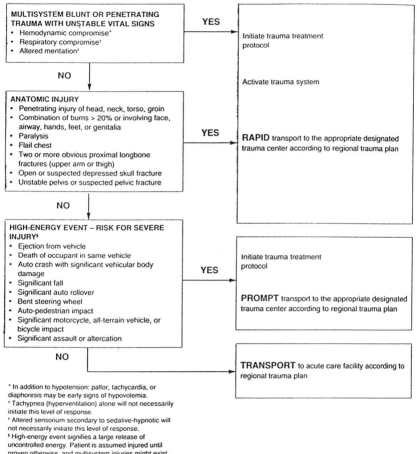

Figure 11. American College of Emergency Physicians. Guidelines for Trauma Care Systems. Model Trauma Triage Algorithm-Prehospital. From ref. 63 with permission from the author and publisher.

varies, and the staffing of a particular EMS (especially whether or not physicians are part of the team) may be important in this respect.

The quality of an EMS and the treatment given by the prehospital anesthesiologist may be described in many aspects. From the point of view of the public or prospective patient it may be divided into (1) accessibility of the service, (2) availability of the service, (3) response times, (4) appropriateness of diagnosis and treatment, and (5) correct triage and assignment. In addition, it would be in the interest of the patient that the service conduct regular audits of these components. Many of these components are not under the authority of the medical director or EMS. To the public, it is, therefore, necessary that the EMS be improved and surveyed as a whole, and by agencies taking responsibility for multiple service.[64,65]

From the viewpoint of medical responsibility, the following elements are critically important: (1) response time, (2) safety of transportation of the team, (3) protocols and adherence to them, (4) knowledge in recognition of correct diagnoses, (5) skills in performing indicated procedures, (6) accuracy and compliance in documentation and reporting, (7) correct triage and assignment, (8) ability to choose the correct vehicle and mode of transportation, and (9) maintainance of a high level of safety for patients and crew.

The definition of what is correct may not be obvious. Some services are relying on written protocols, defined after thorough discussion with appropriate authorities in their fields, and recognized by all parts involved. Strict adherence to these protocols allows the delivery of "correct" care. When a service employs prehospital anesthesiologists or other specialist physicians, protocols often are less developed, as each professional is presumed to be able to evaluate the situation and choose the right therapy. The prehospital working environment differs greatly from the in-hospital environment. The anesthesiologist most often works literally, on his own, and cases seldom have the routine appearance of the operating suite/CCU. It is thus easy to ascribe unwanted incidents to factors unaccessible to the anesthesiologist, and to some anesthesiologists it may be tempting to document such incidents in terms that reduce the possible influence from the anesthesiologist.

Medical directors may find it easier to review, and if necessary, correct nurses and paramedics compared to professional colleagues. Several important points are raised. The medical profession should develop an open, understanding, and supporting environment for incident reporting (as our colleagues in the cockpit have had for years). Even for colleague anesthesiologists, we should define current standards of care in terms of protocols as for paramedics and nurses. We should adapt the evolving in-hospital quality assurance/ improvement activities, where specialist anesthesiologists are reviewed by peers, with respect to the prehospital environment.[66,67]

The process of securing and improving the quality of prehospital services has changed from quality assessment and assurance where certain indicators are identified (e.g., the number of failed intubations)[68–70] to quality improvement.[71] This last trend is based on the fact that a good thing may always be made even better, turning the attention to attempts to find areas where patient treatment may be improved, even though one particular service may have "acceptable" results in that area. Several techniques are used.[72–74] Prospective methods evaluate training, certification, continuing education, and supervised practice. Concurrent methods include on-line medical control, immediate review in the emergency department and, if possible, field observation. Retrospective review includes medical debriefings, critique sessions, and audits where certain categories of missions and incident reports are reviewed. Outcome measures may also be evaluated.[59] Each service must choose suitable, appropriate techniques.

The prehospital working environment may be physically and psychologically exhausting. It is dangerous, as compared to the in-hospital environment, and carries a higher risk of being forced to deviate from safe standards. It is, however, also rewarding. These strains may be part of the explanation of the low average age among prehospital anesthesiologists and other specialist physicians. Experience in the prehospital setting is often bought expensively, and the subsequent draining of experienced colleagues to strict in-hospital service is troublesome and represents a danger to maintaining the quality of prehospital care. Psychological debriefing after distressing incidents should, therefore, be a natural part of the medical director's work toward a high quality of service.

Areas to Be Improved in the Future

In an epidemiological study it was found that 69% of patients with cervical spine injury as the main cause of death actually succumbed either at the scene, or were declared dead on arrival (DOA) to the emergency department.[75] Death due to head injury appeared to occur at the scene or as DOA in 38% of all head injury deaths.

These figures may indicate, that the prehospital EMS still has a need for improvement.

As the first prerequisite, the EMS must be accessible. The public needs simple, efficient ways to get in touch with qualified operators. Uniform emergency phone numbers, e.g., 911 or 113, are expanding, often in combination with the use of nurses or other professionals as operators, allowing operator instructions to bystanders in CPR or other lifesaving procedures.

Second, the specialized EMS units, such as the prehospital anesthesiologists, must be available. Regionalized dispatch centers, with on-line control of all units, may secure the appropriate use of prehospital anesthesiologists. Little attention has been focused on differences between urban, semi-urban, and rural areas in this respect. It is important to develop strategies for each administrative district, with multi-institutional involvement in planning, staffing, deployment, and reviewing services.[64,65,76]

Third, it may be time to define the content of proper prehospital advanced care of injured patients. An intense debate has continued for years concerning treatment strategies at the scene. This fruitless debate has created two directions of thought, the "load and go" versus the "stay and play." Common sense would tell (almost) everyone that the condition of each single patient has to decide to what extent procedures should be performed at the scene.[77] "EMS is more than just a ride to the hospital with fanfare."[76]

Fourth, it should be remembered, that many head-injured patients need transferral to other institutions. This transfer is a dangerous period.[3,5,78] The need for expertise during transfer is no less than during the primary scene response, and intimate coordination with the receiving neurosurgeon is vital.[78]

Still, certain areas of the prehospital treatment may be improved.[79–81] We need the ideal muscular relaxant drug that has rapid onset, short duration, and no side effects. Several pharmacological approaches to central nervous tissue injury have been evaluated, but few have been able to fulfill expectations when assessed in a scientific manner. Monitoring may be improved with portable $ETCO_2$ analyzers. The impact of these refinements on the final outcome for the neurologically injured patient remains, however, to be proven.

Finally, we as prehospital anesthesiologists must behave as responsible citizens, not only focusing on prevention of secondary brain injury, but remembering that brain injury starts with a very often preventable primary injury, and we all have a common obligation to reduce the likelihood of such injury.

Summary

The prehospital management of neurological trauma aims at: precluding the occurrence of "avoidable factors" and thus reduction of the danger of secondary neurological injury; prompt recognition and treatment of associated injuries, protection of the spinal cord from damage by unstable fractures, and careful transportation to a proper institution without *undue* delay. Initial care is achieved by a rather uniform approach to all patients, based on the Advanced Trauma Life Support concept, where airway (including cervical spine protection), breathing, circulation, disability, and exposure forms the backbone of primary examination and resuscitation. Neurological examination is performed repeatedly, by scoring the patient with the Glasgow Coma Scale. When competence permits, early induction of anesthesia and intubation of the trachea is recommended. Circulatory resuscitation is performed to secure adequate perfusion of the injured brain. A meticulous immobilization of the cervical spine is necessary to protect the spinal cord. When spinal cord injury is suspected, prompt intravenous treatment with methylprednisolone is recommended. The treatment of intracranial hypertension rests primarily on securing adequate ventilation and cerebral perfusion, but in certain situations the use of mannitol may be advocated. Monitoring during prehospital treatment ideally consists of all in-hospital monitoring equipment, but prehospital environmental and working conditions may dictate special considerations. Prehospital anesthetic management of trauma patients is difficult, but rewarding. Proper documentation and quality assurance is an essential part of the service.

References

1. Rose J, Valtonen S, Jennett B: Avoidable factors contributing to death after head injury. BMJ 2:615–618, 1977.
2. Berman JM, Prough DS: Neurological injuries. In Grande CM (ed): Textbook of Trauma Anesthesia and Critical Care. Mosby-Year Book, St. Louis, 1993, pp 883–920.
3. Gentleman D: Causes and effects of systemic complications among severely head-injured patients transferred to a neurosurgical unit. Int Surg 77:297–302, 1992.
4. Baxt WG, Moody P: The impact of advanced prehospital emergency care on the mortality of severely brain-injured patients. J Trauma 27:365–369, 1987.
5. Gentleman D, Jennett B: Hazards of inter-hospital transfer of comatose head-injured patients. Lancet II:853–855, 1981.

6. Seelig JM, Becker DP, Miller JD, Grenberg RP, Ward JD, Choi SC: Traumatic acute subdural hematoma: Major mortality reduction in comatose patients treated within four hours. N Engl J Med 304: 1511–1518, 1981.
7. Frost EAM: Neurological trauma. In Grande CM (ed): Textbook of Trauma Anesthesia and Critical Care. Mosby-Year Book, St. Louis, 1993, pp 510–528.
8. Pepe PE, Kvetan V: Field management and critical care in mass disasters. Crit Care Clin 7:401–420, 1991.
9. Teasdale GM, Murray G, Anderson E, Mendelow AD, MacMillan R, Jennett B, Brookes M: Risks of acute traumatic intracranial hematoma in children and adults: Implications for managing head injuries. BMJ 300:363–367, 1990.
10. Bayless P, Ray VG: Incidence of cervical spine injuries in association with blunt head trauma. Am J Emerg Med 7:139–142, 1989.
11. Williams J, Jehle D, Cottington E, Shufflebarger C: Head, facial, and clavicular trauma as a predictor of cervical-spine injury. Ann Emerg Med 21:719–722, 1992.
12. Riggins R, Kraus J: The risk of neurological damage with fractures of the vertebrae. J Trauma 17:126–133, 1977.
13. Hastings RH, Marks JD: Airway management for trauma patients with potential cervical spine injuries. Anesth Analg 73:471–482, 1991.
14. American College of Surgeons, Committee on Trauma: Advanced Trauma Life Support Student Manual. American College of Surgeons, Chicago, 1989.
15. Meyer S, Gibb T, Jurkovich GJ: Evaluation and significance of the pupillary light reflex in trauma patients. Ann Emerg Med 22:1052–1057, 1993.
16. Luerssen TG, Klauber MR, Marshall LF: Outcome from head injury related to patient's age. J Neurosurg 68:409–416, 1988.
17. Teasdale G, Jennet B: Assessment of coma and impaired consciousness: A practical scale. Lancet 2:81–83, 1974.
18. Teasdale G, Knill-Jones R, van der Sande J: Observer variability in assessing impaired consciousness and coma. J Neurol Neurosurg Psychiatry 41:603–610, 1978.
19. Bouillon B, Schweins M, Lechleunthner A, Vorweg M, Troidl H: Assessment of emergency care in trauma patients. Acta Neurochir Suppl (Wien) 57:137–140, 1993.
20. Champion HR, Sacco WJ, Carnazzo AJ, Copes W, Fouty WJ: Trauma Score. Crit Care Med 9:672–676, 1981.
21. Champion HR, Gainer PS, Yackee E: A progress report on the Trauma Score in predicting a fatal outcome. J Trauma 26:927–931, 1986.
22. Moreau M, Gainer PS, Champion HR, Sacco WJ: Application of the Trauma Score in the prehospital setting. Ann Emerg Med 14: 1049–1054, 1985.
23. Champion HR, Sacco WJ, Copes WS, Gann DS, Gennarelli TA, Flanagan ME: A revision of the Trauma Score. J Trauma 29:623–629, 1989.
24. Champion HR, Copes WS, Sacco WJ, Lawnick MM, Keast SL, Bain LW,

Flanagan ME, Frey CF: The major trauma outcome study: Establishing national norms for trauma care. J Trauma 30:1356–1365, 1990.

25. Baxt WG, Berry CC, Epperson MD, Scalzitti V: The failure of prehospital trauma prediction rules to classify trauma patients accurately. Ann Emerg Med 18:1–8, 1989.

26. Parr MJA, Grande CM: Concepts of trauma care and trauma scoring. In Grande CM (ed): Textbook of Trauma Anesthesia and Critical Care. Mosby-Year Book, St. Louis, 1993, pp 71–92.

27. Morray JP, Tyler DC, Jones TK, Stuntz JT, Lemire RJ: Coma scale for use in brain-injured children. Crit Care Med 12:1018–1020, 1984.

28. Pfenninger EG, Lindner KH: Arterial blood gases in patients with acute head injury at the accident site and upon hospital admission. Acta Anaesthesiol Scand 35:148–152, 1991.

29. Erler CJ, Lafayette W, Rutherford WF, Rodman G, Mounts J, Schutz D, Eccles B: Inadequate respiratory support in head injury patients. Air Med J 12:223–226, 1993.

30. Abrams KJ, Nolan JP, Grande CM: Trauma anesthesia: Anesthesiology's oldest specialty reborn. Anesth Clin North Am 9:393–421, 1991.

31. Lord SA, Boswell WC, Williams JS, Odom JW, Boyd CR: Airway control in trauma patients with cervical spine fractures. Prehosp Disaster Med 9:44–49, 1994.

32. O'Malley RJ, Rhee KJ: Contribution of air medical personnel to the airway management of injured patients. Air Med J 11–12:425–428, 1993.

33. Fiser DH: Intraosseous infusion. N Engl J Med 322:1579–1581, 1990.

34. Velasco AL, Delgado-Paredes C, Templeton J, Steigman CK, Templeton JM: Intraosseous infusion of fluids in the initial management of hypovolemic shock in young subjects. J Pediatr Surg 26:4–8, 1991.

35. Halvorsen L, Bay BK, Perron PR, Gunther RA, Holcroft JW, Blaisdell W, Kramer GC: Evaluation of an intraosseous infusion device for the resuscitation of hypovolemic shock. J Trauma 30:652–658, 1990.

36. Naess CE, Aabyholm FE, Bonska TE, Nordli B, Oftedal TA: Infusions in a cold environment. Tidsskr Nor Laegeforen 105:2055–2056, 1985 (English summary).

37. Nordli B, Oftedal TA, Bonska TE, Naess CE, Aabyholm FE: Newly developed personal heater: Function and use. Tidsskr Nor Laegeforen 105: 2057–2060, 1985 (English summary).

38. Bickell WH, Bruttig SP, Millnamow GA, O'Benar J, Wade CE: Use of hypertonic saline/dextran versus lactated Ringer's solution as a resuscitation fluid after uncontrolled aortic hemorrhage in anesthetized swine. Ann Emerg Med 21:1077–1085, 1992.

39. Bickel WH, Bruttig SP, Millnamow GA, O'Benar J, Wade CE: The detrimental effects of intravenous crystalloid after aortotomy in swine. Surgery 110:529–536, 1991.

40. Stern SA, Dronen SC, Birrer P: Effect of blood pressure on hemorrhage volume and survival in a near-fatal hemorrhage model incorporating a vascular injury. Ann Emerg Med 22:155–163, 1993.

41. Bickell WH: Are victims of injury sometimes victimized by attempts at fluid resuscitation? Ann Emerg Med 22:225–226, 1993.

42. Cline JR, Scheidel E, Bigsby EF: A comparison of methods of cervical immobilization used in patient extrication and transport. J Trauma 25: 649–653, 1985.
43. Swain A, Dove J, Baker H: Trauma of the spine and spinal cord. In Skinner D, Driscoll P, Earlam R (eds): ABC of Major Trauma. British Medical Journal, London, 1991, pp 38–45.
44. McGuire RA, Neville S, Green BA, Watts C: Spinal instability and the log-rolling maneuver. J Trauma 27:525–531, 1987.
45. Roye WP, Dunn EL, Moody JA: Cervical spinal cord injury—a public catastrophe. J Trauma 28:1260–1264, 1988.
46. Bracken MB, Shepard MJ, Collins WF et al: A randomized, controlled trial of methylprednisolone or naloxone in the treatment of acute spinal-cord injury. N Engl J Med 322:1405–1411, 1990.
47. Bracken MB, Shepard MJ, Collins WF, et al: Methylprednisolone or naloxone treatment after acute spinal cord injury: 1-year follow-up data. J Neurosurg 76:23–31, 1992.
48. Feldman JA, Fish S: Resuscitation fluid for a patient with head injury and hypovolemic shock. J Emerg Med 9:465–468, 1991.
49. Freshman SP, Battistella FD, Mattcucci M, Wisner DH: Hypertonic saline (7.5%) versus mannitol: A comparison treatment of acute head injuries. J Trauma 35:344–348, 1993.
50. Bruce DA: Head trauma management. In Newfield P, Cottrell JE (eds): Handbook of Neuroanesthesia: Clinical and Physiological Essentials. Little, Brown & Co, Boston, 1983, pp 283–301.
51. Simon C, Scheidegger D: Primary treatment in severe head injury. In Vincent JL (ed): Update in Intensive Care and Emergency Medicine. Springer-Verlag, Berlin, 1990, pp 529–34.
52. Walls RM: Rapid-sequence intubation in head trauma. Ann Emerg Med 22:1008–1013, 1993.
53. DeJarnette R, Holleran R, Von Rotz NP, Downing C, Willhite J, Storer D: Pulse oximetry during helicopter transport. Air Med J 4:93–96, 1993.
54. Aughey K, Hess D, Eitel D, Bleecher K, Cooley M, Ogden C, Sabulsky N: An evaluation of pulse oximetry in prehospital care. Ann Emerg Med 20:887–891, 1991.
55. Oranto JP, Shipley JB, Racht EM, Slovis CM et al: Multicenter study of a portable, hand-size, colorimetric end tidal carbon dioxide detection device. Ann Emerg Med 21:518–523, 1992.
56. Rhee KJ, Strozeski M, Burney RE, Mackenzie JR, LaGreca-Reibling K: Is the flight physician needed for helicopter emergency medical services? Ann Emerg Med 15:174–177, 1986.
57. Stone CK: The air medical crew: Is a flight physician necessary? J Air Med Trans 10:7–11, 1991.
58. Baxt WG, Moody P: The impact of a physician as part of the aeromedical prehospital team in patients with blunt trauma. JAMA 257:3246–3250, 1987.
59. Wisborg T, Guttormsen AB, Soerensen MB, Flaatten H: The potential of an anaesthesiologist-manned ambulance service in a rural/urban district. Acta Anaesthesiol Scand 38:657–661, 1994.

60. Harris BH: Performance of air medical crew members: Training or experience. Am J Emerg Med 4:409–411, 1986.
61. Thomas SH, Stone CK, Bryan-Berge D, Hunt RC: Effect of an in-flight helicopter environment on the performance of ALS interventions. Air Med J 13:9–12, 1994.
62. Gilman JI: Carrier and vendor selection. Int Anesth Clin 25:117–137, 1987.
63. American College of Emergency Physicians: Guidelines for trauma care systems. Ann Emerg Med 22:1079–1100, 1993.
64. American College of Emergency Physicians: Trauma care system quality improvement guidelines. Ann Emerg Med 21:736–739, 1992.
65. National Association of Emergency Medical Services Physicians: Position Paper: Air medical dispatch: Guidelines for scene response. Prehosp Disaster Med 7:75–76, 1992.
66. Mackenzie CF: Simulation of trauma anesthesia. In Grande CM (ed): Textbook of Trauma Anesthesia and Critical Care. Mosby-Year Book, St. Louis, 1993, pp 1180–1191.
67. Fasting S, Gisvold SE: Problems with technical equipment during anaesthesia: A prospective recording of 70,000 cases. Acta Anaesthesiol Scand 37(Suppl)100:227, 1993.
68. Quality assurance in the Connecticut Helicopter Emergency Medical Service: J Air Med Trans 10:(8)7–11, 1991.
69. Dagher M, Lloyd RJ: Developing EMS quality assessment indicators. Prehosp Disaster Med 7:69–74, 1992.
70. Salerno SM, Wrenn KD, Slovis CM: Monitoring EMS protocol deviations: A useful quality assurance tool. Ann Emerg Med 20:1319–1324, 1991.
71. Eastes L: Implementing quality improvement for air medical services. J Air Med Trans 10:(8)12–14, 1991.
72. McCarthy P: Implementation of a regional medical control audit system. Prehosp Disaster Med 7:167–174, 1992.
73. Swor RA: Quality assurance in EMS systems. Emerg Med Clin North Am 10:597–610, 1992.
74. Polsky SS, Weigand JV: Quality assurance in emergency medical service systems. Emerg Med Clin North Am 8:75–84, 1990.
75. Daly KE, Thomas PRS: Trauma deaths in the South West Thames Region. Injury 23:393–396, 1992.
76. Johnson JC: Prehospital care: The future of emergency medical services. Ann Emerg Med 20:426–430, 1991.
77. McSwain NE: Controversies in prehospital care. Emerg Med Clin North Am 8:145–154, 1990.
78. Gentleman D, Dearden M, Midgley S, Maclean D: Guidelines for resuscitation and transfer of patients with serious head injury. BMJ 307: 547–552, 1993.
79. Garcia JH: Prehospital management of head injuries: International perspectives. Acta Neurochir Suppl (Wien) 57:145–151, 1993.
80. Sefrin P: Current level of prehospital care in severe head injury—potential for improvement. Acta Neurochir Suppl (Wien) 57:141–144, 1993.
81. Blackwell TH: Prehospital care. Emerg Med Clin North Am 11:1–14, 1993.

2

Interhospital Transport of Neurotrauma Patients

Gilles A. Orliaguet, MD, Pierre A. Carli, MD

Introduction

When a patient needs services that exceed the available resources of a facility, the patient should be transferred to a facility with the required resources.[1] Interfacility patient transfer should occur when the benefits to the patient exceed the risks of the transfer. The goal of management for the head-injured patient during transport is to provide optimum surveillance, serial assessment, and support of the organ system's function during transport to a facility that can provide evaluation and definitive care of the central nervous system (CNS) insult.

Indications for Interhospital Transport

For many patients, the initial trip to the emergency department is the only medical transport, but further transportation will be re-

From *Trauma Anesthesia and Critical Care of Neurological Injury,* edited by K. J. Abrams and C. M. Grande. © 1997, Futura Publishing Co., Armonk, NY.

quired for those who need specialized care in a referral center, and for those who are injured in rural areas and taken to small community hospitals with limited resources. In fact, the basic reason for moving a head trauma patient, like any other critically ill patient, is the need for additional care (either technology and/or specialists) not available at the patient's current location. Head-injured patients often require transport to neurointensive care units, where they can benefit from the most appropriate care and monitoring, as well as from surgical procedures if needed. Moreover, these patients frequently need neuroradiological assessment, such as computerized tomography (CT) and magnetic resonance imaging (MRI), which are not always available in community or general hospitals.

Pathophysiology of Transport

As with any other critically ill patient, the neurotrauma patient's physiological status, which may already be severely deranged, can deteriorate further during transport. There have been few investigations of the acute physiological changes during transport of neurotrauma patients. The general physiological changes and their consequences for the CNS trauma patient will be considered.

Cardiovascular Changes

Cardiovascular changes during transport occur relatively often,[2,3] and depend on the adequacy of sedation, analgesia or anesthesia, and the hemodynamic status. The hemodynamic status depends on how well blood volume is maintained and the degree of dependence on vasoactive therapy. In a retrospective study over 5 months, involving 86 intensive care transports, it has been found that one patient per month suffered major cardiorespiratory collapse or death as a direct consequence of movement which caused renewed bleeding or arrhythmias.[2] In another retrospective study, the same author also found a significant change in blood pressure in 41% of cases: 13% had hypertension and 15% delayed hypotension, the delayed hypotension probably due to the initiation of intermittent positive pressure ventilation (IPPV).[3] Another author from the same center has shown minimal changes in pulse and blood pressure during intrahospital transport, the most common change being a mild rise in blood pressure, which responded to an increase in sedation or analgesia.[4] It should be noted that these studies were retrospective, and did not refer specifically to head trauma patients. In a recent prospective study, involving the intrahospital transport of 50 head-injured patients, Andrews et al.[5] found a global incidence of cardiovascular events of 24% during transportation, including hypotension (8%), hypertension (14%), and tachycardia (2%). Moreover, the number and duration of insults during transfer correlated significantly with the number and duration of insults both before and after the move. Thus, cardiovascular events are relatively frequent during transport of head trauma patients, and may contribute to morbidity and mortality. This particular susceptibility to hemodynamic changes, especially to hypotension,[6,7] of severe head trauma patients is due to an impairment in cerebral autoregulation, and there is some evidence that cerebral perfusion pressure (CPP) should be maintained above 70–80 mm Hg.[8,9] It has been suggested that early and aggressive treatment, aimed at preventing secondary insults such as hypotension, could decrease mortality and improve neurological outcome after severe head injury.[10]

Respiratory Changes

Respiratory changes during the transport of head trauma patients range from difficulties in airway control in nonintubated patients to inadequate ventilation in those already intubated. In fact, a high incidence of airway obstruction during interhospital transfer of comatose patients has already been shown, with 42% having had no airway or endotracheal tube inserted.[11] Gentleman et al. have documented a 22% incidence of hypoxia in 150 head trauma patients after ambulance transfer from another hospital.[12] Andrews et al.[5] studied the rate of occurrence of adverse factors in unconscious head-injured patients during interhospital transfer. They found the airway to be compromised on arrival at the neurosurgical unit in 23% and hypoxia ($PaO_2 < 70$ mm Hg) in 15% of the patients. Hypoxia was more common among those with a compromised airway than among those without (32% versus 9%). Only 7% of those who were both intubated and ventilated arrived hypoxic, but there was no significant difference in occurrence of hypoxia between those with no airway protection (20%) and those who were intubated but breathing spontaneously (26%). Indeck et al.[13] found that 20% of post-trauma patients had a change in respiratory rate of ±5 ventilation per min, and 17% had a decrease in oxygen saturation of 5% or more in his series of 103 transports. A rise in $PaCO_2$ ranging from 12–31 mm

Hg was found by Waddel et al.[2] in 6 out of 13 transportations. The use of a portable ventilator has been shown by Braman et al.[14] and Hurst et al.[15] to be associated with less variation in blood gases than is seen during manual ventilation, with an increase or decrease of approximately 10 mm Hg $PaCO_2$ occurring frequently in the latter group.

Thermoregulation

Patients with an abnormal body temperature, whether hyperthermia or hypothermia, may not tolerate transport well, mainly due to the cardiovascular, respiratory, and metabolic consequences of temperature changes. If possible, they should be made normothermic before transfer. Minimal changes in core temperature during transport can often be obtained, despite large changes in ambient temperature, using isotherm blankets and duvets.[16]

Metabolic Changes

Metabolic changes during transport are not well documented. Sudden changes in minute volume caused by obstruction or changes in ventilation may cause rapid changes in cardiac output and in serum potassium.[16]

Gastrointestinal Changes

The frequency of gastrointestinal complications during transport is very poorly documented. These complications include vomiting with possible aspiration, and those related to changes in ambient pressure. The latter can cause expansion of any gas-filled space, such as the enlargement of an ileus, and this will create discomfort, colicky pain, and respiratory embarrassment from diaphragmatic splinting caused by the increased intra-abdominal pressure.

Physiological Changes Secondary to Movement

Apart from the secondary lesions due to hypoxia, hypercarbia, and hypotension, some problems are directly due to the transportation of the patient. The position of the patient with cerebral edema in the transporting vehicle, theoretically, may influence changes in intracranial pressure. If the patient is carried feet first, rapid acceleration would cause a rise in intracranial pressure and, conversely, if the patient is carried head first, then a rise in intracerebral pressure could be caused by rapid deceleration. In practice, this does not seem to be a problem. The effects of increase in altitude and dysbarism will be discussed later.

A perfect knowledge of the acute physiological changes during transport of head trauma patients should enable an accurate pre-transport evaluation and stabilization (especially cardiopulmonary stabilization), which only allow the transfer of the most critically ill patients.

Mode of Transport

Transport modality is an important issue that is only now being rationally addressed. There are three modalities of transport: fixed-wing aircraft, rotocraft, or ground vehicles, but it is often difficult to set definitive guidelines as to which is optimal because each of these three modalities has its own advantages and disadvantages. The relative indications, advantages, and disadvantages of each mode of transport will be examined in detail.

Ground Ambulance

There are many advantages in using surface ambulance systems.[17,18] They can provide door-to-door service. They are always available and usable (day or night), whatever the weather. If an emergency situation arises, the medical team can stop the vehicle to provide care or perform a procedure.[19] In considering ground ambulance transport, certain limitations must be acknowledged.[20,21] Apart from the possibility of motion sickness of the patient or the medical staff, which also exists with other modes of transport, other drawbacks are more specific to this kind of transportation. Despite the use of lights and sirens, traffic congestion, road conditions, and construction areas can slow or halt a ground transport. The ride in the back of an ambulance is generally rough due to the suspension system used, the narrow wheel base, and the high center of gravity, which result in increased sway and bounce.[22] The repetitive acceleration and deceleration in the ambulance causes irregular increases and less uniform head-to-toe force, but they are of a lower magnitude than those seen in a helicopter. Other negative aspects of the transport environment include the effects of noise and vibration. Moreover, in the transport setting, constant movement increases the risk of disconnection of patient lines and equipment. The importance of anticipating such occurrences cannot be overemphasized, and all intravascular lines and medical equipment must be secured. Moreover, constant scrutiny of the patient and equipment settings is essential.

Fixed-Wing Aircraft

Fixed-wing aircraft are fast but are expensive to operate, provide a cramped workspace, and cannot be parked to restabilize the patient. A major question to be posed before deciding on an air transfer is: When is air transport better than ground transport? This question can be answered only on a case-by-case basis, by balancing two critical points. First, will air transport save enough time to affect the patient's outcome? It seems that unless distances are more than several hundred miles, or ground congestion is excessive, ground transport is often as fast from hospital to hospital as air transport. Second, will the level of training of the transport team make a difference? And for the unstable patients the personnel may be more important than the vehicle.

Moreover, the transport of head-injured patients by air may give rise to special problems associated with the change in altitude, increased noise, and turbulence. With an increase in altitude, the ambient atmospheric pressure falls and even with cabin pressurization, which is normally between 2,000 and 2,500 meters, the inspired oxygen partial pressure falls to 112 mm Hg, the alveolar PO_2 to 65 mm Hg, and in a healthy person, arterial saturation falls to about 90%.[23] In the head trauma patient with already impaired pulmonary function, this situation can deteriorate further unless measures are taken to increase arterial oxygenation, i.e., increase inspired oxygen concentration or the addition of PEEP.

Another problem during air transport is dysbarism. With a fall in ambient pressure, gases expand (Boyle's law) and at routine cabin pressure a 30% expansion of gas is likely to occur. This can cause physiological changes in the patient as well as potential problems with equipment. Any gas-filled space will enlarge, and thus, for example, any patient with a pneumothorax, fractured skull, or air in the middle ear or sinuses is at risk for a tension situation developing. If a patient is being ventilated with an oxygen/nitrous oxide mixture, these dysbaric problems can all be potentiated, due to nitrous oxide's solubility compared to nitrogen, as any gas-filled space increases further in volume. If intravenous fluids are in rigid containers, i.e., bottles, expansion of gas above the liquid during ascent causes increases in the drip flow. This effect can be prevented by the use of a large-bore needle, venting the container. Theoretically, the cuffs of endotracheal tubes may expand and contract with changing altitude, causing increased tracheal pressure and a possible air leak on increasing and decreasing altitude, respectively. The use of low-pressure, high-volume cuffs usually ensures that this is not a practical problem. Water instead of air within the cuff also circumvents the problem. In the same way, the use of pneumatic limb splints can theoretically cause tissue ischemia as the gas expands at altitude and the pressure in such splints should be readjusted with changing altitude. If intravascular or intracerebral pressures are monitored by the use of transducers, the equipment must be rezeroed to the new ambient pressure.

The noise during flight, especially in smaller aircraft, causes distress and anxiety to conscious patients, as well as making the use of stethoscope and auditory monitoring very difficult.

The last problem due to air transport is that of turbulence. Excessive turbulence may cause pain to the conscious patient if he is not adequately immobilized by the use of splints and restraints. Moreover, motion sickness can be a problem not only to the patient, but also to the staff. The head-injured patient should be positioned with head raised, "cross-cabin" if possible, or at least head toward the front of the aircraft to avoid additional venous pooling.[24]

Rotocraft

Rotocraft occupy a midposition between ground and fixed-wing aircraft. Rotocraft are very quick for short flights (under 100–150 miles), and transport time is one-half or one-third that of a ground ambulance. Thus, the helicopter is beneficial when time is critical for the patient's arrival at the receiving center, such as for patients with acute epidural hematoma. The flight is generally smooth and has fewer vibrations and bumps, which can be beneficial for certain patients (e.g., associated spinal cord trauma). It seems that only the most critically injured patients benefit from transport by helicopter.[25]

Disadvantages are that rotocraft are even more expensive to operate than fixed-wing aircraft and tend to be smaller and noisier. For example, it is impossible to hear heart or breath sounds during the flight.[26] The use of a helicopter requires an adequate helipad or unobstructed landing space, which may not exist in general hospitals. Weather may limit flights because of decreased visibility in fog, rain, sleet, heavy snowfall, and severe thunderstorms. Helicopters, especially those not specifically adapted for medical transport, can also have limitations in electrical systems and the ability to use medical equipment that requires electrical backup.

In fact, despite the respective advantages and disadvantages of each mode of transport, the definitive choice depends on the length and duration of the transport, the clinical status of the patient, and mainly on the availability of the mode of transport.

Pretransport Evaluation

Neurological Assessment

Of the three major immediate threats to life that result from trauma (the other two being respiratory insufficiency and hypoperfusion due to blood loss), central nervous system disruption is the least susceptible to assessment and intervention during transport.[27] Therefore, it is vital to quickly establish a baseline assessment of neurological function to provide a basis for comparison during the transport. Initial neurological examination of head trauma victims has been standardized somewhat by the use of the Glasgow Coma Scale, which summarizes a limited neurological examination with a numeric score. By itself, the GCS is not a very accurate prognostic indicator and is best used to identify changes in the patient during transport. The GCS is not a complete neurological examination, neglecting brain stem function, and should be coupled with a cranial nerve assessment and search for any focal neurological signs.

Vital Function Assessment

The goal of the initial assessment is to determine which physiopathological conditions can be exacerbated by transport, and to prevent or correct them by treatment prior to transport. Most of these problems involve the cardiovascular and respiratory systems and can be diagnosed with appropriate monitoring. Thus, a careful baseline assessment of cardiopulmonary status is mandatory in order to provide a basis for comparison during the transport.

Detection of Untreated Life-Threatening Injuries

Pretransport evaluation is also aimed at detecting untreated life-threatening extracranial injuries. In fact, major injuries missed due to deficiencies in assessment and resuscitation before transfer, sometimes leading to the death of the patient during transport, have already been observed.[28,29] In a prospective study, the authors found that 4 of the 43 patients (9%) transferred to a major trauma center because of head injury had untreated life-threatening extracranial injuries, which resulted in two deaths.[29] Therefore, pretransport evaluation is an important part of the transfer procedure, and it should never be underestimated, even in the rush to transfer the patient to a neurosurgical facility.

Pretransport Stabilization

The key to successful transport of the head trauma patient is stabilization before transport is attempted. It is clinically useful to consider traumatic brain damage as being either primary (occurring at the moment of injury), or secondary (developing later because of evolution of the initial injury or a complicating process). Since secondary damage is potentially preventable or reversible, this concept provides a rational basis for aggressive care of the head trauma patient. After the initial assessment, stabilization is therefore aimed at preventing worsening or progression of the initial injury. Although it is impossible to reverse damage to the brain that results from mechanical forces at the moment of injury, the injured brain remains extremely susceptible to additional insults during the following minutes or hours.[30] Among the additional insults that may occur after head trauma and further adversely affect brain function, some are particularly important: hypoxemia, hypercarbia, hypotension, and intracranial hypertension. The pretransport stabilization of respiratory, hemodynamic, and ICP status are detailed.

Respiratory Status Stabilization

Respiratory insufficiency combined with head injury results in a particularly pernicious scenario because of the influence of ventilation and oxygenation on cerebral blood flow and hence intracranial

pressure (Fig. 1). Patients with the combination of intracranial hematoma and respiratory insufficiency may have a mortality rate as
high as 80%.[24] All nonintubated patients should have high-flow oxygen delivered by face mask, with careful observation of the rate and
depth of breathing, suction with a large-bore catheter available, and
assistance in keeping the mandibular block off the pharynx with the
chin lift, jaw thrust, or adjunctive airway devices. When the airway
is being evaluated, the possibility of cervical spine injury must always be kept in mind because specific airway maneuvers may aggravate preexisting lesions. In fact, the most important single early intervention for the head injury victim, and the most important initial
decision to be made, is whether to perform endotracheal intubation.
Early intubation and airway control are correlated with increased
survival and functional outcome.[31-34] Intubation should be realized
in any head-injured patient with a GCS score less than 8. But, because stabilization of the airway may be very difficult during transport (especially via helicopter), it may be wise to err on the side of
intubation in making this decision, even in patients with a GCS score
higher than 8. In many cases, the use of neuromuscular blockade
and sedation can greatly increase the ease and success of intubation,
and avoid trauma, hypoxia or hypercarbia, and resultant intracranial pressure spikes associated with coughing and fighting the procedure.[32-34] One must be aware of the risks of drug-assisted intubation,
however. Neuromuscular blockade during transport of intubated patients will also help avoid accidental extubation en route, a potentially disastrous scenario.[32,35]

Hemodynamic Stabilization

The cardiovascular status of the head-injured patient typically
reflects a state of sympathetic overdrive, with elevations in blood
pressure, heart rate, and vascular tone.[36-38] Mild to moderate hypertension therefore is common in the patient with severe head injury
and may conceivably be protective in the face of elevated intracranial
pressure (to preserve CPP), so emergency antihypertensive treatment is rarely indicated and may be harmful.[35] Conversely, shock
and hypotension result in increased morbidity and mortality and
should be treated aggressively, because of the resulting fall in CPP.
The trend to absolutely avoid hypotension and to enable mild hypertension is sustained by some evidence that cerebral CPP should be
maintained above 70–80 mm Hg.[8,9] As for any patient, proper fluid

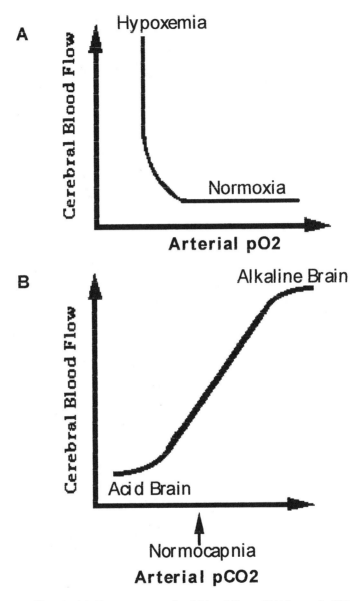

Figure 1. Chemical influence on cerebral blood flow of (**A**) hypoxia (**B**) arterial carbon dioxide level.

administration is the mainstay of circulatory support, with the goal of achieving and maintaining normovolemia and cerebral perfusion, responding to early signs of hypovolemia and hypoperfusion. The best way to detect these early signs is by invasive monitoring, because clinical signs of hypovolemia are often elusive and misleading.

Treatment of Increased ICP

As many as 50% of unconscious head-injured patients may have elevations in intracranial pressure. For patients with intracranial mass lesions, this figure rises to roughly 66%.[39] According to the cerebral compliance curve of Langfitt (Fig. 2), any elevation in intra-

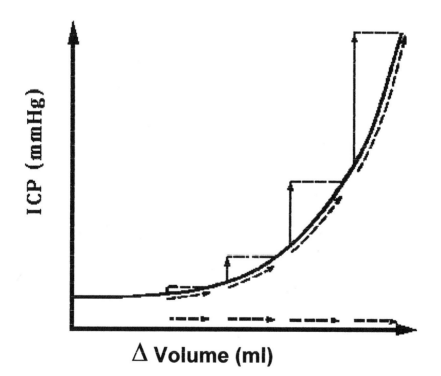

Figure 2. Cerebral compliance curve. Because the skull is rigid, an increase in the volume of one of the components of the intracranial contents (cerebral blood volume for example, i.e., intracranial hematomas) tends to increase intracranial pressure. The effect becomes greater as the volume increases and the compensatory mechanism fails.

cranial volume (intracerebral mass lesion, epidural or subdural hematoma) will be, at least initially, compensated and result in a minimal increase in ICP. But when the "critical point" is reached, ICP rises very rapidly with even a small additional increase in the size of the lesion.[39,40] Uncontrolled elevations in ICP have pernicious effects on cerebral perfusion, and may result in CNS destruction via one of the herniation syndromes. Thus, elevation in ICP (>20–30 cm H_2O) is clearly a cause of secondary brain injury following head trauma and predicts poor outcome. Therefore, for the head-injured patient undergoing stabilization and transport, identification of increased ICP is important and should be treated before transport. It has been shown that all patients with elevated ICP during transport had raised ICP before transfer.[5] It appears that treatment of raised ICP in the 2 hours before transfer prevented ICP insults during transfer in all cases and post-transport increases in ICP in 60% of patients.[5]

Monitoring During Transport

Most problems during transport involve the cardiovascular and respiratory systems and can be diagnosed with appropriate monitoring. Therefore, based on clinical judgment, it is sometimes necessary to institute specific monitoring before transport, which may be invasive (continuous measurements of arterial, central venous, pulmonary arterial or intracranial pressure) or not (pulse oxymetry, end-tidal CO_2, and airway pressure monitoring). The risk-benefit ratio of the institution of this monitoring should be accurately evaluated for each patient and should not delay an emergency transfer. Apart from clinical monitoring, which is always mandatory, head-injured patients, like any other critically ill patients being transported, should have as a minimum level of monitoring: continuous ECG monitoring and intermittent measurements of blood pressure and respiratory rate.[41] Continuous monitoring by pulse oximetry is strongly recommended.[42] Selected patients, based on clinical judgment, may benefit from monitoring by: continuous measurements of arterial, central venous, pulmonary arterial, or intracranial pressure. Unfortunately, intracranial pressure monitoring is rarely available, especially for patients originating from a general hospital lacking a neurosurgical unit. Therefore, identification of intracranial hypertension must be attempted from physical signs and symptoms, which are frequently poorly specific. In fact, a regular assessment of neurological function, should detect any worsening. As previously stated, GCS coupled with a cranial nerve assessment and evidence of any focal neurological findings are used to identify changes in the patient during transport. For example, a sudden dilatation of one or both pupils is presumptive evidence of herniation, and this finding must lead to a quick treatment of raised ICP. Another useful monitoring for these patients is end-tidal CO_2 monitoring. It can be realized either by capnometry, capnography or by the Easy Cap (Nellcor Incorporated, Hayward, USA), which is a colorimetric detector enabling a semiquantitative evaluation of $ETCO_2$ during transport.[43] Airway pressure should be monitored in ventilated patients. If a transport ventilator is used, it should have alarms to indicate disconnections or excessively high airway pressures. Special attention must be given to intravenous lines (e.g., for central venous pressure monitoring) to ensure that they do not accidentally become dislodged and that air is not accidentally entrained. The latter could result in systemic air embolism. Systemic air embolism, which is affected by pressure volume changes, as can occur during air transport, would be disastrous when superimposed on a head injury. A medical record documenting the patient's status and management during transport is required.

Critical Care During Transport

Care of the head-injured patient during transport should proceed as it would in the neurotrauma unit of a sophisticated trauma center. In fact, post-transfer instability may be due to inadequate therapy (intravenous fluid replacement, analgesia, or a change in ventilation) during transfer.[44] Resuscitation and stabilization before transfer should prevent emergency interventions during transport, but still some problems may arise and need immediate treatment. The monitoring instituted before transport should permit detection of these problems very early and immediate treatment. Therapy includes: intubation of a patient developing respiratory insufficiency (as evaluated by physical signs and pulse oxymetry or if neurological status worsens, ventilation parameters change), volume or vasopressor therapy (or both), treatment of an increase in ICP.

Several modalities to decrease ICP are appropriate for transport. Patients should be positioned with the head in the midline position to prevent possible obstruction to jugular venous outflow and resultant increase in ICP. Elevation of the head of the bed to

30° is universally recommended for patients with potentially elevated ICP, although the effects on measured ICP may be largely related to standard practices in transducer calibration. The most immediately effective and useful treatment for transport is induced hyperventilation, most reasonably accomplished via an endotracheal tube. Hyperventilation is aimed at decreasing $PaCO_2$ to 25–30 mm Hg. More pronounced hyperventilation could result in reduced cerebral blood flow with cerebral ischemia. Sedation with drugs such as benzodiazepines, barbiturates, or opiates may markedly reduce ICP in patients who are agitated and "fighting," but these drugs all cause cardiovascular and respiratory depression and may compromise either ventilation or perfusion of the brain. Neuromuscular blockade, preferably with intermediate-acting agents such as vecuronium or atracurium, may also be effective for short-term reduction of ICP by aiding hyperventilation. Osmotherapy with mannitol is another major method of ICP control. In doses of 0.25–0.5 g/kg, mannitol reduces ICP but because it is an osmotic diuretic, it may reduce blood volume and adversely affect circulation and decrease cerebral perfusion pressure. Volume replacement is essential. During patient transport, mannitol is best reserved for desperate situations, such as when herniation appears imminent or when there is obvious and progressive deterioration in neurological status. Other modalities of ICP control probably have no place during transport.

System Organization

The decision to transfer a patient is the responsibility of the attending physician at the referring hospital. He must contact a physician at the receiving hospital who is authorized to admit patients, to describe the patient's condition, and to obtain advice about stabilization and transport. The admitting physician at the receiving hospital must have accepted the patient and confirmed that appropriate resources are available at the receiving hospital before transport begins. Once the decision to transfer has been made, it should be effected as soon as possible. But according to national health system organization, there are some differences concerning the next steps of the transfer organization that need explanations.

Interhospital Transport in the US[33]

Referring and accepting physicians should agree as to who will assume responsibility for on-line medical control during transport if a physician is not in attendance. The mode of transportation (ground or air) used for transport is determined by the transferring physician after consultation with the receiving physician, based on time, weather, medical interventions necessary for ongoing life support during transfer, and availability of personnel and resources. The transport services are contacted to confirm availability, to inform them of the patient's status and anticipated medical needs during transport, and to coordinate the timing of the transfer. A nurse-to-nurse report is given by the referring facility to the unit at the accepting hospital, as well as a copy of the medical record (including a discharge summary and all radiographs). A minimum of two people, in addition to the vehicle operator, accompany the patient. At least one of the accompanying personnel is a registered nurse, physician, or advanced emergency medical technician capable of providing airway management including endotracheal intubation, intravenous therapy, dysrhythmia interpretation and treatment, and basic and advanced cardiac and trauma life support. When a physician does not accompany the patient, there should be a mechanism available to communicate with a physician concerning changes in the patient's status and to obtain additional orders. If this is not technically possible, the registered nurse or advanced emergency medical technician accompanying the patient should have preauthorization by standing orders to perform acute lifesaving interventions.

Interhospital Transport in Europe

In some European countries (France, Germany, Spain), there are several specialized emergency medical services (SAMU in France, i.e., Service d'Aide Médicale Urgente) in charge of extrahospital emergencies and interhospital transfers. The difference between the US system and the SAMU system, is that it is not the referring or accepting physicians who assume responsibility for on-line medical control during the transport, but a physician belonging to the SAMU. The organization of the transfer is then somewhat different. In fact, once the decision of transfer has been made, the physician of the SAMU is contacted to organize the transfer, after being informed of the patient's status by the referring physician. Then, he coordinates the timing of the transfer, determines the level of training of the accompanying personnel (always including a physician) and level of monitoring, as well as the mode of transportation. The other steps of the transfer are the same as for the US system.

The main advantage is that there is always an emergency physician (specially trained in the care of critically ill patients) included in the accompanying team, avoiding the need to communicate with a medical controller to obtain additional orders or preauthorization by standing orders to perform therapeutic interventions. In France, there is a growing need for medical interhospital transfer of head trauma patients, since there are few tertiary hospitals with neurosurgical units. For example, for Paris and its suburbs (approximately 7 million inhabitants) there are only seven referral neurosurgical units that assume the management of all head trauma patients. Therefore, there are some differences in the management of patients, compared to the US, inducing the possibility to hospitalize head trauma patients in a Surgical Intensive Care Unit without a neurosurgical team, which explains the frequent need for interhospital transfer of head trauma patients.

Recently, the French Society of Anesthesiology and Critical Care has edited national recommendations concerning the medical interhospital transfer of critically ill patients. These guidelines define the background of interhospital transfer, the modalities of organization of the transfer, the level of monitoring and critical care before, during, and after transport, the minimum equipment that should be available for transport (Table 1), the mode of transport, and the accompanying personnel.

Conclusion

Head trauma is a frequent problem responsible for significant morbidity and mortality in young patients. Interhospital transfer of head trauma patients to referral neurosurgical intensive care units, where sophisticated evaluation, monitoring, and eventually neurosurgical intervention can be provided, should improve outcome because definitive management of these patients is not possible in general hospitals. The transport itself must be organized in anticipation of intervention that may be required to treat the deteriorating patient. Pretransport evaluation and stabilization are major steps in the transfer, and they should enable prevention of secondary CNS injury and worsening during transport. The emphasis of care during these steps should be on the stabilization of the airway and circulation, and on detection of untreated life-threatening injuries. Some attempts at recognition and control of raised ICP may also be tried during transport, but should not delay the transfer to the referral

Table 1
Minimal Transport Equipment of a Mobile Intensive Care Unit of the SAMU
(France) in 1993

Airway Management	Hemodynamic Management
Bag/valve system with oxygen reservoir	Stethoscope
Adult masks	Cardiac monitor/defibrillator
Intubation kit	Blood pressure cuffs
Oxygen tubing	Non-invasive blood pressure monitor
Suction device and catheters	Arterial line tubing and monitoring equipment
Oxygen source for the expected duration of transport, with 1-hr reserve in addition	Intravenous administration sets
Heimlich valve	Infusion pumps
Chest tubes	Intravenous solutions (colloids and crystalloids)
Automatic transport ventilator	Drugs for ACLS
Positive end-expiratory pressure valve	Inotropic support and vasopressor drugs
Pulse oxymeter	Blood pumps bags
ETCO2 monitor	

Miscellaneous	If appropriate for the patient
Spinal immobilization device	MAST
Temperature monitor	External pacer
Salem sumps	Drugs for sedation

neurosurgical intensive care unit. Thus, it is very important that the transport team includes a medical doctor well trained in the field of emergency care of head trauma patients, such as a trauma anesthesiologist. In fact, rapid and safe transport of patients to definitive care should optimize survival and neurological recovery from severe head trauma.

References

1. Task Force on Guidelines Society of Critical Care Medicine: Guidelines for categorization for services for the critically ill patient. Crit Care Med 12:279, 1991.
2. Wadell G: Movement of critically hill patients within hospital. Br J Med 2:417, 1975.
3. Wadell G, Scott PDR, Lees NW, Ledingham I McA: Effects of ambulance transport in critically ill patients. Br Med J 1:386, 1975.

4. Hanning CD, Gilmour DG, Hothersall AP, et al: Movement of the critically ill within hospital. Intens Care Med 4:137, 1978.
5. Andrews PJD, Piper IR, Dearden NM, Miller JD: Secondary insults during intrahospital transport of head-injured patients. Lancet 335:327, 1990.
6. Shackford SR, Mackersie RC, Davis JW, Wolf PL, Hoyt DB: Epidemiology and pathology of traumatic deaths occuring at a level I trauma center in a regionalized system: The importance of secondary brain injury. J Trauma 29:1392, 1989.
7. Chesnut RM, Marshall LF, Klauber MR, Blunt BA, Balwin N, Eisenberg HM, Jane JA, Marmarou A, Foulkes MA: The role of secondary brain injury in determining outcome from severe head injury. J Trauma 34: 216, 1993.
8. Rosner MJ, Daughton S: Cerebral perfusion pressure management in head injury. J Trauma 30:933, 1990.
9. Chan KH, Miller JD, Dearden NM, Andrews PJD, Midgley S: The effect of changes in cerebral perfusion pressure upon middle cerebral artery blood flow velocity and jugular bulb venous oxygen saturation after severe brain injury. J Neurosurg 77:55, 1992.
10. Baxt WG, Moody P: The impact of advanced prehospital emergency care on the mortality of severly brain-injured patients. J Trauma 27:365, 1987.
11. Jennet B, Carlin J: Preventable mortality and morbidity after head injury. Injury 10:31, 1978.
12. Gentleman D, Jennet B: Hazards of interhospital transfer of comatose head injured patients. Lancet 2:853, 1981.
13. Indeck M, Peterson S, Smith J, Brotman S: Risk, cost, benefit of transporting ICU patients for special studies. J Trauma 28:1020, 1988.
14. Braman SS, Dunn SM, Amico CA, Millman RP: Complications of intrahospital transport in critically ill patients. Ann Intern Med 107:469, 1987.
15. Hurst JM, Davis KJr, Branson RD, Johannigman JA: Comparison of blood gases during transport using two methods of ventilatory support. J Trauma 29:1637, 1989.
16. Edlin S: Physiological changes during transport of the critically ill. Intens Care Med 3:131, 1989.
17. American Academy of Pediatrics: Committee on hospital care: Guidelines for air and ground transportation of pediatric patients. Pediatrics 78:943, 1986.
18. McClosky KA, Orr RA: Pediatric transport issues in emergency medicine. Emerg Med Clin North Am 9:475, 1991.
19. McClosky KA, Johnston C: Pediatric critical care transport survey: Team composition and training, mobilization time, and mode of transportation. Pediatr Emerg Care 6:1, 1990.
20. McClosky KA, Orr RA: Pediatric transport issues in emergency medicine. Emerg Med Clin North Am 9:475, 1991.
21. Lachenmyer J: Physiological aspects of transport. Intern Anesthesiol Clin 25:15, 1987.
22. Frew SA: Patient transfers: How to comply with the law. American

College of Emergency Physicians, Dallas, Texas, 1991, pp 15–18, 23–28, 29–31.

23. Oxer HE: Carriage by air of the seriously ill. Med J Aust 1:537, 1977.
24. Grande CM: Critical care transport: A trauma perspective. Crit Care Clin 6:165, 1990.
25. Boyd CR, Corse KM, Campbell RC: Emergency interhospital transport of the major trauma patient: Air versus ground. J Trauma 29:789, 1989.
26. Hunt RC, Bryan DM, Brinkley VS, Whitley TW, Benson NH: Inability to assess breath sounds during air medical transport by helicopter. JAMA 265:1982, 1991.
27. Vernon DD, Woodward GA, Skjonsberg AK: Management of the patient with head injury during transport. Crit Care Clin 8:619, 1992.
28. Lambert SM, Willet K: Transfer of multiply-injured patients for neurosurgical opinion: A study of the adequacy of assessment and resuscitation. Injury 24:333, 1993.
29. Henderson A, Coyne T, Wall D, Miller B: Aust N Z J Surg 62:759, 1992.
30. Miller JD, Sweet RC, Narayan R, et al: Early insults to the injured brain. JAMA 240:439, 1978.
31. Ampel I, Hott KA, Sielaff GW, et al: An approach to airway management in the acutely head-injured patient. J Emerg Med 6:1, 1988.
32. Copass MK, Oreskovich MR, Badergroen MR, et al: Prehospital cardiopulmonary resuscitation of the critically injured patient. Am J Surg 148:20, 1984.
33. O'Brien DJ, Danzl DE, Sowers MB, et al: Airway management of aeromedically transported trauma patients. J Emerg Med 6:49, 1990.
34. Pepe PE, Stewart RD, Copass MK: Prehospital management of trauma: A tale of three cities. Ann Emerg Med 15:1484, 1986.
35. Cottrel JE, Patel K, Turndorff H, et al: Intracranial pressure changes induced by sodium nitroprusside in patients with intracranial mass lesions. J Neurosurg 48:329, 1978.
36. Rosner MJ, Nesome HH, Becker DP, et al: Mechanical brain injury: The sympathoadrenal response. J Neurosurg 61:76–81, 1984.
37. Millen JE, Clauser FL, Zimmerman M: Physiological effects of controlled concussive brain trauma. J Appl Physiol 49:856–861, 1980.
38. Payen D, Quintin L, Plaisance P, Chiron B, Lhoste F: Head injury: Clonidine decreases plasma catecholamines. Crit Care Med 18:392–395, 1990.
39. Borel C, Hanley D, Diringer MN, et al: Intensive management of severe head injury. Chest 98:180, 1990.
40. Wosters PS, LeBlanc KL: Management of elevated intracranial pressure. Clin Pharmacol 9:762, 1990.
41. Guidelines Committee of the American College of Critical Care Medicine, Society of Critical Care Medicine and American Association of Critical-Care Nurses Transfer Guidelines Task Force: Guidelines for the transfer of critically ill patients. Crit Care Med 21:931, 1993.
42. Société Francaise d'Anesthésie et de Réanimation: Guidelines for the medical interhospital transfer of critically ill patients (Recommandations concernant les transferts interhospitaliers médicalisés). Paris, 1992, pp 1–8.

43. Carli P, Rozenberg A, Bousquet M, Lamour O, Derossi A: Evaluation colorimétrique du CO_2 expiré au cours des transferts interhospitaliers des patients de réanimation. Colorimetric evaluation of $ETCO_2$ during interhospital transport of critically ill patients. JEUR 5:31–34, 1992.
44. Ehrenwerth J, Sorbo S, Hackel A: Transport of critically ill adults. Crit Care Med 14:543, 1986.

3

Priorities in Initial Resuscitation and Perioperative Management:
Multitrauma Patients with Head, Chest, and Other Major Injuries

Thomas E. Knuth, MD, MPH,
Charles B. Watson, MD

Introduction

Epidemiology

Roughly 12% of the 60 million injuries estimated to occur in the United States per year require hospitalization.[1] In contrast with other leading causes of mortality that have declined in the past three decades (heart disease, cancer, and stroke), trauma-related deaths have increased.[2] Trauma is also the fifth leading cause of mortality

From *Trauma Anesthesia and Critical Care of Neurological Injury,* edited by K. J. Abrams and C. M. Grande. © 1997, Futura Publishing Co., Armonk, NY.

in those over 65 years of age. In the elderly population, the death rate from injury exceeds that in the younger population.[3]

Traffic accidents account for the majority of injury-related deaths in the older population.[4] Recent experience in urban trauma centers has demonstrated a shift from blunt trauma to penetrating trauma, largely due to firearms. In 1982, of the 147,884 injury-related deaths reported, 32,988 (22%) were gun-related, while 47,423 (32%) were related to motor vehicle accidents.[5] In 1992, the percentage of penetrating trauma-related death recorded by the Bridgeport Hospital's trauma registry was 54%; in 1993, this figure climbed to 63%.[6] National data parallel this tendency toward increased mortality caused by gunshot wounds: in the years from 1968 to 1991, firearm-related deaths exceeded motor vehicle crash-related deaths in the District of Columbia and Alaska; in 1990, five states demonstrated this trend; and, in 1991, seven states reported such data.[7] Additionally, in 1991, motor vehicle-related deaths exceeded only firearm-related deaths by 10% or less in eight other states. Penetrating injuries present more often as single-system or multiple, localized injuries than blunt trauma; however, the wide availability of automatic weapons has increased the frequency of admissions for multiple wounds in recent years.

Trunkey reported a triphasic death pattern associated with major trauma. Immediate deaths [at the scene or dead on arrival to hospital (DOA)] reported by his group were generally associated with severe central nervous system (CNS) and cardiac insults or tears of one of the great vessels.[3] Hemorrhagic events caused most of the early deaths (within 4 hours of admission). Of "late deaths," brain injury accounted for about 20%. Sepsis and multiple organ failure were the predominant causes. Recently, the issue has been reassessed by Sauaia et al., with a review of 292 deaths reported from data collected in Denver during 1992.[8] Of these, only 38% were due to motor vehicle accidents and 59% were due to penetrating trauma. Forty-five percent died at the scene, and 75% of those who made it to the hospital died within 24 hours: 50% of exsanguination and about 50% of brain injury. Sixty-one percent of the "late" deaths (26 patients) were due to progressive multiple organ failure. Their conclusion was that the first two peaks of Trunkey's trimodal distribution have combined: the trimodal distribution has shifted to a bimodal distribution with early deaths due to massive hemorrhage and severe brain injury and late deaths due to multiple organ system failure syndrome.

Traumatic brain injury is the leading cause of death and disability in young adults.[9] Forty-four percent of injury-related deaths were attributed to CNS insults in 1990.[10] Additionally, spinal cord injury, a subset of traumatic CNS insults that has a high mortality (50%) contributes approximately 4,000 traumatic quadriplegic and 8,000 paraplegic patients to the national "pool" each year.[11] The majority of CNS injuries are associated with motor vehicle accidents. Falls and other accidental trauma account for the remainder; but gunshot wounds are, as in other categories of trauma, an increasingly significant cause of CNS injury.

Frost notes that while only 20% of head injury patients require surgery, all patients with significant head injury (GCS <12) require airway evaluation and many require immediate airway intervention.[9] It follows that since brain-injured and spinal cord-injured patients present very difficult airway management problems and effective resuscitation protocols include maneuvers that protect the cervical spine and limit post-traumatic increases in intracranial pressure (neuroanesthesia), the anesthesia team is routinely called in most centers for neurotrauma as an essential part of the triage and resuscitation effort.

For the last three decades, between 25% and 50% of automobile deaths have been associated with thoracic injury.[12,13] Mechanisms include severe contusion, deceleration, and direct crush injury. In one series of over 600 consecutive chest injuries, chest wall insults presented with flail chest (20%), pneumothorax (35%), and hemothorax (30%).[14] Most patients with blunt chest trauma, sufficient to cause rib fractures, demonstrate signs of pulmonary contusion with progressive, adjacent lung infiltrates, hypoxemia, and tachypnea. Sudden death is most commonly due to direct penetration of, or shearing of, one or more great vessels with immediate exsanguination. One quarter of all exsanguinating trauma deaths are directly due to vascular injury in the thorax.[15]

Penetrating wounds of the chest are most often caused by gunshot or stab wounds. Interestingly, only a small percentage of wounds that were incurred in battle during the Arab-Israeli war in 1967 were thoracic (<5%),[16] a pattern noted during other modern wars. An increase of "street crime" associated with the illicit drug trade and concomitantly increased access to hand guns and assault weapons for "recreational" use catches more unshielded individuals than on the battlefield where defensive posture and apparel tend to limit gunshot injury to more exposed areas.

As multitrauma patients with major injuries are increasingly triaged directly to trauma centers where a team approach to care is essential, anesthesia and surgical staff must work together in a range of settings. The anesthetic requirement for trauma support may range from analgesia for treatment of an isolated extremity fracture to management of complex multisystem injuries requiring extensive resuscitation or penetrating injuries requiring emergency department (ED) thoracotomy. All of these patients require complementary surgical and anesthetic techniques. Since resuscitative support often leads to surgical anesthesia for key operative interventions, the anesthesiologist who is involved in the process from the start has a better opportunity to stay ahead of evolving problems and to contribute to improved overall outcome. Whether support means reversing critical processes such as hypovolemic shock or limiting secondary insults to damaged organ systems, it is only by understanding the injury, probable consequences, and known management strategies that the anesthesiologist can design the best anesthetic technique and avoid classic pitfalls.

In this chapter we review initial management priorities for multitrauma patients from combined surgical and anesthetic points of view. Also, we strive to tie together material covered in greater depth elsewhere in the book and provide a comprehensive overview of the way these topics interlock with one another. Life-threatening conditions that compromise the airway, breathing, circulation, and CNS are discussed first because all successive triage/management strategies are predicated on establishing a viable patient.

A number of management decisions depend on an assessment of the "stability" of the patient and, since the resuscitating anesthetist may have the best grasp of this issue, he or she must be able to interact effectively in management decision-making. On the other hand, the surgeon must be able to integrate the status reports from the anesthetist into an overall plan that will minimize morbidity and mortality for the patient. Consequently, it is most important that both specialties share an understanding of common goals and have the "drill" down right from the beginning.

Immediate Management

Immediate Recognition: The History

When a trauma call comes into the ED, the information reported usually relates to the vital signs and obvious injuries. Emphasis is placed on prompt, deliberative assessment and action seems at odds with a recommendation to obtain a thorough history of the event. The real story of the event may actually arrive hours or days later as witnesses or other involved parties come forward or as time permits discussion with initial responders. A member of the trauma team should always interview the emergency medical technicians (EMTs), paramedics, relatives, police, and any other sources that can serve to provide first-hand data. This team member should directly inform both anesthesia and surgical team members as soon as is appropriate.

The anesthesiologist's primary focus in trauma resuscitation is on establishing airway, ventilatory, and circulatory support (A, B, Cs). Surgical priorities are initially the same with emphasis on controlling blood loss. Even though priorities are appropriately focused on acute lifesaving interventions, good information about the mechanism of injury serves to focus attention on the most likely problems and can be critically important in setting initial management priorities.[17] In blunt injury, the force of impact over a broad area as acute deceleration is converted into shear, compression (bursting), and decompression (shock wave) vectors that can disrupt the chest wall, contiguous and adjacent viscera, and conduction airways or vessels. A useful history of a motor vehicle injury will include the speed and direction at impact, and the location, size, and extent of damage to the vehicle. The victim's location in the vehicle together with the use (or disuse) of restraint devices is important. If the victim was thrown outside the vehicle, one should know the trajectory, distance, and landing position. For penetrating injuries, one should identify the size, location, force, and trajectory of penetration. High-velocity projectiles create a shock wave that creates adjacent blunt trauma. Explosive shells combine penetrating injury with local blast and shock insults. For managing the shooting victim, entry vectors, position of the patient at impact, type of weapon and shells used, and distance from the assailant to the victim become most useful pieces of information.

The mental exercise of visualizing the actual traumatic forces will help predict the most likely combination of injuries. It can reduce wasted time, energy, and expense devoted to unproductive tests or counterproductive interventions, and facilitate more prompt and accurate action.

Immediate Concerns

Management of the multiply injured patient must begin with immediate treatment of life-threatening conditions. Rapid visual assessment is almost all the evaluation that is necessary to initiate lifesaving interventions that should never be delayed for further diagnostic tests. Airway, breathing, and circulation should be addressed in this specific order according to time-tested and widely accepted guidelines.[13]

Airway

Identification of apnea, airway obstruction or disruption, and inadequate protective reflexes is the most immediate concern for the trauma team. Most trauma teams assign an anesthesiologist as the primary responder for this responsibility. Look, listen, and feel the airway first. Evaluation and intervention must be performed expeditiously with a conscientious attempt to limit motion of the neck. Always assume that the cervical spine is injured.

A lower threshold for intubation is appropriate in multitrauma patients who have increased risk of progressive deterioration (i.e., in patients with rib fractures and pulmonary contusion) and in intoxicated and/or combative patients who cannot or will not cooperate with a possible life-saving evaluation or therapy. Although effective ventilation and oxygenation can frequently be achieved with bag/valve/mask ventilation, the high incidence of gastric aeration, distention, and subsequent regurgitation followed by pulmonary aspiration make this unacceptable for any length of time. If effective oxygenation cannot be achieved within 2 to 3 minutes (i.e., because of maxillofacial injuries or airway obstruction), a surgical airway should be created. If a surgeon is not immediately available to perform an emergent cricothyroidotomy, the anesthesiologist should not hesitate to perform a temporary needle cricothyroidtomy. A secure airway should be placed as soon as possible following catheter cricothyrotomy. Finally, it is important for the trauma anesthesiologist to realize that the vast majority of surgeons do not have significant experience in performing emergency surgical airways (i.e., most of their previous experience has been limited to elective situations), and thus will not necessarily be more adept at performing these techniques under duress than would the properly prepared anesthesiologist.

For multitrauma patients who are not in extremis, evaluation of the airway should include assessment of mental status, dyspnea, and/or chest pain and the position and movement of the jaw, tongue, larynx, trachea, and suprasternal region should be observed during breathing and maneuvers such as coughing and swallowing. Obvious facial trauma and/or upper airway bleeding can be disconcerting but is not an immediate threat, provided that blood and debris from the mouth are not aspirated, and should not prevent a brief evaluation of the neck and airway. Midface fractures and nasal bleeding are contraindications for nasal intubation of any type but should not preclude oral intubation attempts. The anesthesiologist should be alert for the findings of stridor, tracheal deviation, distended neck veins, expanding hematoma, and crepitus in the neck. Alert patients can identify neck or chest pain and provide other clues that aid the anesthesiologist; simply the ability to answer such questions provides an immense amount of information, not only about the airway but about the mental status as well. As airway evaluation proceeds, a pulse oximeter should be placed.

Level of Consciousness

Even if the patient spontaneously ventilates and oxygenates adequately, a Glasgow Coma Score (GCS) of <8 is usually associated with inadequate protective glottic reflexes. Somnolence, lethargy, and "delayed" protective reflexes as noted during gentle pharyngeal or oral suctioning suggest a need for airway protection by endotracheal intubation, and this may occur in patients even with a GCS above 13. Unless significant CNS injury is obvious, the most expeditious approach is direct translaryngeal intubation. When closed head trauma is the most likely cause of CNS depression, controlled ventilation by endotracheal tube (ETT) or tracheotomy tube allows hyperventilation as the first step to control rising intracranial pressure (ICP). We recommend a "neuroanesthetic" for tracheal tube placement when elevated ICP is suspected, provided that the patient's hemodynamics will support it. Remember that prior to administration of paralytics and sedatives, a quick neurological assessment should be documented: extremity motor function, pupillary reflexes, and general response to commands or to painful stimuli should be specifically noted.

Application of cricoid pressure (Sellick's maneuver) will reduce the risk of pulmonary aspiration. Cricoid pressure may be especially helpful during paralysis. Rigid cervical collars interfere with cricoid pressure. More recent versions of the rigid cervical collar have either an anterior plate attached by Velcro fasteners that can be removed or an anterior fenestration that allows access for cricoid pressure, palpation of carotid pulses, and needle cricothyroidotomy. An assistant should always stabilize the head and neck until the intubation is completed and the cervical collar is replaced.

Obstruction

Tracheobronchial obstruction from foreign body aspiration (i.e., teeth, food, chewing gum) should be suspected in patients who are stridorous, tachypneic, and using accessory respiratory muscles. Chin lift and jaw thrust maneuvers will displace most obstructing soft tissues and can be performed without neck extension. Suction for removal of pharyngeal blood, secretions, and debris will prevent iatrogenic aspiration. A simple finger sweep or Magill forceps extraction may be all that is needed to clear obstruction in most adults. Before use of nasopharyngeal, oropharyngeal, or laryngeal mask airways, one should always ensure that the airway is clear.

If partial obstruction due to a foreign body persists and the patient is oxygenating adequately, intubation over a flexible fiberoptic bronchoscope (FFB) or removal of the obstructing object is advisable as the initial step. Blind airway insertion and intubation approaches are more dangerous not only because a foreign body can be pushed further into the airway and cause total obstruction but also because false tissue passages encouraged by the partially obstructing object can traumatize mucosa and cause airway hemorrhage.

Tracheal Disruption

Direct laryngotracheal trauma is most commonly caused by steering wheel or clothesline injury, but is possible with any direct blow to the neck. Subcutaneous emphysema, mobile laryngeal elements, and obvious contusion over the larynx and upper trachea should suggest laryngeal crush injury in the multitrauma setting. Total (or near-total) airway disruption should be anticipated: extreme caution must always be used during attempts at intubation. Conversion of a partial tear to a complete disruption is possible when the trachea is instrumented.[18] If the distal segment of the transected trachea retracts into the chest, an emergent tracheostomy will be difficult or near impossible. Thus, there may be only one chance to obtain an airway. The first attempt should use FFB guidance for direct visual placement.[19,20] If the patient is stable and the proper equipment is available, the FFB can serve as a placement guide for tracheal positioning of the tube.[21] The FFB helps gain medically relevant information about the site and character of the tracheal injury in the process.[22]

Oral translaryngeal intubation must proceed with extreme caution, if fiberoptics are unavailable. In some settings, urgent tracheostomy is the best initial option to safely secure the airway and to prevent further damage to the larynx. Occasionally, the cut trachea presents a convenient transcervical opening for immediate external intubation.

Ventilation

Physical examination of the chest must be rapid and goal oriented to ensure equal air entry into both sides of the chest. Auscultation is among the first steps and should identify symmetry of breath sounds and then focus on adventitious sounds and cardiac sounds. More subtle findings such as mediastinal crunch, gallop, or very focal wheezing (suggestive of foreign body aspiration) may be difficult to appreciate in the noisy trauma room. Important visual assessment includes chest wall excursion (rhythm and symmetry), obvious sternal and/or intercostal retractions, surface contusions, abrasions, lacerations, and open wounds. Clues about the patient's preexisting health status (barrel chest, wasting, clubbing of nail beds, a prominent precordial heave, venous spiders, etc.) should be noted as factors in predicting both immediate and long-term ventilatory needs.

Palpation of the chest will verify the integrity of the rib cage and clavicles, symmetry of ventilatory movement, and presence or absence of subcutaneous emphysema; percussion will identify obvious dullness or hyperresonance. Repeated percussion of the chest and auscultation of the neck and thorax at periodic intervals will detect evolving pathology. The conscious patient should be questioned about chest pain, pleuritic symptoms, and other important history as the examination continues.

Capnometry is essential to care for patients whose minute ventilation requirement is difficult to predict. Real-time ventilatory data can be generated by most ventilators. Graphic displays of airway pressure/flow/volume relationships are also available on some ICU ventilators. These monitors and ICU-quality ventilators should be "first-line" equipment in the emergency department and diagnostic areas where trauma patients are managed after initial triage. At least one set of arterial blood gases (ABGs) is necessary to "calibrate" capnographic systems for initial and continuous monitoring through the resuscitation period.

When basic ventilatory requirements are met, the mechanics of lung function can be addressed. Ventilatory support should be designed to restore lung mechanics to baseline and to limit the pain experienced and work requirement for spontaneous breathing.

Tension Pneumothorax

A shift in the trachea, jugular venous distention (JVD), hyper-resonance of a hemithorax, chest "lag," and unilateral absence of breath sounds (localizing signs) during either spontaneous or assisted ventilation implies presence of an air-filled, pressurized cavity—a tension pneumothorax. As soon as tension pneumothorax has been suspected, a #18 (or larger) gauge angiocath should be placed in the midclavicular line of the second intercostal space. Normally, an audible rush of air will identify decompression of the mediastinum sufficient to reestablish venous return to the heart. The catheter should be left in place (underwater seal) until a thoracostomy tube can be placed. Formal tube thoracostomy can wait for management of other high-priority issues if the pneumothorax is demonstrated to be adequately decompressed by physical examination and chest x-ray.

Open Pneumothorax

An occlusive dressing over an obvious penetrating stab, gunshot wound, or laceration of the chest wall should be followed immediately by placement of a large (36–40 Fr) thoracostomy tube into the side of the injury. Reexpansion of the lung will often tamponade minor chest wall and/or parenchymal bleeding. It can also "stent" a pleural tear, thus controlling minor "air leaks." The thoracostomy tube will drain associated blood loss and prevent tension hemothorax after the wound is covered. The open wound should be primarily closed after irrigation when time and patient stability permit.

Flail Chest and Pulmonary Contusion

Multiple fragmented ribs can easily be recognized by palpating the chest wall and finding one or more unstable segments. Underlying pulmonary contusion is the rule rather than an exception when chest trauma is significant enough to break the flexible chest wall in more than one place to create a "flail." Often, paradoxical movement of the flail segment can be appreciated as the patient breathes spontaneously.

A major challenge arises when contralateral thoracotomy is needed in the lateral position. Because overall V/Q matching will deteriorate as the lung with the highest blood flow (dependent) in the lateral position will have deranged ventilation, hypoxemia with or without hypercapnea is likely. On this account, lung isolation and selective ventilation with differential tidal volumes and PEEP make good sense. Many anesthesiologists advocate use of either high- frequency jet ventilation (HFJV) via a single-lumen jet tube (Hi-Lo Jet™, Mallinckrodt, Glynns Falls, NY) or selective blockade with the single-lumen Univent™ (Fuji Systems Corp., Tokyo, Japan) tube. They should be available in the trauma receiving room so they can be used for tracheal intubation from the start. Unfortunately, both HFJV and selective blockade fail to allow effective dual lung ventilation with differential settings in the perioperative period. For this reason, a majority of anesthesiologists continue to use double-lumen endobronchial tubes despite the inconvenience of changing them for postoperative ventilatory support.[23,24]

Hemodynamic Support

As the airway and ventilation are controlled, attention is rapidly, if not simultaneously, directed toward control of ongoing blood loss and circulatory support. Two #16-gauge (or larger) intravenous catheters should routinely be placed in all multitrauma patients, even those who initially appear stable. Since venous integrity is uncertain in chest and abdominal injuries, a specific effort should be made to ensure effective placement of resuscitative lines. When peripheral catheters are not available, the central venous route is often the best way to rapidly infuse large volumes of warmed blood products or fluid. Since this is often the quickest and most easily obtained access in hypovolemic patients, it is reasonable to insert large-bore femoral, subclavian, or jugular venous catheters or introducer sheaths (8–9 French) as a first priority.

The goal is to obtain "adequate" perfusion pressure and not necessarily "normal" pressure since raising blood pressure in patients with an open circulation (uncontrolled bleeding) will effectively increase blood loss. On the other hand, determination of "adequate" perfusion pressure is difficult and the risk of underresuscitation is generally worse than that of liberal volume infusion, especially in young trauma patients. Even brain-injured patients at risk for edema and intracranial hypertension have restoration of brain and other organ perfusion as the first priority. Consequently, the focus should be on stopping the bleeding (close the circulation) so that blood pressure and tissue perfusion can be restored to normal levels.

Sources of hemorrhage can usually be determined after a quick work-up that includes physical examination, chest and abdominal x-rays, and diagnostic paracentesis/lavage. In the absence of obvious bleeding, hypotension should suggest cardiac tamponade or neurogenic vasomotor paralysis due to spinal cord injury.

Intrathoracic Bleeding

Refractory hypotension after penetrating chest injury warrants urgent thoracotomy for direct evaluation and control.[25] Once bleeding has been controlled in the ED, the patient should be transferred to the operating room (OR) for definitive care and closure of the thoracotomy. If hypotension is readily stabilized with volume infusion and either the physical examination or chest film suggests thoracic bleeding, tube thoracostomy, and expectant observation are appropriate and allow the trauma team to address other priorities. An initial hemothorax containing more than 2 liters of blood, and initial drainage of 300–500 mL/hour or greater than 200 mL/hour over 5–6 hours is an indication for thoracic exploration and surgical control.[26]

The fact that a chest tube is in place does not ensure that drainage will be adequate and totally eliminate the risk of tension hemothorax or pneumothorax; the trauma team or anesthesiologist should repeatedly evaluate the chest and drainage system by direct examination and chest film for several hours. This is especially important for the anesthesiologist if later surgical procedures on other organ systems or the extremities are needed. During surgery, the surgical team may be distracted by other problems.

Blunt trauma with injury to the neck, upper ribs, and clavicles are indications for serial differential blood pressure measurements and neurological examinations. Abnormalities in either blood pressure, neurological exam, or asymmetrical venous distention with evidence of penetrating injury near the great vessels warrants arteriography, thoracic CT, and/or transesophageal echocardiography (TEE). Typically, blunt trauma to the carotid artery will present several days later with signs and symptoms of stroke. Arteriography is indicated at this time to rule out intimal disruption and thrombosis.

Penetrating trauma below the clavicles (including zone I of the neck), between the nipples, and above the epigastric area always warrants a pericardial window to exclude injury to the heart and possibly an arteriogram to exclude injury to major blood vessels. TEE can be of tremendous help because it can detect both pericardial fluid and clot. In the OR, the anesthesiologist can facilitate monitoring and assessment with intraoperative TEE, provided esophageal penetration has been ruled out. Early use of TEE will allow a complete, thorough study of the heart, whether the patient undergoes thoracotomy or laparotomy. TEE is more likely to produce a good study than transthoracic echocardiography and is more sensitive than either enzymes or the ECG.[27]

Abdominal Bleeding

For abdominal exsanguination, some surgeons advocate ED thoracotomy and aortic cross-clamping.[28] After ED thoracotomy, the patient is moved rapidly to the OR for celiotomy for definitive assessment and management of the injury before closure of the thoracotomy. Other surgeons prefer to expedite transfer to the OR where rapid entry into the abdomen is followed by aortic control below the level of the diaphragm. The estimated extent of blood loss, the ability to immediately transfer to the OR and to enter the abdomen, and the response to initial resuscitative efforts should dictate which technique is most appropriate. Whether immediate thoracotomy is performed in the ED or in the OR, the anesthesia team needs to be involved from the "ground floor" so that key ventilatory support, vascular access, and hemodynamic drugs can be continuously coordinated.

Refractory hypotension with increasing abdominal distention and/or tenderness warrants immediate transfer to the OR for celiotomy without further diagnostic work-up. In cases where the source of bleeding is not obvious (benign abdominal exam) but intra-abdominal bleeding is suspected because of unstable vital signs, paracentesis, diagnostic peritoneal lavage (DPL), or abdominal CT may be indicated. The appropriate diagnostic step depends on the patient's hemodynamic stability. In a relatively unstable patient, paracentesis is the more appropriate test and if more than 10 mL of frank blood is found, urgent celiotomy is warranted. If less than 10 mL of grossly bloody fluid is obtained, DPL is indicated, and if the results are positive, the patient is moved to the OR with an urgency that is dependent on the clinical status and associated injuries. If the DPL is indeterminant by cell count (>20,000 but <100,000 cells per high-powered microscopic field), the life-threatening hemorrhage is not in the abdomen and other sources should be sought.[29]

Retroperitoneal Bleeding

Most retroperitoneal bleeding in blunt trauma patients is related to pelvic fractures. Gross pelvic instability by examination or disruption found by x-ray should raise suspicion of retroperitoneal hemorrhage. Most retroperitoneal hematomas are discovered and evaluated intraoperatively because abdominal examination, paracentesis, or DPL have warranted celiotomy. Treatment depends on exactly where the hematoma is located and whether it is expanding. Retroperitoneal hematomas from pelvic fractures should almost never be unroofed because the small vessels that are likely to be bleeding are nearly impossible to locate and ligate. The tamponading effect of the intact retroperitoneum is more effective. On the other hand, all retroperitoneal hematomas from penetrating injuries should be explored since there is likely to be a major vessel that can be ligated.

When ceilotomy is not warranted, retroperitoneal hematomas are most often discovered and evaluated by CT scanning. Signs such as flank discoloration and patient discomfort are either nonspecific or late in onset. One must recognize that anywhere from 6 units to several blood volumes can be lost in the retroperitoneal space with no immediate signs other than clinical evidence of hypovolemia. Massive retroperitoneal hematoma can impair pulmonary, renal, bowel, and liver function as well as disrupt circulation in the lower half of the body.

A temporizing but effective acute measure may be inflation of the abdominal compartment of MAST trousers. This should be followed by expeditious orthopedic consultation for application of pelvic external fixation devices that are effective in 95% of cases.[30] If bleeding continues (in the absence of coagulopathy), at a rate arbitrarily set to exceed 4 units over 24 hours, after celiotomy or after placement of the external fixator in the postresuscitative period, arteriography is indicated. Arteriographic embolization is about 90% successful in controlling bleeding pelvic vessels.[31]

Extremity Bleeding

Diffuse pressure as applied to bleeding extremity wounds by gauze dressings or wraps is often inadequate to control direct vascular bleeding following penetrating, lacerating, or rotational/degloving injuries to the extremities. Blood-soaked dressings should be removed so blood loss rate can be appreciated and so that direct finger-control pressure can be applied. Pressure-point compressions (i.e., by inflatable splints) are useful adjuncts in the field, but should be removed in the ED to allow more precise control of bleeding. Like tourniquets, inflatable splints may eliminate perfusion to viable tissue surrounding the injured major vessel. Clamps and ligatures that crush the vessel may compromise repair and are also not advised. Atraumatic vascular surgical clamps are the only devices other than the finger that should be used to control an open vessel and this should be maintained until the patient is taken to the OR for surgical repair. Obviously, diffuse bleeding from abrasions or crush injuries should be adequately controlled by diffuse pressure.

Cardiac Tamponade

After penetrating chest or epigastric injury, cardiac tamponade should be anticipated. Surgical treatment comprises urgent thoracotomy, pericardiotomy, and repair of the heart wound. A pericardiocentesis should never be relied upon to exclude cardiac injury and is as likely to cause myocardial injury as it is to diagnose or treat one. Furthermore, if the rent from the penetrating injury is insufficient to decompress the pericardial sack, a small-bore pericardiocentesis catheter will also be inadequate. Both will clot. The pericardium needs to be widely opened to relieve tamponade and then the patient needs immediate thoracotomy or sternotomy to repair the myocardial injury.

Anesthetic concerns include maintenance of filling pressures at supranormal levels (greater than intrapericardial) and support of blood pressure and circulation while these interventions are performed. Anesthetic management should emphasize volume infusion, control of the airway, paralysis and small doses of amnestic drugs such as scopolamine or a benzodiazepine. Because the patient's sympathetic tone is a major compensatory mechanism, even small doses of ketamine can be followed paradoxically by profound hypotension in the acute setting. There is no "safe" anesthetic agent that will substitute for adequate volume replacement and effective venous return.[32]

Pericardial tamponade is usually not suspected after blunt trauma until large volume infusion, out of proportion with obvious and estimated blood losses, fails to raise the blood pressure. Beck's triad (jugular venous distention, muffled heart sounds, and decreased pulse pressure) is quite nonspecific and often difficult to identify in the acute setting, but may be considered as supporting evidence for pericardial tamponade.

In life-threatening hypotension, pericardiocentesis may be of value as a temporizing resuscitative measure until a definitive subxyphoid pericardial window can be performed, but again should not be relied upon for diagnosis or treatment. When patients are unstable, it is better to avoid general anesthesia in favor of local anesthesia until the pericardial cavity is decompressed. Usually patients with this problem are in extremis so they rarely remember the events if they survive. If the blood pressure can be maintained with volume infusion and pressors, the risk of pericardiocentesis weighs unfavorably against open drainage by a surgical window. General anesthesia for this procedure, if elected, should be provided in a "staged" fashion with small increments of an amnestic drug such as midazolam followed by a relaxant and, after stability is demonstrated or achieved, increments of narcotic and an inhalational agent.

Delayed tamponade is a rare event that can occur at a later time in the OR or ICU. It is usually due to atrial bleeding after a penetrating injury, but may be associated with severe myocardial contusion and transmural rupture.[33] In the latter setting, significant ECG changes are obvious from the time of injury. Postresuscitation/ICU management should include ICU monitoring with this eventuality in mind. In either case, one normally has time for either angiography or TEE, followed by pericardiocentesis guided by TEE and surgical exploration.[34]

Myocardial Injury

Severe myocardial infarction as a cause of hypotension in the trauma setting is not uncommon in the high-risk, elderly population. The heart attack may have been the cause of the accident.[35] When de novo ischemic events occur, stress, pain, hypotension, and direct contusion may all be factors. If the patient is deemed to be at risk, an ECG in the ED is reasonable. If the diagnosis is suspected or confirmed, pulmonary artery catheterization should be undertaken as part of the secondary resuscitation, after the basics have been dealt with. Although the frequency of contusion is variably reported after blunt trauma because mild contusions of no significance are not often documented, the major problem, arrhythmias in the recovery period, is picked up during routine rhythm monitoring. Contusion is not often a primary cause for hypotension; it must be so severe that key structures, such as the mitral valve, are injured before hypotension ensues.

Neurotrauma

Neurogenic Hypotension

Spinal cord injuries can result in loss of peripheral and cardiac sympathetic function. Hypotension is caused by peripheral vasodilation and loss of compensatory cardiac reflexes with unopposed parasympathetic function. When cervical or thoracic films demonstrate vertebral injury, and shock is either unrelated to or out of proportion with demonstrable bleeding, "spinal" shock should be suspected. Assessment of the conjunctival perfusion is helpful in these cases since pink mucous membranes and/or conjunctivae suggest that the problem is more likely neurogenic than hemorrhagic in origin. Restoration of preload is necessary to maintain perfusion and either a central venous pressure (CVP) or pulmonary artery occlusion pressure (PCWP) monitor is helpful to prevent fluid overload. We prefer to use a pulmonary artery catheter placed immediately after resuscitation in the OR or ICU.

Patients with spinal shock can be shown to have progressive cardiac dilatation with both systolic and diastolic dysfunction. Since withdrawal of sympathetic tone can be gradual, the anesthesiologist should have a low threshold for considering neuroreflex shock in the OR and ICU settings, hours after resuscitation in the ED. Dopamine is probably the most widely used vasopressor for addressing both cardiac and peripheral sympathetic denervation in the post-traumatic period. If the patient fails to respond to dopamine and volume expansion, epinephrine is the next best choice because it does not rely upon endogenous catecholamine stores. Meanwhile, other causes for hypotension must be reinvestigated.

Neurotrauma

Closed Head Injuries

Closed Head Injury without Herniation Syndrome

Any patient with head trauma and a GCS <13 needs a cranial CT. CNS evaluation is often difficult because of prior drug or alcohol intoxication. When neurological evaluation is altered or difficult because of intoxication or sedation, CT evaluation is indicated even for head-injured patients with a GCS >13. Since combativeness can be a sign of both head injury and/or intoxication, combative patients, especially when paralytic and sedative medications are required, should have CT scans. If sedation and/or paralysis is needed for some time following admission, either frequent follow-up CTs or an ICP monitor is also indicated. Fluid management and nursing maneuvers such as position, suction, tracheal tube securing systems, etc. will have a significant effect on ICP if delayed edema develops. Thus, fluid balance should be closely monitored with plans made for careful CNS monitoring and prophylactic nursing care.

Herniation Syndrome

In the event that routine medical measures do not prevent progressive signs of uncal herniation, as manifested by anisocoria and lateralizing neurological findings, immediate decompression must be undertaken to decompress the cranium.[36] Burr holes will reverse this process if it is due to epidural hematoma. They should be performed in the OR with the help of experienced staff. Since shock and hypoperfusion may cause a secondary brain injury that can be at least as detrimental to patient survival as the initial traumatic insult, medical measures instituted to correct these should be continued while burr holes are placed.

Burr holes usually will not help patients with subdural and intracerebral hematomas and a formal craniotomy will be required to completely evacuate the clot and find the source of bleeding. Consequently, without a definitive diagnosis, immediate burr holes should be placed only when dramatic signs of progressive brain stem compression are evident and death is imminent. Otherwise, patients should be stabilized as much as possible and taken for immediate CT scanning while medical measures to control ICP are continued.

Setting Priorities

Ideally, all immediate concerns amenable to surgical intervention can be managed simultaneously and multiple teams including neurosurgical, general, and thoracic, as well as orthopedic services can work to stabilize a multitrauma patient. An intracranial hematoma can be evacuated or an intracranial pressure monitor placed when chest and/or intra-abdominal hemorrhage is being addressed, and fractures can be stabilized while vascular repairs are performed. Unfortunately, this high level of trauma care is unrealistic in all but the busiest and most sophisticated trauma centers. Setting difficult management priorities is the norm and must be done when two or more immediate or urgent concerns present simultaneously. Conceptually and practically, both anesthesia and surgical teams manage conflicting priorities as a matter of routine in their daily practices. Typical anesthesia examples include the full stomach/open globe problem or working with the ear, nose, and throat, or thoracic surgeon in the shared airway. There is no setting, however, such as management of the serious multitrauma patient, where the importance of teamwork and a systematic approach pays bigger dividends for the patient.

In general, prioritization is a dynamic, stepwise, and circuitous process during which the resuscitation team must work together. All team members must remain flexible since priorities often change as critical conditions evolve or new problems are discovered. Temporary treatment measures are taken to stabilize immediate injuries. These injuries are continually reevaluated until definitive treatment is possible. For example, a patient with a tension pneumothorax that has been adequately decompressed by needle/catheter thoracostomy is best treated by moving on to other priorities rather than by taking the time to immediately place a definitive thoracostomy tube. A chest tube can be placed as time and clinical status allow, and even this may prove to be temporary if open thoracotomy becomes necessary.

The following dilemmas are typical of issues that need to be worked out in advance. Both anesthesia and surgical staff need a clear understanding of evaluation and treatment options in these situations and should support each other's efforts on behalf of the patient.

Combined Head and Chest Injuries

It is clear that early diagnosis and surgical treatment of an acute extradural hematoma or an acute subdural hematoma results in decreased mortality[37,38] and that delays in the treatment lead to increased morbidity. Delays in treating associated injuries can be equally devastating to the patient's overall outcome if blood loss and hypotension contribute to malperfusion of the head injury. Also, secondary brain injury due to continued hypoxia, with or without hypercapnea and hypotension, can potentiate the initial injury.[39]

When celiotomy or thoracotomy is urgently indicated and there is a question of intracranial hematoma, the surgical dilemma is whether to take the time to evaluate the extent of the closed head injury with a CT scan on the way to the OR.[40] The alternative is to obtain the study after surgery, which may be a few hours later. It is imperative that priorities are set to minimize poor outcome and followed in order to evaluate and treat both injuries as expeditiously as possible.

In the event that both thoracic and head injuries cannot be addressed simultaneously, the decision as to which to treat first can be based on statistical probabilities. Gutman et al.[41] determined that hypotension associated with increasing age (>70), low GCS, fall as the mechanism of injury, and pupillary inequality are predictive of an intracranial mass lesion. At a younger age (>30), vehicular crash as the mechanism, tachycardia, and hypotension are more likely to be associated with a severe torso injury than a head injury. Wisner et al.[42] identified lateralizing signs on initial presentation and a need for intubation in the field as independent indicators for urgent craniotomy. They also pointed out that although as many as 70% of blunt trauma victims suffer some degree of head injury, most require close monitoring and medical management but few have surgically correctable lesions. They concluded that initial priorities in the unstable patient should, therefore, be to perform the celiotomy (or thoracotomy) first and obtain the head CT postoperatively.

Prioritization of this dilemma depends largely on availability of resources. Ideally, a surgical closed head injury can be adequately evaluated in less than 5 minutes by a few correctly placed cross-sectional views produced on the CT scan. Realistically, however, the total procedure, including patient transport and movement time plus the time to obtain and interpret the test, often takes 30 to 45 minutes or longer. The information gained by CT evaluation will determine whether craniotomy or an ICP monitor is indicated at the time of the thoracic or abdominal procedure but this may not be worth the wait.

Some trauma intensivists would place an ICP monitor in any case, if the presentation strongly suggested significant head trauma, and begin medical management immediately. The need for craniotomy and evacuation of a hematoma is determined later. In this case, the patient would be moved from the OR to the radiology suite and back into the OR for definitive management.

Resuscitative management should include controlled ventilation, maintenance of normal oxygenation and perfusion, careful fluid management, pharmacological ablation of abnormally amplified cerebromotor reflexes, pharmacological reduction of cerebral oxygen consumption, and elevation of the head. Immediate mannitol infusion would have debatable benefit because it may cause either volume expansion with subsequent diuresis or progressive hypovolemia. Unguided mannitol therapy should be avoided.

In the more stable patient, and in patients with a negative paracentesis (even if DPL is positive), celiotomy can be delayed briefly for CT scan evaluation of the closed head injury enroute to the OR. When there are localizing signs on neurological examination, however, thoracotomy or celiotomy should be delayed for the head CT on the way to the OR so that simultaneous craniotomy can be performed, if necessary.

In the event that a neurosurgeon is not available for immediate consultation, the most appropriate intervention is even more problematic. Management considerations must include the optimal time to transfer the patient to a neurosurgical facility. If the patient is unstable, a better option is to obtain a neurosurgeon from another institution and manage to have neurosurgical evaluation or intervention available by the completion of the thoracoabdominal procedure. The least desirable option is to transport the patient with both injuries untreated.

Maxillofacial and Chest

Although commonly the most dramatic and attention-attracting injuries, maxillofacial injuries take a low priority in the evaluation and treatment of the multiply injured patient. Except when they compromise the CNS or airway, facial fractures and soft tissue injuries are rarely life-threatening. They can often be treated 4–5 days after the injury.

Noting that 52% of patients with facial fractures also suffered closed head injury, Derdyn[43] found that when ICPs were less than 15, there was no significant difference in survival between patients who underwent early (0–3 days), middle (4–7 days), or late (>7) surgical repair of their facial fractures. With intracranial hypertension, the picture is different. Although aesthetic and functional results were improved by immediate and full correction of facial fractures, poor chances for survival also made patients with a GCS <5, evidence of intracranial hematoma including midline shift or basal cistern effacement, and ICP >15 poor candidates for early maxillofacial surgery. Similarly, plastic procedures designed to improve external appearance should not be considered until all other organ system injuries are stable and/or are definitively controlled.

Pitfalls in Anesthetic Management

There are a number of recurrent problems for the anesthesia team as the initial management and prioritization of multitrauma patients proceeds. The basic approach follows Advanced Trauma Life Support (ATLS) guidelines formulated by the American College of Surgeons. Following these guidelines, we recommend key resuscitation steps that give the greatest survival for the majority of patients. Some issues are beyond negotiation. For example, immediate control of the airway and restoration of effective ventilation are consistent priorities that leave little room for judgment. There are controversies regarding the methods, but all agree on the goal. We shall discuss approaches to difficult airway interventions and review several anesthesia decision-making areas that present recurrent difficulty.

Transport to Outlying Areas

In some trauma receiving centers, diagnostic facilities are remote from the OR, ED, and ICUs. A recurrent issue is lapse of attention to patient care because the patient has been sent to a remote location with no one specifically monitoring the patient or is enclosed within a room where radiation risk limits patient access. Generally, resuscitation progresses until acute volume resuscitation has slowed and monitoring frequency is reduced below that typical in the ED, OR, and ICU. This is a controversial issue in many centers; no one admits that the problem exists and everyone is quick to blame someone else when an unaccompanied patient deteriorates in the corridor outside of the x-ray department or during a cranial CT scan. Sometimes this responsibility devolves on the anesthesia team by plan or protocol, sometimes by default.

Roles for anesthesia staff in the transport and stabilization process may differ at various institutions but removal from the ED resuscitation area or the OR to the radiology suite should never be associated with a lapse of monitoring or attention to detail. Since the anesthesia team will invariably need to compensate for any such lapses when the patient is transferred to the OR, it makes good sense for the anesthesia staff to remain with the patient at all times while outside tests including cranial CTs are performed. In most institutions, patients with severe neurotrauma who require CT scanning are given nondepolarizing relaxants, controlled hyperventilation, and osmotic diuretics as a prophylactic measure pending results of the scan. This is comparable with the anesthetic that would be given for a neurosurgical procedure. Standards of patient monitoring and management expectations from the anesthesia staff should be the same if the anesthesia team has initiated the process.

Conclusion

Although airway and acute circulatory management are most commonly the specific tasks managed by the anesthetia team in the initial resuscitation of the multitrauma patient, roles vary from center to center. The anesthesiologist and anesthesia care team are intimately involved in every part of the in-hospital care of the multitrauma patient. Beginning with the initial resuscitation process, supportive management is continued from the ED into the OR, and often maintained into the postoperative ICU phase. Throughout diagnostic and operative procedures, management and monitoring decisions demand considerable understanding of the processes involved in the multitrauma patient and a high level of anesthesia support is needed. A trauma anesthetist who aggressively follows the patient throughout the entire resuscitation, evaluation, operative, and postoperative process is in the best position to provide optimal care and to make a significantly positive difference in the overall outcome of the multitrauma patient.

References

1. Baker SP, O'Neill B, Karpf RS (eds): Injury Fact Book. Lexington, MA, Lexington Books, 1984.
2. Trunkey DD: Trauma. Sci Am 249:28, 1983.
3. Committee on Trauma Research Commission on Life Sciences National Research Council and the Institute of Medicine. Injury in America: A Continuing Public Health Problem. National Academy Press, Washington, DC, 1985, p 19.
4. Council on Scientific Affairs: Automobile related injuries. JAMA 249: 3216, 1983.
5. Injury in America: A Continuing Public Health Problem. National Academy Press, Washington, DC, 1985, p 23.
6. Ryan-Parsch C, Atweh N: Bridgeport Hospital Trauma Registry Data Base, Nov 1993.
7. CDC data from Morbidity and Mortality Weekly Report: Deaths Resulting from Firearm- and Motor-Vehicle-Related Injuries—United States, 1968–1991. JAMA 271(7):495, 1994.

8. Sauaia A, Moore FA, Moore EE, et al: Epidemiology of Trauma Deaths: A Reassessment, abstract, 53rd Annual Meeting, American Association for the Surgery of Trauma, Riverside Hilton, New Orleans, LA, 1993, p 128.

9. Frost EAM: Neurologic trauma. Ch 48 in Textbook of Trauma Anesthesia and Critical Care. Grande C, et al, eds. Mosby, Baltimore, 1993, p 510.

10. Kraus JF. Epidemiology, New Iss Neurosci 2(2): 113–123, 1990.

11. Albin MS, Gilbert JT: Acute spinal cord trauma. Ch 135 in Textbook of Critical Care. Schoemaker W, Thompson WL, Holbrook PR (eds): 2nd ed, WB Saunders, Philadelphia, 1989, pp 1277–1285.

12. Conn JH, Gardy JD, Fain WR, Netterville RE: Thoracic trauma: Analysis of 1,022 cases. J Trauma 3:22–40, 1963.

13. Cohn R: Nonpenetrating wounds of the lungs and bronchi. Surg Clin North Am 52:585–595, 1972.

14. Ashbaugh DG, Peters GN, Galfrimson CG, et al: Chest trauma. Analysis of 685 patients. Arch Surg 95:546–555, 1967.

15. Mattox KL, Feliciano DV, Beall A, et al: Five thousand seven hundred sixty cardiovascular injuries in 4459 patients: epidemiologic evolution 1958–1988. Ann Surg 209:698, 1989.

16. Hedley-White J, Burgess GE, Feeley TW, Miller MG: High speed and blunt injuries. Ch 14 in Applied Physiology of Respiratory Care. Little, Brown, & Co., Boston, MA, 1976, pp 197–198.

17. Grande CM: Mechanisms and patterns of injury. The key to anticipation in trauma Management. Crit Care Clin 6(1):25 & 26, 1990.

18. Kaplan SG: Diagnostic Imaging: Implications for the trauma anesthesiologist. Ch. 105 in Textbook of Trauma Anesthesia and Critical Care. Grande CM, et al (eds): Mosby-Year Book, Baltimore, 1993, pp 1274–1275.

19. Benumof JL: Anesthesia for emergency thoracic surgery. Ch. 16 in Anesthesia for Thoracic Surgery. WB Saunders, Philadelphia, 1987, p 397.

20. Watson CB: Fiberoptic bronchoscopy in thoracic anesthesia. Balliere's Clin Anaesth 1:33–60, 1987.

21. Benumof JL: Anesthesia for emergency thoracic surgery. Ch. 16 in Anesthesia for Thoracic Surgery, WB Saunders, Philadelphia 1987, p 397.

22. Watson CB: Fiberoptic bronchoscopy in thoracic anesthesia. Ballière's Clin Anaesth 1:33–60, 1987.

23. Watson CB, Norfeel EA, Kates RA, Slogoff S: Thoracic anesthesia practice by members of the Society of Cardiovascular Anesthesiologists. Society of Cardiovascular Anesthesiologists' Sixth Annual Meeting Abstracts, May 1984.

24. Pappin JC: The current practice of endobronchial intubation. Anaesthesia 34:57–64, 1979.

25. Boyd M, Vanek VW, Bourguet CC: Emergency room resuscitative thoracotomy: When is it indicated? J Trauma 33:714–720, 1992.

26. Kirsh MM, Sloan H: Blunt chest trauma: General principles of management. Little, Brown, and Co., 1977, pp 74–75.

27. Clements F: The role of transesophageal echocardiography in patients with cardiac trauma, editorial. Anesth Analg 77:1089–90, 1993.

28. Ledgerwood AM, Kazmers, Lucas CE: The role of thoracic aortic occlusion for massive hemoperitoneum. J Trauma 16:610–615, 1976.
29. Demaria EJ: Management of patients with indeterminant diagnostic peritoneal lavage following blunt trauma. J Trauma 31:1627–1631, 1991.
30. Moreno C, Moore EE, Rosenberger A, Cleveland HC: Hemorrhage associated with major pelvic fracture: A multispecialty challenge. J Trauma 26:987–993, 1986.
31. Panetta T, Sclafani SJ, Goldstein AS, et al: Percutaneous transcatheter embolization for massive bleeding from pelvic fractures. J Trauma 25: 1021–1029, 1985.
32. Weiskopf RB, Boyetz MS, Roizen MF, et al: Cardiovascular and metabolic sequellae of inducing anesthesia with ketamine or thiopental in hypovolemic swine. Anesthesiology 60:214, 1984.
33. Del Santo PB, Hurwitz JL, Bull SM, et al: Delayed rupture from blunt trauma: A case report. Conn Med 46:135–137, 1982.
34. Breauz EP, Dupont JB, Albert HM, et al: Cardiac tamponade following penetrating mediastinal injuries: Improved survival with early pericardiocentesis. J Trauma 19:461–466, 1979.
35. Levy RL, de la Chapelle CE, Richards DW: Heart disease in drivers of public motor vehicles as a cause of highway accidents. JAMA 184: 143–146, 1963.
36. Andrews BT, Pitts LH, Lovely MP, Bartowski H: Is computed tomography scanning necessary in patients with tentorial herniation? Neurosurgery 19:408–414, 1986.
37. Mendelow AD, Karmi MZ, Paul KS, et al: Extradural hematoma: Effect of delayed treatment. Br Med J 1:1240, 1979.
38. Seeling JM, Becker DP, Miller JD, et al: Traumatic acute subdural hematoma: Major mortality reduction in comatose patients treated within four hours. NEJM 304:1511, 1981.
39. Pietropaolo JA, Rogers FB, Shackford SR, et al: The deleterious effects of intraoperative hypotension on outcome with severe head injuries. J Trauma 33:403–407, 1992.
40. Thomaston M, Messick J, Rutledge R, et al: Head CT scanning versus urgent exploration in the hypotensive blunt trauma patient. J Trauma 34:40–45, 1993.
41. Gutman MB, Moulton RJ, Sullivan I, et al: Relative Incidence of intracranial mass lesions and severe torso injury after accidental injury: Implications for triage and management. J Trauma 31:974–977, 1991.
42. Wisner DH, Victor NS, Holcroft JW: Priorities in the management of multiple trauma: Intracranial versus intra-abdominal injury. J Trauma 35:271–277, 1993.
43. Derdyn C, Persing JA, Broaddus WC, et al: Craniofacial trauma: An assessment of risk related to timing of surgery. Plastic Reconstr Surg 86:238–247, 1990.

4

Initial Intrahospital Resuscitation of the Patient with Head Trauma

Georges Desjardins, MD, Albert J. Varon, MD

Introduction

The vast majority of head injuries occur secondary to high-velocity motor vehicle accidents. These include pedestrians (12% to 15%), occupants (75%), motorcyclists, and bicyclists.[1] Some studies have shown that the fastest growing external causes of brain injury in certain high-density urban areas in the United States are assaults and the use of firearms.[1] Falls are frequently shown as the second leading cause of injury followed by recreational activities and sports. The use of alcohol is associated with brain injury in 50% to 75% of cases as a causative factor but also as a factor confusing the diagnosis, affecting recovery and decreasing the chances of survival.

Head injury is associated with more trauma deaths than injury

From *Trauma Anesthesia and Critical Care of Neurological Injury,* edited by K. J. Abrams and C. M. Grande. © 1997, Futura Publishing Co., Armonk, NY.

to any other body region.[1] This is a reflection of the high incidence of severe central nervous system (CNS) injuries in our society and the importance of the initial trauma to the brain. Because primary injury to the brain is often not amenable to therapy and because secondary injury may be just as devastating, clinicians must focus their attention on prevention of secondary injury.

The mortality from head trauma is universally high, but several studies have shown differences in survival rates and amount of functional recovery depending on the type of primary injury, the age of the victim, and the accessibility and quality of the trauma care delivery systems.[1]

Forty percent to 70% of initially hypotensive blunt trauma victims have a severe head injury (GCS score of 8 and under), but only 2.5% to 6% of these will need a craniotomy for intracranial pathology. Because most of these patients have injuries elsewhere,[2] and 50% of preventable deaths in trauma result from a failure to identify and stop ongoing hemorrhage (usually intra-abdominal[3]), trauma specialists must have a high index of suspicion and must search for other injuries.

This chapter will focus on the initial care of the head trauma patient, from the first communication with the prehospital team in the field to admission of the victim to the operating room or intensive care unit.

Prehospital Communications

In well-organized trauma care delivery systems, a physician coordinates the care of the multiply injured patient. Most systems in the United States involve a general surgeon in this role, but it is our opinion that a trauma specialist should undertake this responsibility. The trauma specialist may be a surgeon, an anesthesiologist, or an emergency medicine physician, all of whom should have special interest and training in trauma.[4]

Once the need for around-the-clock coverage by a medical coordinator of trauma care (trauma specialist on-call) is recognized, focus should be placed on the ideal point of intervention in the course of the injured patient. Rapid response and early intervention is a tenet quality of trauma care.

A trimodal distribution of mortality among trauma victims has been described. The first peak (50% of deaths) is usually within seconds to minutes of injury, unfortunately. Even in the best circumstances, few patients with these injuries (lacerations to the brain, brain stem, high spinal cord, large vessels, or heart) can be saved. The second peak occurs within minutes to 4 hours after injury (30% of deaths) and this is the group of patients who have sustained injuries considered treatable if brought to the attention of a qualified team in a timely fashion ("the golden hour"). The third peak (20% of deaths) occurs many hours to days after the initial trauma. The mortality rate in this group may also be improved by prompt resuscitation and correction of shock as prolonged hypoxemia and hypotension is associated with an increased incidence of sepsis and multiple organ dysfunction.[5]

Prehospital communication between the trauma specialist on call and the team in the field offers many advantages to the care of all trauma victims (Fig. 1). First, it permits evaluation and supervision of the quality of prehospital care especially when delivered by nonphysician care providers, ensuring that intervention is in accordance with protocols. Second, it allows appropriate triage of patients, ensuring that the arriving patient will indeed need the services of the trauma team. Only about 15% of injured patients require the

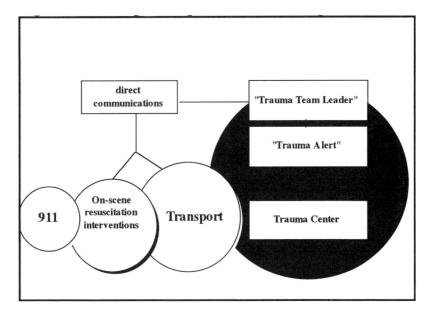

Figure 1. Ideal prehospital trauma set-up.

services of a trauma center; the rest can be treated at the nearest hospital.[5]

Finally, and most importantly, these communications should be used to make preparations for the trauma victim. They should be done in advance of the arrival of the patient in order for the trauma specialist to activate the in-hospital trauma alert system and assemble the trauma team. Doing so permits preparation for needed interventions that were unsuccessfull in the field or for interventions that can be performed only in the hospital.

Therefore, the evaluation and treatment of the patient starts before the victim arrives at the trauma center. The communications should continue at frequent intervals, to report any change in the patient's condition. The communication system should be designed so that the on-scene personnel and trauma center physicians are in direct contact and do not have to relay messages through an intermediary.

The original communication should include the mechanism of injury, estimation of the patient's age, vital signs, Glasgow Coma Scale score, any obvious injuries, and the interventions done by on-scene personnel (airway management, fluid administration, or use of pneumatic garments).

Whether a trauma system is based on "stay and stabilize" or "scoop and run" principles, it should not change the fact that, for the trauma center to be in a state of advance readiness, there should be prehospital communications.

Trauma Team Set-Up

As stated above, in the ideal trauma care system, someone must coordinate the care of the multiple-injury patient: most systems in the United States involve a general surgeon in this important role, but a trauma specialist should undertake this responsibility. No one specialty can claim the exclusive right to leadership. Training, interest, and experience are perhaps more important than the base specialty in selecting a trauma team leader.

The trauma specialist should be involved as early as possible in the care of the injured patient. Ideally, he or she should be the one receiving the communications from the scene and the one activating the "in-hospital trauma alert" (Fig. 1). This should give time for the entire trauma team to gather in the "resuscitation room" ("trauma admitting area," "trauma bay"), waiting for the victim to arrive. The potential for errors is obvious when a patient with multiple injuries is treated by multiple individuals. This is why it is important that the trauma team leader be able to step back, coordinate, and keep control of the resuscitation as a whole, rather than getting too involved in specific technical procedures.

The most effective teams are probably the ones in which team members have preassigned roles and proceed promptly and simultaneously to perform their tasks under the coordination of the team leader. Each team member has responsibilities in clearly defined areas, and they proceed with assessment and management within those limits, leaving the team leader to assess the situation as a whole and to define priorities of intervention (Table 1).

The ideal number of members is debatable. This may vary depending on the organization of the trauma system and the size of the trauma resuscitation rooms. For the care of a multiple-injury patient, a five- to six-member team would be ideal (team leader, one physician for the airway, one other physician for care of the trunk and extremities, and two to three nurses). Other personnel that might be in the room when the injured patient arrives include a radiology technician and a respiratory therapist.

Primary Survey (Initial Assessment)

Prevention of Secondary Injury

There are two stages in the development of brain injury. First, there is the primary injury that results from the biomechanical effect of forces applied to the cranium and its content at the time of insult. Those injuries (diffuse vascular injury, multiple petechial hemorrhages, diffuse axonal and white matter damage, lacerations and contusions) are the ones for which there is no effective medical treatment at this time. Secondary injuries occur later (minutes to hours after the original insult) and are in fact complications of the primary injury. Examples of secondary injury to the brain are intracranial hemorrhage, intracranial hypertension, ischemia, increased cerebral metabolic demand (hyperthermia), decreased cerebral blood flow, and brain edema.

The care of the multiple-injury patient with a head injury must focus not only on support of the patient with primary injury, but more importantly on the prevention of secondary injury. These secondary insults are extraordinarily common, occurring in 57% of patients

Table 1
Responsibilities of the Trauma Team Leader

1. Responsible for prehospital communications, advise any referring hospital at time of referral.
2. Activate "in-hospital trauma alert" if trauma criteria are met.
3. Obtain a history from the paramedics on arrival.
4. Perform primary and secondary assessment.
5. Establish priorities for investigation and intervention.
6. Coordinate team members, ordering procedures, receiving information, and resolving disputes.
7. Maintain an overview, avoiding undue involvement in technical procedures but intervening appropriately in critical situations.
8. Order fluids, blood, and blood products.
9. Order analgesia.
10. Order and interpret investigations in conjunction with team members, the radiologist, and other specialists as needed (example: neurosurgeon).
11. Request surgical intervention, consult with or refer to other specialists when appropriate.
12. Supervise spinal precautions.
13. Supervise patient transfer for radiologic investigation, or transfer to the OR, ICU, or regular trauma ward.
14. Arrange for final disposition, arranging for admission by appropriate primary specialty, handing over care to OR, ICU, or trauma ward, and reviewing subsequently to maintain continuity.
15. Inform the family.
16. Excuse the team members at the end of the resuscitation.
17. Make a record in the notes and dictate a letter to any referring hospital.
18. Provide clinical education for team members during the resuscitation itself and at team meetings.
19. Have no other clinical responsibilities while on duty as team leader.

Modified with permission from Oakley PA: Interface of anesthesiology and emergency medicine in trauma management. In Grande CM (ed): Textbook of Trauma Anesthesia and Critical Care, Mosby, 1993.

suffering severe head injury.[6] Several factors that are found frequently in trauma patients will aggravate the effects of the initial injury on the brain; these include hypoxia, anemia, hypotension, hypercarbia, and hyperglycemia. Of all these factors, it seems that hypotension is the most devastating. A single episode of hypotension occurring at any point between injury and resuscitation is associated with an increase in mortality to 50%, compared to the 27% mortality of patients who did not suffer from a secondary insult.[6] Hypoxia and shock are present in 23% of severe head injuries. Hypotension occurs in 35% of these patients and is associated with an 85% increase in mortality.[6] These data underscore the importance of aggressive treatment of the head-injured patient. Hypotension of any duration and at any time after the primary insult may be devastating for the brain and must be prevented and very aggressively treated if it should occur.

Airway Control and Cervical Spine Stabilization

Although other common practices such as ideal location for placement of intravenous catheters for fluid resuscitation are controversial, the placement of an endotracheal tube in properly selected patients is an area in which there is a more general consensus. Early endotracheal intubation must often be performed before radiographic or clinical clearance of the cervical spine. Hypoxemia and respiratory acidosis are associated with poor outcome after head injury.[6-10] Patients with episodes of hypoxemia have higher mortality rates and lower functional recovery than those without these episodes.[6]

Given the dangers of hypoxemia to the injured brain, clinicians should have a low threshold for implementing early intubation in head-injured trauma patients to prevent secondary injury, provided that intubation can be done rapidly, safely, and reliably. Endotracheal intubation should be considered in patients with inability to adequately protect their airway, or those with airway obstruction, acute respiratory insufficiency, persistent hypoxemia, hemorrhagic shock, severe injuries requiring extensive intervention, coma, and agitation that precludes physical examination and laboratory testing (i.e., CT scan or MRI). Tracheal intubation in the combative patient should not preclude the team leader from searching for the cause of the combativeness: brain injury, hypoxemia, hypercarbia, intoxication with alcohol and/or drugs, or a combination of these factors.

Since the criteria for intubation are imprecise and the consequences of hypoxemia can be devastating to the injured brain, it is probably preferable to intubate some patients who do not prove in retrospect to have required intubation than it is to defer intubation in borderline cases. The Glasgow Coma Scale (GCS) can be used as a tool to help in the decision-making process of who needs intubation. A GCS score under 9 has often been considered an indication for securing the airway in patients with head trauma (Table 2).

Much debate has centered around the safety of oral intubation

Table 2
Glasgow Coma Scale Score

Glasgow Coma Scale		
Eye Opening	Spontaneous	4
	To voice	3
	To pain	2
	None	1
Verbal Response	Oriented	5
	Confused	4
	Inappropriate words	3
	Incomprehensible words	2
	None	1
Motor Response	Obeys commands	6
	Localized pain	5
	Withdraw to pain	4
	Abnormal flexion to pain	3
	Abnormal extension to pain	2
	None	1
Total score (maximum)		15

From Jennett, Teasdale[11] with permission.

in the presence of cervical spine injury. Most of the controversy comes from the theory that blunt injury could create an injury with instability in the cervical spine and that manipulation of the airway during direct laryngoscopy could cause movement of the unstable elements, thus resulting in iatrogenic spinal cord injury. This argument, widely accepted, was one of the principal factors in the adoption of blind nasotracheal intubation as the airway maneuver of first choice in the multiple blunt injured patient. If nasotracheal intubation was not possible, surgical cricothyroidotomy was recommended. There is now an increasing number of reports that argue in favor of the safety of oral intubation.[12-14] Although the controversies of airway management in trauma will be discussed in detail elsewhere in this textbook, certain points must be emphasized:

- All patients with head injuries must be considered as having an unstable injury in the cervical spine until proven otherwise. Up to 15% of patients with a severe head injury will have an associated cervical spine injury.[15]
- Awareness of possible injury and cervical spine in-line immobiliza-

tion/stabilization will decrease the chance of causing cervical spine injury.

- The best initial immobilization of the cervical spine can be obtained with a combination of sandbags taped on each side of the patient's head, a rigid cervical collar, and a spine board (or with plastic foam or vacuum mattress-type immobilizers).
- Orotracheal intubation, nasotracheal intubation, and tracheotomy can all be performed successfully without spinal cord damage as long as the spine is immobilized adequately. It should be remembered that there is always a small amount of movement of the cervical spine with any of the techniques for airway control.[15,16]
- Precise cervical spine in-line immobilization should be maintained throughout the intubation maneuvers. This in-line immobilization, also called manual in-line axial traction, is an active process done by a second individual who is responsible for applying a varying amount of force to counteract the movements of the laryngoscopist, in an attempt to stabilize the cervical spine.
- If time permits, the fiberoptic bronchoscope can be very useful for the control of the airway via the oral or nasal route with minimal movement of the spine.
- Nasotracheal intubation should be avoided in the presence of suspected basal skull fracture, severe facial fractures, or bleeding diathesis. Unfortunately, these disorders are common in patients with severe head injury.
- Rapid sequence induction can be done safely in the trauma resuscitation room when it is performed by an experienced individual in the trauma team (i.e., anesthesiologist). This technique should include preoxygenation, cervical spine precautions, cricoid pressure, use of drugs that would maintain cerebral perfusion pressure, avoiding severe increases in intracranial pressure, and above all, avoiding hypotension. Many drugs or combination of drugs can be used for this purpose, the most important principle being not the drug but the way in which it is used. At times, awake, orotracheal intubation without anesthetic agents may be the safest approach, even in the severe head-injured patient.
- When muscle relaxants are used to control the airway, it is important to do as much of a neurological examination as possible, before pharmacological paralysis. Ensuring the patency of the airway and adequate oxygenation is always the first priority of trauma management; however, even during emergency intubation, the trauma team leader should be able to make a quick observation about

the level of consciousness and whether there is movement of all extremities. When possible, a more detailed neurological examination should be performed, because an initial exam will be needed for comparison with subsequent evaluations and may provide clues on the presence or progression of neurological injuries.

• Clearance of the cervical spine before intubation is ideal. However, this may be impractical in some circumstances. In areas served by a well-trained emergency medical system, most of the severe head-injured patients will require tracheal intubation in the field or immediately upon arrival to the trauma center. Some authors have encouraged obtaining a lateral radiograph of the cervical spine before intubation in all other cases in which the intubation is not an absolute emergency.[17] This principle is based on the theory that a single lateral view of the cervical spine is a reliable means of detecting a cervical spine fracture. In this setting, however, most of these radiographs obtained are inadequate for complete visualization of the entire cervical spine and rule out a fracture. Odontoid fractures and more prevalent fractures, such as the ones at the lower cervical spine and cervicothoracic junction levels, are likely to be missed. Therefore, for practical purposes, the clinician should assume that the cervical spine is injured and unstable in all blunt trauma patients. In-line stabilization and spinal precautions should be maintained until either radiologic or clinical clearance is possible.

Ventilatory Management

When evaluating the ventilation of the multiple-injury trauma patient, the trauma team should focus on early diagnosis of life-threatening chest injuries that require immediate intervention (Table 3). The "look, listen, and feel" techniques are used for this primary survey. Monitoring hemoglobin oxygen saturation with pulse oximetry is a rapid way to assess adequate oxygenation. A member of the trauma team should place a pulse oximeter probe on the patient as soon as he or she arrives in the resuscitation room. Supplemental oxygen at high inspired fraction should be provided to all trauma patients until the actual PaO_2 or hemoglobin saturation is measured by arterial blood gas analysis or pulse oximetry.

Because some life-threatening chest injuries may have a subtle presentation, a high index of suspicion based on the mechanism of

Table 3
Life-Threatening Chest Injuries

Tension pneumothorax
Open pneumothorax
Massive hemothorax
Large vessel injury
Severe blunt cardiac injury
Severe flail chest with pulmonary contusion
Major tracheobronchial injury
Pericardial tamponade
Pulmonary venous air embolism
Esophageal disruption
Traumatic diaphragmatic hernia

injury, previous history, initial examination, and evolution of the patient is required for their diagnosis.

Although a chest radiograph is considered part of the initial evaluation procedures, therapeutic interventions in unstable patients should be performed on clinical grounds and should not be delayed until the radiographs are obtained. For example, in the hemodynamically unstable patient who is difficult to ventilate, and in whom a tension pneumothorax is suspected, a large-bore needle or a chest tube should be inserted for decompression without waiting for a confirmatory chest radiograph.

Hemodynamic Management

Hypotension and hypovolemia are generally regarded to be detrimental for the brain and other organs, and are also associated with worse outcome, particularly when there is severe head injury. In recent reports, there is speculation that hypovolemia and associated hypotension are beneficial in some circumstances where there is uncontrolled hemorrhage.[18,19] The most frequently stated example is a lacerated major artery, when the administration of fluid and associated increase in blood pressure might dislodge a clot from the area of injury, increase the hemorrhage, and turn stable hypotension into a lethal recurrent hemorrhage. The evidence for the occurrence of these theoretical effects from fluid resuscitation is stronger for penetrating trauma than for blunt trauma, which is more common in patients with head injuries. Currently, there is general support for fluid administration as a mainstay of initial resuscitation after blunt trauma. The initial hemodynamic stabilization is still intravenous access, correction of hypovolemia, and hemorrhage identification and control.

The route for fluid administration in trauma is also a source of controversy. There is general consensus that the first choice for cannulation is a vein that is visible, which means most often a peripheral vein on the upper extremities of the patient. Two large-bore peripheral intravenous catheters (16-gauge or larger) should be placed as quickly as possible for the administration of fluids and blood. Using 14- or 16-gauge 2-inch peripheral catheters should allow a flow rate of 300 mL/min of crystalloid or 150 mL/min of blood when used in combination with a pressure bag.[20] In areas with well-developed emergency medical systems, most trauma victims arrive with these intravenous catheters already in place.

If peripheral intravenous access was unsuccessful in the field or in the resuscitation room, or if hypotension persists, additional sites should be considered to ensure immediate intravenous access. Some authors suggest, as a second choice, the cannulation of the external jugular vein; as a third choice, the use of the femoral vein; and as last choices, venous cutdown and catheterization through the internal jugular or subclavian veins.[21]

In the clinical setting where the injured patient does not have adequate IV access, spinal precautions are still being applied (C-collar, backboard, triple fixation of the cervical spine), and if unstable vital signs are present, several problems can be anticipated. Moving the head and neck or opening the C-collar would be necessary to perform easy and timely cannulation of either the external or the internal jugular veins. Removing some of the spinal precautions before clinical or radiological clearance would not be ideal and waiting for radiological evaluation would be impractical. We believe that in these circumstances, the femoral vein could be an excellent second choice for venous access because of its large size and easy access. However, a major concern with the use of the femoral vein as the "main IV" in the acute phase of resuscitation is the possibility of vascular injuries from the original trauma in the pelvic and/or the abdominal regions, especially in penetrating trauma to the abdomen and in patients who have sustained major pelvic fractures where associated vascular injuries are frequent. Relying mainly on the femoral access in this situation might lead to loss of the resuscitation fluid in the extravascular space. Use of a venous cutdown in the lower extremities has the same limitations. Although a venous cutdown in

Table 4
Intravenous Access in the Multiple-Injury Patient

---

1. Peripheral IV × 2 in visible vein of the upper extremities.
2. If unsuccessful, suggested second choice:
   A. If C-spine injury unlikely: external or internal jugular vein access with large-bore IV catheter.
   B. If abdominal or pelvic injuries unlikely: femoral vein access with large-bore IV catheter or venous cutdown in the lower extremities.
   C. If suspected abdominal or pelvic injuries: Subclavian vein with large-bore IV catheter.

---

the upper extremities would avoid this problem, it is technically more difficult, and therefore, more time-consuming. When there is inadequate intravenous access in the severely injured patient with suspected intra-abdominal injuries, it is our practice to use the subclavian vein as our second choice for fluid administration (Table 4).

The use of an 8.5 or 9.0 French introducer allows a flow rate higher than 500 mL/min with the use of a pressure bag and large-caliber IV tubing.[20] Strict aseptic technique should be used even in emergency situations. As a general rule, all intravenous catheters placed in the prehospital phase and in the resuscitation room setting should be changed in the first 24 hours after insertion, because they may have been inserted under less than ideal conditions.[22] Our practice is to provide the history of all IV lines to the ICU or ward teams, who will then change all central catheters over a guidewire, culture the intracutaneous segments with a semiquantitative technique, and remove the prehospital and resuscitation peripheral lines.[22] These should be done only after relative hemodynamic stability has been established and/or additional "clean" intravenous access has been secured.

All intravenous fluids and blood products should be warmed. The H1000 infusion system (Level One Technologies, Inc., Rockland, MA) is capable of infusing and heating 800 mL/min of crystalloid or 500 mL/min of blood.[21] This system is extremely useful in the management of exsanguinating hemorrhage. The use of blood-warming/high-volume infusion systems in addition to warming up the resuscitation room to temperatures as high as 25°C is essential if hypothermia is to be prevented effectively during the resuscitation of the trauma patient.

The notion that fluid resuscitation is a priority in the initial management of blunt trauma victims is in contradiction with the common dogma that fluids should be minimized in patients with head injury.[23] The rationale behind fluid restriction is that fluid administration may increase cerebral edema formation and intracranial pressure, and thus produce secondary brain injury. The trauma team leader faces the dilemma of two conflicting concepts. The dilemma is resolved if one considers data showing that hypotension and hypovolemia are as deleterious for the brain as they are for the rest of the body.[7-9] There is a correlation between hypotension and poor outcome in patients with severe head injury. In order to avoid critical ischemia and to maintain adequate cerebral perfusion pressure, the brain is dependent on adequate circulating blood volume and oxygen delivery. For these reasons, fluid administration, at least in the early stages of resuscitation, is universally warranted even in patients with obvious signs of head injury.

Although there is agreement that maintenance/optimization of oxygen delivery, and the fluid resuscitation necessary to reach that goal, are crucial in the initial care of the blunt trauma patient with severe head injury, the type of fluid that should be administered remains a matter of great debate.

Although colloid-containing fluids have the ability to normalize hemodynamic parameters faster and in smaller volumes than crystalloid solutions,[24] recent studies were unable to demonstrate a difference in intracranial pressure (ICP) or outcome when different amounts and types of fluid were compared in the early postinjury period.[25] There is further evidence that efforts to minimize free water administration by the use of colloid rather than crystalloid solutions are of minimal benefit with respect to measurable effects on the brain.

There is a great deal of interest in fluids that contain large amounts of sodium and chloride. These hypertonic saline solutions are capable of normalizing hemodynamic parameters in much smaller volumes than those required for isotonic solutions (lactated Ringer's or normal saline (NaCl 0.9%).[26] Theoretically, interstitial and cellular edema formation are minimized with the use of hypertonic solutions. Minimizing cerebral edema formation would also minimize the amount of secondary injury after brain trauma. Researchers continue to investigate this hypothesis and the effect of hypertonic solutions on patient outcome.

The ideal resuscitation fluid for the multiple-injury patient with head injury would be one that resuscitates the cardiovascular system by correcting the blood pressure and oxygen delivery, while at the same time providing protection for the brain. If this fluid increases blood pressure while simultaneously minimizing increases in intracranial pressure, cerebral perfusion pressure is maximized. Numerous studies seem to indicate that hypertonic saline solutions minimize increases in the intracranial pressure during resuscitation of the cardiovascular system.[26-30]

A time-honored tradition has been the administration of glucose to prevent hypoglycemia, provide energy, conserve protein, and prevent ketosis. However, studies have shown that hyperglycemia existing before an ischemic or toxic event enhances ischemic damage. Withholding glucose or giving it in moderation to maintain blood glucose levels below 150 mg/dL is recommended whenever brain ischemia may occur.[31]

Another area of discussion in fluid resuscitation of the multiple-injury patient with neurological injury is the timing for administration of blood products. Even if there are no absolute guidelines to follow, the threshold to administer blood in this type of patient should probably be lower to prevent severe anemia with the associated low oxygen delivery to the injured brain and possible cerebral ischemia.

Secondary Survey (Trauma Team at Work)

The secondary survey is, as described in the Advanced Trauma Life Support course of the American College of Surgeons,[17] a detailed topographic examination of the trauma patient from head to toe after he has been completely exposed. This must include, in blunt trauma victims, examination of the head and face, cervical spine and neck, chest, abdomen, rectum and perineum, pelvis, back, extremities, and nervous system. The secondary survey, using the "look, listen, and feel" technique, should also include "tubes and fingers in every orifice" (placement of a gastric tube and urinary catheter) and basic radiographic evaluation, which includes chest and pelvic radiographs, a cervical spine series to visualize all seven cervical vertebrae, and a thoracolumbar spine series. To avoid delaying urgent care, considerable judgment is required concerning the timing of this important evaluation.

Prioritization of Care

A CT scan of the cranium and brain plays a critical role in the detection of intracranial pathological conditions arising from head

Table 5
Indications for CT Following Head Injury

History of loss of consciousness.
Neurological deficit on physical examination.
Head injury in combination with drug or alcohol intoxication.
Glasgow Coma Scale score of less than 15.

trauma. The primary objective of the examination is the early recognition of a surgically correctable lesion. CT scanning of the brain and cranium will also permit early diagnosis of nonsurgical injuries and permit effective monitoring of such lesions.[32] A patient with minimal or no findings on the initial CT may require sequential scans when neurological dysfunction persists or worsens. A lesion not present on the first CT scan may be seen on a subsequent scan several hours to days later.

A history of loss of consciousness and a decreased mental status are indicators that there might be underlying intracranial pathology, and these signs are known to be reliable indications for obtaining a CT scan of the brain.[33–35] In the trauma patient, a CT scan should be performed if there is a history of loss of consciousness, a neurological deficit, a head injury in combination with drug or alcohol intoxication, or a Glasgow Coma Scale score of less than 15[34] (Table 5).

As stated above, measures to combat hypotension and hypovolemia should be taken as soon as possible. This would mean that ongoing hemorrhage into a major cavity should be controlled as quickly as possible. Major thoracic hemorrhage is relatively rare after blunt trauma and can be diagnosed readily by physical examination and a chest radiograph. Major pelvic hemorrhage can usually be found with the help of physical and radiologic examinations of the pelvis. However, making the diagnosis of major intra-abdominal hemorrhage can be extremely difficult. Physical examination is often not possible or reliable. The peritoneal cavity is capable of storing a large amount of blood without obvious physical findings. Before the advent of modern diagnostic techniques, up to 17% of patients with abdominal trauma died secondary to unrecognized intra-abdominal bleeding.[36] The evaluation of blunt abdominal trauma remains a significant challenge because clinical assessment alone is only 55% to 84% accurate.[37] Associated head injury, spinal cord injury, or altered mental status due to alcohol or drugs may decrease the accuracy of the physical examination to as low as 30%.[37] Delaying the diagnosis by waiting for the development of peritoneal signs or complications of an intra-abdominal injury leads to unacceptable morbidity and mortality.[38] The diagnosis and treatment of intra-abdominal hemorrhage are important early priorities in the initial management of the trauma victim.

A problem in clinical practice appears when the priority of diagnosis and treatment of truncal injuries is in conflict with the priority of diagnosis and treatment of head injury. This may occur in patients with a high risk of intra-abdominal injuries. These include high-speed motor vehicle accidents, motorcycle accidents, ejection from a vehicle, fall from heights greater than 15 feet, pedestrians struck by car, associated major chest injury, pelvic fractures, and a history of hypotension either in the field or on admission in the resuscitation room.[39] To help determine priorities, the trauma team leader must take into account the relative incidence of surgical intra-abdominal and intracranial injuries. A recent study reported that in initially hypotensive blunt trauma patients, only 2.5% to 6% of patients with severe head injuries will need craniotomy for the treatment of intracranial hemorrhages, whereas 21% will undergo urgent laparotomy.[40] The combination of an intracranial lesion requiring craniotomy and an intra-abdominal lesion requiring therapeutic laparotomy in the same patient is very rare (0.25% of cases). If patients have lateralizing signs (hemiparesis, hemiplegia, or asymmetrical posturing), they have a 39% chance of requiring a craniotomy.[41]

Some authors have tried to simplify the decision-making process by suggesting that patients with the possibility of both head and abdominal injury should undergo emergent abdominal exploration shortly after admission if they are unstable, have hypotension unresponsive to fluid administration, and do not have a large hemothorax on chest radiography.[41] Hemodynamically stable patients on whom an adequate physical examination of the abdomen cannot be performed should undergo early diagnostic paracentesis followed by lavage and chest radiography, prior to other diagnostic procedures or operative intervention. If the paracentesis is grossly positive and the patient does not have lateralizing signs, abdominal exploration should be the next step. If lateralizing findings are present and the patient remains hemodynamically stable, a CT scan of the head should be done before abdominal exploration. If an intracranial mass lesion is found on CT, craniotomy and laparotomy can be conducted simultaneously.[41]

A standard cerebral CT scan for a trauma patient consists of 10 to 14 axial noncontrast images made parallel to the skull base. Slice thickness in the adult is generally 5 mm through the posterior fossa and 10 mm through the supratentorial region. The time required to complete a study has been reduced with the introduction of new scanners but the average CT of the head requires between 1 and 8 seconds per CT slice. A study is usually completed in less than 5 minutes.[42] This time does not include transportation and transfer of the uncooperative patient to the CT scanner. This is why an unstable patient should avoid the CT suite. If a decision is made to transfer the patient for CT scanning, he or she should be monitored with an electrocardiogram, automated blood pressure measurements, and pulse oximetry. Ideally, the trauma patient should be accompanied by a nurse and a physician capable of continuing resuscitative interventions.

Evaluation of Other Injuries

After securing the airway, insuring proper oxygenation and ventilation, treating hypotension and hypoperfusion, and stabilizing the cervical spine, the trauma team leader's attention should be focused on the remainder of the physical examination. As stated before, this examination should be performed in an orderly fashion, from head to toe. Particular attention should be given at this time to the cardiovascular, gastrointestinal, neurological, and musculoskeletal systems. Obvious areas of blood loss should be controlled by applying direct pressure; gross deviations or dislocations should be reduced and immobilized immediately.

The team leader should keep a high index of suspicion and, when one injury is identified, he or she should look for other commonly associated injuries (Table 6).

The threshold for radiographic examination of possible injuries should be low. Some authors recommend, as a minimum, an initial radiographic examination of the unconscious blunt trauma victim; an anteroposterior chest radiograph; anteroposterior, cross-table lateral, and odontoid cervical spine views; anteroposterior pelvis; and anteroposterior view of injured extremities.[43] Other authors have also suggested adding routine radiographs of the thoracic and lumbar spine because of the high incidence of multiple vertebral fractures occurring in the thoracolumbar area.[44] This attitude appears to be most useful in patients with altered sensorium and high-velocity

Table 6
Commonly Associated Injuries

Obvious Fracture	Associated Injury
Bone and Vascular	
Ribs 1, 2, 3 fractures	Ruptured aorta
Sternum fracture	Blunt cardiac injuries
Pelvic fracture	Laceration of pelvic vascular tree
Distal third femur fracture	Laceration of femoral artery
Knee dislocation	Popliteal artery laceration
Bone and Viscera	
Transverse fracture of the spine (seat belt injury)	Ruptured mesentery or small bowel (15%–20%)
Lower ribs fracture	Laceration of the liver, spleen, kidney or diaphragm
Pelvic fracture	Ruptured bladder or urethra
Pelvic fracture (severe)	Ruptured diaphragm
Bone and Bone	
Spine fracture	Remote additional fractures (5%) particularly thoracolumbar
Chest wall fracture	Scapular fracture
Anterior pelvic arch fracture	Sacrum fracture or dislocated sacroiliac joint
Femoral shaft fracture	Fracture or fracture-dislocation of the hip
Tibia fracture (severe)	Dislocated hip
Calcaneus fracture	Fractured thoracolumbar spine
Distal radius fracture	Scaphoid fracture

Modified with permission from Rogers LF, Hendrix RW: Radiographic imaging in orthopedics. Orthop Clin North Am 1990;21:3.

trauma.[44] It has been reported that in blunt trauma, victims with a Glasgow Coma Scale score less than 10 have a 14% incidence of spine injuries, 10% incidence of pelvic fractures, and 15% incidence of lower extremity fractures.[43–45]

The management of the multiple-injury patient often includes the involvement of many consultant services (neurosurgery, general surgery, maxillofacial surgery, orthopedic surgery). The consultants may not be aware of all the injuries and may be faced with, yet again, conflicting priorities. The complete operative management in patients with maxillofacial or multiple orthopedic injuries can lead to the need for extensive and prolonged operative procedures. Someone should determine the appropriateness of prolonged procedures in patients with multiple injuries, including brain injuries. At least initially, this should be the role of the trauma team leader, decisions should not be left to subspecialists alone. The trauma team leader should keep in mind the range of injuries to different areas of the body and coordinate care. Based on this principle, he or she should keep track of the patient's condition during prolonged surgeries and be involved in the decision-making process to determine if all repairs should be completed as initially planned.

Although no firm guidelines exist to help in the decision-making process when managing associated injuries, some general principles can be applied. Maxillofacial injuries are commonly associated with brain injuries. The usual initial operative interventions required in the early postinjury period for this type of trauma are irrigation of contaminated wounds, debridement of devitalized tissue, and repair of lacerations. These procedures should not result in long operative time or in substantial blood loss. Definitive repair of maxillofacial injuries can be deferred until later, when the clinical status of the patient has stabilized and the overall prognosis is clearer. A delay in the operative treatment might be preferred until facial edema caused by the injury has decreased.

For most orthopedic injuries, the ideal timing for definite care of the multiple-injury patient with brain trauma is not as clear. In orthopedic injuries, optimal outcome is achieved by early fracture fixation. These injuries should be reduced and fixed in the immediate post-trauma period when at all possible[46–48]; this is particularly important for victims with major long bone and pelvic fractures. Recent studies indicate that early fixation helps decrease the incidence and severity of pulmonary and multiple organ dysfunction and decrease the mortality in trauma patients.[40–42]

Patients with evidence of severe injury based on an abnormal neurological examination and severely depressed level of consciousness, or those with evidence of severe anatomic disruption on the CT scan should not undergo extensive or complicated procedures in the immediate post-trauma period, but may benefit from some form of long bone fixation.[49] When both pulmonary and neurological function are severely compromised, orthopedic procedures should be kept to the minimum necessary to provide some degree of stability (i.e., limiting stabilization to simple skeletal traction or external fixation). When planning the appropriate operative procedures in the initial post-trauma period, first priority should be given to long bone fractures that interfere with mobilization of the patient (femur fractures, tibial fractures, ankle fractures, and upper extremity fractures, in that order). Any fracture associated with neurovascular compromise requiring operative intervention may change the prioritization of care. Acetabular and other pelvic fractures should be approached with caution in the immediate post-trauma period in patients with severe brain injury, even though they are of major importance with respect to postoperative mobilization. The fixation of these fractures are major operative procedures with long operative time and significant blood loss and fluid shifts.

The best monitor of the head-injured patient is serial neurological examinations.[6] The ability to perform a neurological examination is lost when the patient is under heavy sedation or general anesthesia. For this reason, if there is evidence of severe neurological dysfunction or cerebral edema on the CT scan, serious consideration should be given to placing an intracranial pressure monitor prior to prolonged operative procedures (especially if the CT scan shows a small epidural or subdural hematoma not requiring initial surgical correction). This monitoring device may help evaluate the neurological status, guide therapy to decrease intracranial pressure, and help determine if the planned procedures should be terminated or if a repeat CT scan is indicated.

Monitoring in the Resuscitation Room

The resuscitation trauma room should be viewed as an acute care unit where as much information as possible should be gathered about the patient.

When the multiple-injury patient arrives at the resuscitation suite, the trauma team should place the basic monitoring devices and these should be kept on the patient during diagnostic procedures and transportation to either the trauma intensive care unit or the operating room. The basic monitoring devices include an electrocardiogram, a noninvasive blood pressure device, and a pulse oximeter. Some means of CO_2 detection should be used at least initially to confirm endotracheal intubation either by an end-tidal CO_2 detector (Easy Cap, Nellcor Incorporated, Hayward, CA) or by capnography. Hourly urine output should be measured to monitor renal perfusion, effects of ICP control therapy (osmotic diuretics), or possible complications of trauma (genitourinary tract trauma, central diabetes insipidus, or rhabdomyolysis).

Hypothermia is a common problem among severely injured patients. Data suggest that severely hypothermic trauma victims with an initial body temperature less than 34°C have a worse outcome.[50] Body temperature should therefore be monitored in the resuscitation room and hypothermia aggressively prevented.

Control of Intracranial Pressure (or Secondary Injury) in the Resuscitation Room

There are two different views in the management of secondary injury prevention in the acute and subacute setting. They share many points in common but, it is the end-point in itself that is different. One focuses the attention on cerebral perfusion pressure (CPP) and the other, the traditional approach, on the control of the intracranial pressure (ICP).[51] Although this subject is discussed elsewhere in this textbook, the significant differences are listed in Table 7.

Table 7
Comparison of Traditional (ICP) versus CPP Management

Modality	Traditional ICP Therapy	CPP Management
Position	Elevate HOB >30°	HOB = 0°; Patient flat
Fluids	2/3 maintenance	Hydrate normally
	BUN 35 mg/ml	I = O + losses
Hypertension	Prevent	Facilitate
	• Use sedatives	• Vascular expansion
	• Use antihypertensives	• Vasopressors
	• Use blockers	• Active stimulation
	• Avoid stimulation	
Mannitol	Osmolality 310–320 mOsm	Normal osmolality
	Replace 2/3 diuresis	Replace ml/ml if euvolemic
		I = O + losses
Barbiturates in Selected Cases	Burst suppression	Avoid cardiac depressants
Hyperventilation	$PaCO_2$ 25–28 mm Hg	$PaCO_2$ 35–40 mm Hg
		Hyperventilate acutely only

HOB = head of bed; I = intake; O = output.

Modified with permission from Rosner MJ: Pathophysiology and management of increased intracranial pressure. In Andrews BT (ed): Neurosurgical Intensive Care. McGraw-Hill, 1993.

Transfer to the ICU or OR

Patients with head injuries may undergo emergency operations such as craniotomy for evacuation of an intracranial hematoma (epidural, subdural, or intracerebral); craniectomy and decompressive procedures; elevation of depressed skull fractures; placement of ICP monitoring devices; and, of course, other non-neurosurgical procedures.

As stated above, the trauma victim necessitating surgery should always be monitored during transport and be accompanied by members of the trauma team. The basic monitoring devices for transport should include an electrocardiogram, automated blood pressure device, and pulse oximeter. End-tidal CO_2 monitoring should be considered if the patient is intubated.

Ideally, the trauma team leader should transfer care directly to the anesthesiologist involved in the case. He should discuss mechanism of injury, injuries that have been identified, results and omissions of investigations, past medical history, and allergies. Giving this advance notice to the team in the operating room before the actual arrival of the patient will avoid delays and keep the focus on continuity and quality of care. The same procedure should be followed when the patient is ready to be admitted to the trauma intensive care unit from the resuscitation room or the operating room.

Conclusion

Head injury is associated with more trauma deaths than injury to any other body region. The physician's actions can be summarized as focusing their attention on prevention of secondary injury to the brain. To ensure continuity of care of the multiple-injury patients, the trauma specialist and team leader should coordinate all interventions being performed on the victims.

References

1. Kraus JF: Epidemiology of head injury. In Cooper PR (ed): Head Injury.William and Wilkins, Baltimore, pp 1–25, 1993.
2. Thomason M, et al: Head CT scanning versus urgent exploration in the hypotensive blunt trauma patient. J Trauma 34:40–45, 1993.
3. Cales RH: Trunkey DD: Preventable trauma deaths: a review of trauma care systems development. JAMA 254:1059, 1985.

4. Oakley PA: Interface of anesthesiology and emergency medicine in trauma management. In Grande CM (ed): Textbook of Trauma anesthesia and Critical Care. Mosby, pp 106–119, 1993.
5. Stene JK, Grande CM: Trauma anesthesia: Past, present, and future. In Stene JK, Grande CM (eds): Trauma Anesthesia. Williams and Wilkins, Baltimore, pp 1–36, 1991.
6. Chestnut RM, Marshall LF, Marshall SB: Medical management of intracranial pressure. In Cooper PR (ed): Head Injury, William and Wilkins, Baltimore, pp 225–246, 1993.
7. Pietropaoli JA, Rogers FB, Shackford SR, et al: The deleterious effects of intraoperative hypotension on outcome in patients with severe head injuries. J Trauma 33:403–407, 1992.
8. Miller JD, Sweet RC, Narayan R, et al: Early insults to the injured brain. JAMA 240:439–442, 1978.
9. Rose J, Valtonen S, Jennett B: Avoidable factors contributing to death after head injury. BMJ 2:615–618, 1977.
10. Miller JD: Head injury and brain ischemia: implication for therapy. Br J Anaesth 57:120–129, 1985.
11. Jennett B, Teasdale G: Aspects of coma after severe head injury. Lancet 1:878, 1977.
12. Crosby ET, Liu A: The adult cervical spine: Implications for airway management. Can J Anaesth 37:77–93, 1990.
13. Majernick TG, et al: Cervical spine movement during orotracheal intubation. Ann Emerg Med 15:417–420, 1988.
14. Hastings RH, Marks JD: Airway management for trauma patients with potential cervical spine injuries. Anesth Analg 73:471–482, 1991.
15. Aprahamian C, Thompson BM, Finger WA, et al: Experimental cervical spine injury model: Evaluation of airway management and splinting techniques. Ann Emerg Med 13:584–587, 1984.
16. Heiden JS, Weiss MH, Rosenberg AW, et al: Management of cervical spinal cord trauma in Southern California. J Neurosurg 43:732, 1987.
17. American College of Surgeons: Advanced Trauma Life Support Student manual. Chicago, American College of Surgeons, 1989.
18. Bickell WH, Wall MJ, Pepe PE, et al: Immediate versus delayed fluid resuscitation for hypotensive patients with penetrating torso injuries. N Engl J Med 331:1105–1109, 1994.
19. Martin RR, Bickell WH, Pepe PE, Burch JM, Mattox KL: Prospective evaluation of preoperative fluid resuscitation in hypotensive patients with penetrating truncal injury: a preliminary report. J Trauma 33:354–362, 1992.
20. Milikan JS, Cain TL, Hansbrough J: Rapid volume replacement for hypovolemic shock: A comparison of techniques and equipment. J Trauma 24:428, 1984.
21. Calcagni DE, Bircher NG, Pretto E: Resuscitation: blood, blood component and fluid therapy. In Grande CM (ed): Textbook of Trauma Anesthesia and Critical Care, Mosby, 1993.
22. Palter MD, Cortes V: Secondary triage of the trauma patient. In Civetta JM, Taylor RW, Kirby RR (eds): Critical Care, second edition. Lippincott, Philadelphia, 1992.

23. Shenken HA, Bezier HS, Bovzarth WF: Restricted fluid intake: Rational management of the neurosurgical patient. J Neurosurg 45:432–440, 1976.
24. Wisner DH, Busche F, Sturm J, et al: Traumatic shock and head injury: effects of fluid resuscitation on the brain. J Surg Res 46:49–59, 1989.
25. Schmoker JD, Shackford SR, Wald SL, et al: An analysis of the relationship between fluid and sodium administration and intracranial pressure after head injury. J Trauma 33:476–481, 1992.
26. Battistella FD, Wisner DH: Combined hemorrhagic shock and head injury: effects of hypertonic saline 7.5% resuscitation. J Trauma 31: 182–188, 1991.
27. Shackford SD, Zhuang J, Schmoker J: Intravenous fluid tonicity: Effect on intracranial pressure, cerebral blood flow, and cerebral oxygen delivery in focal brain injury. J Neurosurg 76:91–98, 1992.
28. Walsh JC, Zhuang J, Shackford SR: A comparison of hypertonic to isotonic fluid in the resuscitation of brain injury and hemorrhagic shock. J Surg Res 50:284–292, 1991.
29. Prough DS, Johnson JC, Poole GV, et al: Effects on intracranial pressure of resuscitation from hemorrhagic shock with hypertonic saline versus lactated Ringer's solution. Crit Care Med 13:407–410, 1985.
30. Prough DS, Johnson JC, Stump DA, et al: Effects of hypertonic saline versus lactated Ringer's solution on cerebral oxygen transport during resuscitation from hemorrhagic shock. J Neurosurg 64:627–632, 1986.
31. Sieber FE, et al: Glucose: A reevaluation of its intraoperative use. Anesthesiology 67:72–81, 1987.
32. Kobayski S, Kakazawa S, Otsuka T: Clinical value of serial computed tomography with severe head injury. Surg Neurol 20:25–29, 1983.
33. Stein SC, Ross SE: The value of computed tomographic scans in patients with low risk head injuries. Neurosurgery 26:638–640, 1990.
34. Stein SC, Ross SE: Mild head injury: A plea for routine early CT scanning. J Trauma 33:11–13, 1992.
35. Livingston DH, Loder PA, Koziol J, et al: The use of CT scanning for triage patients requiring admission following minimal head injury. J Trauma 31:483–489, 1991.
36. Perry JF: A five-year survey of 152 acute abdominal injuries. J Trauma 5:53, 1965.
37. Cortes V, Palter M, Kreis DJ: Abdominal trauma: Diagnostic steps and postoperative considerations. In Civetta JM, Taylor RW, Kirby RR (eds): Critical Care, second edition. Lippincott, Philadelphia, 1992.
38. Trunkey DD, Hill AC, Schecter WP: Abdominal trauma and indications for celiotomy. In Moore EE, Mattox KL, Feliciano DV (eds): Trauma, second edition. Appleton and Lange, 1991.
39. Mackersie RC, Tiwary AD, Shackford R: Intra-abdominal injury following blunt trauma. Arch Surg 124:809, 1989.
40. Thomason M, Messick J, et al: Head CT scanning versus urgent exploration in the hypotensive blunt trauma patient. J Trauma 34:40–45, 1993.
41. Wisner DH, Victor NS, Holcroft JW: Priorities in the management of multiple trauma: intracranial versus intra-abdominal injury. J Trauma 35:271–278, 1993.

42. Johnson MH, Lee SH: Computed tomography of acute cerebral trauma. Radiol Clin North Am 30:325–352, 1992.
43. Mackersie RC, Shackford SR, Garfin SR, et al: Major skeletal injuries in the obtunded blunt trauma patient: A case for routine radiologic survey. J Trauma 28:1450, 1988.
44. Pal JM, Mulder DS, Brown RA, et al: Assessing multiple trauma: Is the cervical spine enough? J Trauma, 28:8, 1988.
45. Enderson BL, Reath DB, Meadors J, et al: The tertiary survey: a prospective study of missed injury. J Trauma 30:6, 1990.
46. Johnson KD, Cadambi A, Seibert GB: Incidence of adult respiratory distress syndrome in patients with multiple musculoskeletal injuries: effect of early operative stabilization of fractures. J Trauma 25:375–384, 1985.
47. Bone L, Johnson KD, Weigelt J, et al: Early versus delayed stabilization of femoral fractures. J Bone Joint Surg (Am) 71:336–340, 1989.
48. Latenser BA, Gentilello GM, Tarver AA, et al: Improved outcome with early fixation of skeletally unstable pelvic fractures. J Trauma 31: 28–30, 1991.
49. Wisner DH: Head injury from the general surgeon's perspective. Advances in Trauma and Critical Care, vol. 8. Mosby-Year Book, pp 183–216, 1993.
50. Jurkovick GJ, Greiser WB, Luterman A: Hypothermia in trauma victims: an ominous predictor of survival. J Trauma 27:9, 1987.
51. Rosner MJ: Pathophysiology and management of increased intracranial pressure. In Andrews BT (ed): Neurosurgical Intensive Care. McGraw-Hill, NY, 1993.

5

Airway Management in Neurological Injuries

Steven J. Tryfus, MD, Kenneth J. Abrams, MD, Christopher M. Grande, MD, MPH

Closed Head Injury

Introduction

Management of trauma victims with isolated closed head injury (CHI) is directed toward rapid diagnosis and therapeutic intervention of severe brain injury with concomitant prevention and control of elevated intracranial pressure (ICP) and limitation of secondary brain injury. Miller and associates retrospectively studied the morbidity and mortality associated with raised intracranial pressure.[1] They followed 160 severely brain-injured patients from arrival through the postoperative course, with ICP measurements determined by ventriculostomy. Of the 48 patients who died, 23 died of severe intracranial hypertension (ICP > 40 mm Hg), 12 had moderate elevations (ICP > 20 mm Hg), and 13 patients died with ICP ≤

From *Trauma Anesthesia and Critical Care of Neurological Injury,* edited by K. J. Abrams and C. M. Grande. © 1997, Futura Publishing Co., Armonk, NY.

20 mm Hg. The authors concluded that patients with severe CHI and ICP $\geq$ 20 mm Hg had a four times greater mortality when compared to patients with ICP $\leq$ 20 mm Hg.

Anesthetic Induction Agents

Barbiturates

In an effort to evaluate the efficacy of barbiturate therapy in traumatic brain injury patients with uncontrolled intracranial hypertension, Marshall and co-workers examined 100 consecutive patients with severe head injury.[2] Twenty-five patients had an ICP greater than 40 mm Hg; 19 of them suffered diffuse brain injury with persistently elevated ICP, while six had uncontrolled intracranial hypertension following surgical correction. All 25 failed conventional ICP management, which included positioning, hyperventilation, surgical evacuation, diuretic therapy, and high-dose steroids. Barbiturate therapy was then instituted as a rescue approach to refractory intracranial hypertension. Each of the 25 patients received pentobarbital (3–5 mg/kg) as an IV bolus, followed by an infusion, achieving a therapeutic blood level of 2.5–3.5 mg %. The initial bolus resulted in a 76% reduction of ICP. Infusion therapy with pentobarbital produced a further decline to near normal values (ICP $\leq$ 15 mm Hg) in 13 patients. Consistent with these findings, in a multicenter study of 925 severely head-injured patients, 12% responded favorably to high-dose barbiturate therapy with a reduction in ICP.[3] Despite this encouraging data, both Ward et al. and Schwartz et al. failed to demonstrate a decline in mortality or greater control of ICP with high-dose barbiturate therapy.[4,5]

While improvement in outcome has not been clearly established for treatment of refractory intracranial hypertension, it is the opinion of these authors that barbiturates have an important role in rapid acquisition and control of the airway in acute head-injured patients. In addition to effects on ICP, barbiturates also mitigate the sympathetic response to laryngoscopy and intubation while decreasing cerebral metabolic rate for oxygen ($CMRO_2$) and cerebral blood flow (CBF).[6–8] Thiopental, an ultra-short-acting barbiturate, continues to be a popular induction agent among traumatologists. Its rapid onset and short distribution half-life make it ideal for rapid sequence induction. However, the standard induction doses of 3–5 mg/kg used in elective patients may lead to precipitous alteration of hemodynamics and perhaps unmask the hypovolemia in a trauma victim.

Therefore, the aforementioned reduction of ICP with hypnotic agents, including thiopental, may be secondary to arterial hypotension, leading to an overall decline in cerebral perfusion pressure (CCP).[9] Hence, induction doses should be individualized to hemodynamic, respiratory, and intracranial parameters. In the hemodynamically unstable patient, either incremental repeated administration of reduced doses is recommended (0.5–2.0 mg/kg) or avoiding hypnotic agents under specific clinical situations should be considered.

Etomidate

Etomidate is a carboxylated imidazole hypnotic agent and, like barbiturates, rapidly induces general anesthesia of short duration with beneficial effects on intracranial dynamics.[10] In addition to lowering ICP by decreasing $CMRO_2$ and cerebral blood flow (CBF), etomidate has the distinct advantage of enhanced cardiovascular stability.[11] Arterial blood pressure is well maintained, leading to an overall increase in cerebral perfusion pressure (CPP), which can be beneficial in patients with closed head injury.[12,13] In severely head-injured patients, etomidate decreased ICP while electrical activity was present but was not effective when cortical activity was maximally suppressed.[14] This indicates that the decrease in ICP may be caused by the reduction of CBF that is induced by metabolic depressant effects of etomidate.[15]

For control during endotracheal intubation, Modica and Tempelhoff administered etomidate, until burst suppression, to eight patients with intracranial space-occupying lesions undergoing craniotomy.[16] All patients were monitored for mean arterial pressure (MAP), ICP, CPP, heart rate, EEG, and spectral edge frequency. The initial bolus of 0.2 mg/kg was followed by an infusion of 20 mg/min until early burst suppression was detected; following this, the infusion was discontinued and tracheal intubation ensued. ICP decreased 50% (22 ± 1 to 11 ± 1 mm Hg), while MAP, CPP, and heart rate were unchanged. The authors concluded that use of etomidate to achieve early burst suppression allowed tracheal intubation with minimal hemodynamic alterations and a significant reduction in ICP.

As with many pharmacological agents, etomidate's potential deleterious effects on the severely head-injured must be considered. The most alarming side effect is etomidate's proclivity to activate seizure foci, which may be harmful in severely head-injured patients.[17] Furthermore, reports of myoclonus and tonic-clonic movements may confuse the neurological evaluation of CNS injured patients. Etomidate's utility may be further limited by reports of adrenal suppression of up to 6–8 hours following single bolus injection, although perhaps not clinically significant.[18]

Etomidate's greater cardiovascular stability and beneficial intracranial effects makes it an ideal agent for CHI patients. However, in the presence of significant hypovolemia, which occurs in many trauma victims, etomidate loses its hemodynamic stability and may precipitate injurious hypotension. Therefore, an induction dose of 0.2–0.3 mg/kg should be administered as incremental aliquots to achieve optimal intubating conditions as well as to provide a minimally changing hemodynamic profile.

Propofol

Propofol is an ultra-short-acting, nonbarbiturate induction agent whose utility in the trauma arena is becoming better defined. Apprehension of its application is due primarily to its potentially dramatic untoward effects on blood pressure and cardiovascular stability, much like that seen with barbiturates.[19] Similarly, by using reduced and incremental doses, these undesirable side effects can be attenuated. Propofol appears to have a favorable profile with respect to intracranial dynamics. It decreases CBF and $CMRO_2$ with an increase in cerebrovascular resistance.[20] In CHI patients, propofol affords a reduction in ICP.[21]

Pinaud et al. studied 10 severely head-injured patients (GCS 6–7) undergoing orthopedic repair of extremity fractures.[22] Induction was accomplished with propofol 2 mg/kg IV bolus followed by 150 mcg/kg/min infusion. Hemodynamic parameters, measured at 5-minute and 15-minute intervals following induction, revealed a reduction in ICP (11.3 mm Hg to 9.2 mm Hg) associated with a 25% decline in mean arterial pressure (MAP). The mean regional cerebral blood flow (rCBF) decreased by 25.7% with a concomitant decrease in CPP of 26.7% and 28%, respectively.

There was no evidence of alteration in cerebrovascular resistance or cerebral arteriovenous oxygen difference. The authors concluded that while propofol possesses the beneficial effects of lowering ICP, it accomplishes this by harmfully decreasing CPP and thus compromising intracranial hemodynamics. Further support from Miller et al. reported profound systemic hypotension in both adults and children with intracranial hypertension treated with propofol infusion.[8] CPP did not improve despite a reduction in ICP.

Although the above investigators have demonstrated a limited usefulness for propofol in head injury patients, Heath et al. recently evaluated the utility of propofol as an induction agent in 20 trauma patients requiring intubation.[23] All patients had a complete primary survey and appropriate fluid resuscitation prior to intubation. Nine patients with isolated head injury (IHI) and 11 multiply injured patients with associated CHI were administered propofol in titration until unconsciousness and then they underwent tracheal intubation following succinylcholine administration. There was an average fall in mean arterial pressure of 7% and 11%, respectively. Mean induction doses ranged between 1.18 mg/kg and 1.25 mg/kg. The authors concluded that titration of propofol in this manner does not result in clinically significant hypotension.

The data did not include information regarding intracranial dynamics or additional hemodynamic variables beyond blood pressure. Although propofol may have beneficial effects on cerebral dynamics, its propensity toward reduced blood pressure may limit its utility. Until further information focusing on this delicate balance becomes available, propofol should be used cautiously.

Ketamine

Ketamine is a phencyclidine derivative and is a unique anesthetic because it induces a catatonic state. Ketamine increases CBF by about 60% and reduces cerebral vascular resistance in humans. However, $CMRO_2$ does not change dramatically.[24] Ketamine markedly increases ICP.[25-27] This increase may be attenuated by prior induction of hypocapnia or by the administration of thiopental.[25-27] However, this has not been a consistent finding. Thus, its use in patients with elevated ICP following CHI is not recommended.[28]

Opioids

Along with addressing the issues of hypoxia, hypercarbia, and aspiration potential, the goals of airway management in patients with CHI includes prevention of secondary brain injury as a result of the process of laryngoscopy and intubation, per se. The hemodynamic events are frequently associated with tachycardia and severe hypertension, which may be attenuated by the judicious use of opiates as an adjunct to traditional sedative hypnotics.[29,30] However, the effect of opiates on ICP has not been clearly established. Thus, the utilization of opiates in the severely head-injured patient remains controversial, while leaving traumatologists no clear path when choosing appropriate care plans.[31] The cardiac stability afforded by opioids lend themselves to represent the ideal agent for control and maintenance of both ICP and CPP. While many studies have examined their effect on CHI, further elucidation and investigation is required.[32]

Sperry and co-workers examined the effects of fentanyl and sufentanil on ICP and CPP in nine severely head-injured (GCS 5–7) patients 1–3 days following injury.[33] All patients required mechanical ventilation and supportive therapy that included mechanical hyperventilation, ICP monitoring, head elevation, sedation with midazolam and osmotherapy. None of the patients underwent surgical intervention prior to completion of the study. Each patient received either fentanyl (3 mcg/kg) or sufentanil (0.6 mcg/kg) as an intravenous bolus and 24 hours later they received the other opioid in the same manner. All patients were fully paralyzed with vecuronium bromide. Heart rate, blood pressure, and ICP were continuously monitored.

Although a significant rise in ICP in both groups occurred following administration of fentanyl and sufentanil (8 ± 2 mm Hg), no patient had an initial ICP greater than 20 mm Hg. There was, however, a demonstrated increase in four patients in ICP to above 20 mm Hg following administration of either fentanyl or sufentanil. Three of these patients required intervention for excessive increases in ICP. Furthermore, there was an average decrease in MAP from baseline of 11 ± 6 mm Hg in the fentanyl group and 10 ± 5 mm Hg in the sufentanil group.

In addition, there was a significant decrease in mean CPP following administration of fentanyl and sufentanil (13 ± 4 mm Hg and 10 ± 4 mm Hg, respectively). The authors concluded that modest doses of the synthetic opioids, fentanyl and sufentanil, may lead to significant rises in ICP in severely head-injured patients.

Despite this clinical evidence, animal studies report no change in ICP following administration of narcotics.[34–36] Recently, Sheehan and co-workers developed an acute brain injury model in rabbits and found that fentanyl and sufentanil had no significant effect on ICP.[37] Several other studies on human subjects have found little or no rise in ICP from sufentanil or alfentanil. No clear resolution of this controversy exists to date, and no obvious direction has been taken by the medical community.

Muscle Relaxants

During rapid control of the airway, the choice of muscle relaxant will depend on its rapidity of onset, reliability, and duration of action.

To this end, succinylcholine still represents the ideal choice for rapid sequence intubation. However, questions regarding its effects on ICP have limited its popularity. Investigations have demonstrated a rise in ICP following administration of succinylcholine in patients with known elevations of ICP.[38] Conversely, further evidence has shown that there is a rather transient rise in ICP with succinylcholine, but this is clinically less significant when thiopental is utilized.[39] Finally, Lam and colleagues found no rise in ICP with succinylcholine in acute head injury patients.[40]

Vecuronium represents another popular selection for rapid sequence intubation in closed head injury patients. Vecuronium is devoid of significant hemodynamic disturbances and exhibits no untoward effects on intracranial dynamics.[41] However, at least three times the ED 95 is required to obtain intubating conditions within 90 to 100 seconds.[42] This is still slightly slower in onset than succinylcholine and results in prolonged paralysis. However, the clinical significance of this issue in the seriously injured patient has been challenged.

A new steroidal competitive neuromuscular blocking agent, rocuronium, may represent a good compromise between onset time and duration of action. Rocuronium is a derivative of vecuronium and pancuronium. It is less potent than the parent compounds, but possesses a quicker onset of action. Doses of 0.9 mg/kg to 1.2 mg/kg will provide intubating conditions comparable to succinylcholine in approximately 60 seconds.[43] There are no specific data available at this time regarding the effect of rocuronium on intracranial dynamics.

Benzodiazepines

The benzodiazepines, diazepam, lorazepam, and midazolam are used extensively by anesthesiologists as an adjunct to general anesthesia. These agents provide preoperative sedation, amnesia, and overall decreased anesthetic requirements. Their role in acute airway management of CHI patients is not clearly established. Unlike thiopental, the benzodiazepines do not have a rapid onset and are less predictable.

Benzodiazepines produce a desirable reduction of both CBF and $CMRO_2$. Canine studies by Maekawa et al. and Sari et al. demonstrated that 0.25 mg/kg of diazepam produced a significant decrease in $CMRO_2$.[44,45] Nugent et al. evaluated diazepam and midazolam in a canine model; they found a dose-dependent decrease in CBF and $CMRO_2$, up to a maximum reduction of 50% of controlled values for both CBF and $CMRO_2$.[46] Nugent et al. reported that midazolam had greater protection from hypoxia than diazepam in a hypoxia mouse model. Finally, Hoffman et al., using a rat model, reported a dose-related decline in both CBF and $CMRO_2$ with a 40-45% reduction of CBF from control and a 55% decrease in $CMRO_2$.[47] In patients undergoing craniotomy for resection of tumor, midazolam induction caused no rise in ICP.[48]

Benzodiazepines would be a suitable alternative to rapidly acting hypnotic agents in the management of patients with traumatic brain injury. However, slow induction times may lead to hypoxia and accumulation of CO_2; both are undesirable effects in CHI. Therefore, we recommend a sedative-hypnotic agent for induction and benzodiazepines for continual sedation, with or without opioids.

Midazolam, used alone in relatively small doses (1–2 mg IV) may have some application as an amnestic. In trauma patients, perioperative recall is an important consideration, especially when hemodynamic instability is encountered and/or anticipated difficult airway situations where essentially "awake" techniques will be used.

Adjunctive Therapy

Using adjunctive agents assists in alleviating the harmful surge of catecholamines from laryngoscopy and intubation, which frequently result in undesirable tachycardia and hypertension. This is more commonly encountered during a rapid sequence induction. The synthetic opioids offer one pharmacological option that may lessen these deleterious effects. Beta blockers and lidocaine have also been shown to be effective.[49]

The goal of blunting hemodynamic response to laryngoscopy and intubation can readily be achieved by the judicious use of beta blocking agents. Single-bolus dosing of esmolol or labetalol have been shown to mitigate heart rate and blood pressure alterations associated with airway stimulation.[50] However, esmolol may possess an advantage over labetalol because it has a shorter duration, especially in the face of potential hemodynamic instability in the multiply injured trauma victim.

The role of lidocaine in attenuating hemodynamic responses to airway manipulation is less clear because the available data are contradictory. However, the use of intravenous lidocaine has been shown to prevent a rise in ICP.[51,52] In two separate studies, Yukeoka and co-workers demonstrated the efficacy of IV lidocaine in suppressing cough during endotracheal intubation with 2 mg/kg completely suppressing the cough reflex.[53] Furthermore, the ideal time to administer this dose was 1–5 minutes prior to laryngoscopy and intubation. Although these data do not support a positive effect on ICP or CPP, one may conclude that there would be an indirect benefit on intracranial dynamics.

Management of the Patient with Head Trauma

The trauma victim suffering from CNS injury, either closed head or cervical spine, presents difficult management decisions. All therapeutic modalities must be directed toward optimizing the multiple dynamic pathophysiological states while minimizing secondary injury. Paramount concerns include raised ICP, unstable cervical spine, and associated injuries resulting in hypovolemic shock. In 1978, the American College of Surgeons' Committee on Trauma (ACSCOT) presented the first Advanced Trauma Life Support (ATLS) course.[54] This new approach focused on managing life-threatening injuries first, hence the concept of ABCs, previously developed in the ACLS paradigm, and airway control became the primary focus of acute trauma care. During the "golden hour," the critical initial phase following injury, traumatologists can have the greatest impact on outcome. Gildenberg and Makela studied the outcome of approximately 2,000 severely head injured patients requiring endotracheal intubation.[55] They demonstrated a significant reduction in mortality in patients intubated within the first hour after injury (22.5% vs. 38%).

Initiation of ATLS protocols may prevent secondary brain damage.[56] In the case of the severely head injured, hypoxia and hypercarbia are directly associated with a poor outcome.[57] In addition, CHI patients suffering a hypoxic event prior to arrival in the emergency department also have a much poorer outcome.[58] Therefore, early tracheal intubation, positive pressure ventilation with 100% oxygen, and systemic hemodynamic resuscitation should be initiated promptly (Table 1).

Although it is important to intubate these patients early, the best method and pharmacological support remains uncertain. Rotondo and colleagues recently reviewed the safety of urgent paralysis in 231 trauma patients requiring emergent intubation.[59] Indications for paralysis and intubation included the need for emergency surgery, or airway control, control of combative behavior, and initiation of mechanical ventilation. Twenty-four intubation mishaps occurred,

Table 1
Overall Goals of Anesthetic Management in CHI

Maintenance of oxygenation and ventilation
Protection of cervical spine
Decrease risk of aspiration
Control hemodynamic variables

CHI = closed head injury.

including 14 multiple attempts at laryngoscopy, seven aspirations, and three esophageal intubations. In 194 of 204 patients who survived at least 24 hours, there were 15 pulmonary complications including eight pneumonias, five persistent infiltrates, and two cases of severe atelectasis. No deaths were related to the intubation mishaps or the pulmonary complications. The authors concluded that paralysis and intubation is associated with low morbidity, no mortality, and may be used safely to facilitate intubation in the trauma victim.

In support of Rotondo's findings, Redan et al. evaluated 100 consecutive trauma patients with suspected head injury who underwent emergent intubation in the emergency department utilizing muscle paralysis.[60] Although subsequent evaluation revealed seven patients who had cervical fractures, no patients developed secondary neurological deficit. One patient developed aspiration pneumonia following intubation. The authors contend that paralysis and intubation in the emergency department can be safe and may facilitate the diagnostic workup in the combative trauma patient.

A continuing quality improvement review at our institution (SJT,KJA), over almost 2.5 years, revealed that 17.3% (283/1,644) of all trauma team patients were being intubated and 78.3% (223/283) of these patients underwent rapid sequence induction (induction agents and muscle relaxants) to facilitate endotracheal intubation and control physiological conditions.[61] Our overall complication rate was 2.4% with two surgical airways and two aspirations, with three patients requiring multiple attempts at laryngoscopy. This low complication rate is in the presence of an anesthesiology team consisting of an attending trauma anesthesiologist, a senior anesthesiology resident or trauma anesthesia fellow, and a junior anesthesiology resident. Overall, if performed by skilled personnel, trauma patients can be as safely anesthetized, paralyzed, and intubated in the emergency department as they would be in the operating room.

A recent study by Nakayama and colleagues has underscored the erratic usage of induction agents and muscle relaxants to facilitate intubation of head-injured pediatric trauma patients.[62] Only 8 of 53 patients received an optimal medical regimen. Thiopental was not used in 25 of 35 stable patients with isolated head injury. Intravenous lidocaine was not used in 38 of 50 head-injured patients in whom it would have been an appropriate adjunct to control potential increases in ICP. Eight patients received paralyzing agents alone without sedatives or narcotics. Hence, pharmacological therapy is often inappropriate or underutilized. Administration of anesthetics should be tailored and directed to meet the needs of each individual patient. Management protocols and pharmacological guidelines should be established to aid the traumatologist in acute airway management of the trauma victim (Table 2). Indications for early and rapid intubation of the head-injured patient are listed in Table 3.[63]

The balance between ICP and CPP is difficult to measure and is therefore intimated clinically by the Glasgow Coma Scale (GCS). Stratification consists of mild (GCS 13–15), moderate (GCS 10–12), or severe (GCS <9) CNS injury. Endotracheal intubation is indicated in patients with a GCS score of 8 or less and in those moderately injured with a deteriorating neurological status.

In general, the traumatologist directing airway intervention must be vigilant in avoiding secondary brain injury. Anesthetic considerations include maintenance of oxygenation and ventilation, protection of the cervical spine, minimizing the risk of aspiration, and control of hemodynamic variables.

Recommended Approach to Emergency Endotracheal Intubation in CHI

The trauma patient who cannot maintain a patent airway must have a cuffed endotracheal tube placed. Oral or nasal airways have a very minor role in the initial management of the unstable trauma patient, and are used only for temporary support. Oral tracheal intubation, facilitated by the use of appropriate induction agents and muscle relaxants, by trained personnel, is the technique of choice for intubating trauma patients. Cervical spine stabilization during intubation can be performed with manual immobilization of the head and neck on a long spine board (Fig. 1).

Table 2
Guidelines for Managing Clinical Presentations[1]

Condition	Induction Agent	Muscle Relaxant	Adjunctive Medications
GCS 3, or traumatic arrest	None	None	None
Shock, sys BP < 80 mm Hg	None	Succinylcholine 1.5 mg/kg or Rocuronium 0.9–1.2 mg/kg[2]	Lidocaine 1.5 mg/kg Midazolam 1–2 mg Fentanyl 0.5–1.0 μg/kg
Hypotension, sys BP 80–100 mm Hg	Thiopental 0.5–2.0 mg/kg (incremental dosing) or Etomidate 0.1–0.2 mg/kg	Succinylcholine 1.5 mg/kg or Rocuronium 0.9–1.2 mg/kg	Lidocaine 1.5 mg/kg Midazolam 1–2 mg Fentanyl 1–2 μg/kg
GCS 4–9 with hypertension	Thiopental 3–5 mg/kg or Etomidate 0.2–0.3 mg/kg	Rocuronium 0.9–1.2 mg/kg Succinylcholine 1.5 mg/kg	Fentanyl 1–2μg/kg Lidocaine 1.5 mg/kg Esmolol 10 mg (titrated)
GCS 10–11, uncooperative, BP normal to increased	Thiopental 3–5 mg/kg Etomidate 0.2–0.3 mg/kg Propofol 1–2 mg/kg (titrated)	Rocuronium 0.9–1.2 mg/kg or Succinylcholine 1.5 mg/kg	Fentanyl 3–5 μg/kg Midazolam 2–5 mg

GCS = Glasgow Coma Scale; BP = blood pressure.

[1] Modified from Stene JK, Grande CM: Anesthesia for Trauma. In Miller RD, editor: Anesthesia, New York, 1994, Churchill Livingston.

[2] Magorian T, Flanery KB, Miller RD. Comparison of rocuronium, succinylcholine, and vecuronium for rapid sequence induction in adult patients. Anesthesiology 79:913, 1993.

Traditionally, "classic" rapid sequence induction imposed a period of apnea; and while cricopharyngeal pressure is used, it was not utilized to its maximal benefit. Essentially, it is now appreciated that many seriously injured multi-trauma patients first present with suboptimal or dangerously low levels of oxygen saturation, despite

Table 3
Indications for Endotracheal Intubation in CHI

Respiratory distress
Respiratory rates >30 or <10 breaths/min
Abnormal breathing patterns
Motor posturing or absence of response to pain
$PaO_2 < 70$ torr or $PaCO_2 > 45$ torr
Glasgow Coma Scale score <9
Seizures
Increased intracranial pressure
Need for analgesics or sedatives
Associated significant injuries (e.g., thorocoabdominal)

CHI = closed head injury; GCS = Glasgow Coma Scale.

From Abrams KJ: Airway management and mechanical ventilation. New Horizons 3:479–487, 1995.

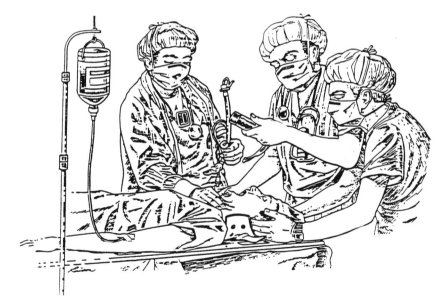

Figure 1. Cervical spine stabilization during intubation can be performed with manual immobilization of the head and neck on a long spine board.

an oxygen nonrebreather device having been placed during transport from the field. For many reasons, it is not possible to achieve normal oxygen saturation in the spontaneously breathing trauma patient.

Many trauma patients exhibit significant degrees of oxygen desaturation as a result of deranged chest wall mechanics and ventilation perfusion abnormalities. Oxygen should be administered via face mask prior to induction of anesthesia, and then positive pressure bag-mask ventilation through cricoid pressure should be used until endotracheal intubation is done.[64] Testing the ability to ventilate also provides the anesthesiologist with the knowledge that the ventilation can be supported if endotracheal intubation proves difficult.

The incidence and occurrence of hypoxia in patients with head injury is much higher than the rate of cervical spine fractures. Hence, the need to establish an airway should take precedence over the concern for cervical instability or aspiration. The goals of pharmacological therapy are to facilitate intubation and oxygenation while preventing further injury.

A "modified" rapid sequence induction for trauma ideally requires three individuals to be performed properly. The modification is that gentle positive pressure ventilation is instituted during the period of apnea using a bag-valve-mask device, prior to intubation, to prevent accumulation of CO_2 and to minimize hypoxia. One individual is dedicated to maintaining manual in-line axial stabilization (MIAS). MIAS is used to counteract the movement associated with performing laryngoscopy. Neither traction nor immobilization should be instituted; stabilization is the goal. Once MIAS is applied, the anterior portion of the cervical collar is removed or released, depending on the type of hard collar used. The front of the collar is removed for three distinct benefits:

1. It allows mouth opening and anterior displacement of the submandibular tissues during laryngoscopy.
2. It permits efficacious application of cricoid pressure.
3. It allows identification of the cricothyroid membrane in case a surgical airway becomes necessary.

The second person is responsible for performing laryngoscopy and ultimately intubation of the trachea. The third anesthesiologist administers induction agents, muscle relaxants, adjunctive medications, and applies cricoid pressure. Once successful intubation has been confirmed by clinical evaluation and capnography, the anterior portion of the cervical collar is replaced and MIAS may be released.

Correctly applied cricoid pressure helps protect the airway from aspiration of stomach contents. The trauma patient with cervical spine stabilization cannot be easily moved to drain gastric contents from the mouth; therefore, prevention of regurgitation is essential. Ultimately, the best protection from aspiration for the trauma patient is a smooth, well-conducted intubation and an extubation delayed until the patient has competent airway reflexes and respiratory dynamics.

The traumatologist must combine knowledge of pharmacology with the complexities presented by the multiply injured victim. Ideally, the use of induction agents and muscle relaxants will aid in rapid intubation and mitigate the rises in ICP. Important information may be obtained from prehospital personnel and initial evaluation must include the mechanism of injury and vital signs prior to arriving at the trauma center.

Patient Profiles

Hemodynamically Stable Patient

In the case of the hemodynamically stable patient, the traumatologist has several pharmacological options. Of primary importance, as with all rapid sequence inductions, a bag-valve-mask device must be available to deliver 100% oxygen, as well as adequate suction and, of course, three well-trained personnel to perform rapid sequence inductions with appropriate MIAS (Table 4).

Once the need to intubate is determined, the patient is preoxygenated with 100% oxygen for 3–5 minutes prior to induction. In circumstances where the patient is combative, this level of preoxygenation may be difficult to achieve and securing the airway should take precedence. During this preoxygenation period, titration of adjunctive agents may proceed.

Lidocaine 1.5 mg/kg to 2.0 mg/kg, and if appropriate fentanyl 3–5 mcg/kg, may be administered as tolerated. Often, smaller doses of fentanyl (1–2 mcg/kg) are given. However, these are less effective in quelling the sympathetic response. Also, fentanyl may cause respiratory depression as well as cause chest wall rigidity and impede one's ability to ventilate. Esmolol in aliquots of 0.5 to 1.0 mg/kg 1–2 minutes prior to laryngoscopy may assist in the induction. Again,

Table 4
Contents of a Trauma Airway Emergency Kit

Essential
- Oral/nasal airways
- Face mask of various sizes
- Self-inflating resuscitator bag
- Endotracheal tubes of various sizes with malleable stylets
- Laryngoscopes with several blade sizes
- Endotracheal tube exchangers
- Laryngeal mask airways
- Jet stylets, gum elastic bougies
- Surgical and needle cricothyroidotomy sets
- Hand-held transtracheal jet ventilatory apparatus
- Combitube

Desirable (Optional)
- Bullard laryngoscope
- Bellscope blades
- Lighted stylet
- Flexible fiberoptic intubating laryngoscope
- Retrograde intubation set
- Augustine guide

Items in this kit may be excluded, substituted, or additional items added depending on individual institutional needs.

caution must prevail with this regimen and any combination of drugs requires expertise, impeccable timing, and vigilance.

Following this phase, an induction agent is delivered to complete hypnosis as well as a skeletal muscle relaxant to facilitate paralysis and intubation. Thiopental (3–5 mg/kg) or etornidate (0.2–0.3 mg/kg) may be administered, always bearing in mind the potential side effects.

The choice of muscle relaxants is not obvious. These authors prefer to avoid succinylcholine secondary to its potential hyperkalemic effects as well as the litany of other untoward possibilities.[65] Vecuronium is a very popular selection in doses of 0.25–0.30 mg/kg, which provides intubating conditions in 90 seconds lasting approximately 100 minutes.

Rocuronium is quickly becoming an agent of choice in the trauma arena. Although not much data are available regarding its use in airway intervention of trauma victims, Magorian and colleagues found that doses of 0.9 and 1.2 mg/kg of rocuronium are similar in onset to succinylcholine for rapid sequence inductions.[43]

Hence, as a result of published studies and our experience, we recommend induction of thiopental followed by rocuronium, but be aware these agents may precipitate.[66,67]

Laryngoscopy and intubation should be limited to minimize the sympathetic response. Endotracheal tube placement is confirmed by direct visualization, auscultation, and detection of end-tidal CO_2. Once the tube is secured, the anterior portion of the C-collar is replaced and the patient is ventilated to normocapnia. Chest x-ray will confirm position above the carina and arterial blood gas analysis will assure adequate ventilation. At this juncture, the injured patient may be sedated with midazolam 0.05 mg/kg and/or fentanyl 1–2 mcg/kg as needed until neuroradiographic studies are complete.

Hemodynamically Unstable Patient

Management of the hemodynamically unstable trauma patient with CHI is a formidable challenge. Airway management of this patient requires a delicate balance in the context of a profound knowledge of traumatic shock and its classification. Unfortunately, patients are not readily confined to one shock class, thus all interventions are titrated in metered doses.

Patients who present in class I shock with CHI may cautiously be considered hemodynamically stable. Adjuvant agents should be used judiciously to avoid abrupt alterations of hemodynamics. Similarly, we recommend titration of either thiopental (3–5 mg/kg) or etomidate (0.2–0.3 mg/kg) with rocuronium (0.9–1.2 mg/kg).

In case of class II–III shock, the flux of this presentation is quite rapid and pharmacological intervention may easily unmask profound hypovolemic hypotension. If only adjuvant treatment would be hemodynamically tolerated, lidocaine 1.5 mg/kg is effective. When using thiopental, we recommend incremental dosing with a total dose of 0.5–2.0 mg/kg. Alternatively, etomidate may be used in doses of 0.1–0.2 mg/kg. If airway deterioration is rapid and uncontrolled, succinylcholine 1.5 mg/kg may be administered. Resuscitation must be ongoing and continued throughout while preparations for transport to the operating room are done expeditiously.

The mortality rate of the class IV shock patient with an associated CHI is quite high. Generally, these patients will not tolerate advanced pharmacotherapy. Typically, only lidocaine 1.5 mg/kg with midazolam 1–2 mg and a muscle relaxant is used to secure the airway, or even a muscle relaxant alone. While patients may recall the event, this is a risk-versus-benefit situation we often face. Either succinylcholine 1.5 mg/kg or rocuronium 0.9–1.2 mg/kg can be used. On occasion, patients may be unconscious and in a condition to allow intubation without medication. The patient is then manually ventilated using 100% oxygen, the endotracheal tube secured, and the patient is rapidly transferred to the operating room. If there are sudden deleterious rises in blood pressure, these may be treated in a variety of ways including midazolam 1–2 mg IV, fentanyl 50–100 mcg IV, or thiopental 25–75 mg IV in incremental doses.

Cervical Spine Injury

Introduction

Cervical spine injuries (CSI) continue to pose major problems in airway management. Virtually all currently available methods of airway manipulation cause movement of the cervical spine to some degree. This includes the chin lift and jaw thrust maneuvers, as well as direct laryngoscopy and other methods of endotracheal intubation.[68]

Approximately 1.5% to 3% of patients have a CSI following major trauma, and at least 50% of these fractures are potentially unstable.[69] Secondary neurological deficit occurs in almost 1.5% to 2.5%, but is seven times more likely to occur when the injury is unrecognized.[70] Although the issue of airway management and the potential for subsequent neurological deterioration remains foremost in the anesthesiologist's mind, there has been only one such published case report of which we are aware.[71] Nevertheless, the goals of airway management in patients with suspected CSI are: a high index of suspicion, diagnosis of the injury, providing a secure airway for ventilation and oxygenation, and the prevention of secondary spinal cord injury.

Epidemiology

With the overall incidence of CSI averaging about 2.5% in severe trauma, there appears to be a greater association in patients concomitantly suffering CHI. Several sources have estimated the frequency of CSI in association with CHI to be approximately 10%.[72,73] Ross and O'Mailey have considered this to be considerably higher than observed in their clinical practice. They concluded that there was a 2.6% overall incidence of CSI in blunt trauma victims and only a

1.8% incidence in patients with CHI.[74] This led Hills and Deane to analyze a series of 8,285 blunt trauma victims to determine the association of CSI with both head injury and facial injury.[75] This study revealed that patients suffering clinically significant head injuries were at greater risk of associated CSIs than those without head trauma. Furthermore, patients with GCS scores of 8 or less were at even greater risk. Interestingly, this study indicated that facial injuries lacked an association with cervical injuries, previously thought to be an issue.

Physical Examination

Evaluation of the patient with potential CSI should follow the principles outlined in the ATLS course.[72] Attention should focus on maintaining a secure airway, adequate oxygenation and ventilation, and hemodynamic stability. Nearly two-thirds of all trauma patients suffer multiple injuries. Significant injuries include pneumothorax, hemothorax, cardiac tamponade, hemoperitoneum, and major orthopedic fractures. As revealed above, the GCS is likely to be a greater indicator of associated CSI than is the presence of associated injuries.

Neurological deficits are present in 30–70% of patients with vertebral injuries. They are even more frequent in patients with fracture dislocations or with C6 to C7 vertebral injuries.[76] Signs of cervical injury may be obvious (Table 5).

Ross and colleagues prospectively identified clinical predictors of unstable CSIs.[74] Significant predictors of unstable injury included

Table 5
Signs of Cervical Spine Injury

Loss of intercostal muscle tone
Diaphragmatic breathing
Hypotension and bradycardia, without evidence of
  hypovolemia
Priapism
Flaccid paralysis
Palpable step-off abnormality
Neck tenderness or pain
Anesthesia below the clavicles

From Abrams KJ, Grande CM: Airway management of the patient with cervical spine injury. Curr Opin Anesth 7:2:184–190, 1994.

loss of consciousness, neurological deficit consistent with cervical cord or nerve root injury, and neck tenderness. In another recent prospective study, 27 patients with cervical spine fractures were identified among 974 blunt trauma patients admitted to UCLA Emergency Medicine Center.[77] All 27 patients had at least one of the following characteristics: midline neck tenderness, evidence of intoxication, altered level of consciousness, or another severely painful injury. Nine hundred forty-seven patients were without cervical spine fractures. Of these patients, 353 had none of the four signs or symptoms. The importance of any of the above findings purports that any neurological deficits must be documented and continually reevaluated to establish a baseline for detecting further neurological deterioration.

Spinal cord injuries of the cervical region are often associated with respiratory and cardiovascular compromise. Primary cardiovascular abnormalities of hypotension and bradycardia (in the absence of hypovolemia) present early in the course of the injury. Hypotension results from the lack of sympathetic innervation to the vasculature, thereby increasing venous compliance. Spinal injury above the first thoracic level denervates the cardiac accelerator nerves, leaving unopposed parasympathetic tone.

Low cervical injuries (C6-C7) will preserve diaphragmatic function since the phrenic nerve roots arise from C3-C5. Patients with lesions above this level usually present in respiratory failure. Manifestations of lower cervical injuries include: reduced ability to cough, decreased intercostal muscle tone, and abdominal distention. Supplemental oxygen should always be administered and careful pulmonary evaluation is mandatory.

Basic Airway Management

In order to prevent secondary injury, the cervical spine should be immobilized until complete evaluation has excluded injury. Properly applied rigid collars reduce flexion and extension to about 30% of normal, and rotation and lateral movement by about 50%.[78] Wide (3″) cloth tape should be applied to a hard backboard, across the forehead and chin to further reduce movement. The combination of rigid collar, backboard, and tape reduces cervical mobility to about 5% of normal.[79] More recently, the Styrofoam-filled vacuum mattresses have been used with the same purpose, but perhaps are more conveniently applied. The airway should first be cleared of blood, secretions, and debris. Airway control can be achieved by simple maneuvers such as chin lift or jaw thrust. Insertion of an oral or nasal airway may be needed to maintain patency until definitive control is obtained. Aprahamian and colleagues demonstrated that both manual maneuvers (jaw thrust and chin lift) caused a greater than 5 mm widening of the disk space in a fresh cadaver with C5-C6 instability.[68] This movement was not eliminated by rigid collars. Interestingly, insertion of oral and nasal airways caused minimal displacement. Despite this, no outcome data are available in patients. Commonly used intubation techniques caused less cervical movement than bag-mask ventilation in cadavers.[80] MIAS will help counteract the effects of these maneuvers.[81]

Advanced Airway Management

The most appropriate technique for performing endotracheal intubation remains controversial.[82–84] The ATLS program recommends either nasal intubation or orotracheal in the spontaneously breathing patient with a suspected CSI.[72] In the apneic patient, the ACS recommends orotracheal intubation with provision of MIAS. Oral intubation may be performed awake or with the aid of sedatives, induction agents, or general anesthesia. Oswalt et al. reported on 64 patients who received oral endotracheal intubation with MIAS, preoxygenation, and cricoid pressure during a rapid sequence induction.[85] They experienced no emergency department deaths attributable to an inability to intubate, and no patient required a surgical airway for failed intubation. In the absence of an experienced anesthesiologist, an emergency medicine physician with suitable training and experience may undertake the responsibility associated with securing a definitive airway when the situation demands.[86] In these circumstances, the responsibility for ensuring that emergency medicine physicians receive adequate didactic and manual skills training for advanced airway management, as well as ongoing quality improvement, rests with the anesthesiology department in a given facility.

Intubation Techniques

A true "standard of care" in the management of the patient with CSI does not currently exist. The airway maneuver selected should be one that will optimize the patient's prospects for a good outcome, minimize the possibility of serious complications, and be capably performed in a timely and efficient manner.[82] In the following section, pertinent issues surrounding various management options are discussed.

Direct Laryngoscopy

Direct laryngoscopy is the most rapid and surest method of tracheal intubation. Rhee et al. retrospectively reviewed 237 blunt trauma patients requiring endotracheal intubation in the emergency department over an 18-month period.[87] Twenty-one patients (8.9%) had cervical injury. Oral intubation with cervical immobilization was the definitive airway management modality in 213 (89.9%) patients. No patients suffered neurological deterioration following airway management in this series.

Wright and co-workers retrospectively reviewed the records of 987 blunt trauma victims requiring emergency intubation.[88] Of 60 patients with cervical spine fracture, 53 were potentially unstable. Twenty-six patients underwent orotracheal intubation, 25 underwent nasotracheal intubation, and two patients required cricothyroidotomy. One patient developed a new neurological deficit following nasotracheal intubation. The authors concluded that commonly used methods of precautionary airway management rarely lead to neurological deterioration.

Some of the most extensively reported experience with orotracheal intubation comes from The Shock Trauma Center in Baltimore, Maryland. They have successfully intubated more than 3,000 trauma patients with suspected CSI.[89] Ten percent of these patients were subsequently discovered to have CSI; however, none developed neurological compromise following intubation. The authors emphasize the importance of using a "modified" RSI by providing bag-mask ventilation with cricoid pressure during induction to maintain adequate oxygenation in seriously injured patients.

Awake Intubation

Concern over the ability to continue neurological evaluations following intubation has led some workers to advocate awake intubation. Meschino et al. reviewed 454 patients with critical cervical spine and/or cord injuries.[90] One group of patients required intubation and the control group did not require intubation. Patients requiring intubation during the hospitalization were intubated awake by either fiberoptic bronchoscope, blind nasal, or direct oral laryngoscopy. The details of the intubation are not available. A comparison of spinal neurological status revealed no statistical significance in neurological deterioration between the two groups. The authors, therefore, conclude that awake tracheal intubation is safe.

Nasotracheal Intubation

The use of nasotracheal intubation in the spontaneously breathing patient is recommended by the ACS COT in the ATLS course. Despite this recommendation, there is no evidence that this method is safer than orotracheal intubation with MIAS in patients with CSI.

Holley et al. retrospectively reviewed 113 patients with unstable injuries requiring operative fixation.[91] Nasal intubation was performed in 86 patients. There were no new neurological deficits noted. The authors felt that nasotracheal intubation in the operating room was safe but they cautioned against extrapolating their findings to the acute situation in the emergency department.

Nasotracheal intubation has additional associated problems. It should not be used in patients with basilar skull fractures because of the risk of intracranial instrumentation. The blind technique has a variable success rate and frequently causes epistaxis. Blind nasal intubation requires patient cooperation and is therefore inappropriate for combative patients. Also, blind techniques should be avoided in cases of concomitant maxillofacial trauma with soft tissue lacerations of the nasopharynx and hypopharynx. This may lead to creation of false tissue passages, the first evidence of which may be subcutaneous emphysema, oxygen desaturation, etc.

The Bullard Laryngoscope

The Bullard laryngoscope incorporates fiberoptic technology in a rigid anatomically shaped blade. By design, it promotes intubation in the neutral position and has been used successfully in patients with potential CSIs.[92] The development of a dedicated intubating stylet that attaches directly to the laryngoscope has improved its ease of use and virtually eliminated the need for the previously utilized intubating forceps.[93] Hastings et al. evaluated cervical spine movement during laryngoscopy with the Bullard, Macintosh, and Miller laryngoscopes.[94] They found that the Bullard laryngoscope caused less head extension and cervical spine extension and resulted in better visualization. Set-up time is minimal; supporting its use in acute situations. Multiple trauma patients with suspected CSI may be ideal candidates for Bullard intubation.

Failed Intubation Alternatives

The American Society of Anesthesiologists Task Force on Management of the Difficult Airway suggests several potential options for managing failed intubations.[95] The recommendation is that practitioners become familiar with as many alternative methods as possible to ensure optimal outcome. Three of the more commonly used modalities will be discussed.

Laryngeal Mask Airway (LMA)

There are case reports on the use of the LMA in patients with CSI.[96,97] Logan reports on the use of the LMA in a patient with an unstable CSI during anesthesia.[97] The LMA has been used in other cases where tracheal intubation has proved impossible.[98] An additional benefit is that endotracheal intubation can proceed through a properly placed LMA blindly or with flexible fiberoptic guidance. Its ease of use is likely to entice further investigation in cervical spine pathology.

The issue of potential lack of protection against pulmonary soilage by the LMA in these "full stomach" patients remains an unresolved issue.[99] However, the current common thinking seems to be that the risk of complications caused by pulmonary aspiration are minimal compared to similar considerations given to the issue of cerebral hypoxia and hypercarbia.

In addition, this device is currently undergoing evaluation for emergency usage to secure the airway by non-anesthesiologists in the field by paramedical personnel as well as in the hospital by ACLS teams.[100]

Combitube

The tracheo-esophageal combitube is a double lumen tube that is inserted blindly into the patient's esophagus or trachea. Two cuffs are present: a proximal pharyngeal cuff and a distal tracheal/esophageal cuff. A patient may be ventilated adequately when inserted into the trachea or the esophagus as long as a definite position has been confirmed by the presence of breath sounds and/or capnography.[101,102]

Two issues become important after placement of this device. First is the conversion to one of the more conventional methods of securing the airway (i.e., endotracheal intubation or tracheostomy).

The second issue is the risk of vomiting/regurgitation upon removal of the device, despite suctioning the stomach via the gastric port.

A recent report revealed a case of successful airway management in a patient with neck impalement.[103] The authors describe the inability to perform conventional laryngoscopy because of a partially blocked pharynx. The patient experienced a respiratory arrest necessitating emergency intervention. The trachea was successfully intubated with the combitube.

Cricothyroidotomy

Cricothyroidotomy may be either full-scale surgical access to the cricothyroid membrane or percutaneous needle access with connection to a high-pressure (50 p.s.i.) oxygen delivery source. Salvino and colleagues recently reported their review of 30 emergency cricothyroidotomies among 8,320 trauma admissions.[104] Seven were performed as the primary airway maneuver, while 23 were performed after attempts at oral intubation failed. No major complications were reported. Minor complications consisted of minimal subglottic stenosis, local wound infection, and nonthreatening hemorrhage. Fifteen patients were long-term survivors. The use of cricothyroidotomy is safe and effective when performed by experienced personnel if endotracheal intubation fails or is contraindicated. This is a technique with which every anesthetist, working regularly with emergency trauma patients, should be familiar and facile.

Summary

Airway management in patients with neurological injuries presents a significant challenge to even the most experienced anesthesiologist. A thorough understanding of the pathophysiology, potential associated injuries, intracranial dynamics, and currently available pharmacology helps facilitate successful management. Early involvement by trained trauma anesthesiologists, as part of the trauma team, helps expedite delivery of care to the injured patient.

References

1. Miller JD, Becker DP, Ward JD, et al: Significance of intracranial hypertension in severe head injury. J Neurosurg 47:503–516, 1977.
2. Marshall LF, Smith RW, Shapiro HM: The outcome with aggressive treatment in severe head injuries. J Neurosurg 50:26–30, 1979.
3. Eisenberg HM, Frankowski RF, Constant CF, et al: High dose barbitu-

rate control of elevated intracranial pressure in patients with severe head injury. J Neurosurg 69:15–23, 1988.

4. Schwartz ML, Tator CH, Rowed DW, et al: The University of Toronto Head Injury Treatment Study: A prospective, randomized comparison of pentobarbital and mannitol. Can J Neurol Sci 11:434–440, 1984.

5. Ward JD, Becker DP, Miller JD, et al: Failure of prophylactic barbiturate coma in the treatment of severe head injury. J Neurosurg 62: 383–388, 1985.

6. Young WL, McCormack PC: Perioperative management of intracranial catastrophes. Crit Care Clin 5:821–844, 1989.

7. Shapiro HM, Galindo A, Wyte SR, et al: Rapid intraoperative reduction of intracranial pressure with thiopentone. Br J Anaesth 45:1057–1062, 1973.

8. Moss E, Powell D, Gibson RM, et al: Effects of tracheal intubation on intracranial pressure following induction of anesthesia with Thiopentone or Althesia in patients undergoing neurosurgery. Br J Anaesth 50:353–360, 1978.

9. Miller JD, Dearden NM, Piper IR, et al: Control of intracranial pressure in patients with severe head injury. J Neurotrauma 9:317–325, 1992.

10. Gooding JM, Corsen G: Etomidate: an ultrashort acting nonbarbiturate agent for anesthesia induction. Anesth Analg 55:286–289, 1976.

11. Milde LN, Milde JH, Michenfelder JD: Cerebral function, metabolic, and hemodynamic effects of etomidate in dogs. Anesthesiology 63: 371–377, 1985.

12. Dearden NM, McDowall DG: Comparison of etomidate and althesin in the reduction of increased pressure after head injury. Br J Anaesth 57:361–368, 1985.

13. Prior JGL, Hinds CJ, Williams J, et al: The use of etomidate in the management of severe head injury. Intensive Care Med 9:313–320, 1983.

14. Bingham RM, Procaccio F, Prior PF, et al: Cerebral electrical activity influences the effect of etomidate on cerebral perfusion pressure in traumatic coma. Br J Anaesth 57:843–848, 1985.

15. Sakabe T, Nakakimura K: Effects of anesthetic agents and other drugs on cerebral blood flow, metabolism, and intracranial pressure. In: Cotrell JE, Smith DS (eds): Anesthesia and Neurosurgery. Mosby, St. Louis, 1994, p 158.

16. Modica PA, Tempelhoff R: Intracranial pressure during induction of anesthesia and tracheal intubation with etomidate-induced EEG burst suppression. Can J Anaesth 39(3):236–241, 1992.

17. Ebrahim ZY, et al: Effects of etomidate on the electroencephalogram of patients with epilepsy. Anesth Analg 65:1004–1006, 1986.

18. Wagner RL, White PF: Etomidate inhibits adrenocortical function in surgical patients. Anesthesiology 61:647–651, 1984.

19. Sebel PS, Lowdon JD: Propofol: a new intravenous anesthetic. Anesthesiology 71:260–277, 1989.

20. Stephan H, Sonntag H, Schenk HD, et al: Effect of propofol on cerebral

metabolism and on the response of the cerebral circulation to CO_2. Anaesthetist 36:60–65, 1987.

21. Herregods L, Verbeke J, Rolly G, et al: Effect of propofol on elevated intra-cranial pressure: Preliminary results. Anaesthesia 43:107–109, 1988.

22. Pinaud M, Jean-Noel L, Chetanneau A, et al: Effects of propofol on cerebral hemodynamics and metabolism in patients with brain trauma. Anesthesiology 73:404–409, 1990.

23. Heath KJ, Samara GS, Davis GE, et al: Blood pressure changes in head-injury patients during pre-hospital anaesthesia with propofol. Injury 25(Suppl 2):S-B7-8, 1994.

24. Takeshita H, Okuda Y, Sari A: The effects of ketamine on cerebral circulation and metabolism in man. Anesthesiology 37:605–612, 1972.

25. Artru AA, Katz RA: Cerebral blood volume and CSF pressure following administration of ketamine in dogs: modification by pre- or post-treatment with hypocapnia or diazepam. Anesthesiol 1:46–55, 1989.

26. Sari A, Okuda, Takeshita H: The effect of ketamine on cerebrospinal fluid pressure. Anesth Analg 51:560–565, 1972.

27. Wyte SR, Shapiro HM, Turner P, et al: Ketamine-induced intracranial hypertension. Anesthesiology 36:174–176, 1972.

28. Belapavovic M, Buchthal A: Modification of ketamine induced intracranial hypertension in neurosurgical patients by pretreatment with midazolam. Acta Anaesth Scand 26:458–462, 1982.

29. Martin D, Rosenberg H, Aukburg S, et al: Low-dose fentanyl blunts circulatory responses to tracheal intubation. Anesth Analg 61:680–684, 1982.

30. Ebert J, Pearson J, Gelman S, et al: Circulatory responses to laryngoscopy: the comparative effects of placebo, fentanyl and esmolol. Can J Anaesth 36:301–306, 1989.

31. Smith J, King M, Yanny H, et al: Effect of fentanyl on the circulatory responses to orotracheal fiberoptic intubation. Anaesthesia 47:20–23, 1992.

32. Cuillerier D, Manninen P, Gelb A: Alfentanil, sufentanil, fentanyl: effect on cerebral perfusion pressure. Anesth Analg 70:S1–S450, 1990.

33. Sperry R, Bailey P, Reichman M, et al: Fentanyl and sufentanil increase intracranial pressure in head trauma patients. Anesthesiology 77:416–420, 1992.

34. Milde LN, Milde JH, Gallagher WJ: Effects of sufentanil on cerebral circulation and metabolism in dogs. Anesth Anal 70:138–146, 1990.

35. Carlsson C, Smith DS, Keykhah MM, et al: The effects of high dose fentanyl on cerebral circulation and metabolism in rats. Anesthesiology 57:375–380, 1982.

36. Michenfelder JD, Theye RA: Effects of fentanyl, droperidol, and innovar on canine cerebral metabolism and blood flow. Br J Anaesth 43:630–636, 1971.

37. Sheehan P, Zorman M, Scheller M, Peterson B: The effects of fentanyl and sufentanil on intracranial pressure and cerebral blood flow in rabbits with an acute cryogenic brain injury. J Neurosurg Anesth 4:261–267, 1992.

38. Minton MD, Grosslight K, Stirt JA, et al: Increases in intracranial pressure from succinylcholine: prevention by prior nondepolarizing blockade. Anesthesiology 65:165–169, 1986.
39. Crosby G, Todd MM: On neuroanesthesia, intracranial pressure, and a dead horse. J Neurosurg Anesthesiol 2:143–145, 1990.
40. Kovanik WD, Lam AM, Slee TA, Mathisen TL: The effect of succinylcholine on intracranial pressure, cerebral blood flow velocity and electroencephalogram in patients with neurologic disorders. J Neurosurg Anesthesiol 3:A245, 1991.
41. Rosa G, Sanfilippo M, Vilardi V, Orfei P, Gasparetto A: Effects of vecuronium bromide on intracranial pressure and cerebral perfusion pressure. Br J Anaesth 58:437–440, 1986.
42. Ginsberg B, Glass PS, Quill T, et al: Onset and duration of neuromuscular blockade following high-dose vecuronium administration. Anesthesiology 71:201–205, 1989.
43. Magorian T, Flanery KB, Miller RD: Comparison of rocuronium, succinylcholine, and vecuronium for rapid sequence induction of anesthesia in adult patients. Anesthesiology 79:913, 1993.
44. MaeKawa T, Sakabe T, Takeshita H: Diazepam blocks cerebral metabolic and circulatory responses to local anaesthetic induced seizures. Anesthesiology 41:389–391, 1974.
45. Sari A, Fukuda Y, et al: Effects of psychotropic drugs on canine cerebral metabolism and circulation related to EEG-diazepam, clomipramine, and chlorpromazine. J Neurol Neurosurg Psychiatry 38:838–844, 1975.
46. Nugent M, Artru A, Michenfelder J: Cerebral metabolic, vascular and protective effects of midazolam maleate. Anesthesiology 56:172–176, 1982.
47. Hoffman W, Miletich D, Albrecht R: The effects of midazolam on cerebral blood flow and oxygen consumption and its interaction with nitrous oxide. Anesth Analg 65:729–733, 1986.
48. Giffin JP, Cotrell JE, Shwiry B, et al: Intracranial pressure, mean arterial pressure, and heart rate following midazolam or thiopental in humans with brain tumors. Anesthesiology 60:491–494, 1984.
49. Helfman S, Gold M, DeLisser E, Herrington C: Which drug prevents tachycardia and hypertension associated with tracheal intubation: lidocaine, fentanyl, or esmolol? Anesth Analg 72:482–486, 1991.
50. Bernstein JS, Ebert TJ, Stowe, DF, et al: Partial attenuation of hemodynamic responses to rapid sequence induction and intubation with labetalol. J Clin Anaesth 1:444–451, 1989.
51. Chraemmer-Jorgensen B, Houilund-Carlsen PF, Marving J, et al: Lack of effect of intravenous lidocaine on hemodynamic responses to rapid sequence induction of general anesthesia: a double blind controlled clinical trial. Anesth Analg 65:1037, 1986.
52. Nagao S, Murota T, Momma F, et al: The effect of intravenous lidocaine on experimental brain edema and neural activities. J Trauma 12:1650–1655.
53. Yukioka H, Yoshimoto N, Nishimura K, Fujimori M: Intravenous lido-

caine as a suppressant of coughing during tracheal intubation. Anesth Analg 64:1189–1192, 1985.

54. American College of Surgeons Committee on Trauma: Advanced Life Support Course for Physicians. American College of Surgeons, Chicago, 1993.

55. Gildenberg PL, Makela ME: The effect of intubation and ventilation on outcome following head trauma. In Symposium of Neural Trauma, Raven Press, New York, 1982.

56. Frost EAM, Arancibia CU, Shulman K: Pulmonary shunt as a prognostic indicator in head injury. J Neurosurg 50:768–772, 1979.

57. Pfenninger E, et al: Blood gases at the scene of the accident and on admission to hospital following cranio-cerebral trauma. Anaesthetist 36:570, 1987.

58. Eisenberg HM, et al: The effects of 3 potentially preventable complications on outcome after severe closed head injury ICPV. Springer-Verlag, Tokyo, 1983.

59. Rotondo MF, McGonigal MD, Schwab CW: Urgent paralysis and intubation of trauma patients: Is it safe? J Trauma 34:242–246, 1993.

60. Redan JA, Livingston DH, Tortella BJ, et al: The value of intubating and paralyzing patients with suspected head injury in the emergency department. J Trauma 31:371, 1991.

61. Koller SR, Abrams KJ, Randazzo AP: Safety of trauma intubation in the emergency department. Anesthesiology 83:A264, 1995.

62. Nakayama DK, Waggoner T, Venkataraman ST, et al: The use of drugs in emergency airway management in pediatric trauma. Ann Surg 216(2):205, 1992.

63. Frost EAM, Neurologic trauma. In Grande CM (ed): Textbook of Trauma Anesthesia and Critical Care. Mosby, St. Louis, 1993.

64. Grande CM, Barton CR, Stene JK: Appropriate techniques for airway management of emergency patients with suspected spinal cord injury. Anesth Analg 67:714–715, 1988.

65. Iwatsuki N, Kuroda N, Amaha K, et al: Succinylcholine induced hyperkalemia in patients with ruptured cerebral aneurysms. Anesthesiology 53:64–67, 1980.

66. Njoku DB, Lenox WC: Use care when injecting rocuronium and thiopental for rapid sequence induction and tracheal intubation. Anesthesiology 83:222, 1995.

67. Molbegott L: The precipitation of rocuronium in a needleless intravenous injection adapter. Anesthesiology 83:223, 1995.

68. Aprahamian C, Thompson B, Finger W, Darin J: Experimental cervical spine injury model: examination of airway management and splinting techniques. Ann Emerg Med 13:584–587, 1984.

69. Woodring JH, Lee C: Limitation of cervical radiography in the evaluation of acute cervical trauma. J Trauma 34:32–39, 1993.

70. Reid DC, Henderson R, Saboe L, Miller JDR: Etiology and clinical course of missed spine fractures. J Trauma 27:980, 1987.

71. Hastings RH, Kelley SD: Neurologic deterioration associated with airway management in a cervical spine injured patient. Anesthesiology 78:580–583, 1993.

72. American College of Surgeons Committee on Trauma: Advanced Trauma Life Support Course for Physicians. American College of Surgeons, Chicago, 1993.
73. Kirshenbaum KJ, Nadimpalli SR, Fantus R, Cavallino RP: Unsuspected upper cervical spine fractures associated with significant head trauma: role of CT. J Emerg Med 8:183–198, 1990.
74. Ross SE, O'Malley KF, DeLong WG, Born CT, Schwab CW: Clinical predictors of unstable cervical spine injury in multiply injured patients. Injury 23:317–319, 1992.
75. Hills MW, Deane SA: Head injury and facial injury: Is there an increased risk of cervical spine injury? J Trauma 34:549–554, 1993.
76. Guthkelch AN, Fleischer A: Patterns of cervical spine injury and their associated lesions. West J Med 147:428–431, 1987.
77. Hoffman JR, Schringer DL, Mower W, Luo JS, Zucker M: Low risk criteria for cervical spine radiography in blunt trauma: a prospective study. Ann Emerg Med 21:1454–1460, 1992.
78. Gajraj NM, Pennant JH, Giesecke AH: Cervical spine trauma and airway management. Curr Opin Anesth 6:369–374, 1993.
79. Podolsky S, Baraff L, Simon R: Efficacy of cervical spine immobilization methods. J Trauma 23:461–465, 1983.
80. Hauswald M, Sklar DP, Tandberg D, Garcia J: Cervical spine movement during airway management: cinefluoroscopic appraisal in human cadavers. Am J Emerg Med 9:535–538, 1992.
81. Majernick TG, Bieniek R, Houston JB, Hughes HG: Cervical spine movement during orotracheal intubation. Ann Emerg Med 15:417–420, 1986.
82. Walls RM: Airway management in the blunt trauma patient: How important is the cervical spine? Can J Surg 35:27–30, 1992.
83. Hastings RH, Marks JD: Airway management for trauma patients with potential cervical spine injuries. Anesth Analg 73:471–482, 1991.
84. Wood PR, Lawler PGP: Managing the airway in cervical spine injury: a review of the advanced trauma life support protocol. Anaesthesia 47:792–797, 1992.
85. Oswalt JL, Hedges JR, Soifer BE, Lowe DK: Analysis of trauma intubations. Am J Emerg Med 10:511–514, 1992.
86. McBrien ME, Pollok AJ, Steedman DJ: Advanced airway control in trauma resuscitation. Arch Emerg Med 9:177–180, 1992.
87. Rhee KJ, Green W, Holcroft JW, Mangli JAA: Oral intubation in the multiply injured patient: the risk of exacerbating spinal cord damage. Ann Emerg Med 19:511–514, 1990.
88. Wright SW, Robinson GG, Wright MB: Cervical spine injuries in blunt trauma patients requiring emergent endotracheal intubation. Am J Emerg Med 10:104–109, 1992.
89. Grande CM, Barton CR, Stene JK: Appropriate techniques for airway management of emergency patients with suspected spinal cord injury. Anesth Analg 67:714–715, 1988.
90. Meschino A, Devitt JH, Koch JP, Szalai JP, Schwartz ML: The safety of awake tracheal intubation in cervical spine injury. Can J Anaesth 39:114–117, 1992.

91. Holley J, Jorden R: Airway management in patients with unstable cervical spine fractures. Ann Emerg Med 18:1237–1239, 1989.
92. Abrams KJ, Desai N, Katsnelson T: Bullard laryngoscopy for trauma airway management in suspected cervical spine injuries. Anesth Analg 74:623, 1992.
93. Cooper SD, Benumof JL. Evaluation of the Bullard laryngoscope using the new intubating stylet: comparison with conventional laryngoscopy. Anesth Analg 79:965–970, 1994.
94. Hastings RH, Vigil AC, Hanna R, et al: Cervical spine movement during laryngoscopy with the Bullard, Macintosh, and Miller laryngoscopes. Anesthesiology 82:859–869, 1995.
95. American Society of Anesthesiologists Task Force on Management of the Difficult Airway: Practice guidelines for management of the difficult airway. Anesthesiology 78:597–602, 1993.
96. Calder I, Ordman AJ, Jackowski A, Crockared HA: The brain laryngeal mask airway: an alternative to emergency tracheal intubation. Anaesthesia 45:137–139, 1990.
97. Logan A, St C: Use of the laryngeal mask in a patient with an unstable fracture of the cervical spine. Anaesthesia 46:987, 1991.
98. Pennant JH, Pace NA, Gajraj NM: Use of the laryngeal mask airway in the immobilized cervical spine. Anesthesiology 77:A1063, 1992.
99. Brimacombe J, Berry A: The laryngeal mask airway as an aid to intubation in patients at risk of aspiration? Anesthesiology 78:1197–1198, 1993.
100. Shearer V, Giesecke AH, Pennant J: Personal communication. Parkland Hospital, November, 1993.
101. Frass M, Rodler S, Frenzer R, et al: Esophageal tracheal combitube, endotracheal airway, and mask: comparison of ventilatory pressure curves. J Trauma 29(11):1476–1479, 1989.
102. Frass M, Johnson JC, Atherton GL, et al: Esophageal tracheal combitube (ETC) for emergency intubation: anatomical evaluation of ETC placement by radiography. Resuscitation 18:95–102, 1989.
103. Eichinger S, Schreiber W, Heinz T, Kier P, Dufek V, Goldin M, Leithner C, Frass M: Airway management in a case of neck impalement: use of the esophageal tracheal combitube airway. Br J Anaesthesia 68:534–535, 1992.
104. Salvino CK, Dries D, Garnelli R, Murphy-Macabobby M, Marshall W: Emergency cricothyroidotomy in trauma victims. 34:503–505, 1993.

91. Holley J, Jorden R: Airway management in patients with unstable cervical spine fractures. Ann Emerg Med 18:1237–1239, 1989.

92. Abrams KJ, Desai N, Katsnelson T: Bullard laryngoscopy for trauma airway management in suspected cervical spine injuries. Anesth Analg 74:623, 1992.

93. Cooper SD, Benumof JL. Evaluation of the Bullard laryngoscope using the new intubating stylet: comparison with conventional laryngoscopy. Anesth Analg 79:965–970, 1994.

94. Hastings RH, Vigil AC, Hanna R, et al: Cervical spine movement during laryngoscopy with the Bullard, Macintosh, and Miller laryngoscopes. Anesthesiology 82:859–869, 1995.

95. American Society of Anesthesiologists Task Force on Management of the Difficult Airway: Practice guidelines for management of the difficult airway. Anesthesiology 78:597–602, 1993.

96. Calder I, Ordman AJ, Jackowski A, Crockared HA: The brain laryngeal mask airway: an alternative to emergency tracheal intubation. Anaesthesia 45:137–139, 1990.

97. Logan A, St C: Use of the laryngeal mask in a patient with an unstable fracture of the cervical spine. Anaesthesia 46:987, 1991.

98. Pennant JH, Pace NA, Gajraj NM: Use of the laryngeal mask airway in the immobilized cervical spine. Anesthesiology 77:A1063, 1992.

99. Brimacombe J, Berry A: The laryngeal mask airway as an aid to intubation in patients at risk of aspiration? Anesthesiology 78:1197–1198, 1993.

100. Shearer V, Giesecke AH, Pennant J: Personal communication. Parkland Hospital, November, 1993.

101. Frass M, Rodler S, Frenzer R, et al: Esophageal tracheal combitube, endotracheal airway, and mask: comparison of ventilatory pressure curves. J Trauma 29(11):1476–1479, 1989.

102. Frass M, Johnson JC, Atherton GL, et al: Esophageal tracheal combitube (ETC) for emergency intubation: anatomical evaluation of ETC placement by radiography. Resuscitation 18:95–102, 1989.

103. Eichinger S, Schreiber W, Heinz T, Kier P, Dufek V, Goldin M, Leithner C, Frass M: Airway management in a case of neck impalement: use of the esophageal tracheal combitube airway. Br J Anaesthesia 68: 534–535, 1992.

104. Salvino CK, Dries D, Garnelli R, Murphy-Macabobby M, Marshall W: Emergency cricothyroidotomy in trauma victims. 34:503–505, 1993.

6

Neuronal Cell Pathophysiology and Modalities of Brain Protection

Ronald A. Kahn, MD, Neal Bodner, MD

Introduction

Before discussing possible modalities of brain protection after neurotrauma, it is important to review the pathogenesis of cerebral injury. A brief summary of the pathogenesis of cerebral ischemia is presented, followed by its application to head trauma. Various pharmacological agents are discussed, including clinically available agents and experimental agents.

Overview of Ischemic Neuronal Damage: Cellular Biology

The pathogenesis of neuronal injury after cerebral insult can be divided into several stages: neuronal adenosine triphosphate (ATP)

From *Trauma Anesthesia and Critical Care of Neurological Injury,* edited by K. J. Abrams and C. M. Grande. © 1997, Futura Publishing Co., Armonk, NY.

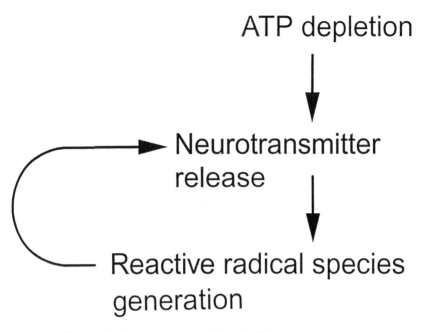

Figure 1. Neuronal insult. Cascade of neuronal injury.

depletion, release of excitatory neurotransmitters, and reperfusion injury (Fig. 1). The first step in the pathogenesis of neuronal injury is energy failure: the inability of cerebral blood flow (CBF) to adequately maintain cerebral metabolic rate (CMR). At some point during this initial insult there is massive release of excitatory neurotransmitters. This energy failure and neurotransmitter release may result in the accumulation of intraneuronal ions, particularly calcium, which may initiate a destructive cascade. During reperfusion, further damage may be produced by free radical production as well as post-ischemia hyper- and hypoperfusion.[1]

Neuronal elements require energy in the form of ATP for the maintenance of cellular integrity and neuronal signal transmission. Since there are only minimal intracerebral ATP stores, ischemia leads to exhaustion of energy reserve within a relatively brief period of time. Normally, CBF is 50 mL/100 gm brain tissue/min. If CBF is reduced to 15–18 mL/100 gm/min, there is failure of electrical transmission resulting in an isoelectric electroencephalogram (EEG) at normothermia. If CBF decreases below 10 mL/100 gm/min, ionic failure and subsequent irreversible neuronal damage are possible.[2]

Tissue ATP depletion occurs within 5–7 minutes after complete ischemia.[3] ATP depletion results in disruption of neuronal membrane integrity, which initially causes ionic leakage with resultant intracellular accumulation of water, calcium, and sodium, and local extracellular accumulation of potassium.[4] The intracellular accumulation of water results in neuronal cell edema, which subsequently depolarizes the cell membrane, leading to additional calcium influx. Local accumulation of potassium results in astrocyte swelling, increasing the distance necessary for oxygen diffusion.[5] Hyperkalemia increases the local CMR for oxygen and glucose.[6] The hyperkalemia-induced increase in CMR in the face of decreased oxygen availability as well as its effect on extraneuronal swelling may possibly enlarge the ischemic penumbra.[7,8]

Differences in neuronal pH are important in the final neuronal outcome. Pre-ischemic hyperglycemia may affect pH. In the presence of ischemia, increased anaerobic metabolism increases lactic acid levels and decreases in tissue pH. Plum suggested that "the level of carbohydrate in the brain is a major factor in determining whether an ischemic insult causes cerebral infarction. . . or results in a more restricted injury that is limited to ischemic neuronal damage."[9] If pre-infarction brain glucose levels are elevated or if glucose delivery continues during ischemia, lactate accumulates. If lactate accumulates above 16–20 mmoles per kilogram, there is a greater chance of astrocyte rupture and endothelial cell necrosis. Injury to these elements may produce edema and infarction of adjacent neurons. The lactate may also produce a greater ion influx through the cell membrane, lipolysis, proteolysis, membrane damage, and cell catabolism[10] (Fig. 2). If hyperglycemia is not present at the time of infarction, astrocytes and endothelial cells may be spared and hence damage may be limited.

Neurotransmitter Release

The Role of Excitatory Amino Acids

Neuronal energy depletion results in massive glutamate release. Neuronal injury by glutamate may occur by direct toxicity or receptor activation, e.g., n-methyl-d-aspartate (NMDA) receptor (see below).[11] Glutamate release excites adjacent neurons and extends the region where elevated levels of excitatory amino acids (EAA) are present extraneuronally. Reperfusion injury causes liberation of free radicals that may stimulate additional EAA release.[12]

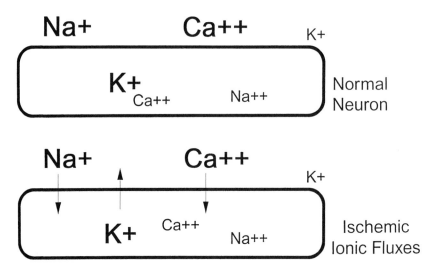

Figure 2. Ischemic ionic fluxes. Before depolarization, sodium and calcium concentrations are higher in the extracellular space compared to the intraneuronal compartment. The converse is true with potassium. With neuronal depolarization, both sodium and calcium enter intraneuronally with entry of potassium into the extracellular space.

The volume of ischemic damage and the amount of EAA released may be related. Butcher et al.[13] compared infarct volume versus EAA release after proximal versus distal middle cerebral artery ligation. They observed that proximal occlusion resulted in a larger infarct volume than distal occlusion. This increased injury was also associated with a greater release of aspartate and glutamate. Baker et al.[14] induced reversible global cerebral ischemia of varying duration in rats and examined the time course of dopamine, glutamate, and aspartate release. There was a progressive increase in glutamate and aspartate concentrations with increasing durations of ischemia. The levels of EAA release returned to pre-ischemic concentrations during reperfusion. Glycine levels also increased during ischemia, but did not return to baseline during reperfusion. The investigators speculated that EAA toxicity is an operant mechanism of cerebral ischemic injury. The rapid return to baseline concentrations implies that EAA do not contribute to the delayed injury but may initiate the cascade. Glycine may modulate the action of glutamate in vivo during and after ischemia.

There is considerable evidence that NMDA receptor activation is involved in the pathogenesis of neuronal injury (Fig. 3). NMDA receptor activation requires presynaptic release and binding of an excitatory neurotransmitter such as aspartate or glutamate, allosteric facilitation by glycine at a separate NMDA receptor site, and sufficient postsynaptic cell depolarization.[15] Activation of the NMDA receptor results in an increase in sodium and calcium conductance. If excessive NMDA receptor activation occurs in the presence of ischemia, the increased ionic conductance results in membrane depolarization and cell swelling. With membrane depolarization, voltage-sensitive calcium and sodium channels are activated, resulting in further ionic fluxes. The calcium influx results in toxic elevations of cytosolic-free calcium. Although the influx of sodium is immediate and its effects on neurons may be reversible, each of these two phenomena may result in irreversible neuronal injury.[16]

In addition to the NMDA receptor, significant ionic fluxes are mediated by the AMPA (α-amino-3-hydroxy-5-methyl-4-isoxazole propionate) receptor. This receptor is activated by glutamate and is classically thought to mediate sodium and potassium currents. Its activation may cause elevation in transmembrane voltages and possibly lead to activation of voltage-sensitive calcium channels. Recent evidence has suggested that the AMPA receptor may also be permeable to calcium, implying that receptor activation may play an important role during the pathogenesis of cerebral ischemia.[17]

The Role of γ-Aminobutyric Acid (GABA)

Increasing GABA activity may have neuroprotective effects. Electrophysiologically, GABA increases the influx of chloride ions into the neuronal cell, causing hyperpolarization of the cell membrane. This hyperpolarization increases the absolute resting membrane potential, and thus inhibits neuronal activation via the NMDA receptor.[11] Administration of γ-vinyl-GABA (GVG), a selective inhibitor of GABA transaminase, produces elevated CNS GABA levels.[18] The administration of GVG prior to bilateral cerebral ischemia decreases the degree of energy metabolism as evidenced by increased energy metabolites (i.e., glycogen, glucose, ATP, and phosphocreatine).[19] Muscimol, a GABA agonist, was able to confer a degree of cerebral protection after ischemic insult using a model of multifocal cerebral ischemia.[20] Other GABA-mimetic agents may also be useful as neuroprotective agents. In summary, GABA receptor activation

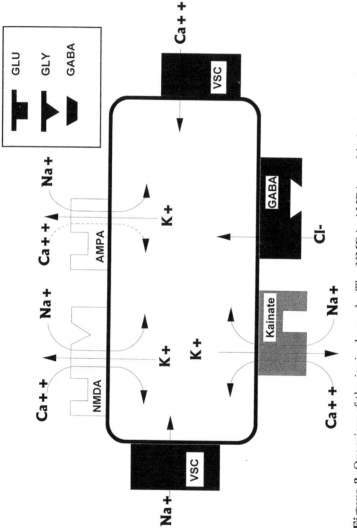

Figure 3. Overview of the ionic channels. The NMDA, AMPA, and kainate receptors are activated by either aspartate and glutamate. In addition, the NMDA receptor requires co-activation by glycine and sufficient post-synaptic depolarization. The neuronal membrane may be hyperpolarized by the activation of GABA receptors causing intraneuronal flow of chloride. In addition, voltage-sensitive channels (VSC) are present that may be opened by membrane depolarization. These channels control the flow of sodium and calcium ions.

increases chloride conductance. Exogenous GABA administration (either directly or indirectly) hyperpolarizes the neuronal membrane, making depolarization by EAA more difficult, thus possibly conferring some degree of neuroprotection.

It may be an oversimplification to attribute ischemic neuronal injury to release of a single neurotransmitter. Globus et al.[21] found that release of glutamate did not correlate with the degree of ischemic neuronal damage. Goskowicz et al.[22] reported that thiopental administration increased glutamate release from the cortex during global ischemia even though there was reduced post-ischemic neuronal injury. Globus et al.[23] examined ischemic insults of variable duration and examined regional CBF, histology, and neurotransmitter release. After a 10- and 20-minute insult, there was a varied degree of damage among neuronal structures. Differences in glutamate release and GABA release alone did not account for the variations in neuronal injury. They suggested that an excitatory index, [glutamate]·[glycine]/[GABA], could predict where injury would occur, presumably due to imbalances between excitation and inhibition causing differences in regional vulnerability.

The Role of Extraneuronal Dopamine

Dopamine (DA) is released in large quantities during anoxia, hypoglycemia, and ischemia.[24–27] In vitro and in vivo preparations demonstrated that high extracellular concentrations of DA are neurotoxic.[28] Extraneuronal DA release also uncouples blood flow and metabolism, which may be a potential mechanism for neuronal injury.[29] Breakdown products of DA may also be involved in neuronal injury. DA is metabolized to 3,4 dihydroxyphenylacetic acid (DOPAC) by monoamine oxidase (MAO) and subsequently to homovanillic acid (HVA) by catechol O-methyl transferase (COMT). During the conversion of DA to DOPAC, hydrogen peroxide, superoxide, and hydroxyl radicals are formed. These byproducts are potentially neurotoxic and may contribute to further neuronal injury during DOPAC production.[30]

Reduction of extraneuronal DA release may attenuate cerebral ischemic injury. Weinberger et al.[31] administered alpha-methyl-para-tyrosine, a tyrosine hydroxylase inhibitor, to gerbils to induce DA depletion. During unilateral irreversible forebrain ischemia, damage to the dopaminergic, serotonergic, and glutaminergic nerve terminals was substantially attenuated in the DA-depleted group compared with the control group. Furthermore, since adjacent non-catecholaminergic neurons were also spared, they hypothesized that the protective effects of decreased extraneuronal DA involved adjacent noncatecholaminergic neurons as well. In a series of experiments, Globus et al.[32,33] induced lesions in the substantia nigra to eliminate dopaminergic input to the corpus striatum in rats and then induced cerebral ischemia. The lesioned animals had an attenuation of ischemic neuronal damage in the striatum compared to the nonlesioned animals. They concluded that dopamine is important in the development of ischemic neuronal injury, and, furthermore, they speculated that dopamine may help modulate the postsynaptic cell depolarization that occurs with NMDA receptor activation.

Intracellular Calcium Accumulation: The Final Common Pathway

The influx of calcium into neurons is hypothesized to be the common final pathway of neuronal injury and destruction.[34] The calcium hypothesis of cell necrosis postulates that the intracellular entry of large amounts of calcium leads to a series of events and ultimately to cellular damage. This increase in calcium conductance can be due to activation of voltage-sensitive calcium channels (VSCC) or agonist-operated calcium channels (AOCC, e.g., the NMDA receptor).

ATP depletion also results in the inability to maintain intracellular homeostasis for calcium. This inability to maintain proper intracellular calcium concentrations may result in irreversible cellular injury.[35] Intracellular calcium can increase by several mechanisms: (1) increased membrane conductance to calcium secondary to membrane depolarization, (2) increased membrane conductance secondary to excitatory neurotransmitter release (see above), (3) release of calcium by mitochondria (stimulated by increased intracellular sodium and free fatty acids), and (4) release by sarcoplasmic reticulum. The increase in intracellular calcium may also activate lipases, proteases, and endonucleases, which further undermines cellular integrity as well as further initiates the prostaglandin cascade.[36] This enzymatic activation results in further insult to membrane integrity, which increases the ionic conductances, resulting in exacerbation of injury. Finally, intracellular accumulation of calcium leads to calmodulin activation, which increases the synthesis of nitric oxide. The enhanced production of nitric oxide probably further contributes to glutamate neurotoxicity.[37]

Reperfusion and Free Radical Formation

Cerebrovascular Instability

During reperfusion, two separate processes occur: abnormalities in the regulation of CBF and the production of destructive oxygen radicals. After restoration of CBF, there is often an early period of hyperemia followed by a later period of hypoperfusion.[38] The latter change is probably the result of an oxygen radical-mediated decrease in prostacyclin metabolism, effectively increasing thromboxane levels, causing vasoconstriction.[39] These changes in local CBF are accompanied by an initial decrease followed by an increase in the $CMRO_2$. These changes often result in a relative mismatching of CBF and $CMRO_2$, leading to relative hyperoxia followed by relative hypoxia.

Excessive Free Radical Formation

Normal cellular processes produce superoxide radicals and smaller amounts of hydrogen peroxide. In nonpathological conditions, these substances are quenched by endogenous chemical scavengers such as ascorbate, glutathione, or α-tocopherol. Alternatively, superoxide may be converted to hydrogen peroxide by superoxide dismutase with subsequent conversation of hydrogen peroxide to water by catalase/peroxidase. After cerebral ischemia, production of oxygen radicals increases. Several sources of this oxygen radical production exist. First, there is an accelerated rate of prostaglandin synthesis, which is fueled by the increased free fatty acids that were formed during the ischemic episode.[8] In the presence of even small amounts of oxygen (e.g., during incomplete ischemia), the prostaglandin cascade generates oxygen free radicals, which further intensifies cellular insult. Next, the increased intracellular calcium level that may be seen after ischemia catalyzes a reaction producing xanthine oxidase. This is significant because xanthine oxidase utilizes molecular oxygen to generate superoxide radicals.[40] It has been suggested, however, that the contribution of free radicals to neuronal injury is significant only during long periods of cerebral ischemia, when there is continued delivery of some oxygen to ischemic tissue or reoxygenation of oxygen-deprived areas.[41]

Free Radical Chain Reaction

Superoxide radicals do not normally react with macromolecules in the absence of a transitional metal catalyst.[42] In vivo this catalyst is iron. The intracellular acidosis that occurs after ischemia causes a delocalization of protein-bound iron (such as from hemoglobin, transferrin, or ferritin). After delocalization, iron may catalyze the conversion of hydrogen peroxide and superoxide radicals (poorly reactive radicals) into hydroxyl radicals (highly reactive).[43] In addition, iron catalyzes the production of a reactive lipid species. In particular, oxygen radicals interact with lipid a lipid-oxygen radical molecule. This molecule can be converted to a lipid alkoxyl radical in the presence of iron. This lipid alkoxyl radical may, in turn, initiate further lipid peroxidation.[44] The free radicals may initiate destructive chain reactions in tissues and cause further damage to lipids, proteins, and DNA.[45] Of these reactions, DNA destruction and lipid peroxidation (rearrangement of the double bonds in the side chain of unsaturated fatty acid side chains by an oxygen radical) is probably associated with the majority of neuronal damage.

The Role of Nitric Oxide (NO)

The role of nitric oxide in the mediation of neuronal damage after cerebral ischemic insult is unclear. NO has two different effects in cerebral ischemia: increased CBF and a direct cellular role in the evolution of neuronal injury.

Regulation of CBF by Nitric Oxide

The maintenance of vascular tone is mediated by a balance of vasoconstrictors such as endothelin-1 and vasodilators such as NO.[46] Nitric oxide increases intracellular cyclic GMP, thus causing vascular smooth muscle relaxation and hence vasodilatation.[47] After administration of a nitric oxide synthase (NOS) inhibitor, Prado et al. observed an increase in mean arterial pressure (MAP) and a decrease in cortical CBF compared to baseline measurements.[48] Induction of global cerebral ischemia using bilateral carotid artery occlusion further reduced cortical blood flow and increased MAP. The decrease in cortical blood flow during ischemia was greater in the NOS-inhibited animals compared to the control animals. After reperfusion, the NOS-inhibited treated animals exhibited a continued low CBF that was not different from that observed during the ischemic period and continued elevation in arterial blood pressure. The investigators concluded that cerebrosvascular resistance is increased by NOS inhibition, and NO may be an important mediator during pathological states. This modulation of CBF was also seen in models of focal cerebral ischemia.[49] After induction of focal cerebral ischemia, there was a significant reduction in CBF of the ischemic cortex in the NOS inhibitor treated group compared to the control group. In addition to modulation of CBF, NO is probably also important in the regulation of cerebral metabolic rate.

Modulation of Neurotransmitter Release by NO

Nitric oxide production and excitatory neurotransmitter release are probably interrelated. Using cell culture techniques, glutamate produced a dose-dependent effect on nitric oxide release.[50] In a separate study, Garthwaite et al. suggested that this release may be mediated by NMDA receptor activation.[51] In a cerebellar brain slice model, addition of NMDA resulted in a substantial rise in cGMP. This rise was inhibited by NOS inhibition and potentiated by l-arginine. NO release may be a direct result of glutamate-mediated intracellular hypercalcemia and the associated activation of calmodulin and NOS.[52]

Similarly, nitric oxide may increase glutamate and aspartate release. Lawrence et al. implanted microdialysis probes in rat medulla oblongata and measured glu and asp recovery.[53] They observed a significant increase in glutamate and aspartate after intracerebral administration of the NO donor S-nitroso-N-acetylpenicillamine (SNAP), which was blocked by methylene blue (guanylate cyclase inhibitor). They concluded that NO acts through cGMP to affect neurotransmitter release.

Buisson et al. examined a possible mechanism for the neuroprotective effects of a NO synthase inhibitor during focal cerebral ischemia.[54] They observed a decrease in NMDA-induced striatal injury after L-NAME pretreatment. Furthermore, L-NAME significantly attenuated glutamate release during both MCA occlusion and potassium-induced depolarization. They concluded that NO may be a major signal or second messenger in the pathogenesis of excitotoxic neuronal death. NO may cause increased neurotransmitter release, resulting in worsened damage.

In addition to modulation of excitatory neurotransmitter release, NO production may promote free radical formation.[55] NO may combine with superoxide to form hydroxyl radicals. Hydroxyl radicals have been implicated in lipid peroxidation and increased edema formation.[56] This reaction also results in peroxynitrite anions (ONOO) production.[57] Peroxynitrite may oxidize sulfhydryl groups and cause lipid peroxidation.[58]

In contrast, other investigators have suggested a mechanism for the neuroprotective effects of NO. Lei et al. suggest free sulfhydryl groups on the NMDA receptor complex form S-nitrosothiois in the presence of NO.[59] In an oxidizing environment, these thiol sites may react with one another producing disulfide bonds, resulting in a persistent block. Hence, NO may downregulate the NMDA receptors and thus reduce neurotoxicity.

Pathophysiology of Neuronal Injury after Trauma

There are four major mechanisms of injury after neurotrauma: loss of calcium homeostasis, free radical formation, massive neuronal depolarization, and mechanical causes. The loss of cellular calcium homeostasis and excessive free radical formation appear to have significant roles in the pathogenesis of traumatic neuronal injury. Acidosis probably plays a secondary role.[60] Trauma increases vascular intra-endothelial calcium concentration leading to microvascular damage. If direct calcium-mediated vascular damage does not occur, damage secondary to diffusion of free radical species through the extracellular space may take place.[61] Following traumatic injury, metabolism of arachidonate by cyclo-oxygenase is increased with concurrent production of oxygen radicals.[62] These free radicals result in loss of vascular autoregulation, enhanced blood-brain permeability, and early vasogenic edema.[60]

Vinc et al. studied the effect of moderate head trauma on high-energy molecules, pH, and magnesium.[63] They observed that there was no reduction in total adenylate energy charge or concentrations of ATP or phosphocreatine. A decrease in intracellular pH and intracellular free magnesium were observed. Although there was no change in the actual energy level, the driving force for many energy-requiring reactions (such as intracellular ionic homeostasis) was reduced. The reduction in energy driving force is not sufficient to cause substantial injury, however, neuronal elements become more sensitive to other aggravating factors.

Closed head trauma results in massive neuronal depolarization.[64] Neuronal depolarization leads to accumulation of extracellular potassium and intraneuronal calcium. This neuronal depolarization may also be potentiated by concomitant intraparenchymal hemorrhage. Release of excitatory amino acids has been documented after head injury.[65] Because of the decreased ability of the neuronal membrane to maintain ionic homeostasis (such as for calcium), even small amounts of excessive EAA release may cause substantial changes in intracellular calcium concentrations.

Mechanical processes may also play a role in neuronal injury. Axonal transection probably does not occur with initial injury.[66] Stretching and kinking of axons and microvesicles may be damaging. In particular, with physical membrane breakage or excessive stimulation in the milieu of partial energy failure, axonal permeability to calcium increases.[60] Povlishock suggested that focal intra-axonal changes in the axonal monofilament causes subsequent impaired axonal transport.[67] This effect on axonal transport may result in axonal swelling and disconnection.

Strategies of Pharmacological Methods of Brain Protection

Protection from neuronal insult may be approached from various avenues, corresponding to the stages of the pathogenesis of injury, including using methods to decrease the imbalance of CBF and CMR, reduction of the effective concentration of excitatory neurotransmitters (such as decreasing total release, blocking the receptor sites, increasing re-uptake), interference with calcium metabolism (calcium channel blockers), or interference with free radical biochemistry (e.g., free radical scavengers or peroxidation antagonists).

Hypothermia

Mechanisms of Protection

In a study of the biochemistry of hypothermia, Michenfelder measured $CMRO_2$ at 37°, 27°, 22°, 18°, and 14° C.[68] Continuous EEG monitoring revealed burst suppression at or below 22° C with some animals still exhibiting burst activity at 14° C. There was a decrease in $CMRO_2$ with decreasing temperatures, and a proportionally greater decrease at less that 27° C. Post-ischemic measurements of phosphocreatine, ATP, ADP, AMP, lactate, pyruvate, and glucose revealed a normal brain energy state. The increased metabolic depression at profound levels of hypothermia highlight the potential beneficial effect of this therapeutic maneuver in providing brain protection. The relationship between CBF and $CMRO_2$ has been confirmed by other investigators.[69,70]

Although it would be easy to attribute the beneficial effects of hypothermia strictly by its ability to lower $CMRO_2$ and brain energy demands, the actual mechanism is not entirely clear. Mild degrees of hypothermia confer substantial degrees of neuronal protection that cannot be explained on the basis of decreased $CMRO_2$ alone.[71] Several potential mechanisms exist. Mild to moderate degrees of hypothermia substantially decrease extraneuronal glutamate and dopamine release.[72] Other studies suggest that hypothermia may lower glycine concentration.[73] This decrease may in turn decrease the activation of NMDA receptors caused by ischemia-induced release of glutamate and aspartate, thus lessening the excitotoxic actions of these amino acids. Furthermore, brain hypothermia during ischemia reduces the post-ischemic inhibition of neuronal protein synthesis[74] and mildly prolongs the time before anoxic depolarization.[75]

Outcome Studies with Hypothermia

Hypothermia has been demonstrated to be protective in models of MCA occlusion.[76] Cooling to 24° C either before or within 15 minutes of arterial occlusion lessened the injury caused by the occlusion in comparison with normothermic animals. Rosomoff examined the effects of induced hypothermia before or after cerebral contusion.[77] Hypothermic animals (25° C) exhibited smaller areas of cerebral edema and hemorrhagic contusion and the inflammatory response was either minimal or absent after 36 hours. Although five of the seven hypothermic animals died, survival times were five times longer than that of normothermic animals. It was concluded that hypothermia limited the brain's deleterious response to trauma.

In another study, infarct size was measured in rats subjected to permanent MCA occlusion and ipsilateral carotid artery occlusion performed at 30°, 33°, 34.5°, and 36.5° C.[78] Twenty-four hours later, the rats were sacrificed and their brains analyzed histologically. The groups at temperatures below 34.5° C had significantly smaller infarct volumes compared to the group at 36.5° C. In another group, within the same study, MCA occlusion was performed at normothermia, and the rats were cooled to 33° C 1 hour later and kept at that temperature for 1 hour. This group also had significantly smaller infarct volumes. Thus, mild hypothermia between 30° and 34.5° significantly decreased brain injury caused by MCA and carotid occlusion, even when the institution of hypothermia was delayed for 1 hour. Similar results were obtained in other studies.[79-86]

Recent clinical observations have demonstrated a beneficial effect of hypothermia on patients who have sustained severe head injuries. Marion et al. randomized patients presenting with severe closed head trauma to induced hypothermia or normothermia.[87] The hypothermic group was cooled to a brain temperature of 32–33° C within a mean of 10 hours after presentation, maintained hypothermic for 24 hours, and then rewarmed over 12 hours. The hypothermic group had a significantly lower ICP over the first 24 hours. A trend toward improved outcome at 3 months was observed with hypothermia, but the differences between the groups did not reach statistical significance. In another study, Shiozaki et al. randomized 33 patients with persistent uncontrollable ICP to either mild hypothermia (34° C) or normothermia.[88] Mild hypothermia significantly decreased ICP and increased cerebral perfusion pressure. These physiological changes were accompanied by a decrease in CBF and $CMRO_2$. Uncontrolled ICP was the cause of death in 31% of the hypothermic group and in 71% of the control group ($P<0.05$). There was a statistically significant increased survival rate in the hypothermic group (50%) compared to the control group (18%).

Anesthetic Agents

The first step in the pathogenesis of neuronal injury is development of ischemia, broadly defined as the insufficiency of supply to adequately serve demand. Generally, anesthetic agents decrease overall CMR and hence forestall the development of a neurotoxic cascade. Realistically, this metabolic suppression would provide only a short window of protection. In a study of focal ischemia, rats were randomized to receive sevoflurane in burst-suppressive doses, halothane, or nothing during the ischemic episode.[89] Theoretically, the burst-suppressive dose of sevoflurane should have significantly decreased the CMR, thus conferring a significant degree of neuroprotection compared to halothane, and the awake animals should have the greatest degree of ischemic damage. The investigators observed, however, a trend toward the least amount of damage with halothane compared with sevoflurane (not statistically significant), and a statistically significantly greater damage in the awake animals. One conclusion of the study was that the decrease in CMR produced by a particular agent could not guarantee cerebral protection as classically described. They stated that the "absence of a difference in outcome between the two anesthetized groups is consistent with a large body of information that has failed to demonstrate that a reduction in the CMR is the primary mechanism by which volatile anesthetic agents might reduce focal ischemic brain damage."

Anesthetic agents such as barbiturates, etomidate, or isoflurane decrease neurotransmitter release during ischemia.[90-92] This strategy of attenuation of neuronal firing may provide an additional avenue for brain protection.

Barbiturates

Thiopental was extensively studied by Michenfelder. In one study,[93] dogs were divided into two groups: one group was subjected to acute hemorrhagic hypotension (27–28 mm Hg) and the other group was subjected to progressive hypoxemia (PaO_2 <5 mm Hg). Half of the animals in each group received thiopental after the physiological insult was administered, and the other half received no additional treatment. In the hypotension group, cerebral ATP concentrations decreased and cerebral lactate increased. After administration of thiopental, ATP levels were sustained higher, and lactate levels were lower compared to the untreated dogs. This difference remained significant for only 5 minutes; at 9 minutes these levels were similar in the thiopental-treated and untreated subgroups. In the hypoxemia group, cerebral ATP decreased and lactate increased in both the treated and the untreated groups. The only difference was the time to appearance of a hypoxia-induced flat EEG; there was a 35-second delay to the flat EEG in the thiopental subgroup compared to the untreated subgroup. Although thiopental has been previously shown to decrease $CMRO_2$ up to 40–50%,[94] significant cerebral protection was not evident from this study.

Functional and metabolic effects of thiopental were also studied by Michenfelder.[95] Dogs were given a progressively increasing infusion of thiopental during partial extracorporeal circulatory support. $CMRO_2$ decreased progressively with the infusion of thiopental until an isoelectric EEG was obtained, leveling off at 58% of control; continued administration of thiopental did not decrease $CMRO_2$ further,

CBF decreased by more than 50%, due both to an increase in cerebral vascular resistance (CVR) and a decrease in MAP. In the face of large but equal reductions in $CMRO_2$ and CBF, there were no changes in the tissue assays of ATP, lactate, and pyruvate when these results were compared to previously obtained values in lightly anesthetized dogs. The conclusion drawn from this and the previously mentioned study was that thiopental protects only brain in which function still exists (EEG activity is still present).

The use of barbituates combined with graded hypothermia (from 28–14° C) was studied by Steen et al.[96] After attainment of the target temperature, the animals were given a bolus of thiopental. The EEG became isoelectric at temperatures below 18° C. $CMRO_2$ was significantly lowered by thiopental only in dogs with EEG activity. The authors speculated that the protective effects of thiopental would be apparent only if given in the face of incomplete ischemia, since profound neuronal ischemia causes cessation of EEG activity.

Clinical studies of barbituate administration in the face of ischemia are not as promising. Nussemeier et al. randomized patients undergoing open-chamber cardiac surgery to perioperative barbituate or to no barbituate administration.[97] They reported a decrease in postoperative neuropsychological complications in the group receiving barbiturates. In a similar study, Zaidan et al. examined neurological outcome after coronary artery bypass grafting surgery in patients receiving thiopental or placebo.[98] This group of investigators did not find a significant difference between the two groups. In yet another study, patients presenting with severe head injury were randomized to pentobarbital or placebo administration.[99] There was no difference between the groups in the incidence of raised ICP or the duration or response of ICP elevation to treatment nor was there a difference in outcome between the two groups. In a study of comatose survivors of cardiac arrest, patients were randomized to thiopental loading.[100] No difference in outcome between the two groups was observed. Further ineffective therapy of barbiturates and hypothermia and its effect on outcome have been demonstrated in survivors of nearly drowned flaccid children.[101]

Etomidate

Etomidate is an imidazole-derivative, anesthetic drug with GABA-mimetic properties, and there is experimental evidence supporting its potential cerebral protectant effect.[102,103] Etomidate has been reported to decrease neurotransmitter release during ischemia.

Koorn et al.[104] examined the effect of etomidate treatment versus chloral hydrate during reversible global forebrain ischemia in the rat. They found a significant reduction in extraneuronal dopamine release from the rat corpus striatum in the etomidate group compared with the control group. Goskowicz et al. examined the effect of etomidate administration on glutamate release from the hippocampus during global ischemia.[22] Although they observed a trend toward decreased glutamate release after ischemia, the differences did not reach statistical significance. Watson reported significant differences in brain in areas supplied by the posterior circulation and watershed areas (i.e., areas of incomplete cerebral ischemia) after temporary forebrain ischemia following etomidate pretreatment.[105] Sano et al.[106] compared the cerebral protective effects of etomidate versus isoflurane during global cerebral damage. There was decreased injury to the ventral CA1 and dorsal CA3 of the hippocampus as well as the temporal-occipital cortex in the etomidate group compared with the control group. Other investigators have observed worsening of cerebral damage after etomidate administration.[107]

Propofol

Propofol has cerebral effects similar to barbiturates. In rabbits, it was shown to cause dose-related decreases in CBF and $CMRO_2$. The decline in EEG activity leading to burst suppression mirrored the decrease of $CMRO_2$.[106] These results were confirmed in other models.[109] With artificially raised ICP, propofol decreased ICP with an accompanying decrease in cerebral perfusion pressure (CPP). No difference in ICP was noted when CPP was returned to normal by use of phenylephrine, proving that the reduction in ICP was not merely from a decrease in blood pressure. This effect on ICP has also been shown in patients with head trauma.[110]

The results of studies examining the potential role of propofol as a neuroprotective agent are contradictory. Rosenberg et al.[111] examined electrophysiological recovery of rat hippocampal slices after anoxic injury. They observed a more rapid return of electrophysiological function in the slices containing propofol and suggested that propofol may protect CA1 pyramidal cells and dentate granule cells from anoxic injury. Kochs et al.[112] found improved neurological outcome and decreased neurological damage following unilateral carotid artery ligation in rats anesthetized with propofol. Ridenour et al.[113] examined reversible right middle cerebral artery ligation during propofol versus halothane anesthesia. They reported no significant decrease in cerebral infarct volume or severity of neurological outcome between the two groups. Comparing the results of these studies is problematic because the variations in experimental design resulted in different degrees of cerebral ischemia.

Isoflurane

Isoflurane has been investigated as an agent to produce cerebral protection. Increasing concentrations of isoflurane from 1.4–6% decreases $CMRO_2$ until the onset of isoelectric EEG at 3% end-expired concentration; further increases in concentration to 6% have no further effect on $CMRO_2$.[114] Rats spontaneously breathing 5% oxygen survived longer when exposed to 1.0% and 1.4% isoflurane than control unanesthetized animals. Those given 2% and 3% isoflurane had shorter survival times, presumably secondary to cardiorespiratory depression.[115] Ruta compared the effects of 1.2 MAC halothane and isoflurane in rats subjected to four hours of left MCA occlusion.[116] The results showed no statistical difference between the two anesthetics in the histological appearance of the brains after MCA occlusion. Similarly, Hoffman et al. found no difference in outcome after incomplete global forebrain ischemia between rats that were anesthetized with isoflurane or with halothane.[117]

Newman studied the cerebral effects of isoflurane-induced hypotension in humans undergoing craniotomy for clipping of cerebral aneurysms.[118] The mean arterial pressure (MAP) was reduced from 79 to 51 mm Hg with a mean inspired concentration of 2.3% isoflurane in 12 patients. CBF remained constant both during and after induced hypotension. The $CMRO_2$ was reduced 25% during hypotension. It was concluded that isoflurane favorably influenced the cerebral oxygen supply/demand balance and that global cerebral oxygenation is maintained during isoflurane-induced hypotension.

In humans, a difference was found in the effects of anesthetics on the critical CBF in patients undergoing carotid endarterectomy under isoflurane anesthesia (critical CBF was defined as that flow below which the majority of patients showed ipsilateral EEG changes indicative of ischemia within 3 minutes of carotid occlusion).[119] The critical CBF was found to be approximately 8–10 cc/100 g/min, which was much lower than a previously obtained value with halothane anesthesia (18–20 cc/100 g/min).[120] Since these data do not examine outcome, no conclusion can be drawn regarding the relative cerebral protective effects of the anesthetics.

Excitatory Amino Acid Antagonists

Theoretically, the increase in transmembrane calcium conductance that occurs during ischemia can be attenuated by blockade at the level of the NMDA receptor complex. This type of blockade can be accomplished with either competitive (e.g., AP7) or noncompetitive (e.g., MK-801) NMDA receptor antagonists. Although early reports of MK-801 treatment during severe global ischemia were promising, later experiments did not confirm a significant degree of neuronal protection.[121] In earlier experiments, animal temperature was not monitored or maintained; it is likely that the earlier cerebral protective effects of the NMDA antagonists were secondary to hypothermia during ischemia and reperfusion and not due to a drug effect per se.[122] Also used in the study were different degrees of cerebral ischemia. With a severe insult, no protection is conferred by NMDA antagonists.

In cases of incomplete global or focal cerebral ischemia, protection may be conferred with NMDA antagonists.[122,123] These differences may be explained by the inability of the NMDA receptor antagonists to prevent calcium influx by receptors other than the NMDA receptor (such as VCSS or AMPA).[122] Alternatively, the extracellular milieu may affect NMDA receptor function. Specifically, acidification reduces NMDA receptor-mediated calcium influx. The lower the pH, the greater the attenuation of this influx. In models of severe global ischemia, there is a greater area of decreased pH, so there are fewer functioning receptors that may be antagonized by NMDA antagonists. Conversely, during focal ischemia (or less severe global ischemia), there are penumbra that are ischemic but not as acidotic as the central ischemic core. Since the acidosis is less severe, more NMDA receptors are functional, so there is greater potential for NMDA receptor activation.[122] In summary, "NMDA antagonists will be cytoprotective in situations where some energy production prevails such as hypoglycemia, epilepsy, and focal ischemia but will prove to be ineffective in experimental paradigms where there is complete energy failure such as global ischemia."[123]

The use of AMPA receptor blockers may be more promising than the NMDA receptor blockers. In a study of both severe global and focal ischemia, AMPA antagonists have demonstrated cerebral protection in excess of that demonstrated by NMDA antagonists.[124,125] This protection was not associated with an increase in regional blood flow and could be demonstrated even after post-ischemic drug treatment.

The use of NMDA antagonists is associated with a myriad of side effects. Exact side effects vary with the class of antagonists.[40] The competitive antagonists may predispose patients to muscle weakness, ataxia, and sedation. Antagonists similar to MK 801 (i.e., noncompetitive antagonists) may induce excitement, anesthesia, respiratory depression, disorientation, or psychotic behavior. Other antagonists may have effects on learning and memory.

Calcium Channel Blockers

Evidence from animal experimentation and clinical trials suggests that calcium channel blockers may be useful in the attenuation of damage after ischemic stroke. The most promising drugs to date are the dihydropyridine calcium channel blockers (e.g., nimodipine, nicardipine, and nilvadipine).[126] These agents have selective and profound cerebral vasodilating effects. The most common side effects of the calcium channel receptor antagonists are cardiovascular.[127] Complications include hypotension, cardiac dysrhythmias, myocardial ischemia, and negative inotropic effects. The protective effect of nimodipine appears not to be effective if it is given after the ischemic insult. Nimodipine probably confers protection by cerebral vasodilatation and increase in CBF to the marginally perfused penumbra.[128] In addition, the drugs may also prevent the large intracellular and intramitochondrial calcium influx that is seen with reperfusion.[129] The benefits of calcium antagonists in models of cerebral ischemia are controversial. The calcium antagonists reduce intracellular calcium entry, thus preserving high-energy phosphates, preventing local acidosis, and attenuating cytoxic and vasogenic edema.[130]

Nimodipine has been shown to be effective in attenuating cerebral ischemic damage in animal models of focal and global ischemia.[128,130] Other experimental studies, however, did not support improved outcome after treatment with calcium antagonists during focal or global ischemia.[127]

In clinical trials, nimodipine has been used successfully in the treatment of subarachnoid hemorrhage.[131] Although there was no difference in the incidence or severity of angiographic vasospasm, there was a significant reduction in the rate of cerebral infarction in the group treated with nimodipine, and a significant improvement in neurological outcome at 3 months. The effect of nimodipine administration to patients presenting with acute ischemic stroke has been investigated in a double blind multicenter study.[132] Patients were randomized to receive either nimodipine 30 mg every 6 hours or placebo. Patients with cerebral ischemia secondary to other causes (e.g., hemorrhage or hematoma) or concomitant severe medical processes were excluded. During the 4-week treatment period, mortality was decreased in the nicardipine group compared to the control group. Survival was increased only in men. During the 6-month follow-up period, there were no differences in mortality between the two groups. Neurological outcome was better in the nimodipine group, and was more pronounced in patients with moderate to severe deficits at the time of admission.

In another study, comatose survivors of cardiac arrest were randomized to receive lidoflazine or placebo.[133] Five hundred and twenty patients were studied. There were no significant differences between the two groups with respect to 6-month survival, recovery of good cerebral function, or survival with severe neurological deficit. When patients were stratified according to depth of coma, the trend was toward improved outcome in patients with less severe neurological insult. The differences, however, did not reach statistical significance. The authors concluded that the administration of lidoflazine after cardiac arrest was not beneficial.

Nitric Oxide Synthase Manipulation

Several investigators have demonstrated a possible protective effect of NO during ischemia by potentiation of CBF, Sancesario et al. described worsening hippocampal neuronal damage after high-dose chronic NOS inhibition.[134] Yamamoto et al. and Kuluz et al. also report worsening of ischemic injury with L-NAME after focal cerebral ischemia.[135,136] Morikawa et al. published further evidence for the protective effect of NO.[137] After administration of l-arginine (a precursor of NO), they observed an increase in regional CBF after MCA occlusion which was associated with a reduction in infarct volume 24 hours after ischemia.

Multiple investigators have suggested a neuroprotective role for NOS inhibition. Trifiletti reported a neuroprotective effect of NOS inhibition after incomplete global ischemia with hypoxemia.[136] Ten days after ischemia, a significant degree of protection was found in the group receiving the NOS inhibitor. Further evidence for a neuroprotective effect of NOS inhibition has been suggested by other investigators.[139,140]

Differences between the outcome of these studies may be explained by the differential effects of NO. There is a beneficial effect of NO in increasing CBF. In models of ischemia where there is a greater ischemic penumbra, the cerebral vasodilation that is mediated by NO may supplement the critical CBF and decrease the degree of cerebral injury. In contrast, the increase in the CBF afforded by NO may not be significant in ischemic models with a smaller ischemic penumbra. The neurotoxic effects of NO may be mediated by neurotransmitter release, excitotoxicity, or free radical production.

Free Radical Scavengers and Lipid Antioxidants

Since lipid peroxidation plays a significant role in the pathogenesis of neuronal injury, compounds that possess lipid antioxidant properties may be useful in the management of neuronal injury (Fig. 4). The prototypical lipid antioxidant is methylprednisolone.

The beneficial effects of methylprednisolone are documented for patients with traumatic spinal cord injuries.[141] The demonstrated neuroprotective mechanisms of methylprednisolone include inhibition of lipid peroxidation, inhibition of lipid hydrolysis (arachidonic acid release) and eicosanoid formation, maintenance of tissue blood flow and aerobic energy metabolism, improved reversal of intracellular calcium accumulation, reduction of neurofilament degradation, and enhanced neuronal excitability and synaptic transmission.[142] Barks et al. examined the influence of dexamethasone in a neonatal rat model of cerebral hypoxia-ischemia.[143] Seven-day-old rats were subjected to incomplete global ischemia with hypoxia. Rats pretreated with dexamethasone in doses of 0.01 to 0.5 mg/kg/day over 3 days had no infarction. Treatment just before or after the ischemic insult or use of lower doses did not prevent infarction; however, a single dose of dexamethasone (0.1 mg/kg) given 24 hours prior to the insult did prevent cerebral infarction. Another study in the same rat model showed complete protection by a similar dose of dexamethasone 6 hours prior to hypoxia-ischemia.[144]

In a study using the same experimental model, the effects of methylprednisolone in brain protection neurons were examined. The treatment group received methylprednisolone 30 mg/kg 40 minutes prior to hypoxia. Controls received saline. After 42 hours, several rats were killed in each group and each control hemisphere was examined for water content. The water content of the 19 methylpred-

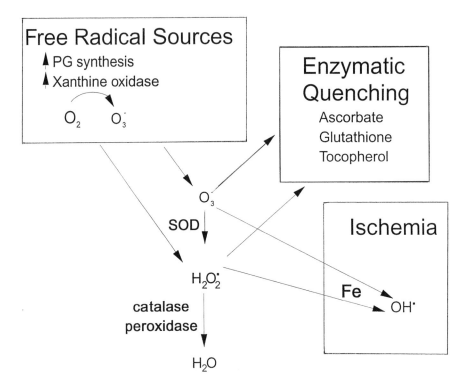

Figure 4. Overview of free radical formation. Free radicals are formed by normal neuronal metabolic processes. With ischemia, there is increased prostaglandin synthesis. This increase in prostaglandin synthesis produces additional free radicals. In addition, the increase in intracellular calcium concentrations will catalyze a reaction producing higher xanthine oxidase levels. Xanthine oxidase converts molecular oxygen into superoxide radical. After production of oxygen radicals, there may be conversion of these radicals into benign species by superoxide dismutase, catalase, and peroxidase. Alternatively, there may be enzymatic quenching of these radicals. After ischemia, there is increased production of these radicals as well as iron dislocation. Iron may catalyze the conversion of oxygen radicals into the very reactive hydroxyl radical.

nisolone-treated rats was significantly lower than was found in the 20 saline-treated rats. At 40 days post-ischemia, the remaining rats were killed and the brains were examined histopathologically. Hypoxic damage was greater in the saline-treated group compared to the methylprednisolone group. It was concluded that methylprednisolone reduces brain edema caused by hypoxic-ischemic insult in 7-day-old rats. The investigators theorized that this drug "stabilizes the membranes and protects them against the toxic effects of free oxygen radicals liberated during hypoxia ischemia."

Of interest is the nonglucocorticoid 21-aminosteroid, U74006F, which has been shown to decrease lipid peroxidation caused by free radicals, to scavenge lipid peroxyl radicals, and to block the release of arachidonic acid from cell membranes.[145] It has enhanced lipid peroxidation inhibitory activity compared to methylprednisolone, but lacks the glucocorticoid effects.[146] The compound inhibits iron-catalyzed lipid peroxidase.[147] In addition, it has been shown to scavenge lipid peroxide radicals.[148] Several studies have documented beneficial effects in rats subjected to forebrain ischemia, fluid percussion injury,[149] and improved neurological outcome following complete cerebral ischemia in dogs.[150]

Enzymatic Quenching of Free Radicals

Oxygen radicals can be quenched by superoxide dismutase (SOD). In a dog model of cerebral ischemia, SOD improved CBF, and decreased edema and histologic damage.[151] In addition, administration of SOD resulted in improved survival and outcome after a fluid percussion injury in a rat model.[152] The use of SOD after ischemic injury has been limited because of its short half-life of 5 minutes. The half-life can be prolonged by conjugation with polyethylene glycol. The use of polyethylene glycol superoxide dismutase (PEG-SOD) has been examined both experimentaly and clinically. In a model of global cerebral ischemia, Helfaer et al., however, failed to demonstrate any difference in post-ischemic hyperemia in PEG-SOD-treated piglets.[153] Armstead et al. demonstrated attenuation of increased blood-brain barrier permeability after cerebral ischemia in piglets pretreated with PEG-SOD.[154] In a model of focal cerebral ischemia, pretreatment with PEG-SOD decreased neuronal injury to the caudate nucleus, but did not affect cortical damage.[155]

Muizellar et al. examined the safety and efficacy of PEG-SOD in head-injured patients.[156] Patients presenting with a Glasgow Coma Scale of 8 or less were randomized to receive a placebo or PEG-SOD. Patients receiving PEG-SOD required less mannitol for control of intracranial hypertension. Neurological outcome was significantly better after 3 and 6 months in patients receiving PEG-SOD. At 3

Table 1
Strategies of Brain Protection

- Improvement of CBF and CMR imbalance
- Reduction of effective neurotransmitter concentrations
  - Decreasing total excitatory neurotransmitter release
  - Blockade of receptor sites
  - Increasing re-uptake of excitatory neurotransmitters
  - Increasing hyperpolarizing neurotransmitters
- Interference with calcium metabolism
  - Calcium channel blockers
  - Calcium chelation
- Interference with free radical biochemistry
  - Free radical scavengers
  - Peroxidation antagonists
  - Iron chelation
  - Xanthine oxidase inhibition
- Modification of nitric oxide production (?)

months, 43% of the patients in the control group were either vegetative or dead compared to 20% of the patients in the PEG-SOD group.

Conclusions

In this chapter the basic mechanisms of neuronal injury have been presented and their relationship to neurotrauma (Table 1). Multiple agents that may or may not be helpful as neuroprotective agents have been discussed. Most of these agents have been tested primarily in animal models, and their use has not been validated in clinical trials. With the exception of the calcium channel blockers after subarachnoid hemorrhage, the clinical use of these agents have not been well defined. Eventually, these agents will probably be used in combination in order to best protect the brain at various stages in the development of cerebral injury.

References

1. Siesjö BK: Cerebral circulation and metabolism. J Neurosurg 60: 883–908, 1984.
2. Murdoch J, Hall R: Brain protection: Physiological and pharmacological considerations. Part I: The physiology of brain injury. Can J Anesth 37:663–671, 1990.
3. Siesjö BK, Folbergrová J, MacMillan V: The effect of hypercapnia upon

intracellular pH in the brain, evaluated by the bicarbonate-carbonic acid method and from the creatine phosphokinase equilibrium. J Neurochem 19:2483–2495, 1972.

4. MacKnight ADC, Leaf A: Regulation of cellular volume. Physiol Rev 57:510–573, 1977.

5. Auer L, Boerke RS, Baron KD, San Fillippo BD, Waldman JB: Alterations in cat cerebrocortical capillary morphometrical parameters following K$^+$ induced cerebrocortical swelling. Acta Neuropathol (Berl) 47:175–181, 1979.

6. Hertz L: Features of astrocyte function apparently involved in the response of the central nervous system to ischemia-hypoxia. J Cereb Blood Flow Metabol 1:143–154, 1981.

7. Messick JM Jr, Milde LM: Brain protection. Adv Anesth 4:47–88, 1987.

8. Raichle M: The pathophysiology of brain ischemia. Ann Neurol 13:2–10, 1982.

9. Plum F: What causes infarction in ischemic brain? The Robert Wartenberg Lecture. Neurology 33:222–233, 1983.

10. Siesjö B, Wieloch T: Cerebral metabolism in ischaemia: Neurochemical basis for therapy. Br J Anaesth 57:47–62, 1985.

11. Rothman S: Synaptic release of excitatory neurotransmitter mediates anoxic neuronal death. J Neurochem 4:1884–1891, 1984.

12. Pellegrini-Giampietro DE, Cherici G, Alsiani M, Carla V, Moroni F: Excitatory amino acid release and free radical formation may cooperate in the genesis of ischemia-induced neuronal damage. J Neurosci 10:1035–1041, 1990.

13. Butcher SP, Bullock, Graham DI, McCulloch J: Correlation between aminio acid release and neuropathological outcome in rat brain following middle cerebral artery occlusion. Stroke 21:1727–1733, 1990.

14. Baker AJ, Zornow MH, Scheller MS, Yaksh TL, et al: Changes in extracellular concentration of glutamate, aspartate, glycine, dopamine, serotonin, and dopamine metabolites after transient global ischemia in the rabbit brain. J Neurochem 57:1370–1379, 1991.

15. Johnson JW, Ascher P: Glycine potentiates the NMDA response in cultured mouse brain neurons. Nature 325:529–531, 1987.

16. Johnson JW, Ascher P: Glycine potentiates the NMDA response in cultured mouse brain neurons. Nature 325:529–531, 1987.

17. Iino M, Ozawa S, Tsuzuki K: Permeation of calcium through excitatory aminoacid receptor channels in cultured rat hippocampal neurons. J Physiol 424:151–165, 1990.

18. Hammond EJ, Wilder BJ: Gamma-vinyl GABA. Gen Pharmacol 16:441–447, 1985.

19. Abel MS, McCandless DW: Elevated γ-aminobutric acid levels attenuate the metabolic response to bilateral ischemia. J Neurochem 58:740–744, 1992.

20. Lyden PD, Hedges B: Protective effect of synaptic inhibition during cerebral ischemia in rats and rabbits. Stroke 23:1463–1469, 1992.

21. Globus MYT, Busto R, Martinez E, Valdes I, Dietrich D: Ischemia induces release of glutamate in regions spared from histopathological damage in the rat. Stroke 21:III 43–46, 1990.

180 • Trauma Anesthesia and Critical Care of Neurological Injury

22. Goskowicz R, Patel P, Drummond J, Sano T, Cole D: Ischemia induced release of glutamate in the rat brain: The effect of etomidate and thiopental. Anesth Analg 76:s123, 1993.
23. Globus MYT, Busto R, Martinez E, Valdes I, Dietrich WD, Ginsberg M: Comparative effect of transient global ischemia on extracellular levels of glutamate, glycine, and γ-aminobutyric acid in vulnerable and nonvulnerable brain regions in the rat. J Neurochem 57:470–478, 1991.
24. Slivka A, Brannan T, Weinberger J, Knott P, Cohen G: Increase in extracellular dopamine in the striatum during cerebral ischemia: a study utilizing cerebral microdialysis. J Neurochem 50:1714–1718, 1988.
25. Globus MYT, Busto R, Dietrich WD, Martinez E, Valdes I, Ginsberg M: Intra-ischemic extracellular release of dopamine and glutamate is associated with striatal vulnerability to ischemia. Neurosci Lett 91: 36–40, 1988.
26. Brannan T, Weinberger J, Knott P, et al: Direct evidence of acute, massive, striatal dopamine release in gerbils with unilateral strokes. Stroke 18:108–110, 1987.
27. Phebus LA, Perry KW, Clemens JA, Fuller R: Brain anoxia releases striatal dopamine in rats. Life Sci 38:2447–2453, 1986.
28. Maker HS, Weiss C, Brannan TS: Amine mediated toxicity: The effects of dopamine, norepinepherine, 5-hydroxytryptamine, 6-hydroxydopamine, ascorbate, glutathione, and peroxide on the in vitro activity of creatine and adenylate kinases in the brain of the rat. Neuropharmacology 25:25–26, 1986.
29. Globus MYT, Ginsberg MD, Harik SI, Busto R, Dietrich WD: Role of dopamine in ischemic striatal injury: Metabolic evidence. Neurology 37:1712–1719, 1987.
30. Maker HS, Weiss C, Silides DJ, Cohen G: Coupling of dopamine oxidation (monoamine oxidase activity) to gluathione oxidation via the generation of hydrogen peroxide in rat brain homogenates. J Neurochem 36:589–593, 1981.
31. Weinberger J, Nieves-Rosa J, Cohen G: Nerve terminal damage in cerebral ischemia: the protective effect of alpha-methyl-para-tyrosine. Stroke 16:864–870, 1985.
32. Globus MYT, Ginsberg MD, Dietrich WD, Busto R, Scheinberg P: Substantia nigra lesion protects against ischemic damage in the striatum. Neurosci Lett 80:251–256, 1987.
33. Globus MYT, Busto R, Dietrich WD, Martinez E, Valdes I, Ginsberg M: Effect of Ischemia on the in vivo release of striatal dopamine, glutamate, and γ-aminobutyric acid studied by intracerebral microdialysis. J Neurochem 51:1455–1464, 1988.
34. Siejö BK: Calcium in the brain under physiological and pathological conditions. Eur Neurol 30(Suppl):3–9, 1990.
35. Farber JL, Chien KR, Mittnacht S Jr: The pathogenesis of irreversible cell injury in ischemia. Am J Pathol 102:271–281, 1981.
36. Orrenius S, McConkey DJ, Jones DP, Nicotera P: Ca^{++} activated mech-

anisms in toxicity and programmed cell death. ISI Atlas Sci: Pharmacology 2:319–324, 1988.

37. Moncada S, Palmer R, Higgs E: Nitric oxide: Physiology, pathophysiology, and phamacology. Pharm Rev 43:109–142, 1991.

38. Kågström E, Smith ML, Siejö BK: Local cerebral blood flow in the recovery period following complete cerebral ischemia in the rat. J Cereb Blood Flow Metab 3:170–182, 1983.

39. Demopulos HB, Flamm ES, Pietronigro DD: The free radical pathology and the microcirculation in the major central nervous system disorders. Acta Physio Scand (Suppl) 492:91–119, 1980.

40. Meldrum B: Protection against ischaemic neuronal damage by drugs acting on excitatory neurotransmission. Cerebrovasc Brain Metab Rev 2:27–57, 1990.

41. Siejö BK, Agardh CD, Bengtsson F: Free radicals and brain damage. Cerebrovasc Brain Metab Rev 1:165–211, 1989.

42. Halliwell B, Gutteridge JMC: Oxygen toxicity, oxygen radicals, transition metals, and disease. Biochem J 219:1–14, 1984.

43. Rehncrona S, Nielson H, Siejö BK: Enhancement of iron-catalyzed free radical formation by acidosis in brain homogenates: Difference in effect by lactic acid and CO_2. J Cereb Blood Flow Metab 9:65–70, 1989.

44. Aust SD, Morehouse LA, Thomas CE: Role of metals in oxygen radical reaction. J Free Radic Biol Med 1:3–25, 1985.

45. Fridovich I: The biology of oxygen radicals. Science 201:875–880, 1978.

46. vanHoutte PM: The endothelium—modulator of vascular smooth muschle tone. N Engl J Med 319:512–513, 1988.

47. DeRubertis FR, Craven PA: Calcium-independent modulation of cyclic GMP and activation of guanylate cyclase by nitrosamines. Science 193: 879–899, 1976.

48. Prado R, Watson BD, Wester P: Effect of nitric oxide synthase inhibion on cerebral blood flow following bilateral carotid artery occlusion and recirculation in the rat. J Cereb Blood Flow Metab 13:720–723, 1993.

49. Wei HM, Chi OZ, Liu X, Sinha Ak, Weiss H: Nitric oxide sythase inhibition alters cerebral blood flow and oxygen balance in focal cerebral ischemia in rats. Stroke 25:445–449, 1994.

50. Garthwaite J, Charles SL, Chess-Williams R: Endothelium-derived relaxing factor release on activation of NMDA receptors suggests reole as intercellular messenger in brain. Nature 336:385–389, 1988.

51. Garthwaite J, Garthwaite G, Plamer RMJ, Moncada S: NMDA receptor activation induces nitric oxide synthesis from arginine in rat brain slices. Euro J Pharmacol 172:413–416, 1989.

52. Choi DW: Glutamate neurotoxicity and diseases of the nervous system. Neuron 1:623–634, 1988.

53. Lawrence AJ, Jarrott B: Nitric oxide increases interstitial excitatory amino acid release in the rat dorsomedial medulla oblongata. Neurosci Lett 151:126–129, 1993.

54. Buisson A, Margaill I, Callebert J, Plotkine M, Boulu RG: Mechanisms involved in the neuroprotective activity of a nitric oxide synthase inhibitor during focal cerebral ischemia. J Neurochem 61:690–696, 1992.

55. Hogg N, Darley-Usmar VM, Wilson MT, Moncada S: Production of

hydroxyl radicals from the simultaneous generation of superoxide and nitric oxide. Biochem J 281:419–424, 1992.

56. Watson BD, Ginsberg MD: Ischemic injury in the brain: Role of oxygen radical-mediated processes. Ann NY Acad Sci 559:269–281, 1989.

57. Blough NV, Zafiriou OC: Reaction of superoxide with nitric oxide to form peroxynitrite in alkaline aqueous solutions. Inorg Chem 24: 3504–3505, 1985.

58. Radi R, Beckman JS, Bush KM, Freeman BA: Peroxynitrite induced membrane lipid peroxidation: the cytotoxic potential of superoxide and nitric oxide. Arch Biochem Biophys 288:481–487, 1991.

59. Lei SZ, Pan ZH, Aggarwal SK, Chen HS, Hartman J, Sucher NJ, Lipton SA: Effect of nitric oxide production on the redox modulatory site of the NMDA receptor-channel complex. Neuron 8:1087–1099, 1992.

60. Siejö BK: Basic mechanisms of traumatic brain damage. Ann Emerg Med 22:959–969, 1993.

61. Kontos HA, Wei EP: Superoxide production in experimental brain injury. J Neurosurg 64:803–807, 1986.

62. White BC, Krause GS: Brain injury and repair mechanisms: The potential form pharmacological therapy in closed head trauma. Ann Emer Med 22:970–979, 1993.

63. Vink R, Faden AL, McIntosh TK: Changes in cellular energetic state following graded traumatic brain injury in rats: Determination by phosphorus 31 magnetic resonance spectroscopy. J Neurotrauma 5: 315–330, 1988.

64. Takahashi H, Manaka S, Sano K: Changes of extracellular potassium concentration in the cortex and brain stem during the acute phase of experimental closed head injury. No To Shinkei 33:365–376, 1981.

65. Faden AI, Demediuk P, Panter SS, et al: The role of excitatory amino acids and NMDA receptors in traumatic brain injury. Science 244: 798–800, 1989.

66. Povlishock JT, Kontos HA: Continuing axonal and vascular change after experimental brain trauma. Cent Nerv Syst Trauma 2:285–298, 1985.

67. Povlishock JT: Pathobiology of traumatically induced axonal injury in animals and man. Ann Emerg Med 22:980–986, 1993.

68. Michenfelder JD, Milde JH: The relationship among canine brain temperature, metabolism, and function during hypothermia. Anesthesiology 75:130–136, 1991.

69. Rosomoff HL, Holiday DA: Cerebral blood flow and cerebral oxygen consumption during hypothermia. Am J Physiol 179:85–88, 1954.

70. Michenfelder JD, Theye RA: Hypothermia: effect on canine brain and whole body metabolism. Anesthesiology 29:1107–1112, 1968.

71. Sano T, Drummond J, Patel P, Grafe M, Watson J, Cole D: A comparison of the cerebral protective effects of isoflurane and mild hypothermia in a model of incomplete forebrain ischemia in the rat. Anesthesiology 76:221–228, 1992.

72. Busto R, Globus MY-T, Dietrich WD Martinez E, Valdes I, Ginsberg M: Effect of mild hypothermia on ischemia-induced release of neurotransmitters and free fatty acids in rat brain. Stroke 20:904–910, 1989.

73. Simpson RE, Walter GA, Phillis JW: The effects of hypothermia on amino acid neurotransmitter release from the cerebral cortex. Neurosci Lett 124:83–86, 1991.

74. Widmann R, Miyazawa, Hossmann KA: Protective effect of hypothermia on hippocampal injury after 30 minutes of forebrain ischemia in rats is mediated by postischemic recovery of protein synthesis. J Neurochem 61:200–209, 1993.

75. Kristian T, Katsura K, Siesjo BK: The influence of moderate hypothermia on cellular calcium uptake in complete ischaemia: implications for the excitotoxic hypothesis. Acta Physiol Scand 146:531–532, 1992.

76. Rosomoff HL: Hypothermia and cerebral vascular lesions. I. Experimental interruption of the middle cerebral artery during hypothermia. J Neurosurg 13:332–343, 1956.

77. Rosomoff HL: Experimental brain injury during hypothermia. J Neurosurg 16:177–187, 1959.

78. Kader A, Brisman MH, Maraire N, Huh JT, Solomon RA: The effect of mild hypothermia on permanent focal ischemia in the rat. Neurosurgery 31:1056–1061, 1992.

79. Baker CJ, Onesti ST, Solomon RA: Reduction by delayed hypothermia of cerebral infarction following middle cerebral artery occlusion in the rat: A time-course study. J Neurosurg 77:438–444, 1992.

80. Hoffman WE, Werner C, Baughman VL, Thomas C, Miletich DJ, Albrecht RF: Postischemic treatment with hypothermia improves outcome from incomplete cerebral ischemia in rats. J Neurosurg Anesthesiol 3:34–38, 1991.

81. Goto Y, Kassell NF, Hiramatsu K, Soleau SW, Lee KS: Effects of intraischemic hypothermia on cerebral damage in a model of reversible focal ischemia. Neurosurgery 32:980–985, 1993.

82. Xue D, Huang ZG, Smith KE, Buchan AM: Immediate or delayed mild hypothermia prevents focal cerebral infarction. Brain Res 587:66–72, 1992.

83. Coimbra C, Wieloch T: Hypothermia ameliorates neuronal survival when induced 2 hours after ischaemia in the rat. Acta Physiol Scand 146:543–44, 1992.

84. Kuluz JW, Gregory GA, Yu ACH, Chang Y: Selective brain cooling during and after prolonged global ischemia reduces cortical damage in rats. Stroke 23:1792–1797, 1992.

85. Miyazawa T, Bonnekoh P, Widman R, and Hossman KA: Heating of the brain to maintain normothermia during ischemia aggravates brain injury in the rat. Acta Neuropathologica 85:488–494, 1993.

86. Clifton GL, Jiang JY, Lyeth BG, Jenskins LW, Hamm RJ, Hayes RL: Marked protection by moderate hypothermia after experimental traumatic brain injury. Journal of Cereb Blood Flow Metab 11:114–121, 1991.

87. Marion DW, Obrist WD, Carlier PM et al: The use of moderate therapeutic hypothermia for patients with severe head injuries: a preliminary report. J Neurosurg 79:354–362, 1993.

88. Shiozaki T, Sugimoto H, Taneda M, et al: Effect of mild hypothermia

on uncontrollable intracreanial hypertension after severe head injury. J Neurosurg 79:363–368, 1993.

89. Warner D, McFarlane C, Todd M, Ludwig P, McAllister A: Sevoflurane and halothane reduce focal ischemic brain damage in the rat: Possible influence on thermoregulation. Anesthesiology 79:985–992, 1993.

90. Bhardwaj A, Brannan T, Weinberger J: Pentobarbital inhibits extracellular release of dopamine in the ischmic striatum. J Neural Transm 82:111–117, 1990.

91. Koom R, Brannan T, Martinez-Tica J, Weinberger J, Reich DL: Effect of etomidate on in vivo ischemia-induced dopamine release in the corpus striatum of the rat: A study using cerebral microdialysis. Anesth Analg 78:73–79, 1994.

92. Koom R, Kahn R, Brannan T, Martinez-Tica J, Weinberger J, Reich D: Effect of isoflurane and halothane of in vivo ischemia-induced dopamine release in the corpus striatum of the rat: A study using microdialysis. Anesth 79:827–835, 1993.

93. Michenfeider JD, Theye RA: Cerebral protection by thiopental during hypoxia. Anesthesiology 39:510–517, 1973.

94. Pierce EC, Lambertsen CJ, Deutsch S, et al: Cerebral circulation and metabolism during thiopental anesthesia and hyperventilation in man. J Clin Invest 41:1664–1671, 1962.

95. Michenfelder JD: The interdependency of cerebral function and metabolic effects following massive doses of thiopental in the dog. Anesthesiology 41:231–236, 1974.

96. Steen PA, Newberg L, Milde JH, Michenfelder JD: Hypothermia and barbiturates: individual and combined effects on canine cerebral oxygen consumption. Anesthesiology 58:527–532, 1983.

97. Nussmeier NA, Arlund C, Slogoff S: Neuropsychiatric complications after cardiopulmonary bypass: Cerebral protection by a barbiturate. Anesthesiology 64:165–170, 1986.

98. Zaiden JR, Klochany A, Martin WM, Ziegler JS, Harless DM, Andrews RB: Effect of thiopental on neurologic outcome following cononary artery bypass grafting. Anesthesiology 74:406–11, 1991.

99. Ward JD, Becker DP, Miller JD, Choi SC, Marmarou A, Wood C, et al: Failure of prophylactic barbiturate coma in the treatment of severe head injury. J Neurosurg 62:383–388, 1985.

100. Brain Resuscitation Clinical Trail I Study Group: Randomized clinical study of thiopental loading in comatose survivors of cardiac arrest. N Engl J Med 314:397–403, 1986.

101. Nussbaum E, Maggi JC: Pentobarbital therapy does not improve neurologic outcome in nearly drowned, flaccid-comatose children. Pediatrics 81:630–634, 1988.

102. Ashton D, van Reempts J, Wauquier A: Behavioral, electroencephalographic and histological study of the protective effect of etomidate against histotoxic dysoxia produced by cyanide. Arch Int Pharmacodyn 254:196–213, 1981.

103. Van Reempts J, Borgers M, Van Eyndhoven J, Hermans C: Protective effects of etomidate in hypoxic-ischemic brain damage in the rat: A morphologic assessment. Exp Neurol 76:181–195, 1982.

104. Koom R, Brannan T, Martinez-Tica J, Weinberger J, Reich DL: Effect of etomidate on in vivo ischemia-induced dopamine release in the corpus striatum of the rat: A study using cerebral microdialysis. Anesth Analg 78:73–79, 1994.

105. Watson JC, Drummond JC, Patel PM, Sano T, Akrawi W, Sang H: An assessment of the cerebral protective effects of etomidate in a model of incomplete forebrain ischemia in the rat. Neurosurgery 30:540–544, 1992.

106. Sano T, Patel P, Drummond J, Cole D: A Comparison of the cerebral protective effects of etomidate, thiopental, and isoflurane in a model of forebrain ischemia in the rat. Anes and Analges 76:990–997, 1993.

107. Cole DJ, Patel PM, et al: A comparison of the effects of thiopental, isoflurane, and etomidate on focal cerebral ischemic injury in rats. Anesthesiology 79:A184, 1993.

108. Ramani R, Todd MM, Warner DS: A dose-response study of the influence of propofol on cerebral blood flow, metabolism and the electroencephalogram in the rabbit. J Neurosurg Anesthesiol 4:110–119, 1992.

109. Artru AA, Shapira Y, Bowdle TA: Electroencephalogram, cerebral metabolic, and vascular responses to propofol anesthesia in dogs. J Neurosurg Anesthesiol 4:99–109, 1992.

110. Weinstabl C, Mayer N, Plattner H, Spiss CK, Hammerle AF: Impact of propofol on intracranila dynamics in head trauma ICU patients. Anesthesiology 73:A1217, 1990.

111. Rosenberg R, Kass I, Cottrell J: Propofol improves electrophysiological recovery after anoxia in the rat hippocampal slices. Anesthesiology 75:A606, 1991.

112. Kochs E, Hoffman W, Werner C, Thomas C, Albrecht R, Schulte am Esch J: The effect of propofol on brain electrical activity, neurological outcome, and neuronal damage following incomplete ischemia in rats. Anesthesiology 76:245–252, 1992.

113. Ridenour T, Warner D, Todd M, Gionet T: Comparative effects of propofol and halothane on outcome from temporary middle cerebral artery occlusion in the rat. Anesthesiology 76:807–812, 1992.

114. Newberg LA, Milde JH, Michenfelder JD: The cerebral metabolic effects of isoflurane at and above concentrations that suppress cortical electrical activity. Anesthesiology 59:23–28, 1983.

115. Newberg LA, Michenfelder JD: Cerebral protection by isoflurane during hypoxemia or ischemia. Anesthesiology 59:29–35, 1983.

116. Ruta TS, Drummond JC, Cole DJ: A comparison of the area of histochemical dysfunction after focal cerebral ischaemia during anaesthesia with isoflurane and halothane in the rat. Can J Anesthesia 38:129–135, 1991.

117. Hoffman WE, Thomas C, Albrecht RF: The effect of halothane and isoflurane on neurologic outcome following incomplete cerebral ischemia in the rat. Anesth Analgesia 76:279–281, 1993.

118. Newman B, Gelb AW, Lam AM: The effect of isoflurane-induced hypotension on cerebral blood flow and cerebral metabolic rate for oxygen in humans. Anesthesiology 64:307–310, 1986.

119. Messick JM, Casement B, Sharbrough FW, Milde LN, Michenfelder

JD, Sundt TM: Correlation of regional cerebral blood flow (rCBF) with EEG changes during isoflurane anesthesia for carotid endarterectomy: critical rCBF. Anesthesiology 66:344–349, 1987.

120. Sharbrough FW, Messick JM, Sundt TM: Correlation of continuous electroencephalograms with cerebral blood flow measurements during carotid endarterectomy. Stroke 4:674–683, 1973.

121. Buchan A, Li H, Pulsinelli W: The n-methyl-d-aspartate antagonist, MK-801, fails to protect against neuronal damage caused by transient, severe forebrain ischemia in adult rats. J Neurosci 11:1049–56, 1991.

122. Buchan A: Advances in cerebral ischemia: Experimental approaches. Neurology Clinics 10:49–61, 1992.

123. Buchan AM: Do NMDA antagonists protect against cerebral ischemia: Are clinical trials warranted? Cerebrovasc Brain Metab Rev 2:1–26, 1990.

124. Buchan AM, Li H, Cho SH, et al: Blockage of the AMPA receptor prevents CA_1 hippocampal injury following severe but transient forebrain ischemia in adult rats. Neurosci Lett 132:255–258, 1991.

125. Buchan AM, Xue D, Huang ZG, et al: Delayed AMPA receptor blockage reduces cerebral infarction induced by flocal ischemia. Neuro Report 2:473–476, 1991.

126. Oparil S, Calhoun DA: The calcium antagonists in the 1990s: An Overview. Am J Hypertens 4:396S–405S, 1991.

127. Wong MCW, Haley EC: Calcium Antagonists: Stroke therapy coming of age. Stroke 21:494–501, 1990.

128. Gotoh O, Mohamed AA, McCulloch J, et al: Nimodipine and the hemodynamic and histopathological consequences of middle cerebral artery occlusion in the rat. J Cereb Blood Flow Metab 6:321–331, 1986.

129. Kucharczyk J, Mintorovich J, Sevick R, Asgari H, Moseley M: MR evaluation of calcium entry blockers with putative cerebroprotective effects in acute cerebral ischemia. Acta Neurochir Suppl (Wein) 51:254–5, 1990.

130. Alps BJ, Hass WK: The potential beneficial effects of nicardipine in a rat model of transient forebrain ischemia. Neurology 37:809–814, 1987.

131. Allen GS, Ahn HS, Preziosi TJ, Battye R, Boone SC, et al: Cerebral arterial spasm: A controlled trail of nimodipine in patients with subarachnoid hemorrhage. N Engl J Med 308:619–624, 1983.

132. Gelmers HJ, Gorter K, de Weerdt CJ, et al: A controlled trial of nimodipine in acute ischemic stroke. N Engl J Med 318:203–207, 1988.

133. A randomized clinical study of a calcium-entry blocker (lidoflazine) in the treatment of comatose survivers of cardiac arrest. Brain Resuscitation Clinical Trial II Study Group. N Engl J Med 324:1225–1231, 1991.

134. Sancesario G, Iannone M, Morello M, Nisticò G, et al: Nitric oxide inhibition aggravates ischemic damage of hipoocampal but not of NADPH neurons in gerbils. Stroke 25:436–443, 1994.

135. Yamamoto S, Golanov EV, Berger SB, Reis DJ: Inhibition of nitric oxide synthesis increases focal ischemic infarction in rat. J Cereb Blood Flow Metab 12:717–726, 1992.

136. Kuluz JW, Prado RJ, Dietrich WD, Schleien CL, Watson BD: The effect

of nitric oxide synthase inhibition on infarct volume after reversible focal cerebral ischemia in conscious rats. Stroke 24:2023–2029, 1993.

137. Morikawa E, Moskowitz MA, Huang Z, Yoshida T, Irikura K, Dalkara T: L-arginine infusion promotes nitric oxide-dependent vasodilation, increases regional cerebral blood flow, and reduces infarction volume in the rat. Stroke 25:429–435, 1994.

138. Trifiletti RR: Neuroprotective effects of N^G-nitro-L-arginine in focal stroke in the 7-day-old rat. Eur J Pharmacol 218:197–198, 1992.

139. Buisson A, Plotkine M, Boulu RG: The neuroprotective effect of a nitric oxide inhibitor in a rat model of focal cerebral ischaemia. Br J Pharmacol 106:766–767, 1992.

140. Nishikawa T, Kirsch JR, Koehler RC, Miyabe M, Traystman RJ: Nitic oxide synthase inhibition reduces caudate injury following transient focal ischemia in cats. Stroke 25:877–885, 1994.

141. Bracken MB, Shepard MJ, Collins WF *et al:* A randomized, controlled trial of methylprednisolone or naloxone in the treatment of acute spinal-cord injury: Results of the second National Acute Spinal Cord Injury Study. New England Journal of Medicine 322:1405–1411, 1990.

142. Hall ED: The neuroprotective pharmacology of methylprednisolone. J Neurosurg 76:13–22, 1992.

143. Barks JDE, Post M, Tuor UI: Dexamethasone prevents hypoxic-ischemic brain damage in the neonatal rat. Pediatric Res 29:558–563, 1991.

144. Chumas PD, Del Bigio MR, Drake JM, Tuor UI: A comparison of the protective effect of dexamethasone to other potential prophylactic agents in a neonatal rat model of cerebral hypoxia-ischemia. J Neurosurg 79:414–420, 1993.

145. Haraldseth O, Gronas T, Unsgard G: Quicker metabolic recovery after forebrain ischemia in rats treated with the antioxid and U74006F. Stroke 22:1188–1192, 1991.

146. Hall ED, McCall JM, Chase RL, Yonkers PA, Braughler JM: A nonglucocorticoid steroid analog of methylprednisolone duplicates its high-dose pharmacology in models of central nervous system trauma and neuronal membran damage. J Pharmacol Exp Ther 242:137–142, 1987.

147. Braughler JM, Hall ED, Jacobsen EJ, McCall JM, Means ED: The 21-aminosteroids: Potent inhibitors of lipid peroxidation for the treatment of central nervous system trauma and ischemia. Drugs Future 14: 143–152, 1989.

148. Braughler JM, Pregenzer JF, Chase RL, *et al:* Novel 21-aminosteroids as potential inhibitors of iron-dependent lipid peroxidation. J Biol Chem 262:10438–10440, 1987.

149. McIntosh TK, Thomas M, Smith D, Banbury M: The novel 21-aminosteroid U74006F attenuates cerebral edema and improves survival after brain injury in the rat. J Neurotrauma 9:33–46, 1992.

150. Perkins WJ, Milde LN, Milde JH, Michenfelder JD: Pretreatment with U74006F improves neurologic outcome following complete cerebral ischemia in dogs. Stroke 22:902–909, 1991.

151. Schettini A, Lippman R, Walsh EK. Attenuation of decompressive hy-

poperfusion and cerebral edema by superoxide dismutase. J Neurosurg 71:578–587, 1989.

152. Levasseur JE, Patterson JL, Ghatak NR, *et al:* Combined effect of respirator induced ventilation and superoxide dismutase in experimental brain injury. J Neurosurg 71:573–577, 1989.

153. Helfaer MA, Kirsch JR, Haun SE, Moore LE, Traystaman RJ: Polyethylene glycol-conjugated superoxide dismutase fails to blunt postischemic reative hyperemia. Am J Physiol 261:H548–53, 1991.

154. Armstead WM, Mirro R, Thelin OP, Shibata M, Zuckerman SL, *et al:* Polyethylene glycol superoxide dismutase and catalase attenuate increased blood-brain barrier permeability after ischemia in piglets. Stroke 23:755–762, 1992.

155. Matsumiya N, Koehler RC, Kirsch JR, Traystaman RJ: Conjugated superoxide dismutase reduces extent of caudate injury after transient focal ischemia in cats. Stroke 22:1193–200, 1991.

156. Muizellar JP, Marmarou A, Young HF, *et al:* Improving the outcome of severe head injury with the oxygen radical scavenger PEG-SOD: A phase II trial. J Neurosurg 78:375–382, 1993.

7

Fluid Management and Resuscitation in Neurological Trauma

Donald S. Prough, MD, Douglas S. DeWitt, PhD, Mark H. Zornow, MD

Introduction

Brain trauma, produced by closed or penetrating head injuries, is subdivided into *severe* (from which the patient is rendered comatose, i.e., unable to obey a simple verbal command), *moderate* (after which the patient either requires cranial surgery or is rendered comatose, if only briefly), and *minor* (after which the patient neither requires surgery nor loses consciousness). Although primary brain injury may not be remediable, preventable or treatable secondary insults such as hypotension, hypoxemia, or intracranial hypertension may worsen the outcome. Post-injury care, including fluid resuscitation, of the head trauma victim is aimed toward prevention of these secondary insults.

From *Trauma Anesthesia and Critical Care of Neurological Injury,* edited by K. J. Abrams and C. M. Grande. © 1997, Futura Publishing Co., Armonk, NY.

Appropriate fluid management of patients with acute neurological injury is grounded in the landmark studies of Weed and McKibben in 1919.[1] Those studies, which used as end-points only gross pathological examination and protrusion of brain through an experimental craniotomy defect, demonstrated that hypotonic fluids visibly increased brain bulk whereas hypertonic (30%) saline shrunk the brain.[1] The confusion regarding fluid management of patients with neurological disease arises from the common recommendation that such patients be kept "dry," apparently because of failure to distinguish clearly between issues of volume and tonicity. This review will address the physiological principles of fluid resuscitation to answer three questions: What type of fluid is appropriate for hypovolemic, head-injured patients? How much should be given? How should the results of fluid administration be monitored?

Physiological Principles in Fluid Resuscitation

Intravenous fluids vary in osmolarity and tonicity. Osmotically active particles attract water across semipermeable membranes until equilibrium is attained. *Osmolarity,* which quantifies the forces determining the distribution of water, refers to the number of osmotically active particles per *liter* of solution. In contrast, *osmolality* is a measurement of the number of osmotically active particles per *kilogram* of solvent. Serum *osmolality* is estimated by the equation:

$$\text{Osmolality} = ([\text{Na}^+] \times 2) + (\text{glucose} \div 18) + (\text{BUN} \div 2.8)$$

$$[\text{Eq. 1}]$$

where sodium concentration ($[\text{Na}^+]$) is expressed in mEq·L^{-1}, serum glucose is expressed in mg·dL^{-1}, and blood urea nitrogen (BUN) is expressed in mg·dL^{-1}. Alcohol and radiographic dyes may increase measured osmolality, generating an increased "osmolal gap" between the calculated and measured values. Osmotic activity also can be expressed in terms of *osmotic pressure,* a measure of the attraction for water exerted across a semipermeable membrane. The changes (Δ) in osmotic pressure produced by a change in osmolality are approximated by the equation:

$$\Delta \text{ Osmotic pressure (mm Hg)} = 19.3 \times \Delta \text{ osmolality (mOsm·kg}^{-1})$$

$$[\text{Eq. 2}]$$

Table 1

Composition of Commercially Available Intravenous Fluids

Solution	Dextrose $(g \cdot L^{-1})$	Na^+ $(mEq \cdot L^{-1})$	Cl^- $(mEq \cdot L^{-1})$	Osmolarity $(mOsm \cdot L^{-1})$
5% dextrose in water	50	—	—	253
5% dextrose in 0.45% saline	50	77	77	505
Lactated Ringer's solution*	—	130	109	273
0.9% ("normal") saline	—	154	154	308**
3.0% saline	—	513	513	1,026**
6% dextran-70 in 0.9% saline	—	154	154	310
6% HES in 0.9% saline	—	154	154	310
5% albumin	—	~154	~154	~310

* Lactated Ringer's solution also contains (per liter) 4 mEq K^+, 3 mEq Ca^{++}, 28 mEq lactate.
** Calculated osmolarity
HES = hydroxyethyl starch.

A hyperosmolar state occurs whenever the concentration of osmotically active particles is high. Thus, uremia (increased BUN), hyperglycemia, and hypernatremia (increased serum sodium) increase serum osmolality. However, because urea distributes throughout total body water, an increase in BUN, unlike an increase in $[Na^+]$, does not cause *hypertonicity*, i.e., osmotically mediated redistribution of water from the intracellular volume to the extracellular volume. Acute hyperglycemia causes hypertonicity, but the effect is modified by cellular uptake of glucose and by insulin-mediated reduction of blood glucose. The term "tonicity" is also used colloquially to compare the osmotic pressure of a solution to that of plasma. A fluid in which the osmotic pressure is similar to that of plasma is termed *isotonic.* Hypotonic solutions exert lower osmotic pressures than plasma; hypertonic solutions exert higher osmotic pressures (Table 1). Note that in this colloquial usage an "isotonic" fluid may produce serum hypotonicity if glucose rather than sodium salts represents a substantial proportion of osmoles and if, as a consequence, infusion reduces serum sodium.

Although only a small proportion of the osmotically active particles in blood consists of plasma proteins, those particles are essential in determining the equilibrium of fluid between the interstitial and

Table 2
Osmolality and Osmotic Pressure in the Systemic Capillary Beds

Osmoles	Osmolality (mOsm·kg⁻¹) Plasma	IF	Osmotic Pressure (mm Hg) Plasma	IF	Osmotic Pressure Difference (mm Hg)
Total	280	279	5,404	5,385	19
[Na⁺], [Cl⁻], [HCO₃⁻], other nonprotein components	278.8	278.8	5,381	5,381	0
Protein	1.2	0.2	23	4	19
Total	282.6	281.3	5,454	5,429	25

IF = interstitial fluid.

plasma compartments of extracellular volume (Table 2). If serum osmolality is normal, i.e., ~280 mOsm·kg⁻¹, the total osmotic pressure exerted is approximately 5,430 mm Hg (19.3 × 280 mOsm·kg⁻¹). However, in the systemic capillary beds, there is virtually complete equilibration between the plasma and the interstitium of all osmoles other than those resulting from protein. Although serum proteins account for only slightly more than 1 mOsm·kg⁻¹, they do not freely equilibrate across capillary membranes. The reflection coefficient (σ) describes the permeability of capillary membranes to individual solutes, with σ = 0 representing free permeability and σ = 1.0 representing complete impermeability. The σ for albumin ranges from 0.6 to 0.9 in various capillary beds. Because capillary protein concentration exceeds interstitial concentrations, the osmotic pressure exerted by plasma proteins (termed *colloid osmotic pressure*) is higher than interstitial oncotic pressure and tends to preserve plasma volume. The small contribution of serum proteins to osmotic pressure (approximately 24 mm Hg in plasma) is a critical factor in maintaining intravascular volume.

Because the cerebral capillary membrane, the blood-brain barrier, is highly impermeable to protein, clinicians have assumed that administration of colloid-containing solutions should increase intracranial pressure (ICP) less than crystalloid solutions. However, because the blood-brain barrier also is highly impermeable to sodium, small changes in serum sodium generate greater osmotic pressure gradients across the cerebral capillary bed than do relatively large changes in serum protein concentrations. For instance, an increase

Table 3

Acute Effects of Changes in Plasma Sodium and Proteins on Osmotic Pressure in the Cerebral Capillaries

Physiological State	Site (Cerebral Capillary Plasma or Cerebral Interstitium)	Osmolality (mOsm/kg)	Osmotic Pressure Difference (mm Hg)	Net Change (mm Hg)
Baseline, sodium, protein and non-protein osmoles	Plasma	280	5,404	
	Cerebral Interstitium	280	5,404	
Plasma [Na⁺] acutely increased by 5 mEq·L⁻¹	Plasma	290	5,597	
	Cerebral Interstitium	280	5,404	
				193
Protein	Plasma	1.2	23	
	Cerebral Interstitium	0	0	
Plasma protein acutely doubled	Plasma	2.4	46	
	Cerebral Interstitium	0	0	
				23

of 5 $mEq \cdot L^{-1}$ in serum sodium would increase osmolality by 10 $mOsm \cdot kg^{-1}$, or 193 mm Hg of osmotic pressure (Table 3), more than sevenfold greater than the osmotic pressure exerted by all serum proteins. Therefore, when administering fluids to brain-injured patients, one critical question is the amount of *sodium-free* water in the solution. When solutions that contain a [Na⁺] less than that of serum are infused, metabolism or excretion of other components can result in a reduction of serum [Na⁺], a decrease in serum osmolality, and an increase in brain water.

The filtration rate of fluid from the capillaries into the interstitial space is the net result of a combination of forces, including colloid osmotic pressure and the hydrostatic gradient between the intravascular and interstitial spaces. The net fluid filtration at any point within a systemic or pulmonary capillary is represented by the Starling-Landis-Staverman equation:

$$Q = kA [(P_c - P_i) + \sigma(\pi_i - \pi_c)]$$ [Eq. 3]

where Q = fluid filtration, k = capillary filtration coefficient (conductivity of water), A = the area of the capillary membrane, P_c = capillary hydrostatic pressure, P_i = interstitial hydrostatic pressure, π_i = interstitial colloid oncotic pressure, and π_c = capillary colloid oncotic pressure.

Interstitial fluid volume is determined by the relative rates of capillary filtration and lymphatic drainage; homeostatic mechanisms acutely accommodate limited amounts of excess fluid. P_c, the most powerful factor favoring fluid filtration, is determined by capillary flow, arterial resistance, venous resistance, and venous pressure. Increased capillary filtration alters the balance of forces in the Starling equilibrium. Usually, the rate of water and sodium filtration exceeds that of protein filtration, resulting in preservation of π_c, dilution of π_i, and preservation of the oncotic pressure gradient, the most powerful factor opposing fluid filtration. When coupled with increased lymphatic drainage, preservation of the oncotic pressure gradient limits the accumulation of interstitial fluid. If P_c is increased at a time when lymphatic drainage is maximal, edema accumulates. In chronically edematous states, interstitial fluid pressure is reduced by enhanced lymphatic drainage through dilated lymphatic vessels.

Distribution of Infused Fluids

Accurate replacement of fluid deficits necessitates an understanding of the distribution spaces of water, sodium, and colloid (Fig. 1). Total body water, the distribution volume of sodium-free water, approximates 60% of total body weight. Total body water includes intracellular volume, which constitutes 40% of total body weight, and extracellular volume, which constitutes 20% of body weight and serves as the distribution volume for sodium. Plasma volume equals about one-fifth of extracellular volume, the remainder of which is interstitial fluid. Red cell volume, approximately 2 L, is part of intracellular volume.

Sodium concentration is equal in plasma volume and interstitial fluid (approximately 140 mEq·L^{-1}). The predominant intracellular cation, potassium, has an intracellular concentration ([K$^+$]) approximating 150 mEq·L^{-1}. Albumin is unequally distributed in plasma volume (~4 g·dL^{-1}) and interstitial fluid (~1.5 g·dL^{-1}). The interstitial fluid concentration of albumin varies greatly among tissues. Extracellular volume is the distribution volume for colloid, although the concentrations in plasma volume and interstitial fluid are unequal.

For example, assume that a 70-kg patient requires replacement of acute blood loss of 1,000 mL, approximately 20% of the predicted

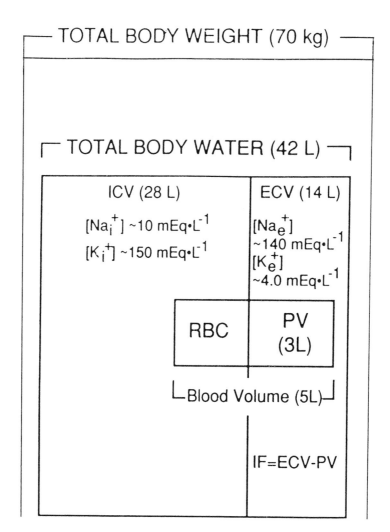

Figure 1. The distribution volume of water, approximately 60% of total body weight, includes both the extracellular and the intracellular volume. Sodium is distributed primarily in the extracellular volume. If capillary integrity is preserved, the concentration of colloid is higher in the plasma volume than in interstitial fluid. $[Na_i^+]$ and $[Na_e^+]$ = intracellular and extracellular concentrations of sodium, respectively; $[K_i^+]$ and $[K_e^+]$ represent intracellular and extracellular concentrations of potassium.

Table 4
Fluid Volumes Necessary to Expand Plasma Volume One Liter

Fluid	ΔPV (mL)	ΔIFV (mL)	ΔICV (mL)	Infused Volume (mL)
D5W	1,000	3,700	9,300	14,000
LRS	1,000	3,700	0	4,700
5% Albumin	1,000	0	0	1,000
25% Albumin	1,000	(−) 750	0	250
7.5% Saline				
Immediate	1,000	(−) 285	(−) 575	140
at equilibrium	170	630	(−) 800	140

PV = plasma volume; IFV = interstitial fluid volume; ICV = intracellular volume; D5W = 5% dextrose in water; LRS = lactated Ringer's solution; "immediate" assumes rapid bolus infusion; equilibrium assumes distribution as proposed by Spital.[14]

5 L blood volume. The formula describing the effects of replacement with intravenous fluids is as follows (Table 4):

$$\text{Plasma volume increment} = \text{volume infused} \times \text{normal plasma volume/distribution volume} \qquad \text{[Eq. 4]}$$

To replace 1 L of blood loss using D5W:

$$1.0 \text{ L} = 14 \text{ L} \times \frac{3.0 \text{ L}}{42.0 \text{ L}} \qquad \text{[Eq. 5]}$$

where 1 L is the desired plasma volume increment, 3 L is the normal estimated plasma volume, and 42 L = total body water in a 70-kg person.

To replace 1 L of blood loss using lactated Ringer's solution:

$$1.0 \text{ L} = 4.7 \text{ L} \times \frac{3.0 \text{ L}}{14.0 \text{ L}} \qquad \text{[Eq. 6]}$$

where 14 L = extracellular volume in a 70-kg person.

If 5% albumin, which exerts colloid osmotic pressure similar to plasma, was infused, the infused volume initially would remain in the plasma volume, perhaps attracting additional interstitial fluid intravascularly. Twenty-five percent human serum albumin, a concentrated colloid, would expand plasma volume by approximately 400 mL for each 100 mL infused, i.e., 1 L of blood loss could be replaced temporarily by 250 mL of 25% albumin.

Solutions for Intravenous Administration

Solutions that could be administered to patients with brain injury can be divided conveniently into crystalloids and colloids. Crystalloid solutions can be further subdivided into hypotonic, isotonic, and hypertonic solutions.

Crystalloid Solutions

Crystalloids are solutions composed solely of low molecular weight solutes (MW<30,000), either ionic (e.g., Na^+, Cl^-) or nonionic (e.g., mannitol). Although the osmolality of crystalloid solutions may vary widely (Table 1), colloid osmotic pressure by definition is zero.

Hypotonic Solutions

Hypotonic solutions (e.g., 0.45% saline, 5% dextrose in water) contain free water which, when infused rapidly in large volumes, can lower plasma osmolality, drive water across the blood-brain barrier into the brain, and increase cerebral water content and ICP. Dextrose-containing solutions should be used with particular caution in patients following traumatic brain injury. In animals, hyperglycemia may aggravate ischemic neurologic injury.[2] In humans, hyperglycemia is associated with worse outcomes in both ischemic[3] and traumatic[4] brain injury. However, separation of cause and effect is difficult because hyperglycemia is a secondary, hormonally mediated response that may vary directly with the severity of the primary injury.[3]

Isotonic Solutions

The most commonly used "isotonic" fluids are lactated Ringer's solution and 0.9% saline. Lactated Ringer's solution is mildly hypotonic when compared to plasma (Table 1). When large volumes of lactated Ringer's solution are infused rapidly, the free water (approximately 114 mL per L) may decrease plasma osmolality and increase brain water.

Hypertonic Solutions

For many years, mannitol, a 6 carbon sugar with a molecular weight of 182 daltons, has been the primary agent used for therapeutic brain dehydration. Excreted unchanged in the urine, mannitol is available as 20% and 25% solutions (osmolarities of 1,098 and 1,372 mOsm/L). Usually given in doses of 0.25 to 1.5 g·kg^{-1}, mannitol cannot pass through the intact blood-brain barrier; hence, intravenous administration acutely increases plasma osmolality and establishes an osmotic gradient favoring the movement of water from the brain's interstitial space into the vasculature. Rapid administration of large doses of mannitol may have a biphasic effect on ICP. Initially, ICP may increase due to an increased cerebral blood volume as a consequence of the vasodilatory effects of the acute increase in plasma osmolarity. Subsequently, ICP will decrease due to the movement of water from the brain interstitial space into the vasculature.

Recently, hypertonic saline solutions have been proposed for the treatment of hemorrhagic shock and control of intracranial hypertension. Although investigators have studied various hypertonic resuscitation solutions for much of this century,[1,5-11] current enthusiasm results from the work of Velasco et al.[6] They used small volumes (4.0 to 6.0 mL·kg^{-1}) of 7.5% hypertonic saline as the sole resuscitative measure in lightly anesthetized dogs that had been subjected to sufficient hemorrhage to reduce mean arterial pressure (MAP) to 45–50 mm Hg for 30 min. Hypertonic saline restored systolic blood pressure and cardiac output and increased mesenteric blood flow to greater than control values for 6 hours after resuscitation.[6] In experimental animals, hypertonic solutions decrease ICP by dehydrating brain tissue in which the blood-brain barrier is intact. Intravenous infusions of small volumes of hypertonic saline solutions have been reported to rapidly restore blood pressure, improve urinary output, and decrease ICP in patients who have failed to respond to large doses of mannitol.[12] These solutions should be administered in judicious amounts and with frequent monitoring of plasma osmolality and sodium concentrations.

The primary mechanism by which hyperosmotic saline increases venous return is plasma volume expansion.[13] Hypernatremic fluids acutely increase plasma volume both by osmotic attraction of water from the intracellular volume into the extracellular volume and by transient translocation of interstitial fluid volume into the plasma volume. Immediately after infusion, the combination of 7.5% saline and 6% dextran-70 increases plasma volume by a volume approximately seven times the original infused volume (Table 4).[13] The immediate effect in part is attributable to the fact that permeability of the systemic capillaries to sodium is not complete ($\sigma = 0.1$); therefore, interstitial fluid volume is translocated into the plasma volume until equilibration occurs.

The effects after equilibration on extracellular volume (ECV) and intracellular volume (ICV) of adding hyperosmotic saline can be calculated as follows[14] (Table 4):

$$\frac{\text{new total extracellular solute}}{\text{new ECV}} = \frac{\text{total intracellular solute}}{\text{new ICV}}$$

$$[\text{Eq. 7}]$$

For instance, assume that a healthy 70-kg patient ($[\text{Na}^+]$) = 140 mEq·L^{-1}) were to receive 2.0 mL·kg^{-1} of 7.5% saline; 173 mEq of sodium would be added as new extracellular solute. Before infusion, total extracellular sodium would be 1,960 mEq (140 mEq·L^{-1} × 14 L) and total intracellular potassium, the predominant intracellular solute would be 3,920 mEq (140 mEq·L^{-1} × 28 L). The equation would then be calculated:

$$\frac{1960 \text{ mEq} + 173 \text{ mEq}}{14 \text{ L} + x} = \frac{3920 \text{ mEq}}{28 \text{ L} - x} \qquad [\text{Eq. 8}]$$

where x = the added extracellular volume. The new total extracellular volume would equal 14.8 L (14 L + 0.8 L), and the new total intracellular volume would equal 27.2 (28 L − 0.8 L). Assuming that the increase in extracellular volume was equal to 0.8 L, the increase in plasma volume would be approximately 170 mL.

The transient effects of hypertonic saline administration represent a major obstacle to wider clinical application. To prolong the therapeutic effects beyond 30–60 minutes, investigators have infused additional hypertonic saline, blood, or conventional fluids, or added colloid to hypertonic fluids. In hemorrhaged animals, adding 6.0% dextran-70 to 7.5% saline increased the duration of hemodynamic improvement when compared with equal volumes of hypertonic saline, sodium bicarbonate, or sodium chloride/sodium acetate.[15]

Because small volumes (relative to shed blood volume) of hypertonic saline, with or without added colloid, rapidly increase blood pressure and cardiac output, clinical trials have evaluated whether rapid infusion of hypertonic solutions might improve outcome when used for prehospital resuscitation. In the largest clinical study of prehospital hypertonic saline resuscitation, Mattox et al. randomized 422 patients, half of whom required surgery, to receive 250 mL of either conventional crystalloid fluid or 7.5% saline in 6% dextran.[16] Although overall survival was unaffected, survival was improved in the patients who required surgery. Vassar et al. compared 250 mL of lactated Ringer's solution to 7.5% saline in 6.0% dextran-70 for prehospital resuscitation of trauma patients.[17] Despite no overall difference in mortality, survival was greater in the subset of patients with severe head injury.[17] In a subsequent randomized multicenter study, Vassar et al. evaluated the effects of 250 mL of sodium chloride with and without 6% and 12% dextran-70 for the prehospital resuscitation of hypotensive trauma patients.[18] A small subgroup of patients with Glasgow Coma Scale scores <8 but without severe anatomic injury seemed to benefit most from resuscitation with 7.5% saline.[18]

The least encouraging observations regarding hyperosmotic resuscitation involve experimental models of uncontrolled hemorrhage,[19] in which hyperosmatic solutions increase bleeding and may adversely affect mortality. In urban trauma patients, Bickell et al. have reported that immediate prehospital resuscitation does not improve mortality in comparison to resuscitation initiated only after arrival at the hospital.[20]

If membrane permeability is normal, fluids containing colloids preferentially expand plasma volume rather than interstitial fluid volume. Each gram of intravascular colloid holds approximately 20 mL of water in the circulation (14–15 mL per gram of albumin; 16–17 mL per gram of hydroxyethyl starch; 20–25 mL per gram of dextran).[21] After equilibration, plasma volume expansion is determined primarily by the number of grams of colloid infused, not by the original volume or concentration of the infusate.[21] Concentrated colloid-containing solutions (i.e., 25% albumin) may exert sufficient oncotic pressure to translocate substantial volumes of interstitial fluid into the plasma volume. Plasma volume expansion unaccompanied by interstitial fluid expansion offers apparent advantages: lower fluid requirements, less peripheral and pulmonary edema accumulation, and reduced concern about the cardiopulmonary consequences of later fluid mobilization.

Table 5
Characteristics of Clinically Useful Colloids

Colloid	Composition	Concentration	Mean Molecular Weight (Range in Daltons)	Percent Intravascular	Colloid Osmotic Pressure (mm Hg)
Albumin	Albumin	5%	69,000	80	20
Hydroxyethyl starch	Amylopectin				
Hetastarch		6%	480,000 (10,000 to 1,000,000)	100	30
Pentastarch		10%	264,000 (150,000 to 350,000)	100	40[89]
Dextran-70	Polysaccharide	6%	70,000 (20,000 to 175,000)	100	40[87]
Dextran-40	Polysaccharide	10%	40,000 (15,000 to 75,000)	100	

Colloidal Solutions

Albumin

A variety of colloidal solutions are available for clinical use (Table 5). Human serum albumin, available in 5% and 25% concentrations, is an effective volume expander that has no intrinsic effects on clotting parameters and has not been associated with allergic-type reactions. Albumin solutions contain no clotting factors. Although derived from pooled human plasma, there is no risk of disease transmission because albumin is heat-treated and then sterilized by ultrafiltration. Albumin can be given without regard to the recipient's blood type as isoagglutinins are removed during processing. Although safe and effective as volume expanders, albumin solutions are more expensive than synthetic colloids.

Plasma

Plasma should be used only when there is an acute need to replace clotting factors and there is evidence of a resulting coagulopathy. Volume expansion and nutritional support are no longer considered valid uses for fresh or frozen plasma. Although all plasma is derived from volunteer blood donors, and careful screening procedures have been implemented, the risk of disease transmission remains a reality. The risk of transmitting hepatitis C is estimated at 1 in 3,300 units, hepatitis B at 1 in 200,000 units, and HIV at 1 in 225,000 units.[22]

Synthetic Colloids

Hetastarch

The synthetic colloid most frequently used in the US is a 6% solution of hydrolyzed amylopectin (hetastarch) dissolved in 0.9% saline (Hespan™). Eighty percent of the molecules range in size from 30,000 to 2,400,000 daltons. The mean molecular weight for hetastarch is approximately 480,000 daltons. The low molecular weight fraction of an administered dose of hetastarch (those hetastarch molecules weighing less than 50,000 daltons) is excreted by renal filtration within 24 hours. Although the incidence of allergic reactions to hetastarch is extremely low, there have been some concerns about the potential for this compound to induce coagulopathies when given in large doses. The mechanism by which hetastarch affects coagulation is multifactorial, including hemodilution of clotting factors, inhibition of platelet function and a direct inhibition of factor VIII.[23] Sporadic case reports of impaired clotting following hetastarch have made many neurosurgeons and neurointensivists hesitant to use this agent in patients at risk for intracranial hemorrhage.

Pentastarch

Pentastarch (Pentaspan™), a new formulation of hydrolyzed amylopectin, has been approved for use during leukophoresis and may have a role as a plasma volume expander. Pentastarch differs from hetastarch in that it has a lower mean molecular weight (264,000 vs. 480,000 for hetastarch), which results in more rapid and complete renal clearance. Seventy percent of pentastarch is excreted in the urine within 24 hours vs. 30% of hetastarch. Preliminary studies also suggest that pentastarch may have fewer adverse effects on coagulation parameters than hetastarch.

Dextrans

Dextran solutions are colloids composed of glucose polymers with mean molecular weights of 40,000 (dextran-40) and 70,000 (dextran-70). While the colloid osmotic pressure of dextran-70 approximates that of plasma, dextran-40 is hyperoncotic and can transiently expand plasma volume by more than the amount infused by recruiting interstitial water into the vascular space. About 50% of dextran-40 and dextran-70 is renally excreted within 24–48 hours of administration. Dextrans have been associated with a variety of adverse effects that have limited their clinical use. Approximately 0.032% of the patients who receive dextrans develop allergic-like reactions. These reactions can be prevented by the prior administration of 20 mL of very low molecular weight dextran (dextran-1) immediately prior to either dextran-40 or dextran-70. Dextran-1 binds to circulating IgG, preventing it from crosslinking with larger dextran molecules and activating complement. An additional problem with dextran solutions is that large volumes (i.e., >20% of blood volume) may interfere with blood typing and crossmatching.

Selection of Fluids in Head-Injured Patients

The effects of clinical fluid administration on cerebral edema and ICP can largely be predicted from the work of Weed and McKibben[1] and from knowledge that the blood-brain barrier, unless disrupted, is highly impermeable to sodium. The effects of fluid choices on cerebral blood flow (CBF) and cerebral metabolism are less easily predicted. Investigation of the effects of fluid infusion on ICP and cerebral edema has generally been carried out in animals, although a few studies have been performed in humans. The studies vary in several critical details. Osmolality, colloid osmotic pressure, and hemoglobin concentration have been altered by fluid infusion, plasmapheresis, fluid infusion as blood is removed (isovolemic hemodilution), or a sequence of hemorrhage followed by fluid infusion (analogous to hemodilution during resuscitation after trauma). Some investigators have studied acute, single-bolus resuscitation, while others have studied more prolonged infusions. In attempting to replicate the features of clinical lesions, studies have been performed both in animals without intracranial pathology and in those with a variety of brain injuries, including focal cryogenic injury (which causes vasogenic brain edema), space-occupying lesions, cerebral ischemia, and concussive brain injury.

Cerebral Effects of Fluid or Blood Infusion (No Hemorrhagic Shock)

The simplest models are those in which fluid or blood is infused in the absence of hemorrhage or shock (Table 6). In such a model, Weed and McKibben[1] showed in cats that hypertonic solutions shrank while hypotonic solutions expanded the brain. They also demonstrated that 0.9% saline had little effect on intracranial volume.

Table 6
Cerebral Effects of Fluid or Blood Infusion (No Hemorrhage or Shock)

First Author	Reference Number	Species (Lesion(s))	Interventions	Observations
Weed	(1)	Cats	30% saline; distilled water; 0.9% saline	30% saline shrank brain; distilled water expanded brain; 0.9% saline had little effect
Wilson	(90)	Dogs	1.0 M sodium lactate or saline; 0.67 M sodium succinate; 2 M glucose	1.0 M salts decreased ICP; after initial decrease, 2.0 M glucose increased ICP
Fisher	(25)	Children (head injury)	3% saline vs. 0.9% saline (crossover design)	3.0% saline decreased ICP; 0.9% did not
Shapira	(27)	Rats (weight drop head trauma)	0.9% saline; 5.0% dextrose (0.25 mL·g^{-1} in 0.5 h)	5.0% dextrose increased edema and impaired neurological outcome; 0.9% saline had no effect
Shapira	(28)	Rats (weight drop head trauma)	10 mL·kg^{-1}·hr^{-1} (for 18 hr) of TPN; D5/0.45% saline; isotonic plasma expander	No difference in brain water or neurological outcome
Morse	(29)	Rats (trethyltin-induced or anoxic cerebral edema)	Dehydration; overhydration; euhydration	No difference in brain water
Albright	(30)	Dogs (cryogenic lesion)	Plasmalyte; 12% HES plus furosemide; 24% HES plus furosemide (6 hours)	Both HES regimens decreased ICP and brain water
Albright	(91)	Dogs (cryogenic lesion)	Plasmalyte plus mannitol; plus furosemide; plus albumin; plus albumin and furosemide	All additions except albumin decreased ICP; only albumin plus furosemide produced normovolemic dehydration
Schell	(32)	Rats (MCA occlusion)	10 mL·kg^{-1} of 10% albumin vs. 10% pentastarch	Blood-brain barrier permeability, brain injury, edema formation better in pentastarch group
Wood	(31)	Dogs (MCA and ICA occlusion)	20% blood volume expansion with dextran-40 × 2	Hypervolemic hemodilution improved perfusion to ischemic brain, increased ICP
Wood	(92)	Dogs (ICA and MCA occlusion)	20% blood volume expansion with blood × 2	Nondilutional hypervolemia did not increase blood pressure, ICP or infarction size

ICP = intracranial pressure; TPN = total parenteral nutrition; HES = hydroxyethylstarch; D5 = 5% dextrose; Plasmalyte = isotonic crystalloid; MCA = middle cerebral artery; ICA = internal carotid artery.

These observations were expanded by Wilson,[24] who demonstrated in dogs that hypertonic salt solutions decreased ICP but that hypertonic glucose solutions actually increased ICP after a transient decrease, presumably reflecting equilibration of glucose across the blood-brain barrier. In head-injured children, Fisher et al. showed, in a double-blind crossover study, that 3.0% saline significantly reduced ICP while 0.9% saline exerted no effect (Fig. 2).[25] It is necessary to note, however, that hypertonic fluids may reduce brain interstitial fluid while only transiently affecting intracellular fluid volume. In cultures of brain glioma cells, after hypertonic challenge cellular volume was quickly restored by a mechanism that was inhibited by loop diuretics[26] (Fig. 3A, B).

However, fluid restriction or less acute administration of fluids of different tonicities to produce dehydration, overhydration, or euhydration has demonstrated little effect on brain water or outcome. Most important among these studies are those of Shapira et al.,[27,28] who demonstrated, in rats subjected to head trauma by weight drop, that marked differences in the volumes of water and electrolytes administered chronically had little effect on brain water or neurological outcome, although 5% dextrose increased edema and worsened neurological outcome.[29] Morse et al. showed similar results in rats with cerebral edema induced by anoxia or triethyltin.[29] In animals, colloids have little ability to change brain water unless combined with diuretics. Albright et al. showed that combinations of hydroxyethyl starch and furosemide[30] or albumin and furosemide[31] decreased ICP and brain water. Perhaps the most interesting data are those of Schell et al.,[32] who studied rats with middle cerebral artery occlusion and demonstrated that 10% pentastarch, in contrast to 10% albumin, reduced edema formation. However, in global cerebral ischemia, pentastarch did not exert similar effects.[33] It is unclear whether pentafraction, a formulation of middle-molecular weight molecules of hydroxyethyl starch that appears to reduce capillary permeability, would influence cerebral edema. From the above, we conclude that rapid administration of hypotonic fluids may increase brain water and ICP, that rapid infusion of hypertonic saline solutions will decrease brain water and ICP, that rapid administration of colloids may reduce brain water only if given with diuretics, but that more gradual administration of fluids markedly blunts these effects.

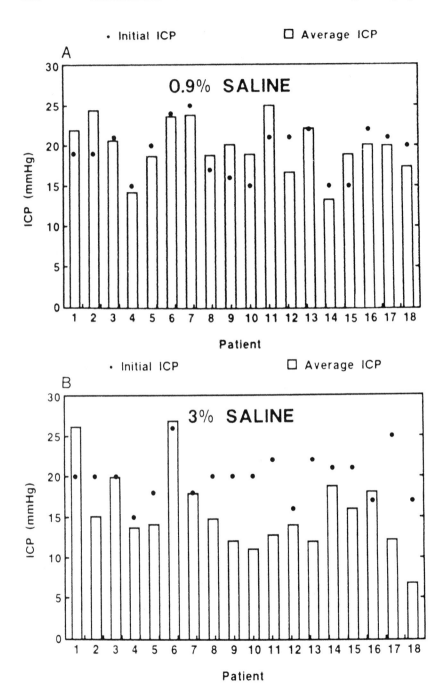

Cerebral Effects of Acute Isovolemic Hemodilution (No Brain Lesion)

Perhaps the most appropriate model of perioperative fluid administration is isovolemic hemodilution (Table 7), since that technique mimics the intraoperative sequence of blood loss and concurrent fluid replacement, without intervening hypovolemia. Isovolemic hemodilution produces several effects. First, in the absence of shock, a reduction in hematocrit increases CBF in animals[34-38] and in humans.[39] The acute effects on ICP depend on the tonicity of the infused fluid. Hypertonic fluids decreased brain water and ICP[35] in rabbits; 0.9% saline increased ICP slightly, but did not change brain water. Lactated Ringer's solution, in which the sodium concentration is 130 $mEq \cdot L^{-1}$, slightly increased brain water; 6% hydroxyethyl starch, dissolved in 0.9% saline (154 $mEq \cdot L^{-1}$), had no effect on either ICP or brain water.[40]

Cerebral Effects of Acute Hemodilution (Brain Injury Present)

In the presence of cryogenic or ischemic brain injury, damage to the blood-brain barrier tends to reduce the differences in CBF, ICP, and brain water produced by acute hemodilution with different solutions (Table 8). In rabbits with cryogenic brain lesions, hemodilution to reduce hematocrit to approximately 23% using hypotonic lactated Ringer's solution or hypertonic lactated Ringer's solution resulted in a greater increase in ICP in the hypotonic group.[41] Brain water was similar in the lesioned hemispheres but less in the non-lesioned hemisphere in rabbits given the hypertonic solution. Hemodilution to a hematocrit of 20% with 0.9% NaCl, 6.0% hydroxyethyl starch, or 5% albumin resulted in similar changes in ICP and brain water in all groups.[42]

Figure 2. A. Intracranial pressure (ICP; vertical axis) in 18 head-injured children (horizontal axis) receiving 0.9% saline (10 mL/kg) over 120 min. The initial ICP is represented by the dots. Average ICP after infusion is displayed by the open bars. Permission from Fisher.[25] **Figure 2B.** Intracranial pressure (ICP; vertical axis) in eighteen head-injured children (horizontal axis) receiving 3.0% saline (10 mL/kg) over 120 min. The initial ICP is represented by the dots. Average ICP after infusion is displayed by the open bars. Permission from Fisher.[25]

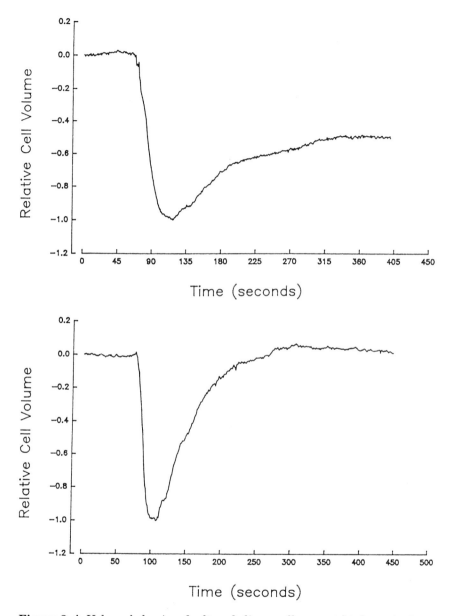

Figure 3. A. Volume behavior of cultured glioma cells exposed to hypertonic saline. Cells were equilibrated in an isotonic solution until the voltage signal remained stable for 15–30 min, then were abruptly exposed to the hypertonic

Table 7
Cerebral Effect of Acute Isovolemic Hemodilution (No Brain Lesion)

First Author	Reference Number	Species	Interventions	Observations
Michenfelder	(93)	Dogs	Hgb decreased from 12.4% to 7.8%, then 5.3%	CBF increased from 77 to 92 to 120 mL·100g^{-1}·min^{-1}
Todd	(35)	Rabbits	0.9% saline; hypertonic LRS (Na$^+$ 252 mEq·L^{-1}); Hct 40% → 20%	Hypertonic LRS decreased brain water and ICP; 0.9% saline slightly increased ICP; increased CBF > 60%
Hurn	(94)	Rats (open cranial window)	Plasma to decrease Hct to 16% to 36%	CBF increased; microvascular pressure unchanged; viscosity correlated with CBF increase
Von Kummer	(38)	Cats	Dextran-40 to decrease Hct 35% to 25%	CBF increased ≤30%; if BP also decreased from ~140 to ~80 mm Hg, CBF ~
Van Woerkens	(37)	Pigs	Dextran-40 to decrease Hct 28% to 9%	CBF increased 170%
Hudak	(34)	Cats (cranial window)	Hct decreased 31% to 17%	CBF increased as Hct decreased; arterioles constricted
Hino	(39)	Humans	Hct decreased 42.5% to 37.2%	CBF increased 45.2 to 47.7 mL·100g^{-1}·min^{-1}; CDO$_2$ decreased
Tommasino	(40)	Rabbits	LRS vs. 6.0% HES to decrease Hct 40% → 20%	ICP and brain water increased with LRS, normalized over 4 hours; HES had no effect on ICP or brain water
Hindman	(95)	Rabbits (CPB)	Hgb decreased 41% to 21% with HES in 0.72% saline or 43% to 29% with 0.9% saline	Brain water unchanged by either fluid
Massik	(36)	Neonatal sheep	Hct increased with oxyhgb or methgb erythrocytes	CBF decreased in both groups although CaO$_2$ remained constant in the methgb group
Muizelaar	(96)	Cats (cranial window)	Hct varied from 60% to 120% of baseline	Arterial caliber changes little with Hct variation; changes in cerebrovascular resistance with hemodilution secondary to change in viscosity

LRS = lactated Ringer's solution; Hct = hematocrit; ICP = intracranial pressure; CBF = cerebral blood flow; CDO$_2$ = cerebral oxygen delivery; CaO$_2$ = arterial oxygen content; oxyhgb = oxyhemoglobin; methgb = methemoglobin; BP = blood pressure; HES = hydroxyethyl starch.

solution. Light-scattering voltages are normalized to the maximal voltage change and presented as relative changes in cell volume. Note the rapid and complete recovery of cell volume despite maintenance of the hypertonic environment. Permission from McManus.[26] **Figure 3B.** Volume behavior of cultured glioma cells exposed to hypertonic saline in the presence of 10^{-4} M bumetanide. The experimental protocol as in Figure 3A. Permission from McManus.[26]

Table 8
Cerebral Effects of Acute Hemodilution (Brain Injury Present)

First Author	Reference Number	Species (Lesion(s))	Interventions	Observations
Zornow	(41)	Rabbits (cryogenic lesion)	Hemodilution with hypotonic or hypertonic LRS to decrease Hct to 23%	ICP increased more in the hypotonic LRS group. Brain water similar in lesioned, more in nonlesioned hemisphere in hypotonic LRS group
Zornow	(42)	Rabbits (cryogenic lesion)	Hemodilution to decrease Hct to ~20% with 0.9% saline, 6.0% HES or 5% albumin	ICP and brain water increased similarly in all groups
Hyodo	(43)	Dogs (ICA and MCA occlusion)	Hemodilution with LRS to decrease Hct to 32% to 33%	ICP increased more in hemodiluted dogs; brain water lower in ischemic hemisphere; hemodilution increased regional CBF in ischemic zone
Tu	(44,97)	Dogs (ICA and MCA occlusion)	Hemodilution with dextran 40 to decrease Hct to 30% to 32%	ICP increased less in dextran-hemodiluted dogs[44]; CBF, neurological status, and infarction better in hemodiluted animals
Cole	(45)	Rats (MCA occlusion and reperfusion)	Hypervolemic hemodilution with albumin (Hct 30%) or diaspirin-linked Hgb (Hct 30% or 9%)	Less brain water in all groups than in blood-infused group; brain injury least in the group with Hct 9%
Perez-Trepichio	(46)	Rats (cerebral embolization)	HES to decrease Hct 46% to 35% for 24 hr	Decreased ischemic and infarct volumes
Korosue	(47)	Dogs (ICA and MCA occlusion)	LRS vs. dextran to decrease Hct to 33% for 1 wk	Worse outcome and larger infarction with LRS
Korosue	(48)	Rabbits (normal or MCA occlusion)	Hemodilution vs. hypoxia	Hemodilution increased CBF in normal and ischemic brain; hypoxia only increased CBF in normal brain
Vorstrup	(49)	Humans (stroke <48 h)	Hemodilution with dextran-40 to decrease Hct from 46% to 39%	CBF increased ~20% in both ischemic and nonischemic areas
Korosue	(50)	Humans (strokes)	Plasma to decrease Hct to 33%	rCBF increased in the ischemia area; CSFP increased 16%; associated neurological improvement

MCA = middle cerebral artery; CBF = cerebral blood flow; ICA = internal carotid artery; LRS = lactated Ringer's solution; Hct = hematocrit; CSFP = cerebrospinal fluid pressure; HES = hydroxyethyl starch; Hgb = hemoglobin.

Isovolemic hemodilution has been used extensively to improve cerebral perfusion in experimental ischemia and in human stroke. In experimental ischemia, hemodilution with lactated Ringer's solution,[43] dextran-40,[44] albumin,[45] hydroxyethyl starch,[46] and di-aspirin-linked hemoglobin[45] resulted in better perfusion in the ischemic regions, decreased infarct volumes,[46] and improved neurological status.[44] Colloids appeared superior to crystalloids.[47] Isovolemic hemodilution influences ICP and brain water in nonlesioned brain as one would predict based on the osmolalities of the infused fluids. In areas of focal ischemia, isovolemic hemodilution improves CBF[48–50] and may limit injury in hypoperfused brain.[50]

Cerebral Effects of Changing Osmolality or Colloid Osmotic Pressure with Plasmapheresis

Plasmapheresis represents an alternative technique for studying the acute effects of changing serum osmolality and colloid osmotic pressure (Table 9). Zornow et al.[51] demonstrated in rabbits that reduction of osmolality by 13 mOsm·kg^{-1} resulted in a marked increase in ICP and in brain water. In contrast, a 13 mm Hg decrease in colloid osmotic pressure (equivalent to a decrease of <1 mOsm·kg^{-1}) produced no significant change. In later studies, Kaieda et al. demon-

Table 9

Cerebral Effects of Changing Osmolality or Colloid Osmotic Pressure with Plasmapheresis (With or Without Brain Lesion)

First Author	Reference Number	Species (Lesion(s))	Interventions	Observations
Zornow	(51)	Rabbits	Osmolality decreased 13 mOsm/kg; COP decreased by 13 mm Hg	ICP and brain water increased with decreased osmolality; no change with decreased colloid osmotic pressure
Kaieda	(52)	Rabbits (cryogenic lesion)	COP decreased ~11 mm Hg (for 45 min); osmolality decreased by ~13 mOsm/kg	ICP increased more with decreased osmolality
Kaieda	(53)	Rabbits (cryogenic lesion)	COP decreased 11 mm Hg (8 hr); COP decreased 3 mm Hg	No effect on ICP or brain water

COP = colloid osmotic pressure; ICP = intracranial pressure.

strated that rapid (45 min) reductions in colloid osmotic pressure produced little if any change after cryogenic injury, but that decreased osmolality continued to exert a substantial effect.[52] In rabbits with cryogenic lesions, reducing colloid osmotic pressure for 8 hours produced no effect on ICP or brain water.[53] These studies demonstrate clearly that changes in osmolality are far more important than changes in colloid osmotic pressure, in part because changes in osmolality produce much greater changes in osmotic pressure. Moreover, they suggest that colloid osmotic pressure is a minor concern in fluid management of patients with brain injury.

Cerebral Effects of Hemorrhage and Resuscitation (No Brain Lesion)

In the absence of brain lesions, the sequence of hemorrhage followed by resuscitation with crystalloid or colloid produces changes in ICP similar to those seen in animals subjected to isovolemic hemodilution (Table 10). However, CBF, which usually is increased after isovolemic hemodilution, often is not increased in the sequence of hemorrhage followed by fluid resuscitation. Slightly hypotonic lactated Ringer's solution produced small increases in ICP after resuscitation[54,55]; resuscitation with colloid, such as 6.0% hydroxyethyl starch, produced somewhat smaller increases in ICP than resuscitation with hypertonic fluids[56]; perhaps because hydroxyethyl starch is dissolved in 0.9% saline. Hypertonic solutions, whether given as boluses or as boluses followed by continued infusion, have been associated with considerably lower ICP[54,55,57-60] and brain water. In general, hypertonic solutions did not improve CBF, although CBF improved in some experimental models.[58,60] Perhaps the most striking observation about the sequence of hemorrhage followed by resuscitation is that CBF may not recover well, despite substantial improvements in mean arterial pressure and cardiac output.[54-56,59,60]

Cerebral Effects and Hemorrhage and Resuscitation (Intracranial Mass Lesion)

Addition of a mass lesion to the sequence of hemorrhage and resuscitation produces similar but exaggerated effects (Table 11). However, if the experimental model produces cerebral ischemia, it is likely that the resulting changes in blood-brain barrier function reduce the differences between fluids in the affected brain. In dogs

Table 10
Cerebral Effects of Hemorrhage and Resuscitation (No Brain Lesion)

First Author	Reference Number	Species	Interventions	Observations
Prough	(54)	Dogs	LRS; 7.5% saline	ICP lower with 7.5% saline; CBF no different
Prough	(55)	Dogs	7.5% saline (4 mL·kg^{-1}); LRS (45 mL·kg^{-1})	ICP lower after 7.5% saline
Poole	(56)	Dogs	LRS (60 mL·kg^{-1}); 6.0% HES (20 mL·kg^{-1})	ICP lower after HES; CBF similar
Gunnar	(57)	Dogs	Resuscitation with shed blood plus 0.9% saline; 3% saline; 10% dextran-40	ICP lower with 3% saline
Schmoker	(58)	Swine	4 mL·kg^{-1} of HSL or LRS as bolus, then HSL or LRS to restore MAP to baseline for 24 hours	ICP lower; brain water lower; CDO$_2$ greater in HSL animals
Whitley	(59)	Dogs	Small volume resuscitation with 7.2% saline; 20% HES	Regional CBF no different; ICP no different
Prough	(60)	Dogs	Small volume resuscitation with 7.2% saline; 20% HES; 20% HES in 7.2% saline	CBF transiently increased with 7.2% saline; no other important differences
Smith	(98)	Rats	HLS vs. LRS (volume-blood loss)	Shock increased brain water; fluid had little additional effect

HES = hydroxyethyl starch; CBF = cerebral blood flow; ICP = intracranial pressure; LRS = lactated Ringer's solution; HSL = hypertonic sodium lactate; CDO$_2$ = cerebral oxygen delivery; MAP = mean arterial pressure; HLS = hypertonic lactated saline.

with subdural mass lesions, 7.2% saline (6 mL·kg^{-1}) decreased ICP and increased CBF in the hemisphere adjacent to the balloon in comparison to 0.8% saline (54 mL·kg^{-1}) after hemorrhagic shock for 30 minutes accompanied by inflation of a subdural balloon (Table 12).[61] In dogs with an epidural balloon, 6.0% hydroxyethyl starch (20 mL·kg^{-1}) was associated with a lower ICP and a similar CBF after resuscitation from hemorrhage in comparison to dogs resuscitated with lactated Ringer's solution (60 mL·kg^{-1}), although the diluent (0.9% saline) for hydroxyethyl starch may have played a role.[62] In animals given a bolus for resuscitation followed by continued fluid

Table 11

Cerebral Effects of Hemorrhage and Resuscitation (Mass Lesion)

First Author	Reference Number	Species (Lesion(s))	Interventions	Observations
Prough	(61)	Dogs (subdural balloon)	0.8% saline (54 mL·kg⁻¹); 7.2% saline (6 mL·kg⁻¹)	7.2% saline decreased ICP, increased CBF in the lesioned hemisphere
Poole	(62)	Dogs (epidural balloon)	RS (60 mL·kg⁻¹); HES (20 mL·kg⁻¹)	Initial ICP lower in HES group, CBF no different
Whitley	(63)	Dogs (subdural balloon)	0.73% saline, with and without 10% pentastarch; 1.46% saline, with and without 10% pentastarch to maintain cardiac output	No effect of fluid choice on ICP or CBF
Gunnar	(64)	Dogs (epidural balloon)	0.9% saline; 3.0% saline; 10% dextran-40 for 2 hours after resuscitation	ICP lower with 3.0% saline; CBF similar in all groups
Gunnar	(65)	Dogs (epidural balloon)	0.9% saline; 3.0% saline; 10% dextran-40 for 2 hours after resuscitation	ICP lower, cerebral edema less with 3.0% saline; no difference in blood-brain barrier function
Ducey	(66)	Swine (epidural balloon)	Blood; 0.9% saline; 6.0% saline; 6.0% HES to normalized O_2	6.0% saline decreased ICP, improved intracranial elastance

ICP = intracranial pressure; CBF = cerebral blood flow; LRS = lactated Ringer's solution; HES = hydroxyethylstarch; DO_2 = systemic oxygen delivery.

infusion, the differences between hypertonic, hypotonic, and hyperoncotic fluids were lost.[63] In dogs subjected to hemorrhagic shock in the presence of a subdural balloon, then resuscitated with 0.73% saline or 1.46% saline, with or without 10% pentastarch, there were no effects noted on ICP or CBF; in fact, ICP rose inexorably throughout the 2 hours of post-insult resuscitation.[63] Gunnar et al.[64,65] resuscitated animals with 0.9% saline, 3.0% saline, or 10% dextran-40 after shock in the presence of an epidural balloon. There were no differences in CBF among the three groups and no differences in blood-brain barrier function, but ICP was lower[64,65] and cerebral edema was less[65] in animals that received 3.0% saline. In swine subjected to shock in the presence of an epidural balloon, Ducey et al. also demonstrated that hypertonic 6.0% saline decreased ICP and improved intracranial elastance.[66]

Table 12
Cerebral Oxygen Delivery (mean ± SEM)

	Group	Baseline	T15	T35	T95	T155
Right frontoparietal cortex (mL·100 g^{-1}· min^{-1})††	1 HS	9.4 ± 1.3	6.5 ± 0.9	9.1 ± 1.9	6.5 ± 0.7	5.1 ± 0.5
	1 SAL	7.7 ± 0.5	5.2 ± 0.3	5.0 ± 0.4	5.0 ± 0.2	5.6 ± 0.5[a]
	2 HS	9.9 ± 1.7	4.1 ± 1.6	4.8 ± 1.1	6.2 ± 2.0	3.9 ± 1.3
	2 SAL[b]	9.8 ± 1.7	2.0 ± 0.4	1.6 ± 0.8[c]	1.2 ± 0.6[c]	1.0 ± 0.6[d]
Right cerebral hemisphere (mL·100 g^{-1}· min^{-1})	1 HS	9.8 ± 1.1	6.7 ± 0.9	9.2 ± 1.8	7.2 ± 1.0	5.7 ± 0.7
	1 SAL	8.2 ± 0.6	5.6 ± 0.3	5.3 ± 0.4	5.5 ± 0.3	6.1 ± 0.5[a]
	2 HS	9.6 ± 1.6	4.5 ± 1.5	5.4 ± 1.1	5.8 ± 1.6	3.9 ± 1.2
	2 SAL[e]	8.8 ± 1.3	2.5 ± 0.5	2.1 ± 0.8[c,f]	1.5 ± 0.7[c,f]	1.2 ± 0.7[d,f]

Cerebral oxygen delivery in the right frontoparietal cortex and right cerebral hemisphere. Group 1 animals were subjected to hemorrhagic shock alone; Group 2 animals were subjected to hemorrhagic shock after inflation of a right hemispheric subdural balloon to 20 mm Hg. All animals were resuscitated with 7.2% saline (HS) or 0.8% saline (SAL).
[a] $P < 0.001$ T155 versus baseline; [b] $P < 0.06$ by ANOVA, group 2-SAL versus group 2-HS; [c] $P < 0.05$ group 2-SAL versus group 2-HS at specific interval; [d] $P = 0.0001$ T155 versus baseline; [e] $P < 0.01$ by ANOVA, group 2-SAL versus group 2-HS; [f] $P < 0.01$ group 1-SAL versus group 2-SAL.
Data from ref. 61 with permission.

Cerebral Effects of Hemorrhage and Resuscitation (Brain Injury)

A variety of investigators have studied a combination of hemorrhage, resuscitation, and brain injury, using models of forebrain ischemia, focal cryogenic injury, and fluid percussion injury (Table 13). In general, there are no differences in brain edema in lesioned brain as a consequence of the choice of resuscitation fluids. In rats subjected to forebrain ischemia, brain edema was similar at 6 and 24 hours in animals resuscitated with blood, hydroxyethyl starch, or 0.9% saline.[67] In animals with focal cryogenic injuries, small boluses of 7.5% saline, followed by hypertonic lactated saline, increased CBF and decreased ICP in comparison to animals that received dextran-70 or lactated Ringer's solution.[68] If lactated Ringer's solution or 7.5% saline were infused for 1 hour following resuscitation from shock to keep mean arterial pressure ≥80 mm Hg, hypertonic saline reduced ICP and brain water in the uninjured hemisphere.[69] In a complex model combining long-bone fractures, crush injury, and focal cerebral cryogenic injury, lactated Ringer's solution in 4.0% albumin resulted in comparable increases in ICP.[70]

In animals subjected to fluid percussion injury, perhaps the

Table 13
Cerebral Effects of Hemorrhage and Resuscitation (Brain Injury)

First Author	Reference Number	Species (Lesion(s))	Interventions	Observations
Warner	(67)	Rats (forebrain ischemia)	40% hemorrhage replaced by blood; HES; 0.9% saline (vol = shed blood)	No difference in edema at 6 or 24 hours
Walsh	(68)	Swine (cryogenic injury)	4 mL/kg bolus of LRS or 7.5% saline in 6.5% dextran-70, then LRS or HSL	7.5% saline/6.5% dextran-70 increased CBF, decreased ICP
Battistella	(69)	Sheep (cryogenic injury)	LRS or 7.5% saline after shock to keep MAP ≥ 80 mm Hg for 1 hr	7.5% saline decreased ICP, brain water (uninjured hemisphere)
Wisner	(70)	Sheep (fracture/crush injury plus cryogenic injury)	LRS or 4% albumin for 2 hr	ICP increased in both groups
Wisner	(71)	Rats (fluid percussion injury)	LRS vs. 6.5% saline	6.5% saline decreased brain water in uninjured, not injured brain
DeWitt	(72)	Cats (fluid percussion injury)	Isovolemic hemodilution with HES vs. resuscitation with shed blood or HES	Trauma, hemorrhage and resuscitation decreased CBF and EEG score
Prough	(73)	Cats (fluid percussion injury)	Resuscitation with 3.0% saline or 10% HES	3.0% saline increased ICP, did not increase CBF

HES = hydroxyethyl starch; LRS = lactated Ringer's solution; HSL = hypertonic sodium lactate; CBF = cerebral blood flow; ICP = intracranial pressure; MAP = mean arterial pressure; HES = hydroxyethylstarch; EEG = electroencephalogram.

best remaining model of closed head injury, hypertonic solutions have been shown to decrease brain water in uninjured but not injured brain. Wisner et al.[71] compared lactated Ringer's solution to 6.5% saline and demonstrated that hypertonic saline decreases brain water in uninjured but not injured brain. DeWitt et al.[72] demonstrated that isovolemic hemodilution with hydroxyethyl starch failed to improve either the CBF or electroencephalographic score.[72] In a similar model, resuscitation with 3.0% saline improved ICP in comparison to 10% hydroxyethyl starch, but did not improve CBF.[73]

Table 14
TCDB Data: Outcome by Secondary Insult at Time of Arrival at TCDB Hospital ER*

Secondary Insults	Number of Patients	Percentage of Patients	Good or Moderate	Severe or Vegetative	Dead
Total Cases	699	100	43	21	37
Neither	456	65	51	22	27
Hypoxia	78	11	45	22	33
Hypotension	113	16	26	14	60
Both	52	7	6	19	75

Hypoxia = PaO_2 <60 mm Hg; hypotension = systolic blood pressure <90 mm Hg; TCDB = Traumatic Coma Data Bank
* Reprinted with permission from Chesnut et al.[75]

Fluid Administration

How Much Fluid?

Hypovolemic hypotension is associated with increased mortality of head-injured patients[74,75] (Table 14). Although shock sometimes occurs in association with an isolated head injury, hypotension due to associated injuries is more common.[76] Such injuries include intra-abdominal hemorrhage (evaluated by CT scan or diagnostic peritoneal lavage), intrathoracic hemorrhage (evaluated by chest radiography, CT scan, or aortography), long-bone fractures (assessed using the skeletal survey), myocardial ischemia or cardiac decompensation (evaluated using electrocardiography or pulmonary arterial catheterization), pericardial tamponade (suggested by a paradoxical pulse, central venous or pulmonary artery pressure monitoring, chest radiography, echocardiography, or pericardiocentesis), and, particularly in children, intracranial or scalp hemorrhage (evident from inspection or CT scan). The outcome of resuscitation from associated injuries may be dependent on the adequacy of resuscitation. Considerable clinical evidence now supports the hypothesis that clinically inapparent tissue hypoperfusion accompanies critical surgical illness[77,78] and that restoration of optimal levels of oxygen delivery improves survival and limits morbidity.[79–81]

The experimentally traumatized brain is uniquely vulnerable to hypotension.[82] In experimentally head-injured cats, hypotension decreases CBF and increases ICP[83,84] (Figs. 4a, b). Rosner has postulated that plateau waves (sustained, severe increases in ICP) may

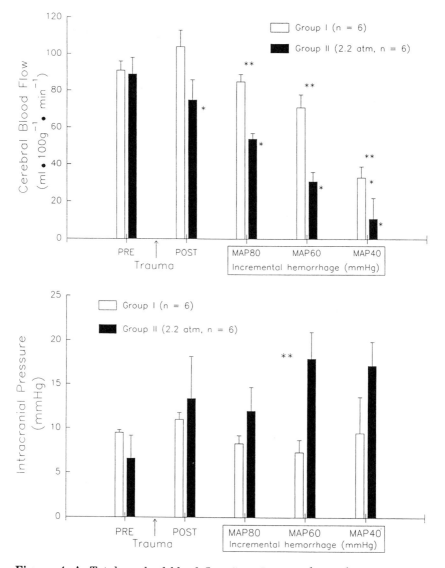

Figure 4. A. Total cerebral blood flow (in mL·100 g^{-1}·min^{-1}) in group I (control) and group II (2.2 atmospheres of fluid percussion head injury) in response to reduction of mean arterial pressure (MAP, in mm Hg) to 80, 60, and 40 mm Hg by hemorrhagic shock. *P < 0.05 in comparison to pretrauma baseline (PRE); **P < 0.05 in comparison to control group I. Permission from DeWitt.[84] **Figure 4B.** Intracranial pressure (ICP; in mm Hg) in group I (control) and group II (2.2 atmospheres of fluid percussion head injury) in

be precipitated by small decreases in mean arterial pressure.[85,86] Consequently, he has proposed that part of the initial treatment of increased ICP in head-injured patients should be to increase mean arterial pressure.[86] Based on available evidence, the viability of the traumatized brain is best served by prompt, effective treatment of hypotension.

How much fluid can be safely administered to a head-injured patient? Current evidence suggests that sufficient fluid should be administered to hypotensive patients to restore adequate blood pressure and systemic oxygen delivery and that maintenance fluids can be administered in sufficient quantities to avoid subsequent hypovolemia and to deliver adequate electrolytes and nutrition.

How Should the Effects of Fluid Administration be Monitored?

Blood pressure, a common end-point used during routine clinical resuscitation, may remain misleadingly high despite progressively declining cardiac output, as intravascular volume declines. Severely traumatized patients with hypovolemia may be monitored with a central venous pressure catheter or a pulmonary artery catheter, either or which provides an estimate of filling pressure. However, central venous pressure and pulmonary aortic occlusion pressure (PAOP) are determined by complex interactions among blood volume, venous capacitance, and ventricular distensibility, contractility, and afterload.

Intermittent determinations of cardiac output with thermodilution have been used to calculate systemic oxygen delivery as a physiological end-point for resuscitation of high-risk surgical patients. Certain data suggest that this approach to hemodynamic management may improve survival and decrease morbidity, compared with conventional management, which uses blood pressure or filling pressures to guide therapy.[79,81]

Clinical estimations of cerebral hemodynamics are difficult. A patient able to follow simple commands, even if stuporous or lethargic, rarely has a raised ICP. Approximately 40% to 50% of head-

◄───

response to reduction of mean arterial pressure (MAP, in mm Hg) to 80, 60, and 40 mm Hg by hemorrhagic shock. **$P < 0.05$ in comparison to control group I. Permission from DeWitt.[84]

injured patients with altered consciousness have intracranial hypertension. The symptoms and signs of raised ICP are not, however, uniformly reliable. In unconscious patients, the probability of increased ICP is lower if the patient withdraws, moans, or grimaces in response to painful stimuli than if motor responses are worse. A frankly raised ICP is likely to be encountered with a Glasgow Coma Scale score of 4 to 6. Severe increases in ICP may present as Cushing's triad of hypertension, bradycardia, and respiratory irregularity; but the absence of Cushing's triad does not rule out intracranial hypertension. Pupillary dilatation may herald transtentorial herniation, but is a late manifestation of central herniation. Herniation, which could be a result of vascular insufficiency or direct compression and infarction of the brain stem, is a major catastrophe, almost synonymous with imminent, extensive, and fatal brain damage.

Monitoring of ICP or other variables related to the adequacy of cerebral circulation in the immediate post-resuscitation interval may exert a favorable effect on outcome after acute head injury in conjunction with multiple trauma. Death in patients with head injuries correlates with the severity of intracranial hypertension. If ICP exceeds 20 mm Hg but can be reduced, the mortality rate approaches 45%; if ICP exceeds 20 mm Hg and cannot be reduced, the mortality rate is 95%.[74] However, current recommendations that ICP be monitored in head-injured patients in whom the Glasgow Coma Scale score is ≤8 require no alteration based on fluid therapy.

Because therapy with fluids of a wide variety of tonicities and colloid concentrations has been associated with intracranial hypertension and gradually declining CBF during resuscitation, other techniques of improving systemic perfusion require further investigation. Particular attention should be paid to the possibility that positive inotropic agents might improve cardiac output and systemic oxygen transport while exerting less deleterious effects than aggressive fluid resuscitation on the cerebral circulation. Rosner et al. have suggested that therapy of head-injured patients should be directed toward maintaining CPP, with proportionately less attention directed at reducing ICP.[86]

Summary

Considerable information is available to guide fluid therapy in head-injured patients. Restoration of systemic hemodynamic stability is essential. Rapid, acute administration of hypotonic fluids should be avoided in patients at risk for intracranial hypertension. Acute resuscitation with 0.9% saline, blood, or colloid dissolved in 0.9% saline is unlikely to aggravate intracranial hypotension. Hypertonic solutions exert favorable effects in most animal models, but have yet to achieve wide clinical use.

References

1. Weed LH, McKibben PS: Experimental alteration of brain bulk. Am J Physiol 48:531–558, 1919.
2. Lanier WL, Stangland KJ, Scheithauer BW, et al: The effects of dextrose infusion and head position on neurologic outcome after complete cerebral ischemia in primates: examination of a model. Anesthesiology 66: 39–48, 1987.
3. Longstreth WT, Jr., Diehr P, Cobb LA, et al: Neurologic outcome and blood glucose levels during out-of-hospital cardiopulmonary resuscitation. Neurology 36:1186–1191, 1986.
4. Lam AM, Winn HR, Cullen BF, et al: Hyperglycemia and neurological outcome in patients with head injury. J Neurosurg 75:545–551, 1991.
5. Traverso LW, Bellamy RF, Hollenbach SJ, et al: Hypertonic sodium chloride solutions: effect on hemodynamics and survival after hemorrhage in swine. J Trauma 27:32–39, 1987.
6. Velasco IT, Pontieri V, Rocha e Silva M, Jr., et al: Hyperosmotic NaCl and severe hemorrhagic shock. Am J Physiol 239:H664–H673, 1980.
7. Jelenko C, III, Williams JB, Wheeler ML, et al: Studies in shock and resuscitation. I. Use of a hypertonic, albumin-containing fluid demand regimen (HALFD) in resuscitation. Crit Care Med 7:157–167, 1979.
8. Monafo WW, Chuntrasakul C, Ayvazian VH: Hypertonic sodium solutions in the treatment of burn shock. Am J Surg 126:778–783, 1973.
9. Shackford SR, Sise MJ, Fridlund PH, et al: Hypertonic sodium lactate versus lactated Ringer's solution for intravenous fluid therapy in operations on the abdominal aorta. Surgery 94:41–51, 1983.
10. Gunn ML, Hansbrough JF, Davis JW, et al: Prospective, randomized trial of hypertonic sodium lactate versus lactated Ringer's solution for burn shock resuscitation. J Trauma 29:1261–1267, 1989.
11. Shackford SR, Fortlage DA, Peters RM, et al: Serum osmolar and electrolyte changes associated with large infusions of hypertonic sodium lactate for intravascular volume expansion of patients undergoing aortic reconstruction. Surg Gynecol Obstet 164:127–136, 1987.
12. Worthley LIG, Cooper DJ, Jones N: Treatment of resistant intracranial hypertension with hypertonic saline: Report of two cases. J Neurosurg 68:478–481, 1988.
13. Schertel ER, Valentine AK, Rademakers AM, et al: Influence of 7% NaCl on the mechanical properties of the systemic circulation in the hypovolemic dog. Circ Shock 31:203–214, 1990.
14. Spital A, Sterns RD: The paradox of sodium's volume of distribution: Why an extracellular solute appears to distribute over total body water. Arch Intern Med 149:1255–1257, 1989.

15. Smith GJ, Kramer GC, Perron P, et al: A comparison of several hypertonic solutions for resuscitation of bled sheep. J Surg Res 39:517–528, 1985.
16. Mattox KL, Maningas PA, Moore EE, et al: Prehospital hypertonic saline/dextran infusion for post-traumatic hypotension. The U.S.A. Multicenter Trial. Ann Surg 213:482–491, 1991.
17. Vassar MJ, Perry CA, Gannaway WL, et al: 7.5% sodium chloride/dextran for resuscitation of trauma patients undergoing helicopter transport. Arch Surg 126:1065–1072, 1991.
18. Vassar MJ, Fischer RP, O'Brien PE, et al: A multicenter trial for resuscitation of injured patients with 7.5% sodium chloride: The effect of added dextran-70. Arch Surg 128:1003–1013, 1993.
19. Gross D, Landau EH, Klin B, et al: Treatment of uncontrolled hemorrhagic shock with hypertonic saline solution. Surg Gynecol Obstet 170: 106–112, 1990.
20. Bickell WH, Wall MJ, Jr., Pepe PE, et al: Immediate versus delayed fluid resuscitation for hypotensive patients with penetrating torso injuries. N Engl J Med 331:1105–1109, 1994.
21. Arfors KE, Buckley PB: Role of artificial colloids in rational fluid therapy. In Tuma RF, White JV, Messmer K (eds): The Role of Hemodilution in Optimal Patient Care. Zuckschwerdt W, Verlag, 1989, pp 100–123.
22. Dodd RY: The risk of transfusion-transmitted infection. N Engl J Med 327:419–421, 1992.
23. Stump DC, Strauss RG, Henriksen RA, et al: Effects of hydroxyethyl starch on blood coagulation, particularly factor VIII. Transfusion 25: 349–354, 1985.
24. Wilson BJ, Jones RF, Coleman ST, et al: The effects of various hypertonic sodium salt solutions on cisternal pressure. Surgery 30:361–366, 1951.
25. Fisher B, Thomas D, Peterson B: Hypertonic saline lowers raised intracranial pressure in children after head trauma. J Neurosurg Anesth 4: 4–10, 1992.
26. McManus ML, Strange K: Acute volume regulation of brain cells in response to hypertonic challenge. Anesthesiology 78:1132–1137, 1993.
27. Shapira Y, Artru AA, Qassam N, et al: Brain edema and neurologic status with rapid infusion of 0.9% saline or 5% dextrose after head trauma. J Neurosurg Anesth 7:17–25, 1995.
28. Shapira Y, Artru AA, Cotev S, et al: Brain edema and neurologic status following head trauma in the rat: No effect from large volumes of isotonic or hypertonic intravenous fluids, with or without glucose. Anesthesiology 77:79–85, 1992.
29. Morse ML, Milstein JM, Haas JE, et al: Effect of hydration on experimentally induced cerebral edema. Crit Care Med 13:563–565, 1985.
30. Albright AL, Latchaw RE, Robinson AG: Intracranial and systemic effects of hetastarch in experimental cerebral edema. Crit Care Med 12: 496–500, 1984.
31. Wood JH, Simeone FA, Fink EA, et al: Hypervolemic hemodilution in experimental focal cerebral ischemia: Elevation of cardiac output, re-

gional cortical blood flow, and ICP after intravascular volume expansion with low molecular weight dextran. J Neurosurg 59:500–509, 1983.

32. Schell RM, Cole DJ, Schultz RL, et al: Temporary cerebral ischemia. Effects of pentastarch or albumin on reperfusion injury. Anesthesiology 77:86–92, 1992.

33. Goulin GD, Duthie SE, Zornow MH, et al: Global cerebral ischemia: Effects of pentastarch following reperfusion. Anesth Analg 79: 1036–1042, 1994.

34. Hudak ML, Jones D, Jr., Popel AS, et al: Hemodilution causes size-dependent constriction of pial arterioles in the cat. Am J Physiol 257: H912–H917, 1989.

35. Todd MM, Tommasino C, Moore S: Cerebral effects of isovolemic hemodilution with a hypertonic saline solution. J Neurosurg 63:944–948, 1985.

36. Coyle JT, Puttfarcken P: Oxidative stress, glutamate, and neurodegenerative disorders. Science 262:689–693, 1993.

37. Putney JW, Jr: Excitement about calcium signaling in inexcitable cells. Science 262:676–678, 1993.

38. von Kummer R, Scharf J, Back T, et al: Autoregulatory capacity and the effect of isovolemic hemodilution on local cerebral blood flow. Stroke 19:594–59, 1988.

39. Hino A, Ueda S, Mizukawa N, et al: Effect of hemodilution on cerebral hemodynamics and oxygen metabolism. Stroke 23:423–426, 1992.

40. Tommasino C, Moore S, Todd MM: Cerebral effects of isovolemic hemodilution with crystalloid or colloid solutions. Crit Care Med 16:862–868, 1988.

41. Zornow MH, Scheller MS, Shackford SR: Effect of a hypertonic lactated Ringer's solution on intracranial pressure and cerebral water content in a model of traumatic brain injury. J Trauma 29:484–488, 1989.

42. Zornow MH, Scheller MS, Todd MM, et al: Acute cerebral effects of isotonic crystalloid and colloid solutions following cryogenic brain injury in the rabbit. Anesthesiology 69:180–184, 1988.

43. Hyodo A, Heros RC, Tu Y, et al: Acute effects of isovolemic hemodilution with crystalloids in a canine model of focal cerebral ischemia. Stroke 20:534–540, 1989.

44. Tu Y, Heros RC, Candia G, et al: Isovolemic hemodilution in experimental focal cerebral ischemia. Part I: Effects on hemodynamics, hemorheology, and intracranial pressure. J Neurosurg 69:72–81, 1988.

45. Cole DJ, Schell RM, Drummond JC, et al: Focal cerebral ischemia in rats. Effect of hypervolemic hemodilution with diaspirin cross-linked hemoglobin versus albumin on brain injury and edema. Anesthesiology 78:335–342, 1993.

46. Raff MC, Barres BA, Burne JF, et al: Programmed cell death and the control of cell survival: lessons from the nervous system. Science 262: 695–700, 1993.

47. Korosue K, Heros RC, Ogilvy CS, et al: Comparison of crystalloids and colloids for hemodilution in a model of focal cerebral ischemia. J Neurosurg 73:576–584, 1990.

48. Korosue K, Heros RC: Mechanism of cerebral blood flow augmentation by hemodilution in rabbits. Stroke 23:1487–1493, 1992.
49. Vorstrup S, Andersen A, Juhler M, et al: Hemodilution increases cerebral blood flow in acute ischemic stroke. Stroke 20:884–889, 1989.
50. Korosue K, Ishida K, Matsuoka H, et al: Clinical, hemodynamic, and hemorheological effects of isovolemic hemodilution in acute cerebral infarction. Neurosurgery 23:148–153, 1988.
51. Zornow MH, Todd MM, Moore SS: The acute cerebral effects of changes in plasma osmolality and oncotic pressure. Anesthesiology 67:936–941, 1987.
52. Kaieda R, Todd MM, Cook LN, et al: Acute effects of changing plasma osmolality and colloid oncotic pressure on the formation of brain edema after cryogenic injury. Neurosurgery 24:671–678, 1989.
53. Kaieda R, Todd MM, Warner DS: Prolonged reduction in colloid oncotic pressure does not increase brain edema following cryogenic injury in rabbits. Anesthesiology 71:554–560, 1989.
54. Prough DS, Johnson JC, Stump DA, et al: Effects of hypertonic saline versus lactated Ringer's solution on cerebral oxygen transport during resuscitation from hemorrhagic shock. J Neurosurg 64:627–632, 1986.
55. Prough DS, Johnson JC, Poole GV, Jr., et al: Effects on intracranial pressure of resuscitation from hemorrhagic shock with hypertonic saline versus lactated Ringer's solution. Crit Care Med 13:407–411, 1985.
56. Poole GV, Jr., Johnson JC, Prough DS, et al: Cerebral hemodynamics after hemorrhagic shock: effects of the type of resuscitation fluid. Crit Care Med 14:629–633, 1986.
57. Gunnar WP, Merlotti GJ, Jonasson O, et al: Resuscitation from hemorrhagic shock: alterations of the intracranial pressure after normal saline, 3% saline and Dextran-40. Ann Surg 204:686–692, 1986.
58. Schmoker JD, Zhuang J, Shackford SR: Hypertonic fluid resuscitation improves cerebral oxygen delivery and reduces intracranial pressure after hemorrhagic shock. J Trauma 31:1607–1613, 1991.
59. Whitley JM, Prough DS, Taylor CL, et al: Cerebrovascular effects of small volume resuscitation from hemorrhagic shock: comparison of hypertonic saline and concentrated hydroxethyl starch in dogs. J Neurosurg Anesth 3:47–55, 1991.
60. Prough DS, Whitley JM, Olympio MA, et al: Hypertonic/hyperoncotic fluid resuscitation after hemorrhagic shock in dogs. Anesth Analg 73: 738–744, 1991.
61. Prough DS, Whitley JM, Taylor CL, et al: Regional cerebral blood flow following resuscitation from hemorrhagic shock with hypertonic saline: Influence of a subdural mass. Anesthesiology 75:319–327, 1991.
62. Poole GV, Jr., Prough DS, Johnson JC, et al: Effects of resuscitation from hemorrhagic shock on cerebral hemodynamics in the presence of an intracranial mass. J Trauma 27:18–23, 1987.
63. Whitley JM, Prough DS, Brockschmidt JK, et al: Cerebral hemodynamic effects of fluid resuscitation in the presence of an experimental intracranial mass. Surgery 110:514–522, 1991.
64. Gunnar W, Kane J, Barrett J: Cerebral blood flow following hypertonic saline resuscitation in an experimental model of hemorrhagic shock and head injury. Braz J Med Biol Res 22:287–289, 1989.

65. Gunnar W, Jonasson O, Merlotti G, et al: Head injury and hemorrhagic shock: studies of the blood-brain barrier and intracranial pressure after resuscitation with normal saline solution, 3% saline solution, and dextran-40. Surgery 103:398–407, 1988.

66. Ducey JP, Mozingo DW, Lamiell JM, et al: A comparison of the cerebral and cardiovascular effects of complete resuscitation with isotonic and hypertonic saline, hetastarch, and whole blood following hemorrhage. J Trauma 29:1510–1518, 1989.

67. Warner DS, Boehland LA: Effects of iso-osmolal intravenous fluid therapy on post-ischemic brain water content in the rat. Anesthesiology 68: 86–91, 1988.

68. Walsh JC, Zhuang J, Shackford SR: A comparison of hypertonic to isotonic fluid in the resuscitation of brain injury and hemorrhagic shock. J Surg Res 50:284–292, 1991.

69. Battistella FD, Wisner DH: Combined hemorrhagic shock and head injury: effects of hypertonic saline (7.5%) resuscitation. J Trauma 31: 182–188, 1991.

70. Wisner DH, Busche F, Sturm J, et al: Traumatic shock and head injury: effects of fluid resuscitation on the brain. J Surg Res 46:49–59, 1989.

71. Wisner DH, Schuster L, Quinn C: Hypertonic saline resuscitation of head injury: effects on cerebral water content. J Trauma 30:75–78, 1990.

72. DeWitt DS, Prough DS, Taylor CL, et al: Reduced cerebral blood flow, oxygen delivery, and electroencephalographic activity after traumatic brain injury and mild hemorrhage in cats. J Neurosurg 76:812–821, 1992.

73. Prough DS, DeWitt DS, Taylor CL, et al: Hypertonic saline does not reduce intracranial pressure or improve cerebral blood flow after experimental head injury and hemorrhage in cats. Anesthesiology 75 (Suppl 3A) :A5441991.

74. Miller JD, Butterworth JF, Gudeman SK, et al: Further experience in the management of severe head injury. J Neurosurg 54:289–299, 1981.

75. Chesnut RM, Marshall LF, Klauber MR, et al: The role of secondary brain injury in determining outcome from severe head injury. J Trauma 34:216–222, 1993.

76. Butterworth JF, IV, Maull KI, Miller JD, et al: Detection of occult abdominal trauma in patients with severe head injuries. Lancet 2: 759–762, 1980.

77. Bland RD, Shoemaker WC: Probability of survival as a prognostic and severity of illness score in critically ill surgical patients. Crit Care Med 13:91–95, 1985.

78. Bland RD, Shoemaker WC, Abraham E, et al: Hemodynamic and oxygen transport patterns in surviving and nonsurviving postoperative patients. Crit Care Med 13:85–90, 1985.

79. Shoemaker WC, Appel PL, Kram HB, et al: Prospective trial of supranormal values of survivors as therapeutic goals in high-risk surgical patients. Chest 94:1176–1186, 1988.

80. Shah DM, Gottlieb ME, Rahm RL, et al: Failure of red blood cell transfusion to increase oxygen transport or mixed venous PO_2 in injured patients. J Trauma 22:741–746, 1982.

81. Boyd O, Grounds RM, Bennett ED: A randomized clinical trial of the effect of deliberate perioperative increase of oxygen delivery on mortality in high-risk surgical patients. JAMA 270:2699–2707, 1993.
82. Ishige N, Pitts LH, Berry I, et al: The effects of hypovolemic hypotension on high-energy phosphate metabolism of traumatized brain in rats. J Neurosurg 68:129–136, 1988.
83. Lewelt W, Jenkins LW, Miller JD: Autoregulation of cerebral blood flow after experimental fluid percussion injury of the brain. J Neurosurg 53:500–511, 1980.
84. DeWitt DS, Prough DS, Taylor CL, et al: Regional cerebrovascular responses to progressive hypotension after traumatic brain injury in cats. Am J Physiol 32:H1276–H1284, 1992.
85. Rosner MJ, Becker DP: Origin and evolution of plateau waves: experimental observations and a theoretical model. J Neurosurg 60:312–324, 1984.
86. Rosner MJ, Daughton S: Cerebral perfusion pressure management in head injury. J Trauma 30:933–940, 1990.
87. Carlson RW, Rattan S, Haupt MT: Fluid resuscitation in conditions of increased permeability. Anaesthesiol Rev 17:14 1990.
88. Rackow EC, Mecher C, Astiz ME, et al: Effects of pentastarch and albumin infusion on cardiorespiratory function and coagulation in patients with severe sepsis and systemic hypoperfusion. Crit Care Med 17:394–398, 1989.
89. Davies MJ: The role of colloids in blood conservation. Int Anesthesiol Clin 28:205–209, 1990.
90. Wilson BJ, Jones RF, Coleman ST, et al: The effects of various hypertonic sodium salt solutions on cisternal pressure. Surgery 30:361, 1958.
91. Albright AL, Latchaw RE, Robinson AG: Intracranial and systemic effects of osmotic and oncotic therapy in experimental cerebral edema. J Neurosurg 60:481–489, 1984.
92. Wood JH, Snyder LL, Simeone FA: Failure of intravascular volume expansion without hemodilution to elevate cortical blood flow in region of experimental focal ischemia. J Neurosurg 56:80–91, 1982.
93. Michenfelder JD, Theye RA: The effects of profound hypocapnia and dilutional anemia on canine cerebral metabolism and blood flow. Anesthesiology 31:449–457, 1969.
94. Martin JB: Molecular genetics of neurological diseases. Science 262:674–676, 1993.
95. Hindman BJ, Funatsu N, Cheng DCH, et al: Differential effect of oncotic pressure on cerebral and extracerebral water content during cardiopulmonary bypass in rabbits. Anesthesiology 73:951–957, 1990.
96. Muizelaar JP, Bouma GJ, Levasseur JE, et al: Effect of hematocrit variations on cerebral blood flow and basilar artery diameter in vivo. Am J Physiol 262:H949–H954, 1992.
97. Tu Y, Heros RC, Karacostas D, et al: Isovolemic hemodilution in experimental focal cerebral ischemia. Part 2: Effects on regional cerebral blood flow and size of infarction. J Neurosurg 69:82–91, 1988.
98. Smith SD, Cone JB, Bowser BH, et al: Cerebral edema following acute hemorrhage in a murine model: the role of crystalloid resuscitation. J Trauma 22:588–590, 1982.

8

Diagnostic Imaging in Neurotrauma

Susan G. Kaplan, MD

Introduction

Trauma is the third most common cause of mortality in the United States, the leading cause of death in adults under the age of 40, and fifth in those over the age of 65. Fifty-four percent of trauma-related fatalities are caused by motor vehicle accidents, 24% by motorcycle accidents, 17% by auto-pedestrian accidents, and 5% from falls, jumps, and assaults.[1]

The leading cause of death in trauma is craniocerebral injury. Smirniotopolis and colleagues[2] report that 8 million cases of head trauma occur annually in the United States. Approximately 500,000 are considered major, and of these, more than 250,000 are considered to have injury severe enough to warrant emergency medical treatment. Peak incidence occurs in young adults from 15 to 24 years of age.[3] Vehicular accidents account for the majority of deaths, while alcohol consumption,[4,5] drugs,[6] missiles, and use of instruments such

From *Trauma Anesthesia and Critical Care of Neurological Injury,* edited by K. J. Abrams and C. M. Grande. © 1997, Futura Publishing Co., Armonk, NY.

Table 1
Imaging Modalities Available for Diagnosis of
Traumatic Brain Injury and Spinal Cord Injury

Plain film radiography
Conventional tomography ("tomos")
Computed tomography (CT)
Angiography
Digital intravenous angiography (DIVA)
Digital subtraction angiography (DSA)
Intraarterial digital subtraction angiography (IADSA)
Intraoperative sonography (IOS)
Intraoperative spinal sonography (IOSS)
Myelography
CT-myelography
Magnetic resonance imaging (MRI)
Radionuclide scanning

as baseball bats,[7] has significantly increased the overall incidence of craniocerebral injury.

Rapid diagnosis and treatment is implicit in improving survival and outcome. Current imaging modalities (Table 1), especially computed tomography (CT), have revolutionized the care of head trauma victims during all phases of management.[8–11] "Ideally, all patients sent to the CT scanner for evaluation of craniocerebral injury are hemodynamically and neurologically stable. In actuality, patients often have multisystem injury in association with head injury and may have ongoing neurologic deterioration." . . . It is *imperative* that adequately trained . . . personnel accompany the patient . . . to monitor vital signs and look for evidence of systemic or neurologic deterioration."[12]

The presence of specially trained traumatologists who are capable of maintaining ongoing resuscitation and monitoring as studies are completed, has allowed adequate evaluation of critically ill patients and has significantly improved the accuracy of surgical intervention and survival in many victims. This chapter is intended to familiarize trauma anesthesiologists with the methods and anesthetic requirements inherent to performing perioperative diagnostic procedures.

Radiological Diagnosis of Neurotrauma

Plain film radiography, computed tomography, and angiography are the primary imaging modalities used in the early evaluation and diagnosis of traumatic brain injury (TBI) and spinal cord injury (SCI). Conventional tomography, magnetic resonance imaging (MRI), radionuclide scanning, and ultrasound are frequently used during the nonacute, subacute, and chronic phases of TBI and SCI.

Initial plain film imaging in acute neurological injury is ideally performed during the "golden hour"[13] of care and consists of a single cross-table lateral view of the cervical spine exposed during ongoing resuscitation (Fig. 1). The anteroposterior (AP) open-mouth view is important as an adjunct to the lateral radiograph to identify abnormalities of C1 and C2 (Fig. 2). If cervical injury is suspected clinically or radiographically, further imaging studies are performed once the patient is hemodynamically stable. The neck is maintained, *at all times,* in a neutral position[14] until all appropriate studies have been completed and interpreted by a qualified radiologist.

In addition to plain films, CT and angiography are often performed on neurotrauma victims. High-quality radiographs are generally obtained in the emergency unit, whereas CT and angiography require patient movement and transport. Ideally, the CT scanner or angiography suite should be adjacent to the emergency unit, although more often than not it is far removed from the triage unit or operating room. A trauma anesthesiologist or certified registered nurse anesthetist should accompany the patient to the CT scanner and angiography suite to provide ongoing monitoring and resuscitation in critical cases.

Imaging of head injuries generally takes precedence over imaging of other acute injuries,[15] although diagnostic imaging of any organ system should **never** take priority over resuscitative efforts. If immediate operative intervention of *any* injury is required, the patient should be transported to the operating suite and imaging studies delayed. The anesthesiologist should assume that intracranial and cervical spine injury has occurred and anesthetic management should proceed accordingly.

CT scanning is generally preferred over MRI in early diagnosis of neurotrauma. During MRI, there is limited visibility of and access to the patient within the bore of the magnet,[16] monitoring equipment frequently causes degradation of MRI images, fresh hemorrhage cannot be adequately differentiated from contiguous cerebral gray matter (signal intensity of unclotted or newly clotted blood is equivalent to that of normal brain),[17] and bone is poorly visualized, making fractures difficult to detect. In addition, valuable time may be wasted while obtaining the necessary history and positioning the patient within the magnet. If further imaging studies are required for diag-

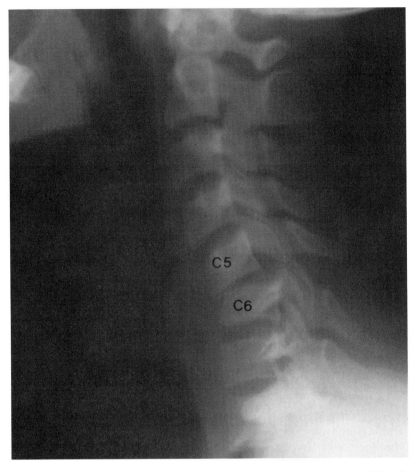

Figure 1. Cervical spine, lateral radiograph. Twenty-eight-year-old male with hyperflexion injury of the neck after a motor vehicle accident. Note the anterior subluxation of C5 on C6. Forces of this magnitude cause severe ligamentous damage. Complete disruption of the posterior longitudinal ligament and interspinous ligament was found at the time of surgery.

nosis, radionuclide scanning, myelography, CT myelography, and intraoperative cranial and spinal cord ultrasonography should be considered.

Although it is not used extensively in the evaluation of acute trauma, MRI is the imaging modality of choice in the evaluation of

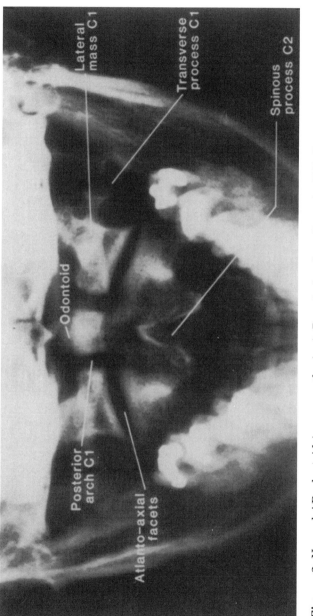
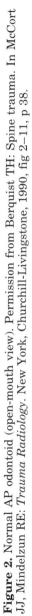

Figure 2. Normal AP odontoid (open-mouth view). Permission from Berquist TH: Spine trauma. In McCort JJ, Mindelzun RE: *Trauma Radiology*. New York, Churchill-Livingstone, 1990, fig 2–11, p 38.

Table 2
Contrast Media for Neurodiagnostic Imaging

Intravenous Agents
  Ionic agents (diatrizoate compounds)
  Nonionic agents (iohexol, iopamidol, iatrol)
  Gadolinium (gadopentatate dimeglumine, Gd-DTPA)
Intrathecal Agents
  Pantopaque (oil-based medium)
  Metrizamide (water-soluble medium)
  Nonionic agents (iohexol, iopamidol, iatrol)
  Gas (air)

subacute and chronic neurological injuries.[18] MRI provides exquisite detail of shearing and diffuse axonal injury, cerebral contusion, subacute and chronic hemorrhage, edema, mass effect, and post-traumatic spinal cysts. There is no ionizing radiation and images can be constructed in multiple planes. The major drawbacks are cost and time.

Contrast Media

Radiopaque contrast media are used to enhance and differentiate adjacent soft tissues (Table 2). Contrast medium is also used to localize hemorrhage and to assess vascular integrity and anatomy. Both intravenous and intrathecal agents are available. Iodinated ionic and nonionic agents are used for CT, angiography, digital angiography, and myelography, while gadopentatate dimeglumine is used for MRI. Air, fat, and fluid act as natural contrast agents.

Intravenous Agents

Iodinated, radiopaque contrast media were introduced in 1929 and are ionic, hyperosmolar derivatives of triiodobenzoic acid.[19] Contrast agents are peripheral vasodilators, and because of significant hyperosmolarity, act as osmotic diuretics. Intravascular injection is by bolus technique, continuous infusion, or by infusion under high pressure for rapid serial examination. Elimination is via the kidney. Patients with limited renal function should not routinely receive intravenous contrast.

Side effects occur frequently after contrast injection and can be mild, moderate, or severe. Hemodynamic alterations are more common in the elderly, and patients medicated with calcium channel blockers present a unique problem. Morris and colleagues[20] report potentiation of the normal hypotensive response to contrast injection by the vasodilatory effects of nifedipine and diltiazem. Heat sensation, caused by rapid vasodilation, localized erythema, nausea and vomiting, and pruritus are frequent side effects and generally require no therapy. Moderate reactions, including mild hypotension, bradycardia, and urticaria, may require symptomatic treatment. Cardiovascular changes usually resolve with intravenous hydration and slight Trendelburg positioning, although intravenous atropine may be necessary. Urticaria usually responds to oral or intravenous diphenhydramine. More serious reactions such as bronchospasm, wheezing, dyspnea, severe hypotension, and tachycardia require aggressive intervention to prevent cardiovascular collapse.[21] Life-threatening reactions are fortunately rare, although cardiac arrest has been reported.[22,23] Pretreatment with steroids and phenothiazines has been met with variable success.

Nonionic contrast agents (iohexol, iopamidol, and iotrol) were introduced in the 1980s and are available for both intravenous and intrathecal use.[24] These newer agents more closely approximate blood osmolality and are associated with fewer adverse reactions than ionic contrast media. The major drawback is cost.

Gadopentatate dimeglumine, formerly called gadolinium-DTPA (Gd-DTPA),[25] enhances contrast for MRI. Gadolinium (Gd^{+3}) is from the lanthanide series of rare earth elements and is highly paramagnetic.[26] It is nontoxic to the human body and is rapidly excreted by the kidneys ($T_{1/2}$ 20 min).[27] Pharmacokinetic behavior is similar to that of the iodinated agents.

Intrathecal Agents

Intrathecal agents are used to enhance contrast studies of the spinal cord. Myelography consists of the injection of a radiopaque contrast substance into the subarachnoid space via cervical[28] or lumbar puncture, and was introduced in the 1940s using Pantopaque,[29] which is an oil-based contrast medium. Pantopaque is not miscible with cerebrospinal fluid (CSF) and is moved throughout the spinal canal by tilting the patient on a specialized fluoroscopy table and allowing gravity-assisted flow. The substance is introduced through a large bore (18-gauge) spinal needle and must be removed via the original lumbar or cervical puncture. It is mildly irritating if left in the subarachnoid space and adhesive arachnoiditis has been reported.[30] Blood in the CSF, which potentiates this irritating effect, is an absolute contraindication to using this agent.[31]

Metrizamide,[32] a water-soluble, iodinated contrast agent, was introduced for intrathecal use in the 1970s and rapidly replaced the oily medium. Metrizamide mixes easily with CSF and can be instilled using smaller caliber needles. Absorption is via spinal and arachnoid granules,[33] eliminating the need for manual removal. Metrizamide is safe to use in the presence of intrathecal hemorrhage. Mild transient reactions are common and include meningeal irritation and visual and auditory disturbances. Seizures have been reported.[34] Phenothiazines lower the seizure threshold and are therefore contraindicated in the treatment of metrizamide-induced nausea and vomiting.[35] There are no know long-term effects associated with the use of metrizamide.

Nonionic contrast agents are gradually replacing metrizamide for intrathecal use. Iopamidol, iohexol, and iotrol are reported to have fewer and less serious adverse reactions[36] than metrizamide, although cost is a limiting factor. The newer agents are significantly more expensive than the other available contrast agents.

Pneumoencephalography uses air as a contrast medium. The procedure is difficult to perform, involves awkward and painful patient positions, is tedious, and requires polytomography for imaging. With the advent of newer techniques, pneumoencephalography has become obsolete as a neurodiagnostic study in the United States and is mentioned for historical purposes only.

Diagnostic Imaging in Acute Neurological Injury

Plain film radiography, computed tomography, and angiography are the primary imaging modalities used in the diagnosis of acute head trauma. Damage to the skull can be readily diagnosed by plain films and CT, while injury to brain parenchyma is diagnosed by CT or MRI. Vascular trauma is best evaluated by angiography.

Plain Film Radiography

Head Injury

Radiographic examination of the head consists of AP and lateral radiographs of the skull. Plain films are used for the diagnosis of fractures in adults and children, for localization of radiopaque foreign bodies such as bullets and aneurysm clips, and for suspected cases of child abuse.[37]

Fractures such as linear, stellate, and eggshell fractures, depressed and nondepressed fractures and "ping-pong" fractures of newborns[38] are easily diagnosed on skull radiographs. Fractures are often better seen on plain films than on CT, especially if a fracture lies parallel to the axial plane of the CT image.[39] Complications of skull fractures, including direct injury to underlying gray and white matter, hemorrhage, pneumocephalus, CSF rhinorrhea and otorrhea, infection, and "growing fractures" of children (leptomeningeal cysts),[40] can only be inferred by radiographs. Diagnosis requires the use of CT or, when equivocal, MRI.

Radiopaque foreign bodies are easily seen on plain films and are localized by exposing radiographs in perpendicular planes. Vascular injury, potential sequelae, and the trajectory course of bullets can be inferred on radiographs. Diagnosis, however, requires CT, MRI, or angiography in conjunction with clinical assessment.

Skull radiography is of critical importance in diagnosing injuries caused by child abuse. The radiographic complex of battered children was first described by Caffey[41] in 1946 and the term "battered-child syndrome" was coined by Kempe et al.[42] in 1962. The battered-child syndrome is characterized by multiple bruises of varying ages, body burns, sullen demeanor, and inconsistent histories provided by caretakers. Radiographic hallmarks include skull fractures, separated cranial sutures, long-bone fractures, multiple fractures of varying ages, and metaphyseal fractures. If child abuse is suspected, radiographic examination of the entire body is mandatory.

Spinal Cord Injury

The cross-table (horizontal beam) lateral view of the cervical spine, also called the lateral cervical view (LCV), has generally been considered the single most important radiograph in the diagnosis of acute cervical spine injury, with a 90% detection rate of significant spinal cord injury reported using this film alone.[43] Although Woodring and Lee[44] have recently challenged this claim, this single radiograph remains valuable as a screening tool in the initial evaluation of cervical trauma.

It is imperative for traumatologists to become well-versed in plain film examination of the cervical spine because the presence or absence of cervical spine pathology may impact significantly on airway management. Of importance is continued stabilization of the neck during resuscitation, radiographic exposure, transport, and surgery until the cervical spine has been cleared of significant injury by a qualified radiologist. If no pain can be elicited in the awake patient on neck palpitation, the spine may be "cleared."

The LCV (Fig. 3), as all radiographs, should be reviewed systematically. Technique (quality, contrast, motion) should be noted initially and all osseous structures should be identified. The atlanto-occipital junction, seven cervical vertebrae, and preferably the C7-T1 interspace should be visible on the LCV. If C7 cannot be seen and the patient is hemodynamically stable, a repeat radiograph should be exposed with emphasis on the C7-T1 interspace. The swimmer's view or traction on the shoulders (with the approval of an orthopedic surgeon or neurosurgeon) can help visualize this interspace. If C7 cannot be adequately visualized, the patient's neck *must* remain immobilized and is considered unstable until appropriate diagnostic studies can be completed.

Vertebral alignment, soft tissue structures, air collections, and foreign bodies should be noted. The cervical spine normally exhibits a slight lordosis. However, muscle spasm, positioning, stabilization devices, and cervical injury can cause loss of this curve. The vertebral bodies should have a smooth contour and should be aligned. The anterior and posterior spinal lines should be smooth, indicating integrity of the anterior and posterior ligaments. Step-offs are indicative of disruption of these ligamentous complexes and generally indicate an unstable spine, although pseudosubluxation at C2-C3[45] may be a normal variant in children under 8 years of age due to inherent laxity of the surrounding ligaments at this level. The lamina and articular processes should be symmetrical, and the spinous processes should be equidistant except at C2-C3 where there is a natural widening. The distance between the anterior arch of C1 (atlas) and the odontoid process of C2 (axis) should not exceed 3 mm in adults.

Soft tissues should be examined for symmetry, swelling, foreign bodies, and air. A narrow air column within the esophagus is normal. The prevertebral soft tissue should closely approximate the anterior aspect of C1 to C5 and should widen slightly at approximately C6. Prevertebral soft tissue measurements of 7 mm or greater are suggestive of underlying cervical injury, while measurements of 10 mm or more are highly suspicious of cervical pathology.[46–48]

Subtle fractures of C1-C3 may not be identified on the LCV alone and missed injuries of the upper third of the cervical spine are com-

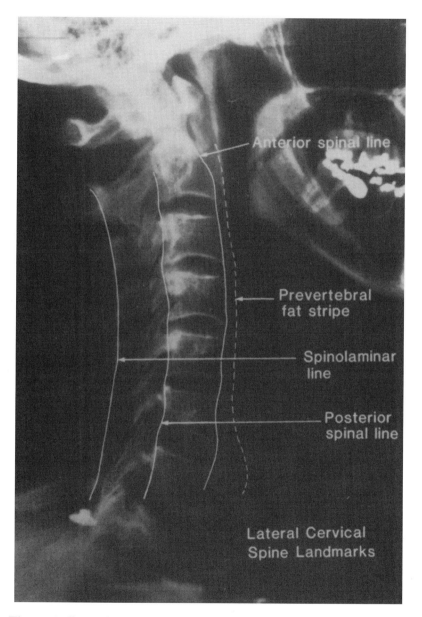

Figure 3. Cervical spine, lateral radiograph. Demonstration of the normal prevertebral fat stripe and spinal lines. See text for details. Permission from Berquist TH: Spine trauma. In McCort JJ, Mindelzun RE: *Trauma Radiology*. New York, Churchill-Livingstone, 1990, fig 2–5, p 35.

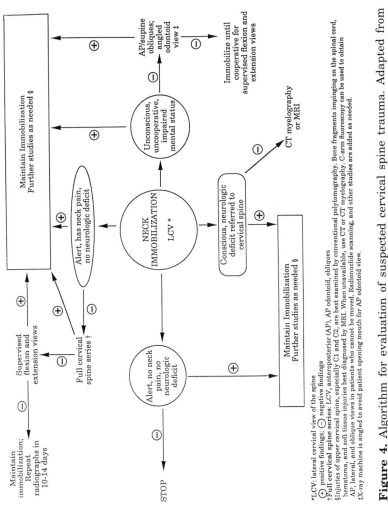

*LCV: lateral cervical view of the spine
⊕ positive findings; ⊖ negative findings
†Full cervical spine series: LCV, anteroposterior (AP), AP odontoid, obliques
§Injuries of upper cervical spine, especially C1 and C2, are best examined by conventional polytomography. Bone fragments impinging on the spinal cord, hematoma, and soft tissue injuries best diagnosed by MRI. When unavailable, use CT or CT myelography. C-arm fluoroscopy can be used to obtain AP, lateral, and oblique views in patients who cannot be moved. Radionuclide scanning, and other studies are added as needed.
‡X-ray machine is angled to avoid patient opening mouth for AP odontoid view.

Figure 4. Algorithm for evaluation of suspected cervical spine trauma. Adapted from Young JWR, Mirvis SE: Cervical spine trauma. In Mirvis SE, Young JWR: *Imaging in Trauma and Critical Care.* Baltimore, Williams & Wilkins, 1992, table 6.1, p 292; Berquist TH: Spine trauma. In McCort JJ, Mindelzun RE: *Trauma Radiology.* New York, Churchill-Livingstone, 1990, table 2–3, p 45.

mon. Further diagnostic imaging studies (Fig. 4) should be obtained as needed. A full cervical spine series should always be obtained if there is clinical or radiographic suspicion of cervical injury. Linear or complex motion polytomography is the study of choice after plain film radiographs are completed to evaluate the atlantoaxial junction and to identify pathology of the odontoid and the body of C2.[49] CT and MRI should be considered as necessary for further evaluation once life-threatening hemodynamic instability has resolved.[50]

Conventional tomography (also known as plain film tomography, body section radiography, polytomography, and "tomos") is a radiographic technique whereby a specific layer of the body is sharply imaged and areas above and below are blurred. X-rays are focused to a specific layer of the body by linking the x-ray source and receiver (generally a film cassette) around a point above the imaging table. Movement of the x-ray source and film cassette in either a linear or a complex motion causes structures other than those at the selected level to be blurred, while the area of interest is kept in sharp focus. Although this technique has largely been replaced by newer methods of imaging, tomography does still offer many advantages, particularly in the diagnosis of vertebral column injury.

Multiple vertebral fractures (Fig. 5) are common. Mirvis and colleagues[51] and Lee, et al.[52] report a 26% incidence of multiple spinal fractures, most involving the atlas and axis (C1 and C2) and the cervicothoracic junction.[53] Computed tomography as well as conventional tomography should be used for diagnosis.

Cervical spine injuries are classified according to mechanism of injury and stability (Table 3). In general, injuries with neurological deficits are considered unstable whereas injuries unassociated with neurological compromise may be considered stable.[54] Four major forces cause cervical fractures and dislocations: flexion, extension, rotation, and axial loading.[55] Flexion injury causes partial or complete rupture of the interspinous, capsular, and posterior longitudinal ligaments and is produced by minimal forces of approximately 700 pounds per square inch.[56] Stronger forces cause retropulsion of bony fragments into the thecal canal (Fig. 1) with sudden and usually permanent quadriplegia. Extension injuries (Fig. 6) that are caused by AP forces striking the head, face, or mandible[57] shear the anterior longitudinal ligaments and crush the posterior elements. These injuries are frequently associated with maxillofacial fractures[58] and laryngeal damage. Neurological deficits range from transient pares-

Table 3
Classification of Cervical Spine Fractures by
Mechanisms of Injury

Hyperflexion
  Bilateral interfacetal dislocation ("locked facets")*
  Flexion-teardrop fracture*
  Anterior subluxation
  Simple wedge fracture (vertical compression)
  Spinous process fracture (clay shoveler)
Hyperextension
  Hangman's fracture*
  Extension teardrop fracture*
  Sprain (whiplash)
  Anterior or posterior arch fracture of C1 (atlas)
  Anteroinferior vertebral chip fracture
Axial or vertical compression
  Jefferson fracture of C1*
  Burst fracture
Flexion-rotation
  Unilateral interfacetal dislocation
Indeterminate
  Odontoid fracture
  Atlanto-occipital dislocation (fatal)
  Dislocation

* Unstable injuries

thesias to complete quadriplegia. Axial compression forces crush vertebrae and cause radial extrusion of the intervertebral discs.

Evaluation of the thoracolumbar (TL) spine[59] is similar to that of the cervical spine. The majority of TL injuries occur from T12 to L2[60] and are caused by flexion injuries secondary to lap belt use.[61] Acceleration of the upper spine over the fixed axis of the lower spine at the level of the lap belt causes shearing of the posterior elements and fracture/dislocation at the L1-L3 levels. These fractures are often accompanied by significant intra-abdominal injuries.[62] Use of the three-point shoulder harness has reduced the incidence of lumbar fractures and abdominal injuries, but thoracic injuries[63] and cerebrovascular injuries[64,65] have increased.

Axial compression, such as is seen in jumps or falls, causes burst and compression fractures of the TL spine as well as fractures of the extremities. Rogers[66] reports that 20% of compression fractures of the calcaneus are associated with fracture/dislocation of the lumbosacral spine.

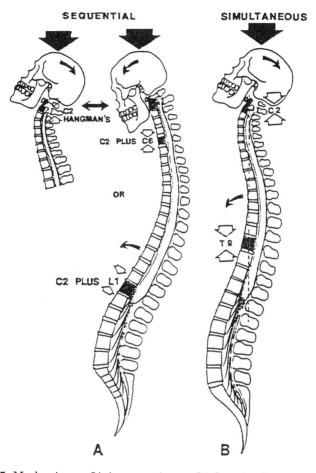

Figure 5. Mechanisms of injury causing multiple spine fractures. **(A)** Sequential fracture mechanism. Neck extension is followed by flexion or flexion is followed by extension. Two fractures of the cervical spine (C2 and C6) or a cervical fracture combined with a distal vertebral fracture (C2 and L1) results. **(B)** Simultaneous fracture mechanism. A solitary axial-compressive force applied to the normal kyphotic curve of the thoracic spine while the neck is extended will produce fractures at C2 and T9. Permission from Lee C, Rogers LF, Woodring JH, Goldstein SJ, Kim KS: Fractures of the craniovertebral junction associated with other fractures of the spine: Overlooked entity? *AJNR* 1984;5:775–781.

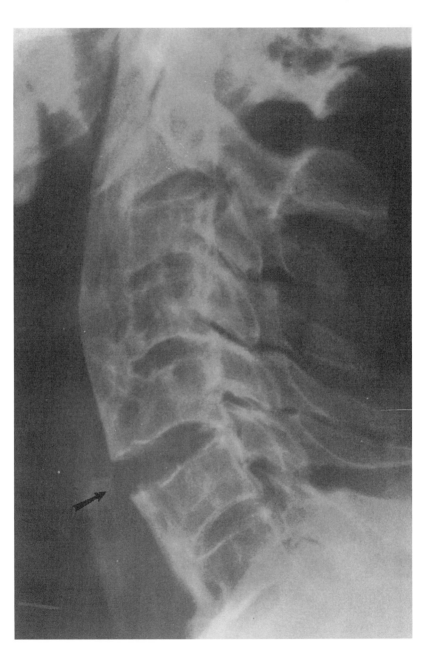

Computed Tomography

Head Injury

Computed tomography has revolutionized the diagnosis and treatment of neurosurgical emergencies.[67] Described by Hounsfield in 1972,[68] CT is currently the most widely used imaging modality for the diagnosis of neurological emergencies. Thornbury and associates[69] and Masters et al.[70] report that the use of CT has reduced surgical intervention of head injuries by 58%, skull radiography by 80%, and cerebral angiography by 84%.

CT scanning is performed by placing the patient within the gantry and exposing the patient to thinly collimated x-ray beams. Radiation is collected and stored by photon detectors located opposite the incident radiation beam and then translated by rapid and complex computer analysis into gray scale images. Normal anatomy, fractures, hemorrhage, mass effect, and other abnormalities can be identified by manipulating the gray scale images.

Minimal CT evaluation of head injury consists of a lateral digital radiograph ("scout view")[71] and four unenhanced axial images examined at both bone and soft tissue window settings. In urgent situations, a single unenhanced axial image taken at the level of the lateral ventricles reveals most surgically treatable lesions. Fresh intracranial hemorrhage (Fig. 7) has a high CT density and appears "white" on scans at soft tissue window settings without the use of intravenous contrast. Subdural hematoma (SDH), epidural hematoma, subarachnoid hemorrhage, and intraparenchymal and intraventricular hemorrhage are usually diagnosed without difficulty on unenhanced images. Tentorial or uncal herniation and massive cerebral edema are also easily recognized.

It is important to emphasize that if CT is performed immediately after traumatic injury, significant pathology may not be radiographically evident.[72,73] This so-called "zero-time" scan may appear normal

---

Figure 6. Cervical spine, lateral radiograph. Hyperextension injury secondary to a motor vehicle accident in a patient with ankylosing spondylitis. Note the fracture of the anterior bridging syndesmophytes (arrow) at C5-C6 and widening of the intervertebral disk space at the same level. Permission from Young JWR, Mirvis SE: Cervical spine trauma. In Mirvis SE, Young JWR: *Imaging in Trauma and Critical Care*. Baltimore, Williams & Wilkins, 1992, fig 6.69, p 328.

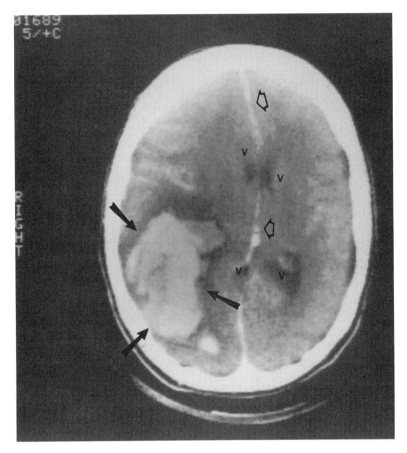

Figure 7. Unenhanced axial CT scan of the brain at the level of the lateral ventricles. A large intraparenchymal hemorrhage is seen (arrows). Mass effect is present with lateral ventricular compression (v) and midline shift (arrowheads).

despite ongoing cerebral insult. In any patient with stable or deteriorating signs, CT scanning should be repeated. Gray and Albert[74] recommend that repeat scanning should be performed 24 hours postoperatively or 3 to 5 days post-trauma regardless of clinical recovery.

Computed tomography is exquisitely sensitive for the diagnosis of air within the cranial vault (Fig. 8). Pneumocephalus, as this entity is called, was originally described by Chiari in 1884[75] and next by Luckett in 1913.[76] Intracranial air occurs in 0.5%–1% of all head

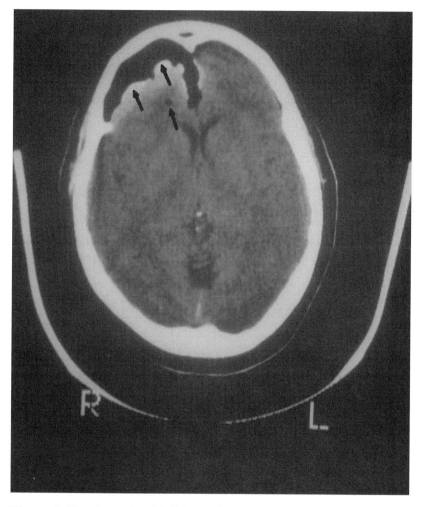

Figure 8. Unenhanced axial CT scan demonstrating pneumocephalus. Air (arrows) is seen within the cranial vault. Courtesy W. Garfinkle, MD, Philadelphia, Pennsylvania.

injuries.[77] As little as 0.5 mL intracranial air can be visualized on CT, while 2 mL is required for visualization on skull radiographs.[78] Diagnosis of pneumocephalus is imperative because its presence is indicative of a meningeal tear and potential contamination of the brain. Mortality from bacterial meningitis still remains at 50% despite the aggressive use of antibiotics.[79] Pneumocephalus often heals spontaneously but complications include pneumatocele,[80] pneumorhachis (air within the spinal canal),[81] and progression from simple, uncomplicated pneumocephalus to life-threatening tension pneumocephalus. The occurrence of the latter complication may be accelerated by the use of nitrous oxide during neuroanesthesia.

Computed tomography of the head has special importance in the diagnosis of child abuse. CT findings compatible with abuse in children under the age of two ("shaken baby syndrome")[82] include bilateral subdural hematomas, interhemispheric SDH, intracranial hemorrhage, and skull fracture. Eighty percent of children with interhemispheric SDH have associated retinal hemorrhage.[83] These findings are highly suspicious of abuse and must be evaluated further.

Shaken baby syndrome is caused by repeated, severe acceleration-deceleration forces applied to a child's unsupported head. Poor myelination, open sutures, a large cranium, and a thin calvarium allow extreme movement of the brain within the skull, causing severe shearing injury and diffuse brain swelling. A syndrome of "malignant cerebral edema"[84] may ensue, resulting in significant and permanent neurological injury. Mental retardation, 100% incidence of cerebral atrophy on follow-up, and 50% incidence of cerebral infarction have been reported.[85]

Soft tissue injuries of the brain such as diffuse axonal injury, contusion, and small petecchial hemorrhage are poorly visualized on CT, especially in the inferior frontal and temporal lobes where streak artifact from adjacent bone may obscure pathology. MRI is superior in detecting these injuries in all parts of the cerebrum, cerebellum, and brain stem.

Spinal Cord Injury

Computed tomography is frequently used in the evaluation of acute spinal cord injury, especially when plain films are inadequate or equivocal or when surgical decompression and stabilization are planned. Fractures and small bony fragments can be easily identified, images can be obtained in several planes, and if intrathecal contrast is instilled, pathology to the cord can be detected. CT is also used postoperatively to identify infection or hemorrhage, to assess the adequacy of fixation devices and surgical decompression, and to delineate spinal cord cyst or syrinx formation.

CT is often superior to plain film radiography and polytomography in diagnosing cervical pathology, but it is not infallible and should not be accepted as a gold standard. Woodring and Lee[86] state that "they have been dismayed by the inability of CT scanning to reliably demonstrate certain types of cervical injuries . . . On numerous occasions we have experienced difficulty in convincing . . . [physicians] that . . . a significant cervical injury [was present] when the CT scan was negative . . . We believe that computed tomography is an excellent means of evaluating cervical trauma and should be liberally employed . . . [However] complex-motion tomography remains the gold standard for the diagnosis of atlanto-occipital dislocations; subluxations of the vertebral bodies; and fractures of the lateral masses, articular processes, vertebral bodies, and dens . . . Whenever a patient has a neurologic deficit that cannot be adequately explained by plain film and CT findings, [further studies such as] TOMOS should be performed."

Arteriography

Four-vessel cerebral arteriography (bilateral carotid and vertebrobasilar arteriography) evaluates the integrity of the cerebral circulation after head injury. Vascular injuries are common after neurotrauma[87] and include carotid artery dissection and occlusion, carotid-cavernous fistula formation,[88] infarction,[89] arteriovenous malformations (AVMs), aneurysms,[90] and vertebral artery injury.[91,92] In addition to diagnosis of head-injured patients, cerebral arteriography is also performed on all patients with suspected vascular injuries in zone III of the neck.[93] Surgical exposure of these injuries may be extremely difficult and interventional occlusive techniques using balloons,[94] coils, and embolic agents[95] have been successful in controlling hemorrhage when surgical intervention has been contraindicated.

Arteriography is usually performed in a suite equipped with a moveable fluoroscopy table, serial film changer, biplane imaging device, image intensifier, automatic high-pressure injector for rapid serial examination, long guide wires, specialized catheters, and water-soluble contrast media. Cerebral vessels are selectively cannulated after femoral artery catheterization using the Seldinger technique.[96] Catheters are introduced into the carotid and vertebrobasilar arteries and serial radiographs are exposed after rapid injection of contrast. Subtraction films are created by neutralizing back-

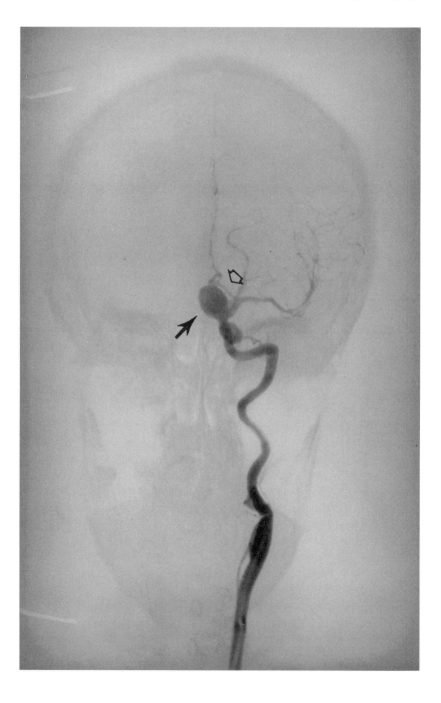

ground anatomy so that the contrast-enhanced vessel is prominent (Fig. 9).

Spinal cord arteriography (SCA)[97] is used to investigate vascular lesions of the spinal cord such as hemangioblastomas, AVMs, and vertebrospinal tumors. SCA is also performed after spinal trauma to evaluate cord ischemia and to demonstrate the artery of Adamkiewicz.[98] SCA is a long procedure and requires large amounts of contrast.

Complications of neuroangiography may be local, systemic, or neurological,[99,100] and include reactions to the contrast medium, infarction secondary to catheter dislodgement of thrombi or plaque, dislodgement of injected embolic agents, air embolism, vasospasm, dissection, perforation, intracranial hemorrhage, stroke, and death.

Anesthesiologists are often asked to assist in the management of patients undergoing cerebrospinal angiography. General anesthesia and invasive monitoring may be required to assure high-quality studies and to provide ongoing resuscitation in trauma victims. Immobilization of apprehensive and uncooperative patients, a prerequisite for high-quality studies, may be possible only under general anesthesia. Special maneuvers such as hyperventilation or apnea may be needed to slow circulation time, to relieve arterial spasm, or to enhance contrast of vessels for subtraction radiography. Cooperation between neuroradiologist and anesthesiologist is obviously imperative for safe patient care.

Digital Subtraction Angiography

Digital subtraction angiography (DSA) utilizes digital technology and subtraction radiographic technique to create computer-generated images of cerebral vessels. Injection is either intra-arterial or intravenous. *Digital intravenous angiography* (DIVA) was originally described as a screening procedure for patients with suspected ischemic cerebrovascular disease.[101,102] In addition to screening, it is now also used as a follow-up study in patients who have undergone carotid endarterectomy or therapeutic embolization, to evaluate pa-

Figure 9. Selective left carotid arteriogram (subtraction film). A large aneurysm is present arising from the distal internal carotid artery (arrow) There is elevation of the A1 segment of the anterior cerebral artery (arrowhead). Courtesy of N. Thompson, MD, Bryn Mawr, Pennsylvania.

tients suffering from cerebral vascular spasm, and to detect abnormal vascularity of intracranial neoplasms, AVMs, and aneurysms. It is safely performed as an outpatient procedure and is less expensive than conventional angiography.[103]

There are several disadvantages to DIVA. It is not a selective arterial study and overlapping of vessels in certain projections may obscure significant pathology. Full patient cooperation is required to ensure high-quality images, a larger quantity of contrast is used than in conventional angiography, and it is contraindicated in patients with significant renal disease. *Selective intra-arterial digital subtraction angiography* (IADSA) has overcome many of the problems. Complications of DIVA include hypersensitivity to contrast medium, vessel perforation, and extravasation of contrast medium at the injection site. Rare complications include infection, dislodgement of thrombi, or plaque, stroke, and death. Although DIVA, DSA, and IASDA have shown promise, they have not replaced conventional arteriography as the gold standard for diagnosing neurovascular pathology in acute trauma.

Ultrasound

Ultrasound has been used extensively in the diagnosis of carotid artery disease,[104] to localize brain tumors in infants,[105] and in evaluating periventricular and intraventricular hemorrhage of neonates.[106] Recently, ultrasound has been used during neurosurgical procedures advantageously. Gooding et al.[107] report excellent results using intraoperative sonography (IOS) for the localization of intracranial neoplasms. Brain biopsy using ultrasound guidance has been described,[108] and IOS localization of intracranial vascular lesions has been reported to significantly reduce surgical localization time.[109]

Ultrasound imaging of the spinal cord via the esophagus using technology based on transesophageal echocardiography has been reported,[110] and ultrasound-guided aspiration biopsies of lytic lesions of the cervical spine have been successfully accomplished.[111] Technical difficulties, such as the need for an adequate acoustic window (Fig. 10) and the need for physician-ultrasonologists to perform the studies still limit the usefulness of this modality in emergent situations. As these limitations are overcome and availability of equipment improves, undoubtedly ultrasound will be used more frequently in acute settings.

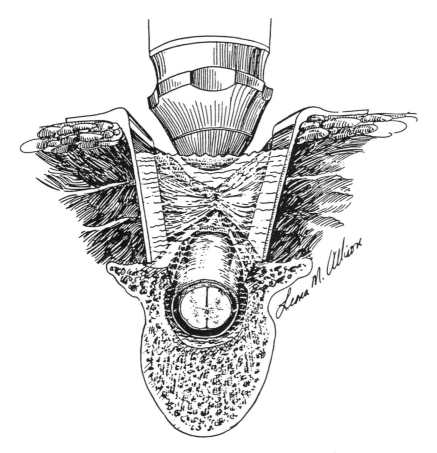

Figure 10. Intraoperative sonography. Technical diagram depicting a cross-sectional view of the thoracic spinal canal and cord. The position of the transducer, dura mater, and spinal cord is shown. Undulations overlying the transducer represent the fluid baths. Permission from Montalvo BM, Quencer RM, et al: Intraoperative sonography in spinal trauma. *Radiology* 1984;153:125–135, fig 1, p 256.

Intraoperative Diagnostic Imaging

In the past, intraoperative diagnostic imaging in trauma has been limited to plain film radiography, C-arm fluoroscopy, and angiography during thoracic, abdominal, and extremity procedures. Recently, IOS (see above) has been described during neurosurgical procedures on the brain and spinal cord, and the use of intraoperative ultrasound for diagnosing neurological injury after spinal trauma shows promise.

Quencer and associates[112] recommend the use of IOS during surgical decompression of post-traumatic spinal cord cysts. Montalvo et al.[113] and Mirvis and Geisler[114] describe intraoperative spinal sonography (IOSS) as a technique for localizing bone fragments impinging on the spinal cord after spinal trauma, for analyzing vertebral body malalignment, for diagnosing cord compression and foreign bodies, and for assessing and aspirating post-traumatic intramedullary and subarachnoid cysts. These authors report a 96.5% detection rate of parenchymal spinal cord lesions by IOSS at the site of fracture or stenosis with technically adequate studies.

Imaging in Nonacute Neurotrauma

Head Injury

All imaging modalities (Table 1) are used in the diagnosis of nonacute neurotrauma. Evolution of intracranial hemorrhage, delayed and recurrent bleeding, and mass effect are easily identified by CT and MRI. Basilar skull fractures, notoriously difficult to assess, require multiple imaging studies, while complications such as middle ear injury[115] and pneumolabyrinth (air in the vestibule and cochlea)[116] have been well documented on single imaging studies. Radionuclide studies are excellent for detecting CSF leaks[117] and chronic subdural collections.[118]

Arteriography is used to diagnose vascular abnormalities and to assess surgical repairs (Fig. 11). Interventional embolic techniques have been used as therapeutic alternatives to surgery for control of intracranial hemorrhage. Transcranial Doppler ultrasound has been useful for intraoperative localization of cerebrovascular lesions as well as for monitoring of intracranial vasospasm.

Spinal Cord Injury

Nonacute spinal cord injury and complications of SCI are best evaluated by plain film radiography, conventional myelography, CT, CT-myelography, and MRI. Long-term sequelae, such as progressive kyphosis, cervical spine instability, syringomyelia, and post-traumatic spinal cord atrophy[119] have been readily evaluated by these imaging techniques. IOSS shows promise for use in neurosurgical procedures after spinal trauma.

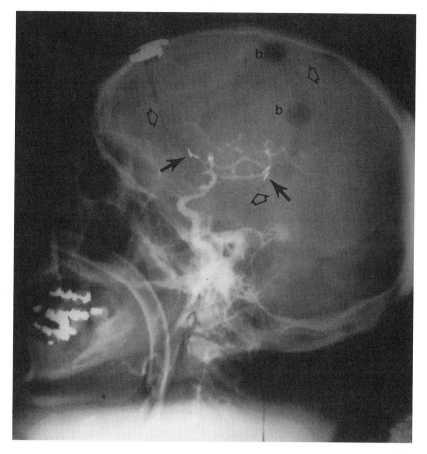

Figure 11. Carotid angiogram after aneurysm repair, lateral view. Surgical clips (arrows), bone flap (arrowheads) and burr holes (b) are seen on this postoperative radiograph. Courtesy of N. Thompson, MD, Bryn Mawr, Pennsylvania.

Myelography

Myelography consists of the injection of a radiopaque contrast substance (see contrast media) into the subarachnoid space using an oil-based or water-soluble contrast agent. The approach for myelography is generally via lumbar puncture at the L2–3 or L3–4 interspace using a 22-gauge spinal needle. Contrast medium is instilled using either metrizamide or the nonionic agents, and radiographs are exposed in multiple projections. If there is a contraindication to lumbar puncture, cervical puncture at C1-2 is performed. CT is often done after intrathecal contrast injection (CT-myelography) to assess integrity of the cord.

Hemodynamic instability, immobilization devices, and technical difficulty performing either lumbar or cervical puncture in trauma victims limits the usefulness of myelography and CT myelography after acute neurological injury.[120] Myelography and CT myelography are valuable, however, during the subacute and chronic phases of neurotrauma. CT-myelography remains the imaging study of choice in evaluating nonacute spinal cord injury, although this study is gradually being replaced by MRI.

Magnetic Resonance Imaging

Magnetic resonance (MR), formerly called nuclear magnetic resonance, was discovered by Purcell and Bloch in the late 1940s. Each was an acknowledged Nobel laureate in 1952 for the discovery.[121] Twenty-one years later Lauterbur suggested that the technique be used for human imaging, and clinical trials for MRI were begun in the 1980s.[122]

MR principles[123,124] dictate that atomic nuclei with an odd number of protons and/or neutrons (H^+, ^{31}P, ^{23}Na, and ^{13}C in the human body) have intrinsic magnetic properties and behave like miniature bar magnets, spinning continuously. If these elements are placed in a strong magnetic field, the nuclei align themselves and rotate, "precessing" to lie parallel to one another within the magnetic field. This precessing occurs at a specific frequency, the Larmor or resonant frequency, which is inherent to each ion and is directly proportional to the strength of the magnetic field in which it lies. If a pulse of radiofrequency (RF) at or near the intrinsic Larmor frequency is directed at a source, the nuclei relax and a radiofrequency signal at the Larmor frequency is emitted. Two time constants, T1 and T2, describe decay of the emitted RF signal. T1 indicates longitudinal relaxation time and T2 signifies transverse relaxation time of the source nuclei.

MRI field strengths are enormous, ranging from 0.5 tesla (T) to 2.0 T. One tesla equals 10,000 gauss. As a comparison, the earth's magnetic field is approximately 1 gauss.[125] Radiofrequency pulses at 5 mT/meter are generated at 1-msec intervals and are directed perpendicularly to the longitudinal axis of the patient and magnet.

Table 4
Magnetic Resonance Imaging: Problems and Hazards

Limited patient visibility and access
Claustrophobia
Noise
Degradation of MRI image quality from monitoring equipment
Attraction of ferromagnetic objects to the static magnetic field causing:
  • Projectile movement of free-standing objects and equipment
  • Dislodgement of aneurysm clips, pacemakers, tympanic implants, microcatheters
Generation of internal electrical currents from the rapidly changing magnetic fields causing:
  • Disruption of pacemaker microcircuitry
  • Local heating

Precessing spins and relaxation of nuclei induce a voltage in receiver coils. These voltage signals are collected, stored, and reconstructed by complex computer analysis, and images are then generated. Intravenous gadolinium may be used to enhance anatomic detail.

Adverse biological effects from static magnetic fields less than 2 T have not been reported,[126] although other serious hazards (Table 4) from the magnet are well documented. Attraction of ferromagnetic objects to the magnet creates dangerous projectiles of free-standing equipment.[127] The magnetic field strength may cause movement of internally placed metallic objects such as aneurysm clips, cardiac pacemakers,[128] middle ear implants, and microcatheters,[129] and MRI may be contraindicated in the presence of these devices.

The advantages of MRI are many and include imaging in multiple planes, lack of ionizing radiation, and excellent soft tissue contrast. These benefits have made MRI a popular choice for neurodiagnosis despite significant technical problems, safety hazards, and disadvantages which, in addition to those previously mentioned, includes the inability to easily detect fresh blood.

Diagnosis of acute hemorrhage by MRI is more problematic than detection by CT. Signal intensity of hemorrhage on MRI is dependent on the presence of paramagnetic elements of hemoglobin.[130] Unclotted and freshly clotted blood contains large amounts of intracellular deoxyhemoglobin, which has signal intensity similar to that of brain parenchyma.[131] Differentiation from adjacent gray and white matter is therefore difficult. Over time, as the hemoglobin molecule changes and breakdown products accumulate, signal characteristics change.

Table 5
Anesthetic Management for MRI

Careful screening for internal ferromagnetic foreign bodies (aneurysm clips, pacemakers, tympanic implants, microcatheters)
Nonferromagnetic tubing and connections
Shielded cables and electrodes
5-meter minimum distance of equipment from bore of magnet
MRI-compatible equipment
Two-person anesthesia team
Induction remote from bore of magnet
Laryngoscope with lithium batteries
RAE endotracheal tube to facilitate placement of breathing circuit
40–50 ft Mapleson D breathing circuit
Medication infusion via microdrip to avoid infusion pumps
"Safe zone" for resuscitation equipment

Subacute and chronic hemorrhage have high signal intensities due to the presence of methemoglobin[132–134] and are well differentiated from adjacent brain.

Examination of uncooperative patients (children, the mentally disabled, and the critically ill) for MRI studies often requires the skills of an anesthesiologist to assure patient safety and high-quality imaging. Technical difficulties such as patient access, limited visualization of the patient while in the bore of the magnet, and magnetic field hazards seriously hinder patient care. Anesthetic management becomes challenging even during routine studies, and may be impossible in critical situations. Image degradation by monitors and anesthesia equipment has been significant.[135] As safety issues are resolved[136] and MRI-compatible equipment becomes more readily available,[137–143] anesthetic management becomes easier (Table 5), and it can be anticipated that management of critical patients will eventually be routine. At the present time, however, CT is faster, more efficient, less expensive, and of greater diagnostic value in acute situations and remains the modality of choice in most institutions in the initial evaluation of neurotrauma victims.

Whereas MRI is of limited value in the acute phase of neurological injury, it is unequivocally superior to CT in evaluating subacute (greater than 48 hours) and chronic neurotrauma.[144] It is especially useful in the diagnosis of shearing injuries[145] and in the examination of the structures of the posterior fossa. Nonacute extradural and

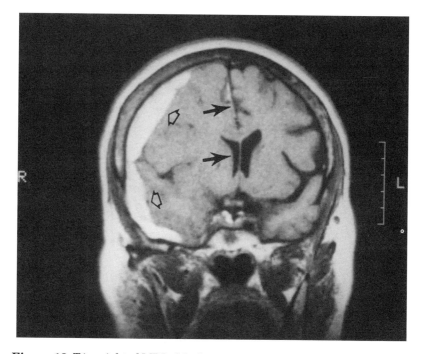

Figure 12. T1-weighted MRI of the brain, coronal view. Subdural hematoma is seen as a crescentic area of increased signal on the right (open arrowheads). Note the mass effect with midline shift and compression of the right lateral ventricle (arrows). Courtesy of N. Thompson, MD, Bryn Mawr, Pennsylvania.

subdural collections (Fig. 12) and nonhemorrhagic contusions are generally well visualized on unenhanced MRI scans regardless of size. Spinal cord injury and disc herniation are exquisitely imaged.[146]

Brain Death

Determination of brain death has become a complex medical and ethical issue due to the use of artificial support devices that are capable of sustaining circulation and respiration even in the absence of adequate brain function. In 1981, guidelines for the determination of death were established by the President's Commission for the Study of Ethical Problems in Medical and Biomedical and Behavioral

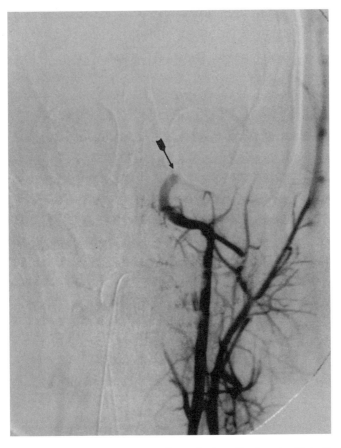

Figure 13. Left carotid arteriogram, frontal view. Contrast within the internal carotid artery, terminating at the level of the carotid siphon (arrow), is indicative of brain death. Courtesy H. Koolpe, MD. Philadelphia, Pennsylvania.

Problems,[147,148] and were adapted by the American Bar Association, the American Medical Association, and the National Conference of Commissioners on Uniform State Laws. Irreversible cessation of all brain function, which is the current definition of whole brain death, is based on those guidelines.

The radiographic standard for diagnosing brain death is absence of blood flow to the cerebral circulation as demonstrated by cerebral angiography[149] (Fig. 13). "Complete cessation of circulation to the normothermic adult brain for more than ten minutes is incompatible with survival of brain tissue. Documentation of this circulatory failure is therefore evidence of death of the entire brain. Four-vessel intracranial angiography is definitive for diagnosing cessation of circulation to the entire brain (both cerebrum and posterior fossa) . . . ",[150] even in the presence of central nervous system depressants. Interventional angiography is gradually being replaced by radionuclide angiography as the standard. Radionuclide scanning is simple to perform, is not contraindicated if organ donation is being considered, and can be performed often at the bedside. Radionuclide angiography is accepted as diagnostic of whole brain death when there is adequate demonstration of arrest of carotid flow at the base of the skull and there is adequate clinical evidence confirming brain stem dysfunction.[151] Radionuclide angiography is not considered valid for diagnosing brain death in patients less than 2 months of age.[152] DSA, xenon CT,[153] and transcranial Doppler[154] have been studied and results are promising.

Conclusion

A variety of imaging modalities are available for the diagnosis of traumatic brain injury and spinal cord injury. Plain film radiography, computed tomography, and neurovascular angiography are the imaging modalities of choice used during the acute phase of traumatic brain injury and spinal cord injury, and polytomography, myelography, CT-myelography, MRI, and radionuclide scanning are used during nonacute and chronic phases. Ultrasound is used intraoperatively during intracranial and spinal neurosurgical procedures.

Skull radiographs detect fractures and foreign bodies and are of primary value in cases of child abuse. Plain film radiography of the cervical spine, specifically the LCV, is performed during initial in-hospital resuscitation and is an excellent screening tool for the early evaluation of cervical spine injury. If indicated, further imaging studies are obtained. CT has revolutionized the early detection and management of neurological emergencies. It is fast, reliable, provides images in multiple planes, and is of significant diagnostic value for multiple organ systems. It is especially useful in the diagnosis of acute, treatable neurosurgical emergencies.

Cerebral angiography is performed after trauma when neurovascular anatomy must be delineated. Interventional, embolic procedures have been successfully used as alternatives to surgery when immediate control of intracranial hemorrhage is necessary and there is a contraindication to operative intervention. Intraoperative ultrasound has been used to detect parenchymal lesions and to guide the surgical approach when intracranial or spinal neurosurgery must be performed.

MRI is still of limited diagnostic value in the acute trauma victim at most institutions. Limitations include magnetic field hazards, cost, technical difficulties in adequately monitoring critical patients, and inability to detect acute hemorrhage. Beyond the 48-hour postinjury period, however, MRI is of unequaled value in the evaluation of neurological injury. It is the imaging modality of choice for the diagnosis of the subacute and chronic phases of neurological injury. MRI provides exquisite anatomic and pathological detail of shearing injuries of the brain, images can be constructed in multiple planes, and there is no risk of ionizing radiation. When MRI is equivocal or not available, polytomography, myelography, CT-myelography, and radionuclide scanning have significant diagnostic value.

Immobility is a prerequisite for imaging studies. Any motion reduces the diagnostic value of the study and increases the risk of complications to the patient by examination repetition. The presence of skilled anesthesiologists and traumatologists has allowed high-quality studies to be obtained safely on uncooperative, critically ill patients. Therapeutic decisions have been made more rapidly and intervention and treatment has been instituted earlier. Although the outcome in serious neurological injury remains dismal in many cases, the presence of the anesthesiologist capable of providing ongoing resuscitation and monitoring has major impact on overall improved patient care and has significantly increased survival and viable outcome in a treatable subset of patients.

References

1. Rogers LF: Radiology of Skeletal Trauma, ed 2. Churchill-Livingstone, New York, 1992, p 149.
2. Smirniotopolis JG, Mirvis SE, Wolf A. Imaging of craniocerebral trauma. In Mirvis SE, Young JWR (eds): Imaging in Trauma and Critical Care. Williams & Wilkins, Baltimore, 1992, p 23.
3. Frost EAM: Neurologic trauma. In Grande CM (ed): Textbook of Trauma Anesthesia and Critical Care. Mosby-Year Book, St. Louis, 1993, p 510.
4. Gurney JG, Rivara FP, Mueller BA, Newell DW, Copass MK, et al: The effects of alcohol intoxication on the initial treatment and hospital

course of patients with acute brain injury. J Trauma 33(5):709–713, 1992.

5. Soderstrom CA, Smith GS: Alcohol's effect on trauma outcome: A reappraisal of conventional wisdom. JAMA 270(1):93–94, 1993.

6. Green RM, Kelly KM, Gabrielsen T, et al: Multiple intracerebral hemorrhages after smoking crack cocaine. Stroke 121:957–962, 1990.

7. Berlet AC, Talenti DP, Carroll SF: The baseball bat: A popular mechanism of urban injury. J Trauma 33(2):167–170, 1992.

8. Seelig JM, Becker DP, Miller JD, Greenberg RP, Ward JD, Choi SC: Traumatic acute subdural hematoma, N Engl J Med 304(25): 1511–1518, 1981.

9. Zimmerman RA, Bilaniuk LT, Gennarelli T, Bruce D, Dolinskas C, et al: Cranial computed tomography in the diagnosis and management of acute head trauma. AJR 131:27–34, 1978.

10. Caron MJ, Hovda DA, Becker DP: Changes in the treatment of head injury. Neurosurg Clin North Am 2(2):483–491, 1991.

11. Johnson MH, Lee SH: Computed tomography of acute cerebral trauma. Radiol Clin North Am 30:325–352, 1992.

12. Smirniotopolis JG, Mirvis SE, Wolf A: Imaging of craniocerebral trauma. In Mirvis SE, Young JWR (eds): Imaging in Trauma and Critical Care. Williams & Wilkins, Baltimore, 1992, pp 28–29.

13. American College of Surgeons: Advanced Trauma Life Support. The American College of Surgeons. Chicago, 1989.

14. Stene JK, Grande CM, Barton CR: Airway management for the trauma patient. In Stene JK, Grande CM. (eds): Trauma Anesthesia. Williams & Wilkins, Baltimore, 1991, pp 64–99.

15. Smirniotopolis JG, Mirvis SE, Wolf A: Imaging of craniocerebral trauma. In Mirvis SE, Young JWR (eds): Imaging in Trauma and Critical Care. Williams & Wilkins, Baltimore, 1992, p 30.

16. Patteson SK, Chesney JT: Anesthetic management for magnetic resonance imaging: Problems and solutions. Anesth Analg 74(1):121–128, 1992.

17. Rogers LF: Radiology of Skeletral Trauma, ed 2. Churchill-Livingstone, New York, 1992, p 309.

18. Kelly AB, Zimmerman RD, Snow RB, Gandy SE, Heier LA, et al: Head trauma: Comparison of MR and CT: experience in 100 patients. AJNR 9:699–708, 1988.

19. Siegle RL, Lieberman P: A review of untoward reactions to iodinated contrast material. J Urol 119:581–586, 1978.

20. Morris LD, Wisneski JA, Gertz EW, et al: Potentiation by nifedipine and diltiazem of the hypotensive response after contrast angiography. J Am Coll Cardiol 6(4):785–791, 1985.

21. Forestner JE: Anesthesia for radiologic procedures. In Murphy CH, Murphy MR (eds): Radiology for Anesthesia and Critical Care. Churchill-Livingstone, New York, 1987, pp 253–254.

22. Wolf GL, Mishkin MM, Roux SG, et al: Comparison of the rates of adverse drug reactions: ionic contrast agents, ionic agents combined with steroids, and nonionic agents. Invest Radiol 26:404–410, 1992.

23. Goldberg M: Systemic reactions to intravenous contrast media: A guide for the anesthesiologist. Anesthesiology 60:46–56, 1984.
24. Katayama H, Yagamuchi K, Kozuka T, Takashima T, et al: Adverse reactions to ionic and nonionic contrast media: A report from the Japanese committee on the safety of contrast media. Radiology 175:621–628, 1990.
25. Ross JS, Masaryk TJ, Schrader M, Gentili AC, Bohlman H, et al: MR imaging of the postoperative lumbar spine: Assessment with gadopentatate dimeglumine. AJR 155:867–872, 1990; & AJNR 11:771–776, 1990.
26. Brasch RC, Weinmann HJ, Wesbey GE: Contrast-enhanced NMR imaging: Animal studies using gadolinium-DTPA complex. AJR 142:625–630, 1984.
27. McNamara MT, Higgins CB, Ehman RL, Revel D, et al: Acute myocardial ischemia: Magnetic resonance contrast enhancement with gadolinium-DTPA. Radiology 153:157–163, 1984.
28. Johansen JG, Orrison WW, Amundsen P: Lateral C1-2 puncture for cervical myelography. Radiology 146:391–393, 1983.
29. Brierre JT, Colclough JA: Total myelography: Complete visualization of the spinal subarachnoid space. Radiology 64:81–84, 1955.
30. Quencer RM, Tenner M, Rothman L: The postoperative myelogram. Radiology 123:667–679, 1977.
31. Sackett JF: The spinal cord and related structures. In Juhl JH, Crummy AB (eds): Paul and Juhl's Essentials of Radiologic Imaging, ed 5. JB Lippincott, Philadelphia, 1987, p 447.
32. Holder JC, Binet EK, Kido DK, Belanger G, Sands MS: Iohexol lumbar myelography. AJNR 5:399–402, 1984.
33. Witwer G, Cacayorin ED, Bernstein AD, Hubballah MY, et al: Iopamidol and metrizamide for myelography: A prospective double-blind clinical trial. AJNR 5:403–407, 1984.
34. Baker RA, Hillman BJ, McLennan JE, Strand JD, Kaufman SM: Sequellae of metrizamide myelography in 200 examinations. AJR 130:499–502, 1978.
35. Wolfson R, Hetrick WD: Anesthesia for neuroradiologic procedures. In Cottrell JE, Turndorf H (eds): Anesthesia and Neurosurgery, ed 2. Mosby, St. Louis, 1986, p 109.
36. Lasser EC, Berry CC: Adverse reactions to contrast media: Ionic and nonionic media and steroids. Invest Radiol 26(5):402–403, 1991.
37. Saulsbury FT, Alford BA: Intracranial bleeding from child abuse: The value of skull radiographs. Pediatr Radiol 12:175–178, 1982.
38. Rogers LF: Radiology of skeletal trauma, ed 2. Churchill-Livingstone, New York, 1992, p 337.
39. Smirniotopolis JG, Mirvis SE, Wolf A: Imaging of craniocerebral trauma. In Mirvis SE, Young JWR (eds): Imaging in Trauma and Critical Care. Williams & Wilkins, Baltimore, 1992, p 25.
40. Lindenberg R: Pathology of craniocerebral injuries. In Newton TH, Potts DG: Radiology of the Skull and Brain: Anatomy and Pathology, vol 3. CV Mosby, St. Louis, 1977, p 3053.

41. Caffey J: Multiple fractures in the long bones of infants suffering from chronic subdural hematoma. AJR 56(2):163–173, 1946.
42. Kempe CH, Silverman FN, Steele BF, Droegemuller W, et al: The battered-child syndrome. JAMA 181(1):17–24, 1962.
43. Kaplan SG: Diagnostic imaging: Implications for the trauma anesthesiologist. In Grande CM (ed): Textbook of Trauma Anesthesia and Critical Care. Mosby, St. Louis, 1993, p 1268.
44. Woodring JH, Lee C: Limitations of cervical radiography in the evaluation of acute cervical trauma. J Trauma 34(1):32–39, 1993.
45. Cattell HS, Filtzer DL: Pseudosubluxation and other normal variations in the cervical spine in children. Bone Joint Surg 47A(7):1295–1309, 1965.
46. Young JWR, Mirvis SE: Cervical spine trauma. In Mirvis SE, Young JWR: Imaging in Trauma and Critical Care. Williams & Wilkins, Baltimore, 1992, p 295.
47. Penning L: Prevertebral hematoma in cervical spine injury: Incidence and etiologic significance. AJNR 1:557–565, 1980.
48. Rogers LF: Radiology of Skeletal Trauma, ed 2. Churchill-Livingstone, New York, 1992, pp 454–456.
49. Anderson LD, Smith BL Jr, De Torre J, Littleton JT: The role of polytomography in the diagnosis and treatment of cervical spine injury. Clin Orthop 165:64–67, 1982.
50. Firoznia H, Rafi MH, Golimbu C, Gulfo VJ: Radiographic diagnosis of fracture-dislocation of the spine. In Errico TJ, Bauer RD, Waugh T: Spinal Trauma. JB Lippincott, Philadelphia, 1991, pp 11–54.
51. Mirvis SE, Young JWR, Lim C, Greenberg J: Hangman's fracture: Radiologic assessment in 27 cases. Radiology 163:713–717, 1987.
52. Lee C, Rogers LF, Woodring JH, Goldstein SJ, Kim KS: Fractures of the craniovertebral junction associated with other fractures of the spine: Overlooked entity? AJNR 5:775–781, 1984.
53. Calenoff L, Chessare JW, Rogers LF: Multiple level spinal injuries: Importance of early recognition. AJR 130:665–669, 1978.
54. Levine AM: Cervical spine injury. In Hurst JM: Common Problems in Trauma. Year Book Med Pub. Chicago, 1987, p 120.
55. Whitely JE, Forsythe HF: The classification of cervical spine injuries. AJR 83:633–641, 1960.
56. Young JWR, Mirvis SE: Cervical spine trauma. In Mirvis SE, Young JWR: Imaging in Trauma and Critical Care. Williams & Wilkins, Baltimore, 1992, p 305.
57. Burke DC: Hyperextension injuries of the spine. J Bone Joint Surg [Br] 53:3–11, 1971.
58. Lewis VL Jr, Manson PN, Morgan RF, Cervilo LJ, et al: Facial injuries associated with cervical fractures: Recognition, patterns, and management. J Trauma 25:90–93, 1985.
59. Nicoll EA: Fractures of the dorso-lumbar spine. J Bone Joint Surg [Br] 31:376–394, 1949.
60. Berquist TH: Spine trauma. In McCort JJ, Mindelzun RE: Trauma Radiology. Churchill-Livingstone, New York, 1990, p 63.
61. Reid AB, Letts RM, Black GB: Pediatric chance fractures: Association

with intra-abdominal injuries and seatbelt use. J Trauma 30(4): 384–391, 1990.

62. Asbun HJ, Irani H, Roe EJ, et al: Intra-abdominal seatbelt injury. J Trauma 130(2):189–193, 1990.

63. Anderson PA, Rivara FP, Maier RV, Drake C. The epidemiology of seatbelt-associated injuries. J Trauma 31(1):60–67, 1991.

64. Reddy K, Furer M, West M, Hamonic M: Carotid artery dissection secondary to seatbelt trauma: Case report. J Trauma 30(5):630–633, 1990.

65. Benito MC, Garcia F, Fernandez-Quero L, et al: Lesion of the internal carotid artery caused by a car safety belt. J Trauma 30(1):116–117, 1990.

66. Rogers LF: Radiology of Skeletal Trauma, ed 2. Churchill-Livingstone, New York, 1992, p 166.

67. Meltzer CC: An imaging approach to the evaluation of head trauma. Appl Radiol, supplement, 3:22–28, 1993.

68. Gifford G: A Handbook of Physics for Radiologist and Radiographers. J Wiley, New York, 1984.

69. Thornbury JR, Masters SJ, Campbell JA: Imaging recommendations for head trauma: A new comprehensive strategy. AJR 149:781–783, 1987.

70. Masters SJ, McClean PM, Arcarese JS, et al: Skull x-ray examinations after head trauma: Recommendations by a multidisciplinary panel and validation study. N Engl J Med 316:84–91, 1987.

71. Cromwell LD, Mark LA, Loop JW: CT scout view for skull fractures: Substitute for scout films. AJNR 3:421–423, 1982.

72. Smith WP, Batnitzky S, Rengachary SS: Acute isodense subdural hematomas: A problem in anemic patients. AJNR 2:37–40, 1981.

73. Bucci MN, Phillips TW, McGillicuddy JE: Delayed epidural hemorrhage in hypotensive multiple trauma patients. Neurosurg 19(1): 65–68, 1986.

74. Gray L, Albert MJ: Neuroimaging. In Ravin CE (ed): Imaging and Invasive Radiology in the Intensive Care Unit. New York, Churchill-Livingstone, 1993, p 10.

75. North JB: On the importance of intracranial air. Br J Surg 85:826–829, 1987.

76. Barth EE, Irwin GE Jr: Traumatic pneumocephalus. Radiology 54: 424–427, 1950.

77. Markham JW: Pneumocephalus. Handbook Clin Neurol 24:201–213, 1976.

78. Osborn AG, Daines JH, Wing SDM, Anderson RE: Intracranial air on computerized tomography. J Neurosurg 48:355–359, 1978.

79. Rogers LF: Radiology of Skeletral Trauma, ed 2. Churchill-Livingstone, New York, 1992, p 355.

80. Orebaugh SL, Margolis JH: Post-traumatic intracerebral pneumatocele: Case report. J Trauma 30(12):1577–1580, 1990.

81. Newbold RG, Wiener MD, Volder JB III, Martinez S: Traumatic pneumorhachis. AJR 148:615–616, 1987.

82. Kleinman PK: Diagnostic imaging in infant abuse. AJR 155:703–712, 1990.

83. Rogers LF: Radiology of Skeletral Trauma, ed 2. Churchill-Livingstone, New York, 1992, p 135.
84. Bruce DA, Alavi A, Bilaniuk L, Dolinskas C, Obrist W, et al: Diffuse cerebral swelling following head injuries in children: The syndrome of "malignant cerebral edema." J Neurosurg 54:170–178, 1981.
85. Zimmerman RA, Bilianiuk LT, Bruce D, Schut L, Uzzell B, et al: Computed tomography of craniocerebral injury in the abused child. Radiology 130:687–690, 1979.
86. Woodring JH, Lee C: The role and limitations of computed tomographic scanning in the evaluation of cervical trauma. J Trauma 33(5): 698–708, 1992.
87. Jinkins JR, Dadsetan MR, Sener RN, Desai S, Williams RG: Value of acute-phase angiography in the detection of vascular injuries caused by GSW to the head: Analysis of 12 cases. AJR 159:365–368, 1992.
88. Bonafe A, Manelfe C: Traumatic carotid-cavernous sinus fistulas. Handbook Clin Neurol 13(57):345–366, 1990.
89. Lee C, Woodring JH, Walsh JW: Carotid and vertebral artery injury in survivors of atlanto-occipital dislocation: Case reports and literature review. J Trauma 31(3):401–407, 1991.
90. Lee J-P, Wang AD-J: Epistaxis due to traumatic intercavernous aneurysm: Case report. J Trauma 30(5):619–622, 1990.
91. Woodring JH, Lee C, Duncan V: Transverse process fractures of the cervical vertebrae: Are they insignificant? J Trauma 34(6):797–802, 1993.
92. Schwarz N, Buchinger W, Gaudernak T, Russe F, Zechner W: Injuries to the cervical spine causing vertebral artery trauma: Case reports. J Trauma 31(1):127–133, 1991.
93. Thal ER: Injury to the neck. In Mattox KL, Moore EE, Feliciano DV: Trauma. Connecticut, Appleton & Lange, 1988, p 305.
94. Scalea TM, Sclafani SJ: Angiographically placed balloons for arterial control: A description of technique. J Trauma 31(12):1617–1677, 1991.
95. Haber DW: Lesson 62: The patient undergoing neuroradiologic procedures. Anesthesiology News March:8–16, 1990.
96. Seldinger S: Catheter replacement of the needle in percutaneous arteriography: A new technique. Acta Radiol 39:368–376, 1953.
97. Sackett JF: The spinal cord and related structures. In Juhl JH, Crummy AB (eds): Paul and Juhl's Essentials of Radiologic Imaging, ed 5. JB Lippincott Philadelphia, 1987, p 453.
98. Lin JP, Kricheff II: Central nervous system and spinal cord neuroradiologic diagnostic tools. In Cottrell JE, Turndorf H: Anesthesia and Neurosurgery, ed 2. Mosby, St. Louis, 1986, p 92.
99. Earnest F IV, Forbes G, Sandok BA, et al: Complications of cerebral angiography: Prospective assessment of risk. AJR 142:247–253, 1984.
100. Dion JE, Gates PC, Fox AJ, Barnet HJM, Blom RJ: Clinical events following neuroangiography: A prospective study. Stroke 18(6): 997–1004, 1987.
101. Sheldon JJ, Janowitz W, Leborgne JM, Sivina M, Rojo N: Intravenous DSA of extracranial carotid lesions: Comparison with other techniques and specimens. AJNR 5:547–552, 1984.
102. Ben-Menachem Y, Fisher RG: Diagnostic and interventional radiology in trauma. In Mattox KL, Moore EE, Feliciano DV: Trauma. Connecticut, Appleton & Lange, 1988, pp 187–211.

103. Lin JP, Kricheff II: Central nervous system and spinal cord neuroradiologic diagnostic tools. In Cottrell JE, Turndorf H: Anesthesia and Neurosurgery, ed 2. Mosby, St. Louis, 1986, pp 98–99.
104. Bashour TT, Crew JP, Dian M, et al: Ultrasonic imaging of common carotid artery dissection. J Clin Ultrasound 13:210–211, 1985.
105. Han BK, Babcock DS, Oestreich AE: Sonography of brain tumors in infants. AJNR 5:253–258, 1984.
106. Bowerman RA, Conn SM, Silver TM, Jaffee MH: Natural history of neonatal periventricular/intraventricular hemorrhage and its complications: Sonographic observations (review article). AJNR 5:527–538, 1984.
107. Gooding GAW, Boggan JE, Weinstein PR: Characterization of intracranial neoplasm by CT and intraoperative sonography. AJNR 5:517–520, 1984.
108. Engmann DR, Irwin KM, Marshall WH, Silverberg GD, et al: Intraoperative sonography through a burr hole: Guide for brain biopsy. AJNR 5:243–246, 1984.
109. Rogers JV III, Shuman WP, Hirsch JH, Lange SC, et al: Intraoperative neurosonography: Applications and techniques. AJNR 5:755–760, 1984.
110. Mugge A, Konitzer M, Gaab M, Haubitz B, Daniel WG: Ultrasound imaging of the spinal cord via the esophagus in conscious patients: Initial experience. J Clin Ultrasound 19:187–190, 1990.
111. Gupta RK, Gupta S, Tandon P, Chhabra DK. Ultrasound-guided needle biopsy of lytic lesions of the cervical spine. J Clin Ultrasound 21:194–197, 1993.
112. Quencer RM, Morse BMM, Green BA, Eismont FJ, Brost P: Intraoperative spinal sonography: Adjunct to metrizamide CT in the assessment and surgical decompression of posttraumatic spinal cord cysts. AJR 142:593–601, 1984.
113. Montalvo BM, Quencer RM, Green BA, Eismont FJ, Brown MY, et al: Intraoperative sonography in spinal trauma. Radiology 153:125–134, 1984.
114. Mirvis SE, Geisler FH: Intraoperative sonography of cervical spinal cord injury: Results in 30 patients. AJNR 11:755–761, 1990.
115. Hough JVD, Stuart WD: Middle ear injuries in skull trauma. Laryngoscope 78:899–937, 1968.
116. Lipkin AF, Bryan RN, Jenkins HA: Pneumolabyrinth after temporal bone fracture: Documentation by high resolution CT. AJNR 6:294–295, 1985.
117. Smirniotopolis JG, Mirvis SE, Wolf A: Imaging of craniocerebral trauma. In Mirvis SE, Young JWR (eds): Imaging in Trauma and Critical Care. Williams & Wilkins, Baltimore, 1992, p 79.
118. Teasdale E, Hadley DM: Radiodiagnosis of brain injury. Handbook Clin Neurol 13(57):165, 1990.
119. Gleason TF, Massey TH: Late sequelae of spinal trauma. In Errico TJ, Bauer RD, Waugh T: Spinal Trauma. JB Lippincott, Philadelphia, 1991, pp 563–580.
120. Young JWR, Mirvis SE: Cervical spine trauma. In Mirvis SE, Young

JWR (eds): Imaging in Trauma and Critical Care. Williams & Wilkins, Baltimore, 1992, p 299.

121. Sanders EG, Martin TW: Anesthesia for magnetic resonance imaging procedures. Problems Anesth 6:40:430, 1992.

122. Nixon C, Hirsch NP, Ormerod IEC, Johnson G: Nuclear magnetic resonance: Its implications for the anaesthestist. Anaesthesia 41:131–137, 1986.

123. Smirniotopolis JG, Mirvis SE, Wolf A: Imaging of craniocerebral trauma. In Mirvis SE, Young JWR (eds): Imaging in Trauma and Critical Care. Williams & Wilkins, Baltimore, 1992, p 432–442.

124. Weston G, Strunin L, Amundson GM: Imaging for anaesthetists: A review of the methods and anaesthetic implications of diagnostic imaging techniques. Can Anaesth Soc J 32:552–561, 1985.

125. Davis PJ, Gillen C, Kretchman E, Davis PL, Cook DR: Experience with anesthesia for children requiring nuclear magnetic resonance imaging. Anesthesiol Rev 17(6):35–40, 1990.

126. Smirniotopolis JG, Mirvis SE, Wolf A: Imaging of craniocerebral trauma. In Mirvis SE, Young JWR (eds): Imaging in Trauma and Critical Care. Williams & Wilkins, Baltimore, 1992, p 431.

127. Fowler JR, terPenning B, Syverud SA, Levy RC: Magnetic field hazard [letter]. N Engl J Med 314:1517, 1986.

128. Pavlicek W, Geisinger M, Castle L, et al: The effects of nuclear magnetic resonance on patients with cardiac pacemakers. Radiology 147:149–153, 1983.

129. Bromage PR, Kozic Z: Magnetic resonance imaging: Implications of metal reinforced spinal catheters. Clin Anesth 3:382–385, 1991.

130. Gray L, Alberts MJ: Neuroimaging. In Ravin CE (ed): Imaging and Invasive Radiology in the Intensive Care Unit. Churchill-Livingstone, New York, 1993, p 11.

131. Smirniotopolis JG, Mirvis SE, Wolf A: Imaging of craniocerebral trauma. In Mirvis SE, Young JWR (eds): Imaging in Trauma and Critical Care. Williams & Wilkins, Baltimore, 1992, p 69.

132. Gray L, Alberts MJ: Neuroimaging. In Ravin CE (ed): Imaging and Invasive Radiology in the Intensive Care Unit. Churchill-Livingstone, New York, 1993, p 9.

133. Smirniotopolis JG, Mirvis SE, Wolf A: Imaging of craniocerebral trauma. In Mirvis SE, Young JWR (eds): Imaging in Trauma and Critical Care. Williams & Wilkins, Baltimore, 1992, p 51.

134. Gomori JM, Grossman RI, Hackney DB, Goldberg H, et al: Variable appearances of subacute intracranial hematomas on high-field spin-echo MR. AJR 150:171–178, 1988.

135. Roth JL, Nugent M, Gray JE, et al: Patient monitoring during MRI. Anesthesiology 62:80–83, 1985.

136. Henneberg S, Hok B, Wiklund L, Sjodin G: Remote auscultatory patient monitoring during magnetic resonance imaging. J Clin Monit 8(1):37–43, 1992.

137. Rao CC, McNiece WL, Emhardt J, Krishna G, Westcott R: Modification of an anesthesia machine for use during magnetic resonance imaging [letter]. Anesthesiology 68(4):640–641, 1988.

138. Kross J, Drummond JC: Successful use of a Fortec II vaporizer in the MRI suite: A case report with observations regarding magnetic field induced vaporizer aberrancy. Can J Anaesth 38(8):1065–1069, 1991.
139. Peden CJ, Menon DK, Hall AS, Sargentoni J, Whitwam JG: Magnetic resonance for the anaesthetist. Part II: Anaesthesia and monitoring in MR units. Anaesthesia 47(6):508–517, 1992.
140. Barnett GH, Ropper AH, Johnson KA: Physiological support and monitoring of critically ill patients during magnetic resonance imaging. J Neurosurg 68:246–250, 1988.
141. Holshouser BA, Hinshaw DB Jr, Shellock FG: Sedation, anesthesia, and physiologic monitoring during MR imaging: Evaluation of procedures and equipment. JMRI 3(3):553–558, 1993.
142. Mirvis SE, Borg U, Belzberg H: MR imaging of ventilator-dependent patients: Preliminary experience. Technical note. AJR 149:845–846.
143. Smirniotopolis JG, Mirvis SE, Wolf A: Imaging of craniocerebral trauma. In Mirvis SE, Young JWR (eds): Imaging in Trauma and Critical Care. Williams & Wilkins, Baltimore, 1992, p 434–438.
144. Hadley DM, Teasdale GM, Jenkins A, et al: Magnetic resonance imaging in acute head injury. Clin Radiol 39:131–139, 1988.
145. Gentry LR, Godersky JC, Thompson B: MR imaging of head trauma: Review of the distribution and radiopathologic features of traumatic lesions. AJNR 9:101–110 & AJR 150:663–672, 1988.
146. Hall AJ, Wagle VG, Raycroft J, Goldman RL, Butler AR: Magnetic resonance imaging in cervical spine trauma. J Trauma 34(1):21–26, 1993.
147. Guidelines for the determination of death: Report of the medical consultants on the diagnosis of death to the President's commission for the study of ethical problems in medical and biomedical and behavioral research. JAMA 246:2184–2186, 1981.
148. Kofke WA, Darby JM: Evaluation and certification of brain death. In Grande CM (ed): Textbook of Trauma Anesthesia and Critical Care. Mosby, St. Louis, 1993, pp 994–1006.
149. Powner DJ: The diagnosis of brain death in the adult patient. Intensive Care Med 2:181–189, 1987.
150. Guidelines for the determination of death: Report of the medical consultants on the diagnosis of death to the President's commission for the study of ethical problems in medical and biomedical and behavioral research. JAMA 246:2186, 1981.
151. Goodman JM, Heck LL, Moore BD: Confirmation of brain death with portable isotope angiography: A review of 204 consecutive cases. Neurosurgery 16:492–497, 1985.
152. Task Force for the Determination of Brain Death in Children: Guidelines for the determination of brain death in children. Arch Neurol 44:587–588, 1987.
153. Black PM: Conceptual and practical issues in the declaration of death by brain criteria. Neurosurg Clin North Am 2(2):493–501, 1991.
154. Payen DM, Lamer C, Pilorget A, et al: Evaluation of pulsed Doppler common carotid blood flow as a noninvasive method for brain death diagnosis: A prospective study. Anesthesiology 72:222–229, 1990.

9

Anesthesia for Neurodiagnostic Evaluation

Irene Osborn, MD, Sharyn Tarricone, MD

Role of Neurodiagnostic Evaluation

The ability to rapidly image the central nervous system has been possible only during the last 15 years. Before the advent of computed tomography (CT) scanning, common radiologic procedures in the management of head-injured patients included skull x-ray, cerebral angiography, ventriculography, and radionuclide brain scanning. Currently, the radiologic procedure of choice in acute trauma is the unenhanced CT scan.[1]

Neurodiagnostic procedures are often noninvasive or without stimulation. Although some are painful, they may often be executed without resorting to general anesthesia. Certain situations require the assistance of anesthesia personnel or others who are skilled in providing sedation, monitoring, and resuscitation. These situations include most pediatric patients, uncooperative adults, or critically ill patients. This discussion will specifically address the anesthetic

From *Trauma Anesthesia and Critical Care of Neurological Injury,* edited by K. J. Abrams and C. M. Grande. © 1997, Futura Publishing Co., Armonk, NY.

management and care of this subset of patients in the acute or post-traumatic setting.

The radiology department is often located in an area remote from the operating room (OR) and post-anesthetic care unit (PACU), which presents the first challenge. Oxygen sources, suction units, and monitoring equipment must be available in the diagnostic suite. Most departments have guidelines and equipment for monitoring of sedated or unstable patients. If monitors and oxygen do not exist, they should be procured before sedation is administered. Access to the patient during the procedure may be difficult due to the equipment used and hazards of radiation exposure.

Considerations for Computed Tomography

With the advent of high-resolution CT scanners, axial cross-sectional images have enabled clinicians to identify and evaluate intracranial parenchymal structures as well as spinal anatomy.[2] CT scans are very reliable when positive. Presently, they are most useful in the evaluation of neurological status in the acute situation but are also used for other innumerable clinical applications.

As with many other radiologic procedures, the CT scan is noninvasive and does not by itself produce any pain. The scan does require immobility of the patient for optimal clarity. If the patient is unwilling or unable to remain still, sedation or general anesthesia may be needed.

The exposure time required for CT scanning has been markedly reduced in recent years, so that time during which the patient must remain immobile has decreased from 20 to 30 minutes to as little as 2 minutes, depending on the diagnosis being sought.[2] The need for contrast enhancement can increase scan time and requires use of a functioning intravenous line.

The Traumatized Patient

Most head-injured patients are sent directly for CT scan after evaluation and stabilization in the resuscitation suite of the emergency department. The condition of the patient (as measured by the Glasgow Coma Scale) will determine whether he/she will be intubated, somnolent, or awake and oriented. The intubated patient should be transported with oxygen and controlled or assisted ventilation as needed. During the scanning procedure, a mechanical ventila-

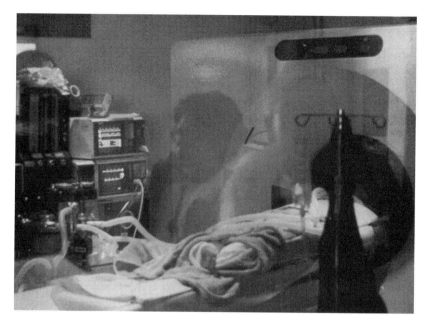

Figure 1. Monitoring of intubated patient for CT scan. The anesthesiologist can remain outside the scanning room with complete view of patient and monitors. Photo by Joseph Lee.

tor is sufficient to maintain respiratory support of the comatose, sedated, or pharmacologically paralyzed patient. These patients should continue to be monitored via pulse oximetry and/or electrocardiogram (ECG) and noninvasive blood pressure, at minimum (Fig. 1).

ECG will allow detection of serious rhythm changes or dysrhythmias but, because of motion artifact or poor monitor resolution, ischemia or ST-T wave changes may be difficult to detect. Patients with arterial lines, central lines, and intracranial pressure (ICP) monitors in place may benefit from continuous monitoring of these parameters. CT scanning may be necessary for the examination of concurrent injuries in the unconscious patient, specifically pneumothorax/hemothorax, visceral injuries of the abdomen, spinal injuries, and injuries involving the extremities. Patients needing emergency procedures, as well as patients who receive contrast agents orally or via a nasogastric tube, should be considered at risk of aspiration.

Once the patient is placed on the scanner table, one should be alert to movement during the procedure which may result in kinking of the endotracheal tube or disconnection from the ventilatory circuit. If the patient begins to move during the study, the scanning can be interrupted and the patient's needs attended to without seriously disrupting the process of data acquisition. When the patient is quiet the scan may begin again.

Patients who received nondepolarizing muscle relaxants to facilitate intubation or transport may begin to cough and struggle when the effects of these agents begin to subside. Unless the patient is truly awake and extubation is planned, excessive straining should not be allowed because it may profoundly aggravate increased ICP.[3] The patient who is semiconscious yet requires airway control may benefit from a number of pharmacological choices (Table 1).

Morphine sulfate 0.05–0.1 mg/kg provides analgesia, tolerance for the endotracheal tube, and sedation. It may be administered if the patient is not hypovolemic. A bolus dose of fentanyl 1–2 μg/kg provides more rapid onset of effect but its duration is limited. Benzodiazepines may be given, particularly if seizures have occurred with the injury. Small doses may be given cautiously to avoid hypotension

Table 1
Agents for Sedation of Intubated Patients

	Advantages	Disadvantages
Opioids:		
Morphine sulfate 0.05–0.1 mg/kg	analgesia sedation reversibility	respiratory depression hypotension
Fentanyl 1–2 μg/kg	same	same, short duration
Benzodiazepines:		
Midazolam 0.01–0.04 mg/kg	anxiolysis amnesia reversible	respiratory depression hypotension opioid interaction
Diazepam 0.1 mg/kg–0.3 mg/kg	similar effect long duration anticonvulsive	not as profound
Lorazepam 2–4 mg	as above as above	as above long duration
Other agents:		
Propofol 1–2 mg/kg + inf–20–50 μg/kg/min	rapid sedation rapid recovery	hypotension resp. depression sepsis ?

and/or interaction with other pharmacological agents already being used.

Propofol has recently been approved for ICU sedation of intubated patients. Its use in the acute setting may be hazardous given the potential for hypotension; infusions have been useful for continuous sedation and control of stress responses.[4] Propofol has been shown to have generally favorable effects on intracranial dynamics as long as cerebral perfusion pressure is maintained.[5,6] Additional doses of muscle relaxants may be administered after it is determined that the patient is still unresponsive to commands and neurological testing is not desired. Relaxants may be given by bolus dose or continuous infusion to facilitate ventilation. Muscle relaxant effect should be monitored with a peripheral nerve stimulator or by careful observation. Exaggerated hemodynamic responses may indicate awakening of the patient or the need for sedation.

The patient who was stable on admission with a Glasgow Coma Scale (GCS) score of 9 to 12 and later deteriorates creates a more distressing situation. This may occur while the patient is awaiting CT scan or shortly after the scan reveals an expanding hematoma, diffuse swelling, or other symptoms that require urgent treatment. Oxygen should be administered while the patient is moved off the scanner and onto a stretcher (if time allows). Endotracheal intubation is performed expediently by the most skilled person available. An obtunded or combative patient should receive a controlled, rapid-sequence (or modified rapid-sequence) induction with thiopental, methohexital, etomidate or propofol with succinylcholine, or nondepolarizing relaxant. Breath sounds are then confirmed and the patient is transported to the operating room or intensive care unit.[7]

The Pediatric Patient

Pediatric patients may require CT evaluation following trauma, falls, or seizures, or in cases of suspected child abuse. The intubated child is managed in a similar fashion to the intubated adult with careful attention to drug dosing. Ventilation of small infants may require a team member to manually ventilate if pediatric ventilators are not available. Patients who are awake or somnolent, but not intubated, may not require sedation. ECG or pulse oximetry may be applied if it does not disturb the child. If no sedation has been given and respiration can be easily observed, the study can begin without monitors.[8]

Table 2
Pediatric Sedation Agents for CT/MRI

Agent	Dose	Comments
Chloral hydrate	75–100 mg/kg	Allow 15–20 min. onset
		Best for infants up to 6 mo.
Pentobarbital	5 mg/kg p.o.	Mix w. conc. Kool-Aid
Pentobarbital	2–3 mg/kg IV up to 9 mg/kg	Give slowly, sedation in 5–10 min
Pentobarbital	4–5 mg/kg i.m.	Painful injection, long duration
Ketamine	4–6 mg/kg i.m.	Fast onset, lasts 20–25 min.
Ketamine	1 mg/kg, slowly divided doses	Analgesia, secretions, good for asthmatics
Methohexital	25–30 mg/kg p.r.	Onset 8–10 min, duration 25 min–1 hr
Methohexital	1–2 mg/kg IV	Give slowly, watch for apnea, repeat bolus or give infusion
Midazolam	0.25–0.75 mg/kg	Give slowly, avoid other agents
Propofol	2–3 mg/kg IV, dilute w. lidocaine inf- 50/100 μg/kg/min	Painful injection, may cause apnea repeat bolus or give infusion

If sedation is required, there are several options (Table 2). Infants up to age 8 months that have not been fed for 4 hours may respond well to chloral hydrate administered orally in a dose range of 50–100 mg/kg. Onset occurs in 10–20 minutes and the infant should be promptly placed in the scanner. Pulse oximetry and "oxygen enrichment" via hose or tubing is recommended. This is often a light form of sedation and excessive handling or the placement of nasal cannulae may disturb the patient. Toddlers and children up to age 5 with no intravenous access may benefit from methohexital administered rectally. A dose of 30 mg/kg has a rapid onset (7–10 minutes) and produces a very somnolent child.[9] Since apnea may occur, it is prudent to administer the dose with oxygen and ventilation equipment at hand.

The child is placed on the scanner and the head positioned with a small roll under the shoulders to facilitate spontaneous respiration and avoid airway obstruction. ECG and/or pulse oximetry should be used in addition to noninvasive blood pressure monitoring at intervals (Fig. 2). Oxygen should be administered to maintain saturation readings above 95%. Following the study, the child should remain in a monitored setting until he/she is awake and following commands.

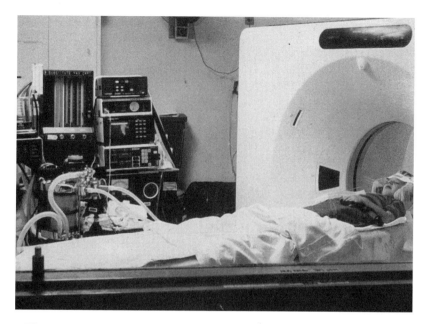

Figure 2. Pediatric patient sedated for CT scan. Photo by Joseph Lee.

Alternatively, ketamine may be administered intramuscularly 4–7 mg/kg in the child without intravenous (IV) access but also without seizure disorder or suspicion of increased ICP (Table 2). Its rapid onset and analgesic properties may benefit the child with multiple injuries devoid of head trauma. Intravenously, it may be given in incremental doses to 1–1.3 mg/kg. Minuscule doses of a benzodiazepine will offset the occasional stormy emergence.

Patients with a flowing IV line may be placed on the scanner and have monitors applied for induction of anesthesia or sedation. Thiopental or methohexital may be given in incremental doses to a total of 3–4 mg/kg or 1–1.5 mg/kg, respectively.[10,11] Oxygen should be administered and the child positioned for the study. If no movement occurs during this period, the study may commence quickly, otherwise be prepared to administer more barbiturate if the patient starts to move excessively. Pentobarbital may be used if a longer study is planned. A dose of 3–4 mg/kg IV or p.o. requires 5–10 minutes for onset but lasts up to 40 minutes with less chance of apnea occurring.

Propofol may be used for sedation in children over age 3. An induction dose of 3–4 mg/kg is often required; however, smaller doses are advised if other agents have been previously given.[12] Pain on injection is a problem that can be alleviated by diluting it to 2.5 mg/cc with 1% lidocaine. Propofol's short duration of action may be sufficient for a brief scan but one should be prepared to give additional doses or begin an infusion (50–100 μg/kg/min) for a longer study. Patients often awaken promptly with little residual drowsiness.

The American Academy of Pediatrics has issued recommendations for the use of conscious sedation of pediatric patients. These guidelines should form the basis for practice in most hospitals whether the sedation is administered by anesthesiologists, other physicians, or nursing staff.[13,14]

Magnetic Resonance Imaging

There is probably no other place in the hospital that provides more challenges to the anesthesiologist than the magnetic resonance imaging (MRI) suite. In addition to working at a considerable distance from the OR and PACU, this area requires the utmost in foresight and vigilance to assure patient and personnel safety.

Currently, MRI is believed to be the best diagnostic tool for many disorders and is now being used increasingly to confirm or further examine pathology discovered by CT scans (Fig. 3). It is frequently used for the evaluation of acute spinal cord compression secondary to tumors. In trauma cases, many of the supposed advantages of high field imaging are outweighed by the practical difficulties of managing the critically ill patient within the magnet[15] (Table 3). MRI is being frequently used for radiologic evaluation after the pa-

Table 3
Computed Tomography vs. Magnetic Resonance Imaging

Computed Tomography	Magnetic Resonance Imaging
rapid study capability	long studies
ionizing radiation	no radiation/magnetic field
routine monitors	MR-compatible monitors/distance
bony structures	soft tissue structures
iodine contrast medium	less noxious contrast
patient visibility	lack of patient visibility

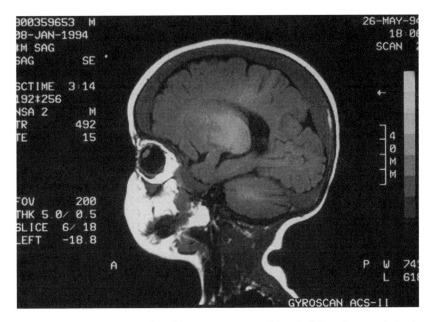

Figure 3. Extensive subdural hematoma caused by shaking of young infant.

tient has stabilized, has undergone surgery, or demonstrates a change in neurological status. Yet with more clinical experience and newer compatible monitoring devices, MRI is increasingly requested for emergency evaluation.[16,17]

The long cylindrical configuration of the MRI tunnel may be frightening to some patients and precludes visual assessment of the patient by personnel (Fig. 4). The presence of the magnetic field contributes to a number of problems: monitoring equipment may malfunction in proximity to the magnet, monitor wires may act as induction coils if looped, causing burns to the patient, and poor scan quality (Table 4). In addition, ferrous objects brought to the scanning room may act as dangerous projectiles, potentially injuring the patient or attendants.

The management of elective patients for MRI sedation has become routine in some university centers. Patients who require airway control, assisted ventilation, supplementary oxygen, invasive monitoring, and cardiovascular support for immobilization pose more challenging logistical problems.[15]

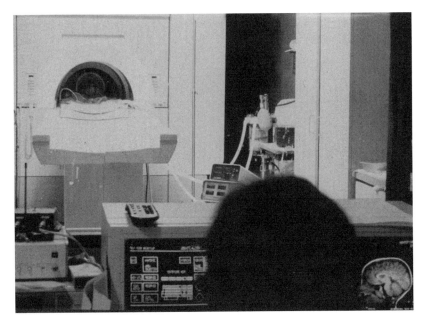

Figure 4. View from the control room. It is difficult to observe the patient. Blood pressure and pulse oximeter reflect patient status.

Monitoring

Adhering to traditional standards for monitoring is difficult in the MRI environment. Many units that function in the OR are not suitable in the MRI suite. Radiofrequency signals can induce currents in ferromagnetic elements in the monitors making them unusable. At the same time there can be a distortion of MR images by

Table 4
Magnetic Resonance Imaging: Anesthetic Considerations

- Magnetic field disables monitoring equipment
- RF interference and risk of burns
- Hazards of ferromagnetic projectiles
- Patient distance/inaccessibility
- Distance from operating room, postanesthesia care unit, etc.
- Prolonged studies

unshielded ferromagnetic materials in the monitors and their cables.[18]

Certain monitors will function adequately from a distance in the scanner or the control room. The Dinamap® (Criticon, Johnson & Johnson) noninvasive blood pressure monitor can be used if placed 5–6 feet from the core of the magnet with long tubing and plastic connectors. Withdrawal-type capnographs placed far from the scanner are very useful for monitoring end-tidal CO_2 in intubated or spontaneously breathing patients.[19]

Electrocardiography is especially difficult to obtain as the lead wires may act as antennae for the radiofrequency field generated during scanning. This may cause a burn if heat is generated and often produces artifact on the cardiac monitor screen. Pulse oximeters may also cause burns if a wire exists in the probe that can heat up and cause injury to the extremity.[20] There has been a proliferation of individual monitors and monitoring systems specifically designed for use in MRI without distortion of image signal (Fig. 5).

Anesthesia machines are available or can be fitted with nonferromagnetic parts and/or aluminum gas tanks. A variety of anesthetic circuits can be used, depending on machine availability and oxygen source. Circle systems with long tubing or a Bain circuit may be used. A Mapleson D-type circuit can be set up with oxygen supply from a large tank outside the scanning room. The presence or lack of an anesthesia machine in the MRI suite will dictate the kind of techniques that one can use.[19]

Anesthetic Techniques

The goal of anesthesia for MRI is to provide immobility and comfort for the patient to achieve the best diagnostic study. MR imaging is obtained in 8- to 10-minute sequences during which data are acquired. If the patient moves during that time, the entire sequence must be repeated (Fig. 6). This produces a longer scanning time than CT and reinforces the need to prevent movement during the study.

Infants and children comprise the largest group of patients requiring anesthesia for MRI. Lying still within a dark tunnel from which "jackhammer" sounds are emitted is also distressing to some adults. The inability of most children to remain perfectly still for 25–50 minutes is common knowledge to parents as well as to physi-

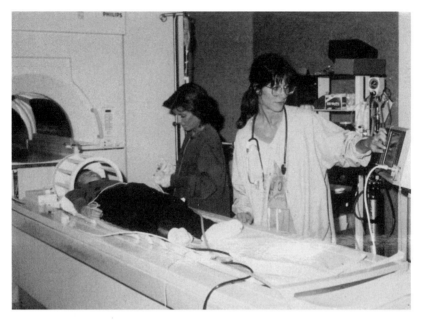

Figure 5. Older child being prepared for scan with spontaneous ventilation and intravenous propofol infusion. Anesthesia machine is MRI-compatible. Monitor from Magnetic Resonance Equipment Corp, provides SpO_2, $EtCO_2$, and NIBP.

cians. The acceptance of this fact and the need for deep sedation or general anesthesia for MRI will save time for many.

Infants under 4 months of age can sometimes be managed with chloral hydrate in doses of 75–100 mg/kg p.o. if a "head scan" without contrast is required.[9] This technique is similar to that described for CT scan, with oxygen enrichment and pulse oximetry being applied if not disturbing. A light plastic object may be placed on the chest to observe movement consistent with respirations.

For older, more vigorous infants and longer studies, general anesthesia is needed. The airway is secured with an endotracheal tube or laryngeal mask airway (LMA). The LMA has proven itself to be most useful in this setting because a laryngoscope is not required for insertion, muscle relaxants are often unnecessary, and it is tolerated at lighter planes of anesthesia[21] (Fig. 7). Endotracheal intubation is recommended for the child with a full stomach, in the prone position, or at risk for aspiration. The child requiring hyperventila-

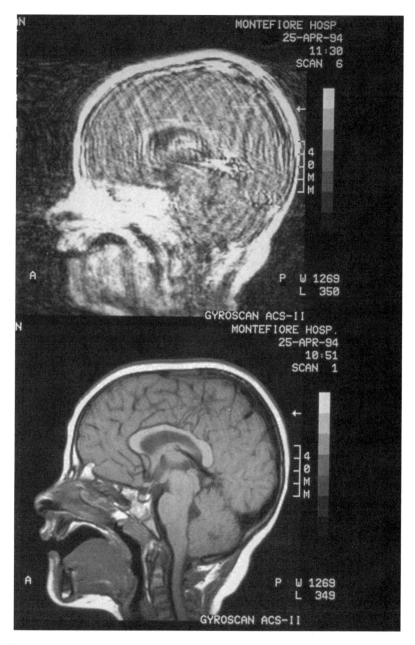

Figure 6. MRI scan with motion artifact; the same patient after receiving intravenous sedation.

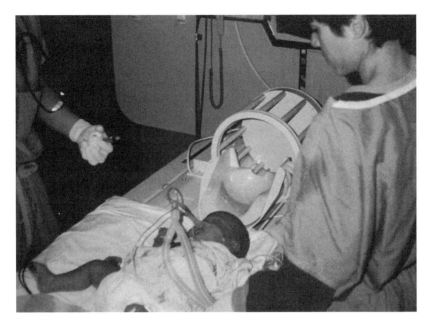

Figure 7. Infant under anesthesia for MRI with laryngeal mask (LMA) in place. Photo by Joseph Lee.

tion is best managed with an endotracheal tube. Once the airway is secure, any anesthetic technique can be used for maintenance. Spontaneous ventilation with volatile agents at low concentrations with or without nitrous oxide is easiest if an anesthesia machine is present. There is no pain or stimulation during the study and light anesthesia is required solely to keep the patient unconscious and immobile but breathing. Intravenous agents may be used for maintenance if there is no anesthesia machine. Patients under general anesthesia should be monitored with pulse oximetry, capnography, ECG, and noninvasive blood pressure measurements (Fig. 8).

Many patients from age 3 to adults can be managed with intravenous infusions and without intubation. Intravenous lines in children may be inserted while awake or following a mask induction with nitrous oxide and halothane is usually as performed in the OR. The latter technique allows for more controlled and efficient placement in children who may have had many previous cannulations. Once IV access is secured, a bolus or infusion of agent is begun.

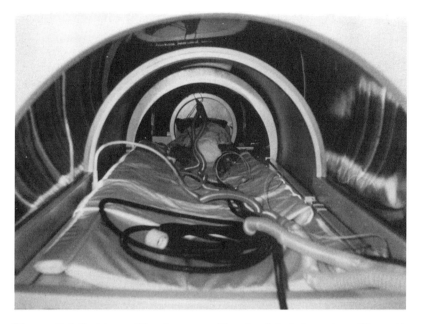

Figure 8. Infant in position for scan with extended circle system, fiberoptic pulse oximeter cable, and blood pressure cables. Photo by Joseph Lee.

Monitors should be in place by this time for assurance of adequate ventilation and heart rate during induction.

Propofol is the most widely used agent for deep sedation/general anesthesia in this setting. It provides a rapid onset and can be maintained by titrated infusion throughout the duration of the scan. Many syringe pumps cannot be used within 10 feet of the scanner due to disabling by the magnetic field. A buret with a calibrated drip chamber may be used and infusion maintained by "counting drops."[22] Spontaneous respiration can be maintained, but it is extremely important at this time to position the patient's head appropriately to prevent airway obstruction. A rate of approximately 100 μg/kg/min will prevent most children from awakening or moving during studies.[23] The infusion is titrated according to heart rate, depth of respiration, and blood pressure. It can be decreased or stopped 5 minutes before scan completion to allow more prompt awakening shortly after completion. The administration of propofol by infusion to spontaneously breathing patients requires constant physician supervision and meticulous technique. Recovery criteria are similar to those for CT scan.

Pentobarbital may also be useful for MRI anesthesia when administered intravenously in incremental doses of 2.5 mg/kg to a maximum of 7.5 mg/kg. It has a slower onset of effect, but when compared with propofol, there was no difference in the physiological response to sedation. Recovery was significantly faster with propofol but instances of transient dips in SpO_2 occurred more frequently.[24]

The Critically Ill Patient

MRI is used increasingly to provide accurate diagnoses, define plans for therapy, and provide new information on physiological changes. In the critically ill patient who may be unable to tolerate numerous invasive studies, it offers an attractive diagnostic alternative. Problems exist because both the static magnetic field and the radiofrequency energy may damage or cause malfunction of electrical or mechanical life-support and monitoring equipment.[25] It is extremely important to search patients carefully for ferrous objects such as pins, buckles, and paper clips. These may cause scan artifact or become projectiles within the scanning suite. Certain conditions and devices are absolute contraindications to entering the MRI suite[15] (Table 5).

Patients with spontaneous respiration via tracheostomy or endotracheal tube may be as described for elective patients. A ventilator specifically designed for MRI is now available. It is a fluidic, pneumatically driven, and volume-cycled ventilator that contains

Table 5
Criteria for Exclusion from MRI Scanning

Unstable vital signs including severely labile intracranial pressure
Permanent cardiac pacemaker
Temporary cardiac pacemaker
Automated internal cardiac defibrillator
Intravascular wire or transthoracic pacing wires
Neuroaneurysmal or vascular surgical clips
Intraocular metallic foreign body
Ferrous endoprostheses
Dependence on technology incompatible with MRI:
    Extracorporeal membrane oxygenator, intra-aortic balloon pump, ventricular
      assist device

aluminum and nonferric components.[26] The ventilator alone may be used or connected to an anesthesia machine. Ventilation can also be maintained manually by someone who remains in the room during the procedure; this can be done without risk of exposure to ionizing radiation. An MRI-compatible anesthesia machine with a long circuit or a Mapleson D circuit with extension can be used.[19] Ventilation can be monitored and modified by end-tidal CO_2 measurement.

Intravenous extension tubing is needed for infusions that must continue during the study. Medications administered by infusion pumps, such as vasopressor agents, antihypertensive drugs, insulin, and sedatives, can be transferred to microdrip burets if needed. A small number of motor-driven pumps are becoming available that require considerable lengths of extension tubing.[19]

The anesthetic technique for critically ill patients is based primarily on the patient's level of consciousness. Comatose patients may require only a dose of nondepolarizing relaxant to prevent movement or coughing on the endotracheal tube. Patients who are responsive to command may receive a sedative or amnestic agent simply to prevent awareness and movement, particularly if intubated. Patients with multiple injuries may receive small doses of opioid for pain relief during the transport and scanning period. Any agent or combination that avoids excessive hypotension is useful.

In the event of an emergency, patients can be removed from the bore of the magnet often in less than 10 seconds. Resuscitation should be performed on a stretcher outside the scanning room to prevent disabling of equipment (defibrillators, ECG machines) and avoid flying projectiles such as pens, clipboards, stethoscopes, name badges, oxygen tanks, laryngoscopes, etc.[9]

Angiography

Spinal or cerebral angiography is performed using retrograde catheterization through the femoral artery or, less commonly, other arteries. Many indications for angiography have been supplanted by noninvasive (CT, MR) radiologic examinations, but studies are still performed for the evaluation of cerebral aneurysm, arteriovenous malformations, and certain tumors.[3] The patient who has suffered head injury may require angiography for evaluation of a concurrent vascular injury or to determine the source of an intracranial hemorrhage. Many emergent cerebral angiographic procedures are performed in the evaluation of subarachnoid hemorrhage. These procedures are often performed with sedation and monitoring without anesthetic assistance; however, unstable patients, uncooperative patients, and children may require additional expertise. The quality of some studies of cerebral circulation is enhanced by hyperventilation, which allows greater concentration of contrast material by the constriction of cerebral vessels.[27]

Considerations for monitoring and sedation are similar to those described for the CT scanner with the addition of noninvasive blood pressure measurements at regular intervals (Fig. 9). Cannulation of the arterial vessel is painful and local anesthetic infiltration is advised, particularly in the heavily sedated patient. Once cannulation has occurred, the patient must remain immobile for the study. Acutely injured patients who are in pain will benefit from the administration of an opioid prior to this point. A burning sensation may occur with contrast injection and this should be anticipated.

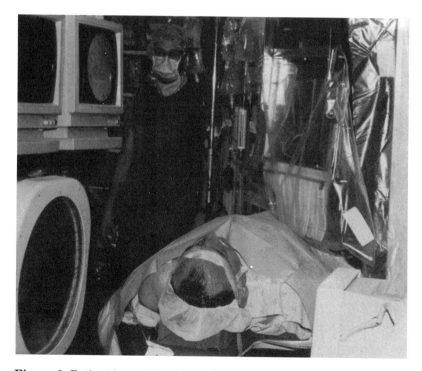

Figure 9. Patient in position for cerebral angiogram. The anesthesiologist is wearing protective covering. Photo by Joseph Lee.

Table 6
Complications of Angiography

Local:	Systemic:
Hematoma	Vasodilation
Infection	Septicemia
Arterial spasm	Cerebral embolism
Subintimal	Anaphylactic
dissection	reactions
	Renal insufficiency

There are several risks and problems associated with angiography; of greatest concern is the reaction to intravenous contrast material[27] (Table 6). The introduction of low-ionic and nonionic contrast material has reduced both the discomfort and the toxicity associated with angiography. High-osmolality contrast media are associated with approximately twice the incidence of adverse reactions, including life-threatening reactions.[28] Because low-osmolality contrast media cost as much as 20 times that of high-osmolality contrast, specific indications are usually listed for the use of the more expensive media.[29] Low-osmolality contrast agents would thus be advantageous in patients with a prior history of contrast agent reaction. Allergic reactions to contrast media range from pruritus, burning on injection, and mild skin rashes to wheezing, dyspnea, syncope, and cardiovascular collapse. These most likely result from nonimmunologic release of histamine and other vasoactive mediators from mast cells and basophils. The incidence of adverse reactions in patients with a history of allergy (particularly to shellfish) is often twice that of the general population.[27] Prophylaxis with steroids and antihistamines is recommended in patients with a history of allergies or specific reaction to contrast media. One should be adequately prepared for all degrees of treatment, including cardiac resuscitation.

To prevent renal complications, fluid management should be aimed at maintaining euvolemia to offset the diuretic effect of the injected contrast. Acutely resuscitated patients may or may not be adequately hydrated prior to the procedure and urine output should be carefully monitored.

The Future of Neurodiagnostic Evaluation

The radiologic armamentarium available for investigation of neurological dysfunction is extensive. The patient requiring acute radiologic diagnosis in the future will likely undergo CT scanning with a faster, more powerful machine. MRI imaging remains exciting as a diagnostic alternative, yet its cost is prohibitive and, unless redesigned to easily accommodate the unstable patient, it is often impractical. It is more likely that adjuncts to CT will be utilized, such as transcranial Doppler evaluation or near-infrared spectroscopy.[30] The latter technique has been useful in localization of intracranial hematomas and would also be used to follow patients postoperatively. Devices for the monitoring of cerebral oxygenation are being developed and used in intensive care. The role of the anesthesiologist may be decreased by newer, even less invasive modalities; however, adequate monitoring, comfort, and resuscitation must be provided by the designated caregivers for successful outcome.

References

1. Gopinath SP, Robertson CS: Management of Severe Head Injury in Anesthesia and Neurosurgery, Third Edition. Cottrell JE, Smith DS (eds): Mosby, St. Louis, 1994.
2. Brann CA, Janik DJ: Anesthesia in the Radiology Suite in Anesthesia for Remote Locations. Romanoff ME, Mirenda JV (eds): JB Lippincott, Philadelphia, 1992, pp 413–424.
3. Tobias M, Smith DS: Anesthesia for Diagnostic Neuroradiology in Anesthesia and Neurosurgery, Third Edition. Cottrell JE, Smith DS (eds): Mosby, St. Louis, 1994.
4. Vezzani A, Barbagallo M: Neurological assessment and ICP control in severe head injury: Use of propofol as a short-acting sedative agent. J Drug Devel 4 (Suppl 3):114, 1991.
5. Farling PA, Johnston JR, Coppel DL: Propofol infusion for sedation of patients with head injury in intensive care: A preliminary report. Anaesthesia 44:222, 1989.
6. Ravussin P, Tempelhof R, et al: Propofol vs. thiopental-isoflurane for neurosurgical anesthesia: Comparison of hemodynamics, CSF pressure, and recovery. J Neurosurg Anesth 3:85, 1991.
7. Smith I, Fleming S, Cernaianu A: Mishaps during transport from the intensive care unit. Crit Care Med 18:278, 1990.
8. Brown TCK, Fisk GC: Anaesthesia for Radiological and Organ Imaging Procedures in Anaesthesia for Children. Blackwell Scientific Publications, Oxford, 1992, p 294.
9. Cote CJ: Anesthesia outside the operating room. In Cote, Ryan, Todres, Goudsouzian (eds): A Practice of Anesthesia for Infants and Children, 2nd Edition. WB Saunders, Philadelphia, 1993, p 401.
10. Varner PD, Ebert JP, et al: Methohexital sedation of children undergoing CT scans. Anesth Analg 64:643, 1985.
11. Strain JD, Campbell JB, et al: IV nembutal: Safe sedation for children undergoing CT. AJR 151:975, 1988.

12. Bready R, Spear R, et al: Propofol infusion: Dose response for CT scans in children. Anesth Analg 74:S36, 1992.
13. Committee on Drugs: Section on anesthesiology. Guidelines for elective use of conscious sedation, deep sedation, and general anesthesia in pediatric patients. Pediatrics 89:1110, 1992.
14. Keeter S, Benator RM, Weinberg SM, et al: Sedation in pediatric CT: National survey of current practice. Radiology 175:745, 1990.
15. Tobin JR, Spurrier EA, Wetzel RC: MRI in critically ill children. Br J Anaesth 69:482, 1992.
16. Hadley DM, Teasdale, GM, Jenkins A, et al: Magnetic resonance imaging in acute head injury. Clin Radiol 39:131, 1988.
17. Sanders EG, Martin TW: Anesthesia for Magnetic Resonance Imaging Procedures in Anesthesia for Remote Locations. Romanoff ME, Mirenda JV (eds): JB Lippincott, Philadelphia, 1992, pp 430–442.
18. Hall S: Anesthesia Outside the O.R.: The Pediatric Patient. ASA Refresher Course Lectures, 1993, p 142.
19. Patteson SK, Chesney JT: Anesthetic management for magnetic resonance imaging: problems and solutions. Anesth Analg 74:121, 1992.
20. Shellock FG, Slimp GL: Severe burn of a finger caused by using a pulse oximeter during MR imaging. AJR 153:1105, 1989.
21. Pennant JH, White PF: The laryngeal mask airway: Its uses in anesthesiology. Anesthesiology 79:144, 1993.
22. Lefever EB, Potter PS, Seeley NR: Propofol sedation for pediatric MRI. Anesth Analg 76:902, 1993.
23. Frankville DD, Spear RM, Dyck JB: The dose of propofol required to prevent children from moving during magnetic resonance imaging. Anesthesiology 79:953, 1993.
24. Bloomfield EL, Masaryk TJ, et al: Intravenous sedation for MR imaging of the brain and spine in children: Pentobarbital versus propofol. Radiology 186:93, 1993.
25. Barnett GH, Ropper AH, Johnson KA: Physiological support and monitoring of critically ill patients during magnetic resonance imaging. J Neurosurg 68:246, 1988.
26. Smith DS, Askey P, Young ML, Kressel HY: Anesthetic management of acutely ill patients during magnetic resonance imaging. Anesthesiology 65:710, 1986.
27. Young WL, Pile-Spellman J: Anesthetic considerations for interventional neuroradiology. Anesthesiology 80:427, 1994.
28. Goldberg M: Systemic reactions to intravascular contrast media: A guide for the anesthesiologist. Anesthesiology 60:46, 1984.
29. Caro JJ, Trindade E, McGregor M: The risks of death and of severe nonfatal reactions with high- vs. low-osmolality contrast media: A meta analysis. Am J Roentgenol 56:825, 1991.
30. Gopinath SP, Robertson CS, Grossman RG: Near-infrared spectroscopic localization of intracranial hematomas. J Neurosurg 79:43, 1993.

$$\boxed{10}$$

Intraoperative Anesthetic Management of Closed Head Injuries

Elizabeth A.M. Frost, MD

Introduction

Given that the severity of head injury may range from mild to life-threatening, it is clear that there must be a similar range for anesthetic techniques from monitored care to general endotracheal anesthesia and from spontaneous to controlled ventilation. Several issues that have been accepted for years have been challenged recently and, in many instances, a different approach to the intraoperative care of the head-injured patient has been explored and even adopted. Some of the controversies that are closer to resolution are described.

Head injury is not a homogeneous disease because many etiologies may be involved. Therapy and prognosis depend on the underlying pathology. Moreover, head injury is a dynamic process with a

From *Trauma Anesthesia and Critical Care of Neurological Injury,* edited by K. J. Abrams and C. M. Grande. © 1997, Futura Publishing Co., Armonk, NY.

variable course that depends on the initial injury and secondary brain damage. The injury caused by the impact is not amenable to treatment and therefore the goals of management are to prevent secondary brain damage due to intracranial or extracranial complications and to provide an optimal physiological environment to maximize the potential for recovery.

Types of Head Injuries

Anesthetic care must be, in part, dictated by the underlying cause of the injury. Several distinct pathological situations are recognized.

Injury to Brain Coverings

Simple depressed skull fractures, most frequently seen in neonates, rarely call for emergency intervention. Time is available to assess the physical status and ensure that conditions are optimal for administration of anesthesia.

Fractures under lacerations are usually compound and should be repaired surgically in under 24 hours to minimize infection.[1] Bony fragments should not be manipulated in the emergency room because they may be tamponading a torn vessel or dural sinus. Similarly, penetrating objects that are still in place should be protected from movement during transportation and removed under controlled conditions in the operating room.

Missile Injuries

Most civilian gunshot wounds are caused by relatively low-velocity bullets whereas military wounds are generally due to shell fragments and high-velocity explosives. However, the pattern is changing as semi-automatic weapons are becoming increasingly available in urban areas.

The bursting fracture of the skull results from a high-pressure wave transmitted from the brain. Epidural, subdural, or intracerebral hematomas result in over 50% of cases.[2] In the absence of a hematoma, devitalized brain tissue may act as a mass lesion and cause extremely high levels of intracranial pressure (ICP) within a few hours.[3] Surgery is aimed at debridement and evacuation of blood clots. The major contaminant is staphylococcus and appropriate antibiotic therapy should be started.

Epidural Hematoma

Traumatic epidural hematoma, usually the result of an automobile accident, is an infrequent complication of head injury. It is associated with laceration of middle meningeal vessels or dural sinuses. Patients are usually in the 15–20 year age group. The clinical course with arterial bleeding is one of rapid deterioration, occasionally, but not invariably, following a lucid interval. Clinical signs of tentorial herniation with ipsilateral third nerve palsy may be elicited. Treatment requires prompt evacuation of the clot. Venous epidural hemorrhages develop more slowly and time for diagnostic evaluation is available.

Subdural Hematoma

The most common cause of subdural hematoma (SDH) is trauma but it may occur spontaneously associated with various coagulopathies, aneurysms, and certain neoplasms. It is considered acute if the patient is symptomatic within 72 hours, subacute if the time interval is 3–15 days, and chronic after 2 weeks.

Acute SDH is the most common intracranial hematoma of traumatic origin requiring surgical evacuation. A lucid interval is frequently seen. Wide craniotomy is indicated to drain the clot and remove devitalized tissue. Subacute and chronic SDH are usually observed in patients over 50 years of age. A history of head trauma is often absent. Clinical presentation varies from focal signs of brain dysfunction to a depressed level of consciousness or development of an organic mental syndrome. ICP is usually elevated. Bedside removal of the liquid under local anesthesia is curative in many instances.[4]

Intracerebral Hematoma

Coup and contracoup injuries usually produce cerebral contusion and intracerebral hematomas. The development of delayed intracerebral hematoma has a poor prognosis. However, some improvement in the neurological state may be achieved by evacuation of the clot.

Control of Intracranial Hypertension

One of the major, recognizable, and easily measured consequences of head injury is raised ICP. The exact relationship between degree of morbidity and level of ICP is unknown. However, generally prolonged increases in ICP are usually associated with poor outcome. Many respiratory maneuvers and anesthetic techniques affect ICP.

Indeed, for decades, head-injured patients have been managed by reducing $PaCO_2$ levels to <30 mm Hg. Hyperventilation may effectively reduce ICP. However, if cerebral blood flow is already reduced because of brain edema, such a maneuver, by further reducing cerebral blood flow, may be deleterious. Arteriovenous oxygen saturation differences across the brain may be used to monitor critical cerebral oxygen delivery and cerebral blood flow (i.e., systemic arterial oxygen content minus jugular venous bulb (JVB) oxygen content.[5] A JDO_2 less than 10 indicates that cerebral blood flow is probably adequate and intracranial hypertension can be treated by mild hyperventilation as is commonly the case in children.[6] Increased oxygen extraction indicates reduced flow and diuretic therapy is indicated with maintenance of normocarbia. This situation is most frequently encountered in adults after blunt trauma. If normal arterial oxygen saturation and hemoglobin concentration exist, JVB oxygen tension may be used alone. Mechanical passive ventilation should be adjusted to levels of JVB oxygen tension over 30 mm Hg.

Thus, ICP is best decreased in most instances by diuretic therapy. Both mannitol and furosemide are effective. Although a bolus of mannitol may initially aggravate intracranial hypertension, the time of elevation of ICP is short and there are apparently no ill effects. Nevertheless, in infants or in elderly patients with cardiac disease, the hyperosmolar effect of mannitol may precipitate cardiac failure. Mannitol also decreases blood viscosity, thus increasing oxygen delivery to the brain.[7] Furosemide lowers ICP and brain water content alone and in combination with mannitol. It does not appear to increase ICP or blood volume, exerts little effect on electrolyte balance, and may be advantageous to infants and in the elderly.[8,9] In large doses, furosemide reduces cerebrospinal fluid formation and may reduce water and ion penetration across the blood-brain barrier.[9] Furosemide prolongs the effectiveness of mannitol.[10] Administration of mannitol 0.5 gm/kg followed after 15 minutes by furosemide 0.5 mg/kg is most effective in causing prompt and adequate brain shrinkage.

Fluid and electrolyte losses are increased. Water excretion of up to 42 mL/min has been reported with the use of both drugs compared to 17 mL/min with mannitol alone.[11] Moreover, the duration of diuresis is prolonged.

A complication of diuretic therapy is hyponatremia, which has also been associated with increased ICP, altered mental status, and pulmonary edema.[12] Close monitoring and appropriate correction of electrolyte balance are indicated. The danger of rapid sodium replacement in increasing neurological abnormalities has been emphasized.[13] Correction of hyponatremia must be slower than 0.55 mmol/L/hr to avoid further complications.

Steroid Administration

Steroid administration does not improve outcome after head injury.[14] Moreover, a study of the effects of steroid administration in children indicated a detrimental effect by potentiation of post-traumatic catabolic response and increased protein breakdown.[15]

Fluid Replacement

Neurosurgeons have often requested that a negative fluid balance be established in the belief that cerebral edema can be reduced. However, such treatment may prove detrimental for the following reasons:

1. Despite complete fluid restriction in animals, cerebral water content decreases minimally or not at all.[16]

2. Hypovolemia may cause hypotension, which increases hypoxia.

3. Hypovolemia decreases oxygen transport, causing cerebral vasodilation and increasing intracranial pressure.

4. A hemodynamically unstable anesthetic course frequently results from perioperative hypovolemia.

A recent review of the literature has shown that the days of keeping the patient "dry" are over and the debate between the neurosurgeon and the orthopedist who demanded replacement for all patients with multiple fractures has resolved in favor of the latter.[17]

Choice of the type of fluid to be given has also changed. A time-honored tradition has been to administer glucose intraoperatively to prevent hypoglycemia, provide energy, conserve protein, and prevent ketosis. However, studies have shown that hyperglycemia existing prior to an ischemic or hypoxic event enhances ischemic damage.[18] This effect is probably due to the failure of oxidative metabolism of glucose in the presence of ischemia or hypoxia. Hence, glycolysis, with lactate as an end-product, increases. Withholding glucose or giving it in moderation to maintain blood glucose levels below 150 mg/dL is recommended whenever brain ischemia may occur.[18]

Recent studies have examined suitable replacement fluids.[19] Low-volume hypertonic sodium lactate solution has been shown to significantly decrease ICP and improve survival. Cerebral blood flow is increased.[17] Maintenance of a hematocrit at 28–32% does not decrease oxygen delivery and decreases viscosity, permitting improved rheologic conditions.[20] Thus, following head injury, it would seem appropriate to avoid sugar-containing solutions, use fewer crystalloids, and to maintain systemic pressure with colloid infusions at a rate adjusted according to central pressures. Comparison of the advantages and disadvantages of colloid and hypertonic saline administration are outlined (Table 1).

Table 1A

• Human serum albumin} • Plasmanate	Minimal infection risk Expensive Support survival Cause dilutional reduction of fibrinogen Bind calcium → negative inotropic effect Rarely necessary (rapid restoration from body pools)

Table 1B

Dextrans	• Dextran-70 • Dextran-40 • Hydroxethyl • Eydroxethyl	Long-term storage Less expensive Support survival 30% invascular retention after 24 hr Reduces ARDS adult respiratory distress syndrome Antiplatelet effect Decreased renal function Hypocoagulability Anaphylaxis (rare)

Table 1C

(7.5% saline in hypertonic saline)	Improves microcirculation 12× volume expanding capacity of crystalloids Half-life 9 hours Hypernatremia Hemolysis

Several advantages and disadvantages of the use of colloids or hypertonic solutions have been identified.

Anesthetic Care

Only about 20% of head-injured patients have lesions requiring surgical intervention that necessitates general endotracheal anesthesia. Key aims of anesthetic management include establishment and maintenance of an impeccable airway, cardiovascular stability, and optimizing of intracranial dynamics.

Controversy continues over what constitutes the preferred anesthetic technique in head-injured victims. Routine administration of preoperative medication is not indicated. Pain is rarely a major complaint and the use of narcotics and sedatives that depress respiration are not justified. Barbiturates and tranquilizers may obscure changing neurological status, and tachycardia caused by belladonna alkaloids may mask excessive blood loss. Phenytoin is the initial drug of choice for seizure control because it causes less sedation. Side effects (hypotension, cardiac dysrhythmias, and central nervous system depression) are minimized if the drug is given at an intravenous rate no faster than 50 mg/min.

In reviewing outcome of head-injured patients at the Albert Einstein College of Medicine, better results were obtained in patients who had sustained blunt trauma when inhalation agents were used.[21] As the pathology of head injury is often one of decreased flow, maintenance of excess flow in relation to metabolic demands may provide better conditions for recovery (i.e., the uncoupling of flow and metabolism provided, for example, by isoflurane). Administration of nitrous oxide alone (i.e., 70% with muscle relaxation) yielded uniformly poor results. Laboratory studies have confirmed these findings.[22] Isoflurane alone improved neurological outcome compared to nitrous oxide alone. However, the addition of lesser amounts of nitrous oxide to the inhalation agent did not worsen outcome. A brief review of some of the more relevant features of several of the currently available anesthetic agents follows.

Inhalation Agents

Isoflurane

Of the presently available agents, isoflurane has shown most promise as a neuroanesthetic agent. Concentrations that produce satisfactory anesthesia for neurosurgical procedures cause little or no depression of myocardial function and no increase in ICP. Thus, cerebral perfusion pressure is maintained. Autoregulation, which ensures constancy of cerebral blood flow throughout a wide range of systemic arterial blood pressure, remains effective during isoflurane anesthesia at concentrations of up to 1.5 MAC (minimum alveolar concentration). Vascular reactivity to CO_2 is also maintained, making possible a rapid decrease in ICP should it be desirable, this may be achieved by hyperventilation. Cerebral metabolic rate is reduced in a dose-related fashion. A cerebral protective effect that is maximal at clinical concentrations has been demonstrated in hypoxic and ischemic animal models.

Isoflurane produces predictable electroencephalographic changes as anesthesia deepens. At subanesthetic levels, frequency and voltage increase; increases in concentration through anesthetic levels produce a progressive decrease in voltage and frequency, and burst suppression occurs at 2 MAC. Above 2 MAC, the EEG becomes isoelectric. Convulsive activity is not provoked by deep levels of isoflurane anesthesia, by decreasing $PaCO_2$ levels, or by auditory or visual stimulation. Metabolism of isoflurane in vivo is extremely low. Thus, the risk of postanesthetic interference with organ function or adverse drug reactions in patients chronically receiving many pharmacological agents is reduced.

Cardiovascular stability is not compromised by standard doses of epinephrine or propranolol. The potency of isoflurane ensures that a stable anesthetic course may be readily maintained without the use of N_2O.

The rapid, precise adjustment of depth that accrues to the low solubility of isoflurane is especially beneficial in neurosurgical procedures because of the great variability of surgical stimulation. Prompt elimination of isoflurane allows fast return to consciousness and permits early neurological examination in the postoperative period. Isoflurane does not appear to alter cerebrospinal fluid dynamics.

Desflurane

Desflurane has recently been introduced to clinical practice and it is, as yet, too early to evaluate its place in neuroanesthesia. Suffice to say that the low solubility allows fine adjustment of depth—an important component of the neuroanesthetic technique. For over 100 years it has been recognized that neurosurgical operations are characterized by short periods of intense stimulation (scalp incision, dural manipulation) and long periods of brain dissection that is pain-free. Prompt elimination of desflurane allows accurate neurological evaluation. However, a recent study has shown that desflurane increases CSF production and significantly increases ICP.[25]

Nitrous Oxide

The use of nitrous oxide in the brain-injured patient is probably not justified.[26] Its addition decreases the amount of inspired oxygen and increases the risks of tension situations developing if pneumothorax (e.g., in cases of multiple trauma) or pneumocephalus (e.g., fractured skull) exists. Cerebral blood flow may increase almost 50% and the electroencephalogram is activated with little change in metabolic rate.[27]

Intravenous Agents

A belief that intravenous drugs had little effect on cerebral dynamics prompted liberal use of these agents in the care of patients after head injury. More recent studies have indicated that not all agents are harmless.

Barbiturates

Long the mainstay of anesthetic induction, thiopental remains a useful agent for the anesthesiologist. However, the dose of thiopental should be adjusted downward. Head injury is usually categorized by hypertension and tachycardia due to catecholamine release. Patients are often hypovolemic—a state that may first be unmasked by a relatively excessive dose of thiopental.

Long-term use of barbiturates has proven less efficacious than was hoped for in the care of severe brain injury.

Joint investigations have shown that, although satisfactory control of otherwise refractory intracranial hypertension may be achieved in 25% of patients by barbiturate infusion, outcome is not improved.[28] Moreover, considerable patient variability exists in clearance of pentobarbital after head injury and daily monitoring of barbiturate levels is indicated.[29]

Opioids

Conflicting results continue to emerge from clinical and laboratory studies of the effects of opioids on intracranial dynamics. A statistically significant increase in ICP and decrease in mean arterial pressure was observed when fentanyl and sufentanil were given to severely head-injured patients in two separate studies.[30,31] However, these effects were not confirmed in a rabbit model of acute brain injury.[32] However, use of low-dose fentanyl (1–2 μg/kg/hr) has not resulted in an increase of ICP in critically injured patients.

Ketamine

Ketamine, a drug known to cause hypertension and hallucinations, has not received acclaim as a major part of the neuroanesthetist's armamentarium. However, a recent study of blunt head injury in rats showed that ketamine decreased cerebral infarct volume and improved neurological outcome.[33] The authors noted that head injury increases concentrations of extracellular excitatory amino acids, which stimulate glutamate receptors in general and the N-methyl-D-aspartate (NMDA) receptor subtype in particular. Calcium influx is increased and a cascade leading to neuronal destruction soon follows. Blockage of NMDA receptors with specific antagonists of noncompetitive ion channel blockers may protect against excitatory amino acid-induced neurotoxicity. Ketamine is an NMDA receptor antagonist. Further clinical use of NMDA antagonists is supported by encouraging results in a variety of in vivo and in vitro models of experimental brain ischemia, hypoxemia, and trauma; and specific antagonists, including dizocilpine maleate, dextromethorphan, and ketamine have been used in low doses in humans for other indications. The time may have come for clinical trials.

Propofol

Propofol was introduced as a short-acting induction agent over a decade ago. Both laboratory and clinical studies indicate that propofol has no obvious adverse effects on intracranial dynamics and may even exert an anticonvulsant effect.[34] Cerebral blood flow decreases approximately 25–50% and cerebrovascular resistance increases approximately 50%. Animal studies have shown that decreases in oxygen requirements exceed the decrease in oxygen delivery secondary to decreased flow, thus increasing reserve and the margin of safety. Initially because of observed hypotensive side effects, propofol was not recommended for neuroanesthesia, especially in patients with increased intracranial pressure. However, a better understanding of the actions of the drug, and expanding options in current practice that coincide with the changing needs of neurosurgeons and neuroradiologists have identified propofol as an interesting and potentially very useful agent for the neuroanesthesiologist.

Etomidate

Etomidate is an intravenous anesthetic agent that provides rapid onset of hypnosis, short duration of action, and good cardiovascular stability. The main effects of the drug on cerebral function seem to pertain to somatosensory evoked potentials (SEPs). Etomidate increases the amplitude of cortically derived median nerve SEPs.[35] Also, introduction of etomidate during a narcotic anesthetic may improve SEP responses from posterior tibial nerve stimulation and allow monitoring of neural function in otherwise unreliable situations. Prolonged myoclonic activity, tonic-clonic movements, and even seizure activity have been associated with etomidate administration. Use of the drug may be relatively contraindicated in patients with head injury because of the propensity for seizures.

Benzodiazepines

Diazepam and midazolam, sedatives frequently used as adjuncts during neuroanesthesia and neuroradiologic testing, may have a long duration of action and interfere with neurological assessment. Benzodiazepines bind to the GABA-ergic receptor complex and enhance the inhibitory action of G-amino-benzoic acid (GABA). Indeed, high doses of midazolam have been shown to exert a protective effect against anoxia in an in vitro model.[36]

Midazolam causes a dose-related decrease in $CMRO_2$ to a maximum of 55% of control and a concomitant decrease in frequency and increase in amplitude on the EEG. Other studies have shown a more limited dose-related decrease in $CMRO_2$, still correlating with decreased neuronal function.[37] A resistance to absorption of CSF has been observed, but there is no alteration of CSF formation.[38]

Administration of the specific benzodiazepine antagonist $RO_{15-1788}$, flumazenil, may cause hypotension. Impaired cerebral autoregulation may also occur, especially if an increased stress response is induced or intracranial damage exists.[39]

Muscle Relaxants

Succinylcholine is often incorporated in rapid-sequence intubation. At least one case of hyperkalemia has been reported after use of this muscle relaxant given to a nonparetic comatose patient.[40]

Also, succinylcholine may increase ICP by central and peripheral actions. Whether or not this is the case, the availability of other agents suggests that succinylcholine should not be used in patients with cerebral damage. Vecuronium, while effective, may be required in increased doses in patients who have been maintained on anti-seizure medications such as dilantin or barbiturates.[41] The break-down product of atracurium, laudanosine, has been implicated as a seizure-provoking agent in animals. However, the dose of atracurium necessary to produce such toxic levels is greatly in excess of that required in neurosurgical procedures.[42]

After compilation of the above data, a reasonable scheme for providing analgesia to the head injury is outlined in Table 2.

Table 2
Scheme for Providing Analgesia to a Head-Injured Patient

The following scheme should allow for prompt reversal especially if the patient was awake preoperatively.

Anesthetic Scheme

Premedication
None or diazepam 5–10 mg orally
Induction
lidocaine 1 mg/kg
fentanyl 1–2 μg/kg
pentothal 2–3 mg/kg
atracurium 0.4 mg/kg
(labetalol 0.2 mg/kg)
(lidocaine spray 4%/4 mL)

Maintenance
O_2
air
isoflurane 0.5–1%
fentanyl 1–1.5 μg/kg/hr
(atracurium 0.2–0.4 mg/kg/hr)
propofol 1 mg/kg or 20–40 μg/kg/hr
labetalol 0.2–0.4 mg/kg
(Neuromuscular blockade reversal only if indicated)

Emergence
Transport with O_2

Emergence

Patients who are conscious or semiconscious preoperatively should be returned to the same state or better postoperatively. Reversal of the anesthetic state and extubation, if at all possible, allow the best conditions for neurological examination. Patients in whom considerable cerebral edema was demonstrated pre- or intraoperatively must be carefully observed for the development of hypercapnia, hypoxia, alteration in the sensorium, and increase in ICP. Should any of these conditions occur, reintubation and assisted ventilation must be performed immediately.

Monitoring

Appropriate intraoperative monitoring (Table 3) requires continuous ECG with the capability of strip recording. Pulse oximetry, capnography, and temperature recordings are invaluable and gas analyses are highly desirable. Arterial cannulation allows frequent blood gas and serum electrolyte (including glucose) analyses and continuous systemic arterial blood pressure monitoring. Trend record-

Table 3
Abnormal Electrocardiograph Findings
in Head-Injured Patients Listed
in Order of Frequency

Finding	Percent
QTc (>440 msec)	60
Tachycardia (>100)	45
ST segment depression	20
QRS prolongation	15
Large U waves	15
ST segment elevation	15
Ventricular extrasystoles	10
Heart block	8
Peaked T waves	8
PR interval prolongation	5
Bradycardia	2

Adapted from Miner ME, Allen SJ: Cardiovascular effects of severe head injury: In Frost E (ed): Clinical Anesthesia in Neurosurgery, 2nd edition. Butterworth, Boston, 1990.

ings and availability of a final hard copy of all parameters provide indications of continued adequate cerebral perfusion. Urinary output and fluid balance must be monitored both to balance fluid shifts caused by blood loss and diuresis and as an early warning of the development of diabetes insipidus.

If the operation is performed in a head-up position or if the injury involves skull fracture, Doppler monitoring is recommended. Placement of a right atrial catheter is ideal. However, several circumstances mitigate against such a maneuver; e.g., time may not be available, placement of the patient in a Trendelenburg position to insert the catheter may prove deleterious to the cerebral status and, interference of cerebral venous drainage may be a consequence of internal jugular cannulation. Moreover, entrained air cannot usually be extracted via this route.

In patients with acute, arterial epidural hematomas, because of the potential for good survival if the clot is released promptly, preanesthetic time should not be devoted to cannulation of vessels other than a peripheral vein. Rather, anesthesia should be induced and invasive monitoring established later. After the surgery has commenced, an arterial route can be established. In the interim, continuous assessment of blood pressure may be obtained by use of finger plethysmography. Pulse oximetry can be used to judge the adequacy of arterial flow.[40]

Summary

The anesthesiologist plays a crucial role in the operative management of the head-injured victim. Establishment of the airway, maintenance of stable intracranial dynamics, appropriate choice of anesthetic agents, and careful perioperative monitoring can all help to ensure maximal neuronal survival.

References

1. Miller JD, Jennett WB: Complications of depressed skull fracture. Lancet 2:991–995, 1968.
2. Barnett JC: Hematomas associated with penetrating wounds. In Coates JB, Jr (ed): Neurological Surgery of Trauma. Office of the Surgeon General, Dept. of the Army, Washington, 1965, pp 131–134.
3. Crockard HA: Early intracranial pressure studies in gunshot wounds of the brain. J Trauma 15:339–347, 1975.
4. Tabaddor K, Shulman K: Definitive treatment of chronic subdural hematoma by twist-drill craniotomy and closed system drainage. J Neurosurg 46:220–226, 1977.

5. Deardon MN: Jugular bulb venous oxygen saturation in the management of severe head injury. Curr Opin Anaesth 4:279–286, 1991.

6. Raphaely R: Central nervous system trauma in children. In Rogers M (ed): Current Practice in Anesthesiology. BC Decker Inc., Toronto, 1988, pp 268–272.

7. Nelson PB, Kapoor W, Rinaldo G et al: Hyponatremia associated with increased intracranial pressure, altered mental status and pulmonary edema following a marathon run. Proc Annu Meet Am Soc Neurol Surg, April 1988, (paper 49).

8. Muiselaar JP, Lutz HA, Becker DP: Effects of mannitol on ICP and CBF correlation with pressure autoregulation in severely head injured patients. J Neurosurg 61:700, 1984.

9. Pollay M, Fullenwider C, Roberts PA, et al: Effect of mannitol and furosemide on blood-brain osmotic gradient and intracranial pressure. J Neurosurg 59:945–950, 1983.

10. Roberts PA, Pollay M, Engles C, et al: Effect on intracranial pressure of furosemide combined with varying doses and administration rates of mannitol. J Neurosurg 66:440–446, 1987.

11. Schetinni A, Stakurski B, Young HF: Osmotic and osmotic loop diuresis in brain surgery: Effects on plasma and CSF electrolytes and ion excretion. J Neurosurg 56:684, 1982.

12. Sterns RH: Severe symptomatic hyponatremia: Treatment and outcome. Ann Intern Med 107:656–664, 1987.

13. Weissman JD, Weissman BM: Routing myelinolysis and delayed encephalopathy following the rapid correction of acute hyponatremia. Act Neurol 46:926–927, 1989.

14. Dearden NM, Gibson JS, McDowall DG, et al: Effect on high dose dexamethasone and outcome from severe head injury. J Neurosurg 64:81–88, 1986.

15. Ford EG, Jennings LM, Andrassy RJ: Steroid administration potentiates urinary nitrogen loses in head injured children. J Trauma 27:1074–1078, 1987.

16. Jelsma LF, McQueen JD: Effect of experimental water restriction on brain water. J Neurosurg 26:35–40, 1967.

17. Frost E: Perioperative management of the head trauma patient. Curr Opin Anesth 6:379–384, 1993.

18. Sieber FE, Smith DS, Traystman RJ, et al: Glucose: A re-evaluation of its intraoperative use. Anesthesiology 67:72–81, 1987.

19. Kreimeier U, Frey L, Messmer K: Small-volume resuscitation. Curr Opin Anesth 6:400–408, 1993.

20. Hint H: The pharmacology of dextran and the physiological background for the clinical use of Rheomaerodex and Maerodex. Acta Anaesth Belg 19:119–138, 1968.

21. Frost E, Kim B, Thiagarajah S, et al: Anesthesia and outcome in severe head injury. Br J Anaesth 53:310, 1981.

22. Baughman VL, Hoffman WE, Albrecht RF, et al: The interaction of N_2O and isoflurane on regional cerebral ischemia in the rat. Anesthesiology 67(Suppl 3A):A578, 1987.

23. Lam AM: Isoflurane and brain protection: Lack of clear-cut evidence is not clear-cut evidence of lack. 2(4):315–18, 1990.
24. McPherson RW, Traystman RJ: Effects of isoflurane on cerebral autoregulation. Anesthesiology 67(Suppl 3A):A576, 1987.
25. Artu AA: Rate of cerebrospinal fluid formation, resistance to reabsorption of cerebrospinal fluid, brain tissue water content, and electroencephalogram during desflurane anesthesia in dogs. J Neurosurg Anesth 5(3):178–186, 1993.
26. Lam AM, Mayberg TS: Use of nitrous oxide in neuroanesthesia: Why bother? J Neurosurg Anesth 4:285–289, 1992.
27. Algotsson L, Messeter K, Rozen I, Hoemin T: Effects of nitrous oxide on cerebral hemodynamics and metabolism during isoflurane anaesthesia in man. Acta Anaesth Scand 36:46–52, 1992.
28. Gokaslan ZL, Robertson CS, Narayan RK, et al: The effect of barbiturates on cerebral blood flow and metabolism. Proc Annu Meet Am Soc Neurol Surg, April 1988 (paper 288).
29. Pentobarbital in patients with severe head injury. Drug Intell Clin Pharm 21:459–463, 1987.
30. Sperry RJ, Bailey PL, Reichman MV, Peterson JC, et al: Fentanyl and sufentanil increase intracranial pressure in head trauma patients. Anesthesiology 77:416–420, 1992.
31. Werner C, Kochs E, Hoffman WE, Bischoff P, et al: Sufentanil does not change cerebral hemodynamics and ICP in head injured patients. J Neurosurg Anesth 4:313, 1992.
32. Sheehan PB, Zorman MH, Scheller MS, Peterson BM: The effects of fentanyl and sufentanil on intracranial pressure and cerebral blood flow in rabbits with an acute cryogenic brain injury. J Neurosurg Anesth 4: 261–267, 1992.
33. Shapira Y, Artru AA, Lam AM: Ketamine decreases cerebral infarct volume and improves neurological outcome following experimental head trauma in rats. J Neurosurg Anesth 4:231–240, 1992.
34. White PF: Propofol: Pharmacokinetics and pharmacodynamics. Semin Anesth 7(Suppl 1):4–20, 1988.
35. Gancher S, Laxer KD, Krieger W: Activation of epileptogenic foci by etomidate. Anesthesiology 61:616–618, 1984.
36. El-Sheikh AM, Lu GP, Frost E, Gibson J, Monell C: Cerebral microcirculatory effects of midazolam in rat model of intracranial hypertension. ASA meeting, San Francisco, 1991.
37. Fleischer JE, Milde JH, Mayer TP, et al: Cerebral effects of high dose midazolam and subsequent reversal with RO 15-1788 in dogs. Anesthesiology 68:234–242, 1988.
38. Artu AA: Dose-related changes in the rate of cerebrospinal fluid formation and resistance to reabsorption of cerebrospinal fluid following administration of thiopental, midazolam and etomidate in dogs. Anesthesiology 69:541–546, 1988.
39. Kochs E, Roever N, Schulte AM, Esch J: Effects of flumazenil on cerebral blood flow and intracranial pressure after incomplete cerebral ischemia in goats. Anesthesiology 69(3A):A586, 1988.
40. Freisen RH: Pulse oximetry during pulmonary artery surgery. Anesth Analg 64:376, 1985.

$\boxed{11}$

Intraoperative Management of Spinal Cord Injury

Joseph P. Giffin, MD, Vance Shearer, MD

Introduction

Each year approximately 10,000 survivors of spinal cord injury (SCI) enter our national health care system: an annual incidence of 12.4–42.8 cases per million.[1–3] Males are involved 2.4 times more often than females and 70% to 80% of the patients are between 11 and 30 years of age.[2,4,5] This latter fact underlines the poignancy of this problem in terms of lost human potential and the urgency of efforts to preserve whatever function remains as well as to foster functional recovery.

In addition to such humanitarian considerations, the demands of handling these patients are increasing due to an expanding pool of long-term survivors.[1] This is a result of advances in resuscitation, supportive care, rehabilitation and chronic care facilities, and methodology, which have reduced mortality. Although mortality before reaching the hospital remains approximately 30%,[2,6] mortality during the first year of treatment is approximately 10%.[1] After this,

From *Trauma Anesthesia and Critical Care of Neurological Injury,* edited by K. J. Abrams and C. M. Grande. © 1997, Futura Publishing Co., Armonk, NY.

survival has improved to such an extent that life expectancy and causes of death are relatively normal. This is especially true of paraplegics and patients treated in specialized care centers.[6] Consequently, the current prevalence of SCI is from 300,000 to 500,000 patients with an economic impact (costs plus lost wages) of greater than one million dollars per case.[6–8]

Surgical decompression or stabilization procedures during the acute phase of SCI are usually indicated only in a subset of patients with complete lesions of less than 48 hours' duration or whose condition is unstable or deteriorating.[9] For these reasons and for a variety of associated injuries or sequelae developing during the course of the illness, 78% of patients admitted to one spinal injury center undergo some type of surgical procedure.[9,10] Clearly, the anesthesiologist should be familiar with spinal cord injury and its management.

In the following discussion, relevant anatomy and fracture patterns, current concepts of the pathophysiology of SCI, and potential resuscitative modalities are described. Principles of the acute management of SCI are briefly reviewed. Finally, the sequelae of SCI that influence medical management and the particulars of anesthetic care are examined in more detail.

Epidemiology of Spinal Cord Injury

Considering the long-term disability and the demands on both the patient's and governmental resources, cervical spinal cord injury poses a major public health problem. Cervical spine injuries occur in about 1.5% to 3% of all major trauma cases that arrive at the hospital alive.[11–19] The victims of fatal blunt trauma have a 16–25% incidence of cervical spine injury.[20,21] In 1981, approximately 6,000 automobile passengers died in the United States from cervical spine injury.[22] The wearing of shoulder-lapbelt restraint systems has been effective in reducing fatal neck injuries.[23] Hopefully these injuries will decrease further with the institution of airbags as a standard feature on all automobiles. The majority of spinal cord injuries result from motor vehicle accidents and account for about 50% of the spinal injuries seen throughout the United States.[21,24] In California, the incidence of spinal cord injuries was estimated at 53 per million population per year, occurring mostly in males 15–35 years of age and in those over 65 years of age.[2,5] Although much focus has been placed on football as a cause of spinal cord injury, water sports (diving, surfing, and water skiing) as well as snow skiing accounted for more than 80% of the athletically related spinal cord injuries seen in California.[23,25] Younger children are less likely to suffer a cervical spine injury as a result of their decreased body weight and cartilaginous cervical spine.[26-28] Children tend to have higher level cervical spine injuries, with those less than 2 years of age almost exclusively suffering C_1 or C_2 injuries as a result of their more horizontal facet joints and lax ligaments.[29]

The Anatomy of the Cervical Spine

Before considering airway management with the abnormal cervical spine, either through trauma or disease, a review of the anatomy of the normal cervical spine is in order (Fig. 1). There are seven cervical vertebrae. Since the first cervical vertebra (C_1, the atlas) and the second (C_2, the axis) are anatomically and functionally different from the lower five cervical vertebrae, they will be discussed separately.

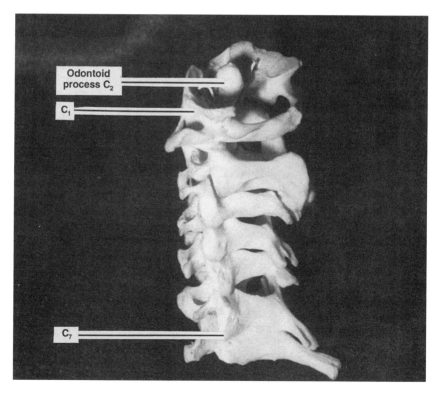

Figure 1. Lateral view of the cervical spine.

Upper Cervical Spine

The function and anatomy of C_1, the atlas, and C_2, the axis, are highly specialized. The atlas supports the head and, therefore, derives its name (Fig. 2) from the mythical Greek character who supported the earth. The vertebral body is normally the major

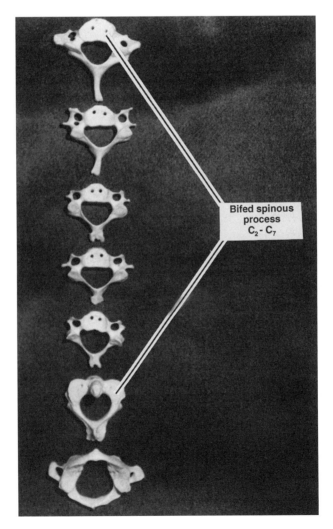

Figure 2. Cervical vertebrae C_1–C_7.

weight-bearing portion of the vertebrae. However, the atlas (C_1) is the only vertebra without a body, and instead consists of an anterior and a posterior arch. Furthermore, instead of articular processes, the atlas has a pair of lateral masses formed at the junction of the anterior and the posterior arches. These lateral masses are the site of the superior and inferior articular surfaces, which articulate with occipital condyles above and the superior facet joints of the axis (C_2) below. Projecting medially from the two lateral masses are bony tubercles to which are attached the transverse ligament (Fig. 2). When the atlas and axis are articulated, the upward projection of the axis, the dens, lies behind the anterior arch of the atlas and is retained in this position by the transverse ligament (Fig. 2). Projecting laterally from the lateral masses on C_1 are the transverse processes. Each transverse process from C_1–C_6 has a foramen through which the vertebral artery passes. The vertebral vein also passes through the foramen in the transverse process of C_7.

The axis (C_2) is the pivot on which the axis and, therefore, the head rotate (Fig. 3). The body of the axis gives rise to the dens (odontoid process), which projects vertically through the atlas and at-

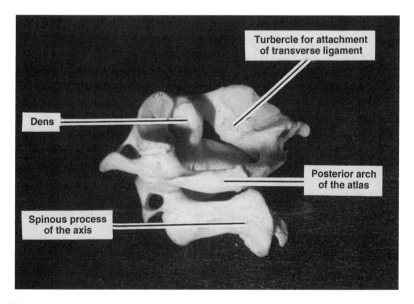

Figure 3. Posterior view of the first cervical vertebrae (the atlas) and the odontoid process.

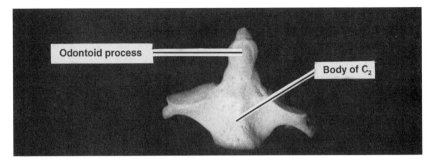

Figure 4. Anterior-posterior view of the second cervical vertebrae (the axis).

taches to the anterior margins of the foramen magnum by the alar and apical ligaments (Fig. 4). This attachment forms the occipitalo-atlantoaxial complex. The lamina of the axis are thicker than any other cervical vertebra and provide attachment to the ligamentum flavum and fuse posteriorly with the large and powerful spinous processes which take the attachment for the muscles that extend, retract, and rotate the head. The spinous processes of C_2 through C_6 are unique in that they are bifid (Fig. 5).

Lower Cervical Vertebrae

The lower five cervical vertebrae are anatomically more typical of the remaining vertebrae. Their transverse processes are unique in that they possess the foramen transversium, which transmits the vertebral artery through most of the cervical spine (Fig. 5). The seventh cervical vertebra, sometimes called the vertebra prominens, has a long spinous process that is visible through the skin at the base of the neck. The ligamentum nuchae is tied to the spinous process of the seventh cervical vertebra.

Ligaments and Articulations

The articulations of the atlas to the occiput and axis are highly specialized. The atlanto-occipital joint is a synovial joint that allows flexion and extension, but no rotation or lateral bending of the head on the atlas. The atlas and axis articulate at three sites to allow rotation of the atlas on the axis and a small amount of flexion and extension. Synovial cavities exist between the anterior arch of the

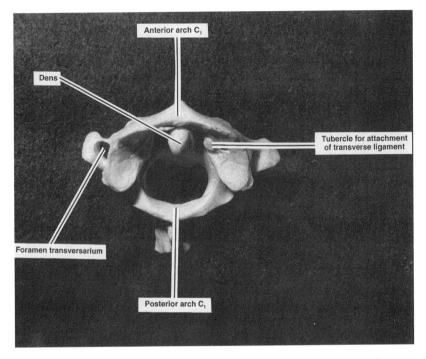

Figure 5. Sagittal view of the alignment of the dens with the atlas.

atlas, the dens, and between the dens and the transverse ligament to allow rotation (Fig. 2). The dens is also held in place by the cruciform ligament complex, which consists of fibers that attach the body of the axis to the occiput (Fig. 4). Apical ligaments attach the dens to the occiput laterally and restrict rotation. The ligamentus attachments of the atlas to the occiput are the anterior and posterior atlanto-occipital membranes, which are the continuations of the anterior longitudinal ligament and the ligamentum flavum, respectively. The superior continuation of the posterior longitudinal ligament is the tectorial membrane.

The articulations of the lower five cervical vertebrae are the vertebral bodies and the superior and inferior pedicles, which articulate horizontally to form the facet joints (Fig. 5). These osseous articulations are synovial joints and are separated by synovial capsules.

The joint between the vertebral bodies consist of two bony surfaces coated with hyaline cartilage. At the periphery, a ring-like epiphysis fuses with the vertebral body in early adult life; however, the cartilage persists and helps to enclose the intervertebral discs. The intervertebral discs are composed of peripheral fibrocartilage arranged in concentric rings, the annulus fibrosis, and the nucleus pulposus, which act as shock absorbers. These discs are thicker anteriorly than posteriorly and give the cervical spine a lordotic curve.

The cervical spine is stabilized anteriorly by the anterior and posterior longitudinal ligaments, which extend the length of the cervical spine. The anterior longitudinal ligament joins adjacent vertebral bodies anteriorly and anterolaterally and travels along the anterior surface of the vertebral bodies and terminates over the anterior arch of the atlas forming the anterior atlanto-occipital ligament, which inserts on the base of the skull. The posterior longitudinal ligament courses upward along the dorsal surface of the vertebral bodies and fans over the body of the axis and the odontoid process and terminates as a tectorial membrane that inserts at the base of the occiput. The anterior longitudinal ligament limits extension and the posterior longitudinal ligament tends to limit flexion.

The spine is stabilized posteriorly by the supraspinous and interspinous ligaments and ligamentum flavum. The supraspinous ligament courses between the tips of the spinous processes and imparts a significant degree of structural integrity to the cervical spine. The weaker interspinous ligaments connect one spinous process to the next along the length of the processes. The ligamentum flavum connects adjacent laminae and consists of paired elastic ligaments. These posterior column ligaments tend to limit flexion of the cervical spine.

Narrow intertransverse ligaments are located between the transverse processes but add little strength to the spine.

Kinematics of the Cervical Spine

Kinematics describe the motion of bodies without the influence of external load forces. The cervical spine is capable of many types and ranges of motion. It is capable of rotary motion about its vertical axis, anterior flexion and posterior extension about its transverse axes, and lateral bending about the vertical axis. The normal range of motion of the occipito-atlantoaxial complex in flexion and extension is about 23.4.[30] Flexion within this complex is limited by the contact between the odontoid process and the anterior border of the foramen magnum, tectorial membrane, and the posterior elements.[31]

Extension is limited by the contact of the occiput, posterior arch of the atlas, and the arch of the axis.[30] A narrow atlanto-occipital gap, and to a lesser extent a short interspace between the posterior arches of the atlas and axis has been associated with difficult intubations due to restricted extension.[32–34]

Up to 50% of the total axial-rotation of the neck is achieved at the atlanto-axial complex. This degree of rotation has been associated with the development of vertebrobasilar ischemia due to kinking of the vertebral arteries. No lateral bending occurs at the C_1–C_2 complex. Lateral displacement of the C_1–C_2 complex greater than 4 mm is abnormal. Anterior-posterior translation greater than 1 mm is abnormal at the occipito-atlantoaxial complex. Movement in the vertical, horizontal, and lateral directions without rotation is called translation. Because of the various angles of the facet joints, a motion in one direction can simultaneously cause a motion in a different direction. For example, the axial rotation at the C_1–C_2 complex is associated with as much as 2 mm vertical translation. Over-rotation can result in the rupture of the alar and occipitodentate ligaments.

The range of motion of the lower cervical spine contributes an additional 66° of flexion-extension.[29] The largest component of this motion occurs between the C_5–C_7 vertebrae. Although the etiology of a decrease is unclear, the range of motion of the lower cervical spine in the adult decreases as much as 25% between the ages of 20 and 80. Most of this decrease occurs at the C_5–C_7 segments.[35]

Stability and Instability of the Cervical Spine

Stability is defined as the ability to maintain normal anatomical relationships between vertebrae under conditions of normal physiological loading.[36] Conversely, instability occurs when normal physiological loads can cause displacement of the vertebral elements, jeopardizing the spinal cord, nerve roots, and/or vasculature.[37]

The stability of the occipito-atlantoaxial complex is secured by the transverse, alar, and apical ligaments and the superior terminations of the anterior and posterior longitudinal ligaments.[36] The vertebral canal is largest at the occipito-atlantoaxial complex. At C_1 this canal is divided into thirds. One-third of the space at C_1 is odontoid, one-third spinal cord, and the other third is empty space.[38] Although no more than 3 mm of anterior-posterior translocation between the dens and the anterior arch of the atlas normally occurs, an isolated rupture of the transverse ligament with intact alar and apical ligaments may allow 5 mm of movement. As much as 10 mm of displacement can occur if all of these ligaments are disrupted.[36] The normal vertebral canal at C_1 is approximately 20 mm and cord compression is not seen when this distance is greater than 18 mm. However, cord compression can occur with a decrease to less than 14 mm.[39] The previously mentioned one-third empty space in the vertebral canal allows for some margin of safety at the level of C_1.

The lower cervical spine consists of an anterior and a posterior column. The anterior column is supported by structures anterior to the posterior longitudinal ligament; likewise, the posterior column is supported by those elements posterior to the posterior longitudinal ligament. Those structures supporting the anterior column are the anterior longitudinal ligament, the intervertebral disc, and the posterior longitudinal ligament as well as the facet joints with the capsular and intertransverse ligaments. The posterior column is primarily supported by the supraspinous, interspinous ligaments, and the ligamentum flavum.[35,40]

Studies on the cadaveric model with extension and flexion under physiological loads found the cervical spine to be unstable when all of the elements of one column were disrupted. Furthermore, if only one element of the motion segments of one column were intact and all of the segments of the other column were intact, either posterior or anterior, the cervical spine remained stable under physiological loads.[39] Clinically, this condition cannot be assumed; therefore, the cervical spine must be considered unstable until proven otherwise.

Specific Injuries and Mechanisms

Atlanto-Occipital Dislocations

Atlanto-occipital dislocation is an extremely rare injury. In 1980, Pang and Wilberger found only 13 case reports in the world literature with only six of these patients reported as surviving after admission to the hospital.[41] Although survivors with this injury are rare, it is the most common cervical spine injury in fatal motor vehicle accidents.[20,42,43] The mechanism of death appears to be transection of the medulla oblongata or of the spinomedullary junction.[42,44] The mechanism of injury appears to be a combination of hyperextension of the head with an associated distraction force on the cranium. Frequently, there are abrasions on the chin, cheeks, or forehead, suggesting that there has been a hyperextension force sufficient to tear the transverse ligament, the tectorial and cruciform membranes, and the alar ligaments. With atlanto-occipital dislocation, the atlas itself remains in position held by the anterior and posterior occipital atlantal membranes and the anterior and posterior longitudinal ligaments. This results in the slippage of the occiput backward upon the atlas. Along with the subsequent damage to the medulla, compression of the vertebral arteries between the condyles and the lamina of C_1 may also occur. The radiologic diagnosis of atlanto-occipital dislocations may not be readily visible on plain lateral cervical films and may be easily missed. The diagnosis can be suggested by the demonstration of retropharyngeal swelling on the lateral cervical spine film. The distance between the anterior edge of the foramen magnum and the tip of the posterior arch of the atlas should be equal to the distance between the anterior arch of the atlas and the posterior edge of the foramen magnum. If this ratio is greater than one, then the head is forward relative to the spine.[45] Atlanto-occipital dislocation is a treacherously unstable injury. Even the slightest amount of traction on the patient's cervical spine can result in cardiorespiratory arrest.[46]

Although the discussion of airway management will be covered elsewhere in this book, special mention should be noted with this injury. If possible, these patients should be kept awake in order to continuously assess their cardiorespiratory and neurological status, and they should be immobilized as soon as possible. Since respiration may be severely impaired, they may need an emergency airway. Any motion of the cervical spine during intubation attempts may be extremely dangerous.

Injuries to the C_1–C_2 Complex

Among the fatalities of traffic accidents that are associated with severe cervical spinal cord injury, 80% involve the articulations among the occiput, C_1, and C_2, and only 20% involve the cervical spine below the level of C_2. Conversely, serious neurological injury is less common in surviving patients sustaining injury to the upper cervical spine than in those sustaining injury to the lower cervical spine. Since the spinal cord occupies only one-third of the vertebral canal at this level, survivors with these lesions rarely have neurological sequelae.[47,48]

Fractures of the Atlas

Fractures of the atlas can be either stable or unstable. Those fractures with an intact transverse ligament are stable, whereas those fractures associated with rupture of this ligament are unstable. If posterior movement of the dens is greater than 3 mm behind the anterior ring of the atlas, significant injury to the transverse ligament is probable.[36] Jefferson's fracture or fracture of the atlas was first described by him in 1920. He described bilateral fractures of the posterior arch of the atlas resulting from a direct vertical blow to the head, causing a "squeeze" of the atlas. As a result of this compression, the lateral masses are displaced outward. Since the bursting fragments are displaced outward, with resulting widening of the spinal canal, the cervicomedullary junction may remain unharmed. Patients present with occipital or neck pain and signs of nuchal rigidity with limitation of motion.[49] The patient may support the forehead in the hands when looking downward and support the head posteriorly when looking upward. Dysphasia and thick speech occasionally may be associated with a rotary dislocation. In cases of fracture of the anterior arch, palpation of the pharynx may detect a protuberance. Computed tomography is useful in demonstrating the Jefferson fracture.

Transaxial Cervicomedullary Injury

Transaxial cervicomedullary injury involves a deadly direct blow to the vertex without the fracture of the skull or the cervical spine. After rebounding from this blow, the brain stem and cervical spinal cord are herniated caudally through the foramen magnum to the level of the C_2 segment; resulting in immediate cardiorespiratory arrest and death. A fatal football accident of this type was caught on motion pictures[48] and the mechanism for this injury was duplicated in monkeys.[50]

Odontoid Fractures

The odontoid process is almost completely interarticular and its close relationship with the atlas makes it susceptible to any injury of the atlas. Although the exact mechanism for odontoid fracture is not known, it may result from high-velocity blows to the face, the side, or the back of the head. Lateral loading combined with other forces may be responsible for this injury. Anterior displacement from flexion forces of the transverse ligament occur in about 80% of these fractures, whereas extension forces the anterior ring on the odontoid with posterior displacement occurring in 20% of these fractures.[51] Odontoid fractures compose about 75% of cervical spine injuries in children and about 10–15% in adults.[52] Clinically, these fractures present with severe high cervical pain and muscle spasm. Pain may also radiate to the back of the head. The diagnosis of odontoid fracture can be made by anterior/posterior plain films or lateral tomograms. This injury can be confused with os odontoideum, which is the congenital nonunion of the dens with the axis.

There are three types of odontoid fractures. Type I fractures involve only the tip of the odontoid. These fractures usually occur from disruption of the apical or alar ligaments. Since the transverse ligament is intact, the cervical spine remains stable and since the blood supply is not disturbed, these injuries have a good prognosis.[53–55]

Type II fractures occur at the base of the dens at the site of its union with the vertebral body. The blood supply is disrupted and except for children, nonunion of this injury is common. Type II fractures are the most common odontoid fracture and this injury can result in displacement of the odontoid.

Type III fractures occur to the body of the axis and heal well since this fracture occurs through cancellous bone. This injury is usually stable; however, displacement can occur.[56]

Fractures of the odontoid process may result in atlantoaxial dislocation. Atlantoaxial dislocation can also occur from congenital deformities of the bones and ligaments as with os odontoideum, and with ligamentus injuries not associated with bony fracture. Tears of the transverse and alar ligaments as well as avulsion of the tectorial and cruciform membranes can occur with severe hyperextension or flexion. Anterior atlantoaxial dislocations are more common with this injury. These patients present with neck soreness and stiffness, with pain later radiating to the shoulders. This injury can be diagnosed on cautious extension flexion during which the anterior ring of the atlas dislocates either forward or backward. These injuries require surgical repair because the soft tissue ligaments will not heal spontaneously.

Bell described the brachial cruciate paralysis syndrome.[57] This syndrome, which mimics central cervical cord syndrome, results from the dens pressing into the base of the medulla, causing pressure on the pyramidal tracks in the midline. This occurs with atlantoaxial dislocation and results in paralysis of the upper extremities. Proper traction and positioning will usually revert this neurological picture to normal.

Traumatic Spondylolisthesis of the Axis ("Hangman's Fracture")

In 1913 Wood-Jones described this fracture, which results from judicial hanging performed by the platform-drop technique.[58] This injury occurs with the avulsion of the laminar arches of C_2 with some dislocation of the vertebral body of C_2 on C_3. In a proper judicial hanging with the knot placed in the submental position using the platform-drop technique, the weight of the body pulls downward. The clivus of the skull and the C_1 and the C_2 vertebral bodies move as a solitary unit avulsing the laminar arches. The resulting mechanism of hyperextension with sudden violent distraction causes complete transection of the cord and vertebral arteries, destroying the cervicomedullary junction and resulting in immediate death.[59] Today the majority of patients with this lesion are injured in either motor vehicle or diving accidents.[58,60] Schneider et al. reported eight cases of "hangman's fracture" that occurred as a result of motor vehicle accidents.[59] Two of the patients in their series did not loose consciousness and described themselves as hanging on the steering wheel or dashboard of the vehicle. Both of these patients had abrasions on their chins and faces.[59] The mechanism of injury in these cases was severe hyperextension; however, unlike judicial hanging, the weight of the body is supported without a further drop, so the avulsed arches decompress the cervicomedullary junction, and neurological deficit may not occur. Neurological injury is probably uncommon because of the large diameter of the vertebral canal at this level. Although a neuroinjury is relatively uncommon in survivors, this injury is the second most common lesion in victims of fatal motor vehicle accidents.[40,41,61] Head trauma and mandibular fractures occur in approximately 70% of these patients and other upper cervical spine lesions are common.[58] The diagnosis of this injury is easily made on lateral or oblique plain films and can be classified into three types. Type I fractures are without angulation and have less than 3 mm displacement. Type II fractures are bipedicular fractures with significant angulation and translation. Type III fractures are characterized by severe angulation and displacement with unilateral or bilateral facet dislocations. This type results in the separation of the skull and the first two cervical vertebrae from the remainder of the cervical spine and is extremely unstable.[62]

Lower Cervical Fractures and Dislocations

The various fractures and dislocations of the lower cervical spine are dependent on the mechanism of injury. Most of these injuries are the result of indirect forces originating in the head or the trunk that subject the cervical spine to forces of flexion, rotation, extension, and vertical compression.

Hyperflexion can cause a strain injury that results from partial tearing of the posterior ligamental structures. Radiographic evaluation of these patients frequently demonstrate a normal spine; however, flexion views may demonstrate separation of the interspinous ligaments. The primary pathological lesion with this injury is the syndrome of chronic neck ache, and involvement of the spinal cord and nerve roots is rare.

Unilateral facet dislocation occurs with the combination of forward flexion and rotation. There is tearing of the interspinous ligaments and the facet capsule on the involved side, resulting in forward displacement over the inferior facet at the level of the dislocation. The most common vertebral levels of facet dislocation are as follows: C_5 on C_6 followed by C_6 on C_7 and C_4 on C_5. Unilateral facet dislocation frequently results in cervical nerve root entrapment and the potential for spinal cord injury at the level of subluxation.

Bilateral facet dislocation occurs when the flexion forces are greater than those contributed by rotation. This injury involves disruption of the interspinous ligaments as well as both facet capsules with the potential for disruption of the posterior and anterior longitudinal ligaments. Greater than 50% subluxation between the vertebral bodies is frequently seen. The spinal canal may be compromised with bilateral facet dislocation, often resulting in severe spinal cord injury.

A wedge compression fracture occurs with the combination of hyperflexion and a compressive force applied to the anterior portion of the vertebral body. This injury causes disruption of the posterior ligamentus structures with separation of the spinous processes and instability of the cervical spine.

A teardrop fracture occurs when major compressive forces are applied with the neck in flexion. This mechanism results in a comminuted fracture of the vertebral body in which the anterior-inferior vertebral fragment is triangular. The posterior fragments of the vertebral body are commonly displaced into the spinal canal, causing major spinal cord damage.

Hyperextension injuries probably account for the majority of cervical spine injuries.[63,64] Hyperextension injuries may be divided into two subgroups: distractive and compressive.[62] With distractive hyperextension injuries, the forces are directed away from the trunk placing the anterior elements of the cervical spine under tension. Either the anterior ligamentus complex fails or the vertebral body fractures transversely. This may be seen radiographically by widening of the disc space; however, these injuries are frequently missed on initial radiographic exams. If the distractive force is more severe, the posterior ligamentus complex fails, allowing for displacement of the superior vertebral body posterially into the vertebral canal. Compressive hyperextension injuries occur when the major force vector is directed toward the trunk while the head is extended, causing compression of the posterior elements. The resulting injury, depending on the degree of force, can vary from unilateral vertebral arch fracture (with or without displacement) to bilateral lamina fracture without other tissue failure, to bilateral vertebral arch fracture with full vertebral body displacement anteriorly.

Penetrating Injuries to the Cervical Spine

Although penetrating injuries to the neck and the cervical spine can occur with industrial and motor vehicle accidents, they are most likely to occur with stab and gunshot wounds. Unfortunately, with the ever-increasing urban violence and gang warfare on the city streets as well as the ready availability of weapons, penetrating trauma to the neck is becoming increasingly common. The authors recently found a 1% incidence of cervical spine injury with penetrating neck trauma.[65] Penetrating trauma to the neck is also frequently associated with injuries to other major structures, namely airway and vascular structures, which further complicates the airway management of these patients.

Pathophysiology of Spinal Cord Injury

Spinal cord trauma results in both primary and secondary injuries. The primary injury, if severe enough, will result in functional or anatomic disruption of the cord at the scene of the accident with a correspondingly dismal prognosis. The uniformly encountered anatomic and histologic findings associated with such primary injury include direct neurilemmal and neuronal disruption and/or destruction, petechial hemorrhages, gross hematomyelia, or even total cord transection, a rare event. The areas rendered nonviable by this primary insult will go on to develop a cavitating necrosis and ultimately glial scar formation.

The observation that areas of the spinal cord not immediately destroyed by traumatic force subsequently undergo progressive hemorrhagic necrosis, edema, and inflammation at a rate proportional to the severity of the lesion has produced the concept of a secondary injury. This injury is perhaps mediated and propagated by mechanisms initiated by, but distinct from, the initial mechanical deformation.

The extension of tissue necrosis from the initial gray matter involvement to include the white matter, producing the clinical picture of quadriplegia or paraplegia, is preceded by endothelial damage with platelet adhesion, platelet aggregation, microvascular occlusion, and embolization of microthrombi. On a macroscopic scale, corresponding vascular stasis, decreased spinal cord blood flow (SCBF), and ischemia are noted. Axonal degeneration (hydropic and then granular), myelinolysis, cell necrosis, inflammatory infiltrate, and neuronophagia ensue. A striking feature is the occurrence of intraaxonal calcium hydroxyapatite crystals and mitochondrial calcification. Similar degenerative changes have been observed following exposure of rat spinal cords to calcium or calcium in the presence of an ionophore.[66]

Biochemical events coinciding with this process of progressive autodestruction include: (1) a massive translocation of calcium from the extracellular to the intracellular space; (2) the loss of intracellular potassium; (3) decreased $Na+ - K+ - ATPase$ activity; (4) activation of phospholipase A_2 leading to arachidonic acid release and its metabolism to lipid peroxides (via free radical attack), prostaglandins (via cyclo-oxygenase), or leukotrienes (via lipoxygenase); (5) increase in total thromboxane (TxA_2) as well as its ratio to prostacyclin (PGI_2); (6) the degradation of axonal and myelin proteins by neutral proteinases; (7) the failure of energy metabolism and protein synthesis; and (8) hypoxia and lactic acidosis.[65,67]

The tantalizing aspect of this wealth of biochemical data is that it is possible to organize these events into a positive feedback cascade mechanism activated by the release of certain catalysts from the blood and their initial intracellular flux caused by the endothelial and neuronal membrane disruption at the initial site of maximal tissue trauma. Calcium,[68] in addition to bradykinin, thrombin, and ferrous ion,[66] have been cast in such a role. Another recent investigator[69] made a case for norepinephrine.

The basic scheme of such a secondary injury hypothesis is the activation of membrane phospholipase A_2 by calcium, thrombin, or bradykinin to catalyze hydrolytic cleavage of arachidonic acid and other free fatty acids from the cell membrane. Metabolism of arachidonic acid to prostaglandins (mostly thromboxane) and leukotrienes can account for microcirculatory thrombosis and stasis, vasogenic edema, ischemia, and chemotaxis. Free radicals generated during hypoxia, by neutrophils, or during prostanoid biosynthesis react with polyunsaturated lipids during oxidative degradation to produce lipid peroxides. Iron catalyzes both free radical generation and lipid peroxidation. Lipid hydrolysis and peroxidation fragment membrane phospholipids, which would have a positive feedback effect on calcium influx and further phospholipase activation. Increased prostaglandin F_2 alpha production and thrombin generation may also augment phospholipase activity. Lipid peroxidation itself tends to be a geometrically progressive chain reaction.[66,67,70]

Calcium overloading of the intracellular space, in particular the mitochondria, secondary to influx through damaged membranes and further membrane lipid destruction as described above should have obvious deleterious effects on cellular energy metabolism and maintenance of integrity and function. $Na+ -K+ -ATPase$ has been shown to be phospholipid-dependent and very susceptible to free radical attack and lipid peroxidation.[68] This enzyme is needed to maintain normal cellular volume and ion content, membrane potential, and cellular function. Cellular swelling secondary to loss of this enzyme and membrane integrity in general can further worsen ischemia and result in enlargement of the area of lipid destruction and necrosis. Finally, the neutral proteinase, which is the predominant source of increased proteolytic activity in experimental SCI, is calcium-activated.[67]

The feasibility of such secondary injury mechanisms is supported by a number of additional observations. The time course of change in tissue concentration of some of the proposed mediators closely matches that of the histological, biochemical, and physiological processes described above. In the case of calcium, neurological deficit scores have also been shown to be proportional to the extent of calcium influx, the rise in phospholipase-generated metabolites, vascular damage, and increased tissue water content.[71] In addition, as mentioned before, exposure of the spinal cord to calcium chloride solution results in similar prostaglandin (thromboxane) generation, proteolysis, and morphological changes in proportion to the solution molarity.[67]

The excitotoxin hypothesis of neuronal injury has been expanded to include trauma in addition to ischemic or degenerative disorders. Excitatory neurotransmitters such as glutamate or aspartate have experimentally documented neurotoxic properties, perhaps acting through such observed effects as acute cellular swelling produced by a depolarization-induced influx of sodium and chlorine and a more delayed influx of calcium. The calcium might conceivably participate in secondary injury models such as those examined above. Faden and Simon[72] found that MK-801, a selective, noncompetitive N-methyl-D-aspartate antagonist, improved neurological recovery in SCI rats while exogenous NMDA worsened it.

Finally, Faden and coworkers had previously demonstrated an increase in the endogenous opioid kappa receptor agonist, dynorphin, as well as an increase in receptor-binding capacity after experimental SCI in rats, which correlates closely with neurological dysfunction. No change in mu or delta receptor binding was found. Since intrathecal dynorphin A, but not other opiate agonists, can produce dose-related hindlimb paralysis in the rat, it has been postulated that this opioid system may contribute to the pathophysiology of secondary spinal cord injury when activated during the beta endorphin surge that occurs after SCI[73,74] and which is believed to also play a role in spinal shock.

However, caution must be exercised in equating close correlation with causation, and further investigation continues. Nevertheless, what has been clearly documented is that in the period following primary spinal cord injury, a progressive decrease in SCBF occurs, resulting in marked ischemia associated with a morphological and biochemical cascade as detailed above.[75] The fact that this sequence may not begin for over an hour, in some cases as much as 4 hours after the primary injury, suggests the possibility of intervention to prevent or alter the ischemic sequence.[76]

The normal mean spinal cord blood flow of 40–50 mL/100 g/min is partitioned in a ratio of 3:1 between gray and white matter, respectively.[77] Autoregulation of SCBF between 60 and 150 mm Hg has been demonstrated in dogs.[78] Spinal cord blood flow has been shown to vary in direct proportion (1:1) to $PaCO_2$.[79] Although conflicting results have been reported,[80] the preponderance of researchers agree that total SCBF decreases significantly from 1 to 4 hours after subtotal experimental injury, with most of the decrease occurring in the central cord region.[74]

Spinal cord injury in cats has been shown to abolish autoregulation with the onset of ischemia.[81] This would be expected to render the spinal cord susceptible to increased hemorrhage and edema in the face of significantly increased blood pressure, as has been shown experimentally in cats.[82] Such a hypertensive phase has been documented for 3–4 minutes after experimental SCI.[83–85] Spinal shock, in which endorphin-mediated parasympathetic stimulation has been implicated, would decrease SCBF in the absence of autoregulation.

Also, vasoconstriction of resistance vessels would more readily result in ischemia. Such vasoconstriction may be secondary to some of the mediators already mentioned: a preponderance of thromboxane over prostacyclin, PGF_2 alpha, and slow reacting substance of anaphylaxis.[65] Although the originally proposed increase in spinal cord catecholamines (as a cause of ischemia and hemorrhagic necrosis)[86,87] has not been verified by subsequent investigators, norepinephrine has been shown to significantly reduce SCBF when the cord-blood barrier had been disrupted.[88] More recent investigations already mentioned have enumerated a number of membrane-damaging factors, operating by way of free radical attack and lipid peroxidation, which may disrupt the cord-blood barrier and which correlate with cord edema. Norepinephrine has been shown to be capable of activating similar membrane lipid peroxidation.[68] Of interest is the finding that acute ethanol intoxication (blood level of 100 mg/dL) worsens spinal cord hemorrhage and the extent of anatomic damage, and impairs recovery of function.[89] Possible reasons for this include the direct effects on neuronal conduction, vascular congestion, and increased permeability (altered blood-cord barrier), increased lactate production, increased free radical peroxidation catalyzed by iron, and toxic aldehyde metabolite effects.

On a gross physioscale, spinal cord impulse transmission, as assessed by evoked potentials, disappears immediately with complete transection and after a variable delay period in less severe lesions. Somatosensory evoked potentials (SSEPs) studied in humans distinguished complete anatomic lesions with little or no hope of recovery from patients with complete or incomplete functional deficits, but could not predict the degree of functional deficit.[90] On the other hand, motor evoked potentials (MEPs) or corticomotor evoked potentials (CMEPs) have been shown in both rat and cat dynamic LSCI models to be more sensitive indicators of the onset of injury[91] as well as good predictors of the extent and anatomic distribution of tissue damage and the prognosis for functional recovery.[92,93]

Resuscitative Modalities in Spinal Cord Injury

A number of pharmacological and physical measures have been used in an effort to limit the progression of secondary spinal cord injury and, hopefully, yield improved neurological recovery. Spinal cord injury may abolish normal autoregulation, causing SCBF and blood volume to vary directly with perfusion pressure. Spinal cord perfusion pressure must be maintained close to the middle of the normal autoregulatory range of 60–150 mm Hg by cautious restoration of a normal circulating blood volume. Although a number of physical modalities of SCI cord resuscitation such as hypothermic irrigation and hyperbaric oxygenation have been attempted sporadically with inconsistant results, a more controlled trial is necessary to evaluate them.[94]

Glucocorticoids and hyperosmolar agents have frequently been used to decrease post-traumatic edema and increase SCBF. Mannitol draws fluid from the interstitial space into the intravascular space and then promotes a net loss of fluid via osmotic diuresis. It has been shown to reduce edema following traumatic canine spinal cord injury.[95] In view of the initially low central venous pressures in the acute phase after SCI and the limited cardiac reserve, allowance must be made for the initial rise and then fall in venous return caused by mannitol.

In a canine model, improved functional recovery after SCI has been demonstrated with dexamethasone therapy.[96] Better recovery of SSEPs and partial restoration of extracellular calcium concentration have been shown in cats receiving 15–30 mg/kg of methylprednisolone 45 minutes after spinal cord contusion.[97] Others have found less axonal degeneration using morphometric analysis when the same steroid dose was given to rats after SCI.[98]

Nonetheless, the first multicenter, double-blind, randomized clinical trial in humans sponsored by the National Acute Spinal Cord Injury (NASCI) Study Group failed to find any improvement in motor or sensory neurological function 1 year after injury as a result of two levels of methylprednisolone therapy.[99]

Having recognized the problems of NASCI I, a second study was initiated that had three study groups[100]: placebo; naloxone (5.4 mg/kg loading dose, followed 45 minutes later by 4 mg/kg/hr for 23 hours); and methylprednisolone (30 mg/kg loading dose, followed 45 minutes later by 5.4 mg/kg/hr for 23 hours). Outcome was based on neurological evaluation, not functional ability. Evaluations were done on admission, at 6 weeks, and 6 months after injury. Patients who received methylprednisolone within 8 hours of injury had significant improvement in motor responses at 6 months and in a follow-up study at 1 year.[101] The study strongly suggests that methylprednisolone, when given within 8 hours of injury, had significant beneficial effects in humans with spinal cord injury.

During the 1980s opiate antagonist therapy was a subject of heated research and debate. Following the demonstration that the opiate antagonist naloxone improved arterial pressure and survival in hemorrhagic and septic shock, investigators studied its effect in spinal shock and in enhancing recovery from spinal cord injury.[102] Intravenous naloxone has effectively prevented or reversed spinal shock in rat and cat cervical cord transection models, significantly increasing mean arterial pressure (MAP) increasing respiratory rate, and decreasing hypothermia.[103] Also, naloxone in doses of 2–10 mg/kg has been shown to yield significant improvement in SSEPs[104] and neurological function.[105] A dose-related improvement in neurological recovery of rats after traumatic SCI when nalmefene, a relatively specific kappa receptor antagonist, was administered 60 minutes after injury has been demonstrated.[106]

Although these and many other animal studies supported naloxone's effectiveness, the results of both the NASCI I and II naloxone groups were less encouraging.[98,99] These trials showed clinical improvement with the highest loading dose of naloxone, but the results fell short of statistical significance. The mortality rate was not greater than expected in similar injuries, but awareness of pain was significantly increased. A possible contributing factor limiting success may be the average interval of 6.6 hours from admission until the start of therapy.[107] A number of recent animal researchers have challenged naloxone's effectiveness.[108–110]

Experimental work on the possible sites and mechanisms of action of opiate antagonists has been reviewed.[101] Briefly summarized, evidence indicates that naloxone interacts stereospecifically at a central site to inhibit opiate receptor-mediated stimulation of the para-sympathetic nervous system in achieving improvement of MAP and SCBF. A central outpouring of beta endorphin following SCI has been found at the time of cord ischemia, and naloxone may antago-nize its effects. In addition, naloxone elevates peripheral dopamine levels 300–400%, partially contributing to naloxone's hemodynamic effects after SCI. Other catecholamine levels remain unaltered. It is postulated to be an indirect effect, possibly mediated by the central parasympatholysis. Finally, because naloxone is effective only in dose orders of magnitude greater than that required for mu receptor agonist reversal, it is possible that it is acting at a receptor, perhaps the kappa receptor, for which it has marginal affinity. Naloxone and a specific kappa receptor antagonist have prevented experimental cord damage induced by dynorphin, a kappa receptor agonist (see above). In fact, some evidence exists that naloxone acts through non-opiod mechanisms, involving its ability to inhibit membrane damage by free radical-induced lipid peroxidation, to act as an antioxidant, to modulate calcium fluxes, and to increase cyclic-AMP activation of prostaglandins. Alpha-tocopherol (vitamin E), selenium (co-factor of glutathione peroxidase), and DMSO have been shown to be experi-mentally beneficial in ameliorating spinal cord injury, maybe as a result of their shared ability to act as antioxidants or reducing agents in scavenging free radicals and interrupting lipid peroxidation reac-tions.[66] Protease inhibitors, such as leupeptin, have shown promise experimentally.[111]

Finally, it should be noted that new physiotherapeutic measures show promise in preserving and enhancing function remaining after spinal cord injury, and initial investigation of chemical and physical stimulation of axonal regeneration is showing some promising re-sults. Functional neuromuscular stimulation has been used to create or enhance knee extension and bicycle ergometer exercises. How-ever, limitation in skeletal strength, the deteriorated condition of the muscles, and lack of cardiopulmonary and other system adjust-ments to exercise have limited its success. Strength and endurance gains have been made, but relatively easy fatigability remains a problem.[112]

Recent studies have demonstrated potential effectiveness of GM-1 ganglioside[113] and a combination of triethanolamine and cyto-sine arabinoside[114] to markedly stimulate axonal growth in spinal cord transected rats. Continuously applied weak electrical fields achieved similar results in guinea pigs.[115] A series of investigations has shown that peripheral nerve grafts or central nervous system implants derived from the embryonal neuroaxis can stimulate axonal outgrowth and may prove useful in repairing disrupted intraspinal circuits.[116]

For example, a small clinical study in humans provided evidence that GM-1 ganglioside enhanced the recovery of neurological function after 1 year. An analysis of the individual muscle recoveries revealed that the increased recovery in the GM-1 ganglioside group was attributable to initially paralyzed muscles that regained useful motor strength rather than to strengthening of paretic muscles.[117] While this is a dramatic study with a drug that may enhance regeneration, the results of a larger trial that is under way must be considered before GM-1 ganglioside is safe in treating patients with spinal cord injury.

Currently, much of this work has proven to be of limited clinical utility except the NASCI II high-dose methyprednisolone group. Nevertheless, understanding and new directions for research, as well as more effective application of existing knowledge, are advancing at an unprecedented and encouraging pace. Prompt initiation of currently accepted therapy or experimental protocols in a specialized care center hold the most hope for preserving or restoring function.

Anesthetic Management of Patients with Spinal Cord Injury

In view of the high percentage of SCI patients with associated injuries, the anesthesiologist may be required to care for these patients during initial diagnostic procedures, during emergency operations aimed at managing life-threatening trauma elsewhere in the body (e.g., closed head injury, hemorrhage), for emergency spinal decompression or stabilization, or for other procedures (e.g., urologic, plastic) during the more chronic phase of illness.

Acutely, maintenance of normal acid-base and blood-gas parameters as well as adequate spinal cord perfusion pressure are paramount in importance. Experimental work in cats has suggested that there is no therapeutic advantage of either hypercarbia or hypocarbia over normocarbia in terms of both neurological recovery and histologic tissue preservation. Although not statistically significant, mortality and tissue preservation results suggested that hypocarbia may be less harmful than hypercarbia in the acute post-injury period.[118] It seems prudent to maintain $PaCO_2$ in the 35–40 mm Hg range for spinal cord injury and for closed head injury.

Hypoxemia must be prevented by careful attention to minimizing significant physiological shunting, which is suggested by the inability to maintain a PaO_2 greater than 60 mm Hg with an FIO_2 of 50%. Possible contributing etiologies such as hemothorax or pneumothorax, pulmonary embolization of fat or thrombi, foreign body or gastric content aspiration, and noncardiogenic pulmonary edema should be searched for and either excluded or treated appropriately. PEEP may be required to decrease shunting and increase oxygenation once pneumothorax or other reversible causes of hypoxemia have been excluded. However, the possible negative effect of PEEP on blood pressure, cardiac output, and intracranial pressure must be considered. In case the patient is not already intubated and this is necessary, it should be carried out as previously discussed.

Cardiovascular management most frequently requires judicious repletion of intravascular volume to restore normal venous return and filling pressures. However, it should be recalled that 4 of 22 patients in the study cited on volume loading in the acute post-injury period actually showed a decrease in SCI accompanying infusion to increase PAOP, which necessitated decreasing halothane concentration from 0.5% to 0.25% to restore the cardiac index (CI) to baseline. However, both before and after infusion and at all halothane concentrations, the CI was at or above normal resting limits and no evidence of organ hypoperfusion was noted.[119] Hence, caution but not exclusion is indicated with the use of potent inhalational agents during the acute stage of SCI, as compared to later when autonomic hyperreflexia is likely (see below). During the phase of spinal shock lasting from 3 days to 6 weeks (average of 3 weeks), the advantages of pulmonary artery catheter monitoring are obvious in maintaining hemodynamics and avoiding pulmonary edema. Also, it allows quantitation of shunt and monitoring of the respiratory and hemodynamic effects of PEEP and continuous positive pressure ventilation. Keeping in mind electrolyte, neuromuscular, and other potential systemic alterations is also necessary, with management as outlined above.

As noted by Schonwald,[120] both a sufficiently deep general anesthetic technique, using halothane or enflurane, and regional anesthesia (subarachnoid or epidural) effectively prevented episodes of autonomic hyperreflexia. An alternative where surgical considerations would require high spinal levels (above T5) is subarachnoid block followed by light general anesthesia with endotracheal intubation and controlled ventilation.

A study[121] using dogs showed consistent statistically significant increases in lumbosacral spinal cord blood flow with a lesser, nonsignificant tendency toward increases in thoracic and cervical cord flow after subarachnoid tetracaine, as long as mean arterial pressure remained 100 mm Hg or more. The favorable effect was blocked by the addition of epinephrine to the tetracaine; in fact, a nonsignificant tendency toward decreased thoracic and cervical cord flows actually occurred. Hence, spinal anesthesia may improve cord blood flow but vasoconstrictors should not be added to the anesthetic. Although spinal or epidural anesthetics have been considered hemodynamically unpredictable in these patients,[122] baseline hemodynamic stability as well as ablation of autonomic hyperreflexia has been verified by many other workers.[119,123] One recent study[124] showed such stability of cardiac output, stroke volume, and heart rate during cystoscopy that it was actually impossible to determine when bladder distention and emptying had occurred from the inspection of the data alone. Also, no ephedrine was required during the study. These authors emphasized the importance of judicious choice of the anesthetic dose and attention to intravascular volume as factors contributing to the noted stability. Low-dose intrathecal morphine 0.2–0.25 mg has, incidently, been shown to be effective in alleviating the symptoms of spastic bladder for up to 24 hours.[125] A note of caution is warranted in patients with subarachnoid block of cerebrospinal fluid circulation because a 14% incidence of neurological deterioration following removal of cerebrospinal fluid or delayed leakage through the puncture site has been reported.[126]

Nitrous oxide/oxygen/narcotic-based techniques seem less recommendable in light of their failure to prevent hyperreflexia in two of nine patients. Regardless of the technique used, direct-acting arteriolar dilators (e.g., nitroprusside), alpha adrenergic blockers (e.g., phentolamine), antiarrhythmics (e.g., lidocaine, propranolol, esmolol), new antihypertensives such as labetalol and nifedipine, and atropine should be readily available.[119] The need to avoid succinylcholine is reiterated. However, the new, short-acting nondepolarizing agents make this constraint clinically feasible since they are a reasonable alternative.

In the case of incomplete spinal cord lesions, somatosensory evoked potentials (SSEPs) and motor evoked potentials (MEPs) can be useful in monitoring cord function (see pathophysiology). This is true during surgery to relieve cord compression or to correct spinal deformity, as well as during the acute phase of spinal cord injury when neurological status may progressively worsen. The usefulness of electrophysiological monitoring is exemplified by a case report of verified iatrogenic posterior SCI which was immediately diagnosed by SSEP, but not by two false negative "wake up" tests, or during the admission evaluation in PACU.[127] The use of transcutaneous corticomotor stimulation with recording of spinal level CMEPs or EMG activity distal to the area at risk has also proven feasible. It often indicates injury when the ascending pathways are normal, and occasionally the reverse is true. SSEPs and CMEPs cover distinct regions of the cord and, used separately or together, can diagnose almost all injuries with more sensitivity and specificity than clinical observations alone.

Of possible utility during surgery in patients with incomplete lesions is the observation that etomidate improved the SSEP in patients receiving neuroleptanesthesia by increasing the latency and amplitude of the short latency cortical responses.[128] A 0.3–0.5 mg/kg bolus of etomidate followed by a continuous infusion of 0.01–0.05 mg/kg/min were used. Further study is needed before widespread acceptance of this technique; however, where SSEP monitoring is considered essential but is technically nonreproducible, etomidate may provide a solution. Another recent report[129] suggests that the use of lower-than-usual stimulus presentation rates (1.1–2.1 Hz compared to 5.1 Hz) resolved problems similar to those found in the first study and may provide an acceptable alternative solution.

Summary

The anesthetic management of the patient with spinal cord injury follows a continuum of care from the initial injury through the chronic phases. At all times, the potential pathophysiological consequences of the injury must be incorporated into the patient's care plan. Therefore, a knowledge of pattern of injuries and the consequences based on level of injury must be appreciated. As the pathophysiology of spinal cord injury is defined, newer resuscitative modalities will be introduced. The effects of specific anesthetic drugs on spinal cord injury require further study, although preliminary study would indicate that they are not harmful.[130] Adjunctive therapy requires further definition.[131]

Acknowledgment: The authors thank Grune and Stratton for giving permission to use information that was previously published in Giffin JP: Spinal cord injury. Semin Anesth 5(4):246–259, 1987. They also thank Adrienne Dansiger for preparation of the manuscript.

References

1. Eisenberg MG, Tierney DO: Changing demographics profile of the spinal cord injury population: implications for health care support systems. Paraplegia 23:335, 1985.
2. Kraus JF, Franti GE, Riggins, et al: Incidence of traumatic spinal cord lesions. J Chronic Dis 28:471–492, 1975.
3. Bracken MB, Freeman DH, Hellenbrand K: Incidence of acute traumatic hospitalized spinal cord injury in the United States, 1970–77. Am J Epidemiol 1:615–622, 1981.
4. Green BA, Eismont FJ, O'Heir Jt: Spinal cord injury. A systems approach: Prevention, emergency medical services, and emergency room management. In Albin MS (ed): Critical Care Clinics—Acute Spinal Cord Injury. 3:471, 1987.
5. Green BA, Eismont FJ, O'Heir JT: Spinal cord injury. A systems approach: Prevention, emergency medical services, and emergency room management. In Albin MS (ed): Critical Care Clinics—Acute Spinal Cord Injury. 3:471, 1987.
6. Kraus JF: A comparison of recent studies on the extent of the head and spinal cord injury problem in the United States. J Neurosurg 53: 35–43, 1980.
7. Young JS: Initial hospitalization cord rehabilitation costs of spinal cord injury. Orthop Clin North Am 9(2), 1978.
8. Young JS, Northup NE: Statistical information pertaining to some of the most asked questions about spinal cord injury. SCI Digest 1:11, 1979.
9. Ransohoff J, Flamm ES, Demopoulos HB: Mechanisms of injury and treatment of acute spinal cord trauma. Cottrell JE, Turndorf H (eds) Anesthesia and Neurosurgery. CV Mosby Company, St. Louis, 1980, pp 361–386.
10. Woolsey RM: Rehabilitation outcome following spinal cord injury. Arch Neurol 42:116–119, 1985.
11. Bachulis B, Long W, Hynes G, Johnson M: Clinical indications of cervical spine radiographs in the traumatized patient. Am J Surg 153: 473–477, 1987.
12. Bryson B, Mulkey M, Murnford B, Schwedhelm M, et al: Cervical spine injury: Incidence and diagnosis. J Trauma 26:669, 1986.
13. Cadoux C, White J, Hedberg M: High-yield roentgenographic criteria for cervical spine injures. Ann Emerg Med 16:738–742, 1987.
14. Bayless P, Ray VG: Incidence of cervical spine injuries in association with blunt head trauma. Am J Emerg Med 7:139–142, 1989.
15. Kreipke D, Gillespie K, McCarthy M, Mail JT, et al: Reliability of indications for cervical spine films in trauma patients. J Trauma 29: 1438–1439, 1989.
16. Talucci RC, Shaikh KA, Schwab CN: Rapid sequence induction with

oral endotracheal intubation in the multiply injured patient. Am Surg 54:185–187, 1988.

17. Ross SE, Schwab CN, David ET, Delong WG, et al: Clearing the cervical spine initial radiographic evaluation. J Trauma 27:1055–1060, 1987.

18. O'Malley KF, Ross SE: The incidence of injury to the cervical spine in patients with craniocerebral injury. J Trauma 28:1476–1478, 1989.

19. Grande CM, Barton RB, Stene JK: Appropriate techniques for airway management of emergency patients with suspected spinal cord injury. Anesth Analg 67:714–715, 1988.

20. Alker GJ, Oh YS, Leslie EL: Postmortem radiology of head and neck injuries in fatal traffic accidents. Radiology 114:611–617, 1975.

21. Bucholz RW, Burkhead WZ, Graham W: Occult cervical spine injuries in fatal traffic accidents. J Trauma 19:768–771, 1979.

22. Huekle DF, O'Day J, Mendelsohn RA: Cervical injuries suffered in automobile crashes. J Neurosurg 54:316, 1981.

23. Watson N: Road traffic accidents, spinal injuries and seat belts. Paraplegia 21:63, 1983.

24. Weiss MH: Cervical spine injuries with and without neurological deficit: Part I. Contemp Neurosurg 2(12):1–6, 1975.

25. Weiss MH, Rosenberg AW, Apuzzo MLJ, Kurze T: Management of cervical spinal cord trauma in Southern California. J Neurosurg 43:732–736, 1975.

26. Rachesky I, Boyce T, Duncan B, Bjelland J, et al: Clinical prediction of cervical spine injuries in children. Am J Dis Child 141:199–201, 1987.

27. Lally K, Senal M, Hardin W, Haftel D, et al: Utility of the cervical spine radiograph in pediatric trauma. Am J Surg 158:540–542, 1989.

28. Roshkow JE, Haller J, Hotson G, Sclafni S, et al: Rachlin S: Imaging evaluation of children after fall from a height: Review of 45 cases. Radiology 175:359–363, 1990.

29. Fesmire F, Luten R: The pediatric cervical spine: Developmental anatomy and clinical aspects. J Emerg Med 7:133–142, 1989.

30. Jafe MH, White AA, Panjab MM: Kinematics. In The Cervical Spine Research Society: The Cervical Spine. JB Lippincott, Philadelphia, 1983, pp 23–35.

31. Ragozzino MW, Deluca SA: Upper cervical spine trauma. Am Fam Physician 32:113–119, 1985.

32. White A, Kander PL: Anatomical factors in difficult direct laryngoscopy. Br J Anaesth 47:468–473, 1975.

33. Zuck D: Difficult tracheal intubation. Anaesthesia 40:1016–1077, 1985.

34. Nichol HC, Zuck D: Difficult laryngoscopy: The "anterior" larynx and the atlanto-occipital gap. Br J Anaesth 55:141–1414, 1983.

35. Hayashi H, Okada K, Harrada M, Tada K, et al: Etiologic factors of myelopathy: A radiographic evaluation of the aging changes in the cervical spine. Clin Orthop 214:200–209, 1987.

36. White AA, Southwick WO, Panjabi MM: Clinical instability in the lower cervical spine. Spine 1:15–27, 1976.

37. Hayashi H, Okada K, Harada M, Tada K, et al: Etiologic factors of

myelopathy: A radiographic evaluation of the aging changes in the cervical spine. Clin Orthop 214:200–209, 1987.

38. Steel HH: Anatomical and mechanical considerations of the atlantoaxial articulations. J Bone Joint Surg 50:1481–1490, 1968.

39. Hensineer RN: Congenital anomalies of the atlantoaxial joint. In Cervical Spine Research Society: The Cervical Spine. JB Lippincott, Philadelphia, 1983, pp 155–160.

40. White AA, Johnson RM, Panjabi MM, Southwick WO: Biomechanical analysis of clinical stability in the cervical spine. Clin Orthop 109: 85–95, 1975.

41. Pang D, Wilberger JE, Jr: Traumatic atlanto-occipital dislocation with survival: Case report and review. Neurosurgery 7:503–508, 1980.

42. Alker GJ, Oh YS, Leslie EV: High cervical spine and craniocervical junction injuries in fatal traffic accidents: A radiologic study. Orthop Clin North Am 9:1003–1010, 1978.

43. Dorr LD, Harvey JP, Jr: Traumatic lesions in fatal acute spinal column injuries. Clin Orthop 157:178–190, 1981.

44. Evarts C: Traumatic occipito-atlantal dislocation: Report of a case with survival. J Bone Joint Surg 52(A):1653–1660, 1970.

45. Powers B, Miller MD, Kramer RS: Traumatic anterior atlanto-occipital dislocation. Neurosurgery 4:12–17, 1979.

46. Gabrielsen TO, Maxwell JA: Traumatic atlanto-occipital dislocation, with case report of patient who survived. Am J Roentgenol Radium Therapy Nuc Med 97:624–629, 1966.

47. Ersmark H, Lowenhielm P: Factors influencing the outcome of cervical spine injuries. J Trauma 28:407–410, 1988.

48. Levine AM, Edwards CC: Treatment of injuries in the C_1–C_2 complex. Orthop Clin North Am 17:31–34, 1986.

49. Fielding JW, Hawkins RJ: Atlanto-axial rotary fixation. J Bone Joint Surg 59:37–44, 1979.

50. Gosch HH, Gooding E, Schneider RC: Distortion and displacement of the brain in experimental head injuries. Surg Forum 20:425–426, 1969.

51. Mouradian WH, Fietti, Cochran GV: Fractures of the odontoid: A laboratory and clinical study of mechanisms. Orthop Clin North Am 9: 985–1001, 1978.

52. Sherk HH: Fractures of the atlas and odontoid process. Orthop Clin North Am 9:973–984, 1978.

53. Anderson LD, D'Alonzo RT: Fractures of the odontoid process of the axis. J Bone Joint Surg 56(A):1663–1674, 1974.

54. Ryan MD, Taylor TK: Odontoid fractures: A rational approach to treatment. J Bone Joint Surg 64(4):416–421, 1982.

55. Schatzker J, Rorabeck CH, Waddell JP: Fractures of the dens (odontoid process): An analysis of thirty-seven cases. J Bone Joint Surg 53(3): 392–405, 1981.

56. Hanssen RD, Cabenela ME: Fractures of the dens in adult patients. J Trauma 27:928–934, 1987.

57. Bell HS: Paralysis of both arms from injury of the upper portion of the pyramidal decussation: "cruciate paralysis." J Neurosurg 33:376–380, 1970.

58. Wood-Jones F: The ideal lesion produced by judicial hanging. Lancet 1:53, 1913.
59. Francis WR, Fielding JW, Hawkins RJ: Traumatic spondylolisthesis of the axis. J Bone Joint Surg 63:313–318, 1981.
60. Schneider RL, Livingston RE, Cave AJE: "Hangman's fracture" of the cervical spine. J Neurosurg 22:141, 1965.
61. Bucholz RW, Burkhead WZ: The pathologic anatomy of fatal atlanto-occipital dislocations. J Bone Joint Surg 61(2):248–250, 1979.
62. Levine AM, Edwards CC: The management of traumatic spondylolisthesis of the axis. J Bone Joint Surg 67(2):217–226, 1985.
63. Allen BL, Ferguson RL, Lehman TR: A mechanistic classification of closed, indirect fractures and dislocations of the lower cervical spine. Spine 7(1):1–27, 1982.
64. Gehweiler JA Jr, Clark WM, Schaaf RE, Powers B, et al: Cervical spine trauma: the common combined conditions. Radiology 130(1):77–86, 1979.
65. Shearer VE, Giesecke AH: Airway management for patients with penetrating neck trauma: A retrospective study. Anesth Analg 77: 1135–1138, 1993.
66. Banik NL, Hogan EL, Hsu CY: Molecular and anatomical correlates of spinal cord injury. Cent Nerv Syst Trauma 2:99–107, 1985.
67. Anderson DK, Demediuk P, Saunders RD: Spinal cord injury and protection. Ann Emerg Med 14:816–821, 1985.
68. Hogan EL, Hsu CY, Banik NL: Calcium-activated mediators of secondary injury in the spinal cord. Cent Nerv Syst Trauma 3:175–179, 1986.
69. Kurihara M: Role of monamines in experimental spinal cord injury in rats: Relationship between Na^+-K^+-ATPase and lipideroxidation. J Neurosurg 62:743–749, 1985.
70. Hall ED, Wolf DL: A pharmacological analysis of the pathophysiological mechanisms of posttraumatic spinal cord ischemia. J Neurosurg 64:951–961, 1986.
71. Hsu CY, Hogan EL, Gadsden KM: Vascular permeability in experimental spinal cord injury. J Neurosci 70:275–282, 1985.
72. Faden AI, Simon RP: A potential role for excitotoxins in the pathophysiology of spinal cord injury. Ann Neurol 3:623–626, 1988.
73. Faden AI, Molineaux CJ, Rosenberger JG: Increased dynorphin immunoreactivity in spinal cord after traumatic injury. Regul Pept 11:35–41, 1985.
74. Krumins SA, Faden AI: Traumatic injury alters opiate receptor binding in rat spinal cord. Ann Neurol 19:498–501, 1986.
75. Sandler AN, Tator CH: Review of the effect of spinal cord trauma on the vessels and blood flow in the spinal cord. J Neurosurg 45:638–646, 1976.
76. Senter HJ, Venes JL: Altered blood flow and secondary injury in experimental spinal cord trauma J Neurosurg 49:569–578, 1978.
77. Rivlin AS, Tator CH: Regional spinal cord blood flow in rats after severe cord trauma. J Neurosurg 49:844–853, 1978.
78. Griffiths IR: Spinal cord blood flow in dogs. II: The effect of the blood gases. J Neurol Neurosurg Psychiatr 36:42, 1973.

79. Griffiths IR: Spinal cord blood flow in dogs. I: The effect of blood pressure. J Neurol Neurosurg Psychiatr 36:914–929, 1973.
80. Kobrine AI, Doyle TF, Martins AN: Local spinal cord blood flow in experimental traumatic myelopathy. J Neurosurg 42:144–149, 1975.
81. Senter HJ, Venes JL: Loss of autoregulation and posttraumatic ischemia following experimental spinal cord trauma. J Neurosurg 50:198–206, 1979.
82. Rawe SE, Lee WA, Perot PL: The histopathology of experimental spinal cord trauma. J Neurosurg 48:1002–1007, 1978.
83. Albin MS, Bunegin L, Wolf S: Brain and lungs at risk after cervical spinal cord transection: Intracranial pressure, brain water, blood-brain barrier permeability, cerebral blood flow, and extravascular lung water changes. Surg Neurol 24:191–205, 1985.
84. Rawe SE, Perot PL: Pressor response resulting from experimental contusion injury to the spinal cord. J Neurosurg 50:58–63, 1979.
85. Young W, DeCrescito V, Tomasula JJ: The role of the sympathetic nervous system in pressor responses induced by spinal injury. J Neurosurg 52:473–481, 1980.
86. Osterholm JL, Mathews GJ: Altered norepinephrine metabolism following experimental spinal cord injury. I. Relationship to hemorrhagic necrosis and post-wounding neurological deficits. J Neurosurg 36:386–394, 1972.
87. Osterholm JL, Mathews GJ: Altered norepinephrine metabolism following experimental cord injury. II. Protection against traumatic spinal cord hemorrhagic necrosis by norepinephine synthesis blockade with alpha methyl tyrosine. J Neurosurg 36:395–401, 1972.
88. Crawford RA, Griffiths IR, McCulloch J: The effect of norepinephrine on the spinal cord circulation and its possible implications in the pathogenesis of acute spinal trauma. J Neurosurg 47:567–576, 1977.
89. Anderson TE: Effects of acute alcohol intoxication on spinal cord vascular injury. CNS Trauma 3:183–192, 1986.
90. Chabot R, York DH, Watts C: Somatosensory evoked potentials evaluated in normal subjects and spinal cord-injured patients. J Neurosurg 63:544–551, 1985.
91. Levy W, McCaffrey M, York D: Motor evoked potential in cats with acute spinal cord injury. Neurology 19:9–19, 1986.
92. Levy WJ, McCaffrey M, Hagichi S: Motor evoked potential as a predictor of recovery in chronic spinal cord injury. Neurosurgery 20:138–142, 1987.
93. Simpson RK, Baskin DS: Corticomotor evoked potentials in acute and chronic blunt spinal cord injury in the rat: Correlation with neurological outcome and histological damage. Neurosurgery 20:131–137, 1987.
94. Albin MS: Resuscitation of the spinal cord. Crit Care Med 6:270–276, 1978.
95. Parker AJ, Park RD, Stowater JL: Reduction of trauma-induced edema of spinal cord in dogs given mannitol. Am J Vet Res 34:1355, 1973.
96. Kuchner EF, Hansebout RR: Combined steroid and hypothermia treatment of experimental spinal cord injury. Surg Neurol 6:371–376, 1976.
97. Young W, Flamm ES: Effect of high-dose corticosteroid therapy on

blood flow, evoked potentials, and extracellular calcium in experimental spinal injury. J Neurosurg 57:667–673, 1982.

98. Iizuka H, Iwasaki Y, Yamamoto T: Morphometric assessment of drug effects in experimental spinal cord injury. J Neurosurg 65:92–98, 1986.

99. Bracken MB, Shepard MJ, Hellenbrand KG, et al: Methylprednisolone and neurological function 1 year after spinal cord injury: Results of the National Acute Spinal Cord Injury Study. J Neurosurg 63:704–713, 1985.

100. Bracken MB, Shephard MJ, Collins WF, et al: A randomized, controlled trial of methylprednisolone or naloxone in the treatment of acute spinal cord injury. N Engl J Med 322:1405, 1990.

101. Brachen MD, Collins WF, Freeman DF, et al: Methylprednisolone or naloxone treatment after acute spinal cord injury: 1 year follow-up data. J Neurosurgery 76:23–31, 1992.

102. Hamilton AJ, Black PM, Carr DB: Contrasting actions of naloxone in experimental spinal cord trauma and cerebral ischemia: A review. Neurosurgery 17:845–849, 1985.

103. Holaday JW, Faden AI: Naloxone acts of central opiate receptors to reverse hypotension, hypothermia and hypoventilation in spinal shock. Brain Res 189:295–299, 1980.

104. Flamm ES, Young W, Demopoulos HB: Experimental spinal cord injury; treatment with naloxone. Neurosurgery 10:227, 1982.

105. Faden AI, Jacobs TP, Holaday JW: Opiate antagonist improves neurologic recovery after spinal injury. Science 211:493–494, 1981.

106. Faden AI, Sackson I, Noble LJ: Opiate receptor antagonist nalmefene improves neurologic recovery after traumatic spinal cord injury in rats through a central mechanism. J Pharm Exp Ther 245:742–748, 1988.

107. Flamm ES, Young W, Collins WF: A phase I trial of naloxone treatment in acute spinal cord injury. J Neurosurg 63:390–397, 1985.

108. Haghighi SS, Chehrazi B: Effect of naloxone in experimental acute spinal cord injury. Neurosurgery 20:385–388, 1987.

109. Wallace MC, Tator CH: Failure of blood transfusion or naloxone to improve clinical recovery after experimental spinal cord injury. Neurosurgery 19:489–494, 1986.

110. Wallace MC, Tator CH: Failure of naloxone to improve spinal cord blood flow and cardiac output after spinal cord injury. Neurosurgery 18:428–432, 1986.

111. Iwasaki Y, Iizuka H, Yamamoto, T: Alleviation of axonal damage in acute spinal cord injury by a protease inhibitor: automated morphometric analysis of drug-effects. Brain Res 347:124–126, 1985.

112. Glaser RM: Physiologic aspects of spinal cord injury and functional neuromuscular stimulation. CNS Trauma 3:49–62, 1986.

113. Bose B, Osterholm JL, Kalia M: Ganglioside-induced regeneration and reestablishment of axonal continuity in spinal cord-transected rats. Neurosci Lett 63:165–169, 1986.

114. Guth L, Barrett CP, Donati EJ: Enhancement of axonal growth into a spinal lesion by topical application of triethanolamine and cystosine arabinoside. Exp Neurol 88:44–55, 1985.

115. Borgens RB, Blight AR, Murphy DJ: Transected dorsal column axons

within the guinea pig spinal cord regenerate in the presence of an applied electric field. Comp Neurol 250:168–180, 1986.

116. Reier PJ: Neural tissue graft and repair of the injured spinal cord. Neuropathol Appl Neurobiol 11:81–104, 1985.

117. Geisler FH, Dorsey FC, Colemena WP: Recovery of motor function after spinal cord injury: A randomized, placebo-controlled trial with GM-1 ganglioside. N Engl J Med 324:1829–1838, 1991.

118. Ford RWJ, Malm DN: Therapeutic trial of hypercarbia and hypocarbia in acute experimental spinal cord injury. J Neurosurg 61:925–930, 1984.

119. MacKenzie CF, Shin B, Krishnaprasad D, et al: Assessment of cardiac respiratory function during surgery on patients with acute quadriplegia. J Neurosurg 62:843–849, 1985.

120. Schonwald G, Fish KJ, Perkash I: Cardiovascular complications during anesthesia in chronic spinal cord injured patients. Anesthesiology 55: 550–558, 1981.

121. Kozody R, Palahniuk RJ, Cumming MO: Spinal cord blood flow following subarachnoid tetracaine. Can Anaesth Soc J 32:23–29, 1985.

122. Desmond J: Paraplegia: Problems confronting the anaesthesiologist. Can Anaesth Soc J 17:435–451, 1970.

123. Verduyn WH: Spinal cord-injured women, pregnancy and delivery. Paraplegia 24:231–240, 1986.

124. Barker I, Alderson J, Lydon M: Cardiovascular effects of spinal subarachnoid anaesthesia. Anaesthesia 40:533–536, 1985.

125. Herman RM, Wainberg MC, del Guidice PF, Wilkscher MK: The effect of a low dose of intrathecal morphine on impaired micturition reflexes in human subjects with spinal cord lesions. Anesthesiology 69: 313–318, 1988.

126. Hollis PH, Malis LI, Zappulla RA: Neurological deterioration after lumbar puncture below complete spinal subarachnoid block. J Neurosurg 64:253–256, 1986.

127. Ben-David B, Taylor PD, Haller GS: Posterior spinal fusion complicated by posterior column injury: A case report of a false negative wake-up test. Spine 12:540–543, 1987.

128. Sloan TB, Ronai AK, and Toleikis RJ. Improvement of the intraoperative somatosensory evoked potentials by etomidate. Anesth Analgesia 67:582–585, 1988.

129. Schubert A, Drummond JC, Garfin SR: The influence of stimulus presentation rate on the cortical amplitude and latency of introperative somatosensory-evoked potential recordings in patients with varying degrees of spinal cord injury. Spine 12:969–973, 1987.

130. Cole DJ, Shapiro HM, Drummond JC, Zivin JA: Halothane, fentanyl/nitrous oxide, and spinal lidocaine protect against spinal cord injury in the rat: Anesthesiology 70:967–972, 1989.

131. Drummond JC, Moore SS: The influence of dextrose administration on neurologic outcome after temporary spinal cord ischemia in the rabbit. Anesthesiology 70:64–70.

12

Critical Care Management of Closed Head Injury

T. James Gallagher, MD, Anne F. Boudreaux, MD

Types of Injuries

Incidence and Etiology

Head injuries occur more often than any other type of trauma. An estimated 2 million to 10 million people suffer head trauma each year in the United States. Approximately 500,000 to 600,000 of these require evaluation and treatment, ranging from observation to medical and surgical interventions. Head injury leads all causes of death among people under the age of 24 years. The largest group includes males 15 to 30 years of age.[1] Blunt trauma to the head occurs more commonly than penetrating trauma. Motor vehicle accidents top the list as the most common etiology of blunt trauma. Falls and assault with blunt objects make up another large group. Gunshot wounds are the most common type of penetrating head trauma in the United States.[2]

From *Trauma Anesthesia and Critical Care of Neurological Injury,* edited by K. J. Abrams and C. M. Grande. © 1997, Futura Publishing Co., Armonk, NY.

Classification (Primary vs. Secondary)

Head injury responses run the spectrum from minor confusion to coma and death. A history and physical examination are the most important means of identifying those at risk for significant head injury. The physician must remain cognizant that often injuries may initially appear deceptively benign. Patients at moderate to high risk of intracranial pathology should undergo immediate CT of the head and be prioritized accordingly. This includes those with even a brief period of loss of consciousness or a history that suggests the likelihood of severe trauma. A high-speed deceleration injury is one example. Focal intracranial lesions carry an improved prognosis over diffuse lesions since focal lesions are often amenable to surgery. Examples of focal lesions are: subdural, epidural, and intraparenchymal bleeds. Diffuse lesions include: concussions, diffuse axonal injury, and edema.

Brain injury classification has progressed to differentiation of primary and secondary brain injury.[3] The primary injury occurs at the time of the initial trauma. Current management emphasizes the prevention of further brain insults, or secondary injuries. Potentially avoidable secondary complications that contribute to death or a poor neurological outcome include: hypoxia, hypotension, hypercarbia, seizures, hyperthermia, anemia, infections, and electrolyte abnormalities. Complications from anesthesia and delays prior to evacuation of intracranial hematomas are less common today. Secondary insults continue to be a common post-traumatic phenomenon. As many as 40% of head injury patients demonstrate evidence of delayed secondary deterioration.[3]

Causes of Poor Outcome

Poor prognostic findings include bilateral intracerebral hemorrhage, combined intra-axial and extra-axial hemorrhage, shift of midline structures, delayed intracerebral hematomas, severe anatomic disruption following a penetrating injury, and brain stem hemorrhage. Bleeding within the corpus callosum, or basal ganglion, and diffuse axonal injury all forecast severe neurological impairment. A focal neurological finding or a Glasgow Coma Score of 8 or less correlates with a 50% to 75% incidence of CT-proven intracranial lesion.[4]

Diffuse Axonal Injury or Shear Injury

Diffuse axonal injury (DAI) is the most common cause of the vegetative state and severe disability after a nonmissile head injury.[5,6] The injury occurs immediately upon impact. The most common etiology is a motor vehicle accident. Fall from heights can generate DAI. Less common precipitating factors include assault, often with a blunt object such as a steel bar or a baseball bat. A human fist or kicks can also create enough force to induce DAI. A detailed explanation of the extensive study into the exact mechanical forces required to produce DAI is beyond the scope of this text.

The severity of DAI depends principally on the magnitude and duration of the acceleration forces as well as the direction of head motion. Acceleration of the same magnitude in the coronal plane produces more severe DAI than brain movement in another plane.[7] The frontal lobes are particularly vulnerable to damage. DAI patients usually do not experience a lucid interval immediately post injury. The cerebral edema produced in DAI patients is more often bilateral than in non-DAI patients.

The common pathological finding of DAI is the destruction of the axonal cytoskeleton. Less serious forms of DAI result in microscopic axonal abnormalities, whereas the more severe types produce gross tissue and blood vessel tears. Pathologically, DAI acutely takes the form of axonal retraction balls and microglial infiltration or clusters in areas of axonal disruption and punctate hemorrhage throughout the brain. Axonal balls are brought on by the extrusion of axoplasm resulting from anterograde axoplasmic flow and characteristic swelling at about 12 to 18 hours.

A CT scan will not delineate DAI, unless it occurs in association with tissue hemorrhages or edema.[8] Magnetic resonance imaging (MRI) provides more sensitivity in identifying DAI in white matter and can better detect these lesions than a CT scan. Patients with deeper white matter tissue lesions, especially in the corpus callosum, have a greater impairment of consciousness on admission. Those with severe DAI have corpus callosal injuries and significantly lower initial Glasgow Coma Scores (GCS).[9–14] The lesion must be between 0.5 and 1.5 cm before it can be detected by CT scan. Two to 4 days post injury the lesion increases in size and a halo of edema forms around the lesions. Tissue tear following hemorrhage can be established by CT scan in approximately 15% of patients.[8]

Severe DAI has a mortality rate of approximately 50%. Less than 25% of patients have an acceptable outcome. The mildest forms of DAI have a 15% mortality rate and a 63% good recovery rate.[15] In this group coma usually lasts only 6 to 24 hours. Moderate DAI is deinged as a coma for more than 24 hours and associated with little or no evidence of brain stem dysfunction. Severe DAI has regularly occurring signs of brain stem dysfunction in patients comatose for longer than 24 hours. Severe DAI will have characteristic findings of hemorrhage in cerebral gray-white matter interface, basal ganglia, corpus callosum, and the dorsolateral part of the brain stem and cerebellum.

A grading system has also been used to describe diffuse axonal injury. Grade 1 has histological evidence of axonal injury in the white matter, the corpus callosum, the brain stem and, occasionally, the cerebellum. This damage can only be identified microscopically. Grade 2 has a focal lesion in the corpus callosum. In addition to the diffuse axonal injury, grade 3 lesions have a focal lesion in the dorsilateral quadrant or quadrants of the rostral brain stem.[16,17] The higher the grade of DAI, the deeper and more prolonged coma, and the residual neurological deficits in survivors are more severe.

The management of patients with DAI does not differ from patients with other types of head injuries. Efforts are directed at prevention of secondary brain injury. Aggressive management of elevated intracranial pressure (ICP) requires the measures discussed later in this chapter.

Hematoma Space-Occupying Lesion

Extra-axial or nonparenchymal hematomas are the most common post-traumatic lesion. Approximately 40% of all extra-axial hematomas are associated with a concomitant intra-axial or parenchymal lesion. Mass effects are generated by large hematomas that cause a shift of midline structures. Extra-axial clots result from subdural and epidural hematomas and subarachnoid hemorrhage. Subarachnoid hemorrhage is the most common intracranial injury resulting from head trauma. It develops due to small tears in subarachnoid vessels. Epidural and subdural hematomas thicker than 1 cm on CT scan require immediate attention.

Subdural Hematoma

A subdural hematoma has blood under the dura and above the brain surface. Acute subdural hematomas are the most common operable lesions that result from closed head injury. Some authors have demonstrated a significant mortality reduction in patients with acute subdural hematoma in whom evacuation takes place within 4 hours of injury. These patients have experienced a 60% to 70% functional recovery with less than 40% mortality rate.[18] However, these results have not always been reproducible. Treatment delay beyond 4 hours has an associated 80% to 90% mortality rate.[19]

Acute subdural hematoma usually results from a venous bleed. Diagnostic criteria on CT scan includes a hyperdensity along the cortex margins (see Chapter 7). It is usually crescent-shaped. A large blood collection may cause a concave appearance. Subdural hematomas are frequently associated with an underlying parenchymal contusion.

Epidural Hematoma

Epidural hematoma is a blood collection between the skull and the dura. A skull fracture accompanies 75% to 90% of such lesions. The fracture is usually linear and along the thinnest portion of temporal-parietal skull, disrupting the middle meningeal artery. *The arterial force of a bleeding dissects the dura from the skull*, frequently producing a true neurological emergency. The posterior meningeal artery can also be disrupted. Not all epidural hematomas result from arterial injury. Approximately 70% also have a venous source.[20] These include dural sinuses, venous tributaries, diploic veins, and meningeal emissary veins. Common locations for epidural hematoma include the temporal, frontal, and occipital regions.

The "classic" history of immediate loss of consciousness followed by a lucid interval is extremely rare. The CT scan has a biconvex or lenticular shaped appearance[21] (see Chapter 7). An acute epidural hematoma does not usually have an underlying parenchymal contusion. An epidural hematoma will become symptomatic within minutes to hours and can be diagnosed earlier than a subdural hematoma. An epidural hematoma usually has a better prognosis than an acute subdural lesion.

Subarachnoid Hemorrhage

Subarachnoid hemorrhage (SAH) is the single most common hemorrhagic lesion after head trauma. A small SAH following trauma does not carry the same serious prognostic implications as a nontraumatic SAH. Increased density within the basal cistern, interhemispheric fissures, and sulci are pathognomonic for SAH.[22]

Other Lesions

Intraventricular hemorrhage occurs in 5% of head trauma patients.[23] Intracranial or intra-axial hemorrhage after head trauma is usually in the form of parenchymal hematoma or contusion. The posterior portion of the frontal lobes and the anterior portion of the temporal lobes are common sites for contusions and require medical therapy. Hematomas are usually found within the white mater and can be surgically evacuated if necessary. "Coup" injuries are contusions at the site of trauma. Opposite to the site of injury is a "contrecoup" injury.

Initial Resuscitation

All patients require rapid assessment of the ABCs (airway, breathing, circulation). Patients should also be rapidly examined for any other potential life-threatening injuries, such as massive bleeding or an open chest wound. Attention should then be turned to the priorities of resuscitation.

Airway

Hypoxemia and hypercarbia need to be prevented or reversed as rapidly as possible. The secondary effects of head trauma including ischemia, cellular injury, and infarction follow hypoxemia or hypercarbia. The goals of oxygenation and ventilation can be accomplished without immediately resorting to intubation. In fact, it is probably better to first use a self-inflating bag and face mask to oxygenate the patient and provide ventilation. Immediate attempts to intubate, particularly if difficult, only result in further exacerbations of hypoxemia. Once the equipment is on hand and the patient is stabilized and oxygenated, intubation can proceed. This should almost always be carried out by direct laryngoscopy.[24] If a neck injury is suspected the head should be stabilized in the position it is currently found, hopefully by an experienced individual. The unconscious patient rarely will require either sedation or muscle paralysis in order to accomplish intubation. Although there may be a transient increase in intracranial pressure during the intubation process, this is usually of limited duration or consequence. It is far more important to intubate the patient and continue oxygenation and ventilation.

On occasion the semi-awake patient requiring intubation may also need sedation but rarely paralysis. We recommend that such sedation be carried out with small doses of a drug such as sodium pentothal, usually in 50-mg increments. Given in this fashion, the drug will not produce hypotension, particularly in the hypovolemic patient. Also, its short action rapidly dissipates. Etomidate in 20- to 40-mg increments works in a similar fashion and with even fewer hypotensive effects.[25] Each agent reduces intracranial pressure and cerebral perfusion pressure (CPP).

In the rare circumstance when paralysis is required, we recommend the use of succinylcholine. This drug, given in a 1.0 mg/kg dose, will provide rapid onset of paralysis and rapid dissipation of action. These kinetics provide a measure of protection if the patient cannot be intubated; return of some form of spontaneous respiration will soon occur. Almost all of the nondepolarizing neuromuscular blockers such as vecuronium and pancuronium, or even rocuronium, last much too long to be of any benefit in an emergent condition. If patients cannot be rapidly intubated, cricothyrotomy should be immediately performed. Kits are now available that aid in this Seldinger-type technique. As soon as possible cricothyrotomy should be converted to a tracheostomy. All authorities, however, agree that tracheostomy is not the procedure of choice for emergency establishment of an airway.[26,27]

The reader should be reminded that some techniques that have not been perfected in a nonemergent situation should not be attempted under these circumstances. These include fiberoptic bronchoscopy or fiberoptic laryngoscopy. Other methods such as retrograde advancement of a transtracheal wire should also not be attempted.

Blind nasal intubation should not even be considered in the acutely head-injured patient. To be successful, the method requires a spontaneously breathing patient. Furthermore, if a patient has a basilar skull fracture, nasal intubation may increase the risk of cerebral spinal fluid (CSF) infection. Long-term nasal intubation generally requires a smaller-diameter tube with a more acute bend. Suctioning becomes more difficult and the work of breathing during spontaneous breathing can significantly increase.[28]

Cardiovascular Considerations

Extremes of blood pressure should obviously be avoided. The severe and moderate head-injured patients require continuous arterial-line hemodynamic monitoring. Hypotension due to a head injury rarely happens. Other causes must be immediately searched for. These might include spinal shock or another injury that produces hypovolemia. Other injuries such as tension pneumothorax can also cause acute hypotension. Uncorrected hypotension leads to further brain ischemia with a worsened outcome and prognosis. Most patients can tolerate at least 500 to 1,000 mL of balanced electrolyte-containing solution as part of the attempt to restore blood pressure. In the patient without obvious hypovolemia, vasopressors may be necessary. We recommend the use of dopamine at between 4 and 12 μg/kg/min. The goal must always be to maintain cerebral perfusion pressure above 70 mm Hg. In fact, as ICP increases and cerebral autoregulation alters, patients may require even higher cerebral perfusion pressures to maintain brain oxygen delivery.[29]

Severe hypertension rarely manifests itself in the head-injured patient. However, pressure may be elevated secondary to agitation or as part of the Cushing response as the brain swells. Systolic pressures in excess of 170 mm Hg may require therapy. However, this will depend on the actual CPP. With an elevated ICP, high systemic pressures may be necessary to maintain an adequate CPP. However, with a normal ICP, an elevated systemic blood pressure may be harmful. The injured brain loses some degree of autoregulation and high pressures can increase overall perfusion to the previously ischemic and injured area. This hyperemic response can result in the release of toxic oxygen radicals and other mediators, all of which have deleterious effects on brain cell function.

When control of elevated blood pressure is required, we have found labetalol an effective agent.[25,31] The drug has both vasodilating and negative inotropic effects and can rapidly reduce blood pressure. Initial dosages range between 5 mg and 40 mg. For ongoing therapy the drug can be infused on a continuous basis at dosages up to 80 mg/hr. Many authorities do not recommend nitroprusside for blood pressure control.[32] They feel that agent's vasodilator properties will, in fact, increase ICP. We have used the drug often and have not seen significant increases in ICP secondary to its use. However, it can also reduce CPP. It requires infusion usually through a central line at rates starting at 0.05 μg/kg/min. When initially started, the patient should be watched carefully since nitroprusside can rapidly cause profound hypotension in the hypovolemic patient. Both labetalol and nitroprusside should be infused with great care. Their vasodilating properties coupled with a significant drop in systemic blood pressure can potentially worsen the effects of an elevated ICP.

The patient with an isolated head injury rarely requires large volume replacement. Under normal circumstances, the blood-brain barrier differs significantly from other interstitial capillary interfaces. The tight endothelial junctions of the capillary endothelium preclude movement of protein and solute. This differs from other areas such as the lung where protein and solute can move more readily between the interstitium and the intravascular compartment. This means that the vast majority of fluid movement in the brain is influenced by osmolarity, primarily related to serum sodium values. Under normal circumstances, balanced electrolyte solutions are preferred as the fluid to maintain the brain in a relatively dry state. The clinician must realize the Ringer's lactate is a hypotonic solution, and, as such, can potentially increase brain water. The most logical solution is normal saline with 154 mEq/L of sodium or an even more hypertonic solution[33-36] (see Chapters 6 and 16).

Probable loss of normal blood-brain barrier function follows brain injury. The endothelial junctions appear to increase in diameter.[37] As such, solutes and proteins may move more readily between the brain and the intravascular space. Because of these concerns and the potential for brain injury, many authorities recommend that colloids be used as the fluid of choice. They reason that the oncotic pressure from protein will tend to pull fluid out of the brain while the endothelial junctions remain small enough to inhibit most protein movement into the brain tissue.[38]

Therefore, we, as do most institutions, tend to use colloid solutions to maintain intravascular volumes. However, we recognize that the serum osmolarity still plays an important role. For that reason, we attempt to maintain serum *sodium close to 140 mEq/L. This helps maintain a normal or slightly elevated osmolarity.*

Many authorities have recommended that patients should be kept "dry." However, in order to assure adequate brain perfusion, the patient needs to be at least euvolemic. Hypovolemia as a method to keep the brain dry may actually contribute to further injury due to ischemia. Whenever we have any question of volume status, we place a pulmonary artery catheter. This permits more objective interpretation of the clinical status and aids in appropriate volume restoration. However, the reader should recognize that a linear relationship between intravascular volume and the pulmonary capillary wedge pressure or central venous pressure does not exist. The wedge and central venous pressures measure intraventricular pressures, which hopefully reflect intraventricular volume.

Most younger patients with head injury do not experience any significant or severe myocardial involvement. However, older patients may already have preexisting myocardial or coronary artery disease, and they may be more susceptible to cardiovascular compromise. Acute brain injury may result in a sudden release of catecholamine. The resultant vasoconstriction can lead to myocardial ischemia, particularly in patients with fixed lesions in the coronary artery system. The ischemia may only be manifested by electrocardiographic (ECG) changes, but can also result in either cardiac arrhythmias or a low-output state.

Myocardial contusion can also result from the initial event that caused the head injury. Myocardial contusion may present itself as tachyarrhythmia, multiple ventricular arrhythmias, or a low-output state.[39]

For all of the above reasons, following head injury, the patient should have a standard 12-lead ECG. Any signs of ischemia or abnormalities should be followed up with echocardiography. Although we normally use transesophageal echocardiography, will provide an even more complete picture of the myocardial status.

Critical Care Treatment of the Head Injury

Simultaneously while attending to the pulmonary and cardiovascular systems, the brain must also be treated. Following injury and/or operative intervention, most of the therapy in the intensive care unit (ICU) is directed at the secondary effects. Most attention has been focused on maintenance of ICP within a reasonable range (less than 25 mm Hg) as well as treatment of agitation and any other problems that may increase brain oxygen requirements or reduce oxygen delivery. After the initial and follow-up assessments and assignment of a Glasgow Coma Score, decisions must be made in regard to further ICP monitoring. If either the CT scan or intraoperative observation demonstrates significant brain swelling, most patients will have ICP monitored. Nonoperated patients usually have a subdural bolt. Operated patients may have a ventriculostomy placed for intracranial pressure monitoring.

Cerebral Hemodynamics and Hyperventilation

If the CT scan, the physical examination, or the surgical review do not indicate significant brain swelling, then ICP monitoring may not be necessary. Under these circumstances we generally tend to mildly hyperventilate these patients, maintaining $PaCO_2$ of 30 to 34 mm Hg. The patient is then simply monitored according to neurological status. Any deterioration would result in further hyperventilation and an emergent CT scan.

Patients have almost universally been hyperventilated when ICP exceeds 20 mm Hg.[40] In the last several years, the entire spectrum of therapy to treat elevated ICP has undergone a reexamination. Some of the more traditional approaches have been questioned, and their clinical relevance has become less clear. An underlying uniform theme evokes the need to maintain a minimum cerebral perfusion pressure (CPP). Furthermore, as brain compliance changes, it may take a higher than normal CPP to perfuse the brain. Despite elevated ICP, the CPP still remains the principal determinant of cerebral blood flow and oxygenation. The reduction in cerebral perfusion following hyperventilation and hypocapnia can and will lead to cellular ischemia.[41] The degree of ischemia and metabolic acidosis increases as $PaCO_2$ and consequently blood flow falls to increasingly lower levels. Some clinicians have begun to essentially eliminate hyperventilation and focus attention on maintaining CPP at a minimum of 70 to 80 mm Hg.[42,43] Despite what may be a severe head injury, cerebrovascular autoregulation can remain relatively intact. Also, the reader should recognize that the space occupied inside the cranium is fixed. Pressures and flow may change, but not volume. If blood pressure and flow fall, the vasculature will vasodilate, which in turn causes an elevation in ICP and concomitant reduction in CPP.[37] When blood pressure increases, the vasoconstriction follows and ICP again decreases.[44]

Mannitol

Mannitol has been indicated to help reduce elevated ICP due to its osmotic effects on the brain. It is generally given in does of 0.5 to 1.0 g/kg. since mannitol pulls fluid into the intravascular compartment, it causes some hemodilution.[39] However, it is doubtful that this improves microcirculatory flow. Mannitol may affect the red blood cell conformation and improve flow secondary to altered viscosity.[45,46] After several days the mannitol molecules will find their way into the brain interstitium and act as a gradient to actually draw fluid back into the brain.[47]

Barbiturate Coma

Traditionally, barbiturates have been advocated as the final tool to control ICP.[42] The barbiturates have two potential benefits: (1)

they can reduce overall brain metabolism and oxygen requirements; and (2) barbiturates cause a decrease in cardiac output and blood brain flow that should lead to a reduction in ICP. However, CPP may also be significantly compromised.[48] Since barbiturates are used only when ICP has been refractory to other therapy, the outcome associated with its use has been abysmal.[48,49] However, despite the data, we will use the drug in a final attempt to save the patient, particularly in the younger population.

The end-point of barbiturate therapy is ordinarily an isoelectric electroencephalogram (EEG). Obviously this requires bedside placement of a portable EEG monitor. Pentobarbital is usually begun at a 4- to 6-mg/kg loading dose. The continuous infusion is maintained at 2 to 4 mg/kg/hr or as guided by the EEG.

Pentobarbital dosages in these range will suppress cardiac output and reduce blood pressure. Often these patients will require inotropic support with either dopamine or epinephrine to maintain blood pressure, cardiac output, and CPP; therefore, at the time of initiation of pentobarbital coma, we place a pulmonary artery catheter to guide management of the cardiovascular system.

It is unclear how long barbiturate therapy should be continued. In our own institution we vary from 3 to 14 days depending on the clinical circumstances.[50] Barbiturate levels must be monitored. Serum levels >30 mg% of pentobarbital can be toxic and severely depress cardiac performance. Once discontinued, the blood levels may not return to below 5 mg% for 24 to 48 hours, primarily depending on renal function.

Positional Changes

Traditionally, patients have been kept in the head position, usually 30°. This promotes venous drainage (if the head is maintained in midline.) However, this may be less important than first thought.[51,52] Although ICP may increase in the supine position, the concomitant increase in CPP more than makes up for any increase.

Induced Hypothermia

Other protective mechanisms following head injury have been directed at reduction of the brain's metabolic demands. Approximately 20 years ago, whole-body cooling was first attempted as a method to reduce metabolic demands;[53,54] however, the results at that time were uniformly poor, with the vast majority of patients dying, many times secondary to sepsis. In retrospect, our increased understanding of the immune system would suggest that hypothermia reduces total body immune response. That, coupled with the poor understanding of measures to prevent sepsis, probably contributed to the dismal outcome at that time. However, better understanding of methods to minimize the risk of sepsis have recently been combined with efforts to reduce brain oxygen requirements. It appears that the earlier these methods are introduced, the more likely they are to succeed.

Prevention of Sepsis

The injured patient will have an extended stay in the ICU. Additionally, they often require long-term mechanical ventilatory support and are at increased risk for developing various infections.

Pneumonia

A head-injured patient, especially when comatose and mechanically ventilated, has the highest risk of any patient group for development of nosocomial pneumonia.[55] No doubt this relates to the inability to cough or mobilize secretions. These patients develop microatelectasis and retention of secretions. Poor pulmonary conditions contribute to an excellent culture media for various organisms and pneumonia or at the very least tracheobronchitis will likely develop. In order to prevent the development of stress ulceration or gastritis, most patients are treated with either H2 blockers or antacid therapy in order to alkalinize the stomach.[56]

Unfortunately, the reduced acid content provides an excellent media for hospital-acquired organisms to grow. The majority are gram-negative. Sufficient data exist to suggest that with gram-negative colonization of the stomach, these bacteria find their way into the upper respiratory tract of the patient. Since almost 80% of intubated patients aspirate to some degree, this no doubt represents the inoculation mechanism.[57] Despite the increase in colonization, and possibly pneumonia, there is little evidence to suggest that these patients have a prolonged stay, more severe complications, or a higher mortality rate. However, in order to mitigate against these problems, we prefer to leave the stomach in an acid state and instead use sucralfate to prophylax against ulceration and gastritis while at the same time maintaining the acid medium to minimize bacterial overgrowth.

On occasion, pneumonia can develop secondary to blood-borne infections from another distant site. However, this rarely occurs in these patients.

Septicemia

The head-injured patient's prolonged ICU stay also means that the use of centrally placed catheters increases. These represent an increased risk for colonization and the potential for the development of a bacteremia. The vast majority of evidence would suggest that line-associated bacteremia are more frequent in those that are not changed on a regular or frequent basis. If patients have a central line and are without other overt signs of sepsis, we change their central lines every 6 days.[58] The new line requires placement in a fresh site.[59]

When patients have a temperature higher than 38.5°C (101.3°F), we draw percutaneous blood cultures. If blood cultures are drawn through an indwelling line and are later positive, it is unclear if the culture represents a true bacteremia or simply line colonization. If cultures drawn through a catheter or the catheter tip grow the same organisms as the percutaneous blood culture, then we presume that the catheter is the source of the bacteremia. That line should immediately be changed to a new site.

Urinary Tract Infection

The requirement for continuous bladder catheterization significantly increases the risk of urinary tract infection. As part of a fever workup, urine should always be cultured. If bacteria grow in urine at colony counts of greater than 100,000, institute appropriate antibiotic therapy. Unlike other infections such as those of the lungs or blood, relatively low doses of aminoglycosides will successfully eradicate the infection. The aminoglycosides concentrate in urine since it is their primary route of excretion.[60] Irrespective of blood levels, the urine aminoglycoside concentration will be sufficiently high to kill any susceptible organisms.

Almost all institutions have noted an increase in the number of fungal urinary tract infections. If the catheter cannot be removed, and because these patients are at increased risk for development of a systemic fungal infection, we institute prophylactic therapy with an agent such as fluconozale, which does not have the renal toxicity of amphotericin B. If at all possible we prefer removal of the indwelling catheter.

Antibiotics

If the patient has an indwelling device, such as an epidural bolt or bentriculostomy drain, we generally continue antibiotic coverage. Depending on the recent history in the particular ICU, this may strictly be gram-positive coverage, but on occasion, gram-negative coverage will also be provided. Once the device is removed, the antibiotics are discontinued.

When signs of sepsis, such as hyperthermia or a white blood cell count elevation with a left shift greater than 10% develop, a complete physical examination should be performed and cultures should be drawn from blood, sputum, and urine. If any central lines sites appear inflamed or have frank pus, the catheter is removed and inserted in a new site. Removal of the catheter for at least 6 hours will allow clearance of any organisms present. Other diagnostic studies as appropriate should be undertaken. These might include a CT scan of the abdomen to attempt to locate a source for the fever. Continued fever elevation may require broad-spectrum antibiotic coverage. If the cultures remain negative after 3 to 4 days or the patient clinically improves, the antibiotics can be discontinued. If the culture becomes positive, antibiotic therapy can be adjusted based on drug sensitivities.

Nutritional Support (See Chapter 14)

All long-term patients in an ICU will require nutritional support. As a general rule, particularly in the head-injured patient, the gut is the preferred route.[61] This helps preserve its function by prevention of mucosal atrophy and potential malabsorption. Although less clear, continued use of the gut probably reduces the likelihood of any bacterial translocation into the mesenteric lymph nodes and potentially into the circulation.[62]

Glucose Homeostasis

There are animal and human data suggesting that high glucose levels at the time of brain injury are associated with a worsened outcome.[63,64] This linkage is not straightforward, and furthermore it is unclear as to whether or not elevated glucose levels contribute to problems during the entire recovery process. We attempt to maintain glucose levels within a normal range, usually less than 125 mg%. This can be readily accomplished with either intermittent or continuous infusions of insulin as necessary and close regular monitoring of blood glucose levels. We see no reason to withhold feedings from these patients since the potential for gut injury and other problems will rapidly increase.

Tube Feeding Regimes

A small-bore, soft silastic catheter can usually be advanced by means of a stylet through the nose or mouth into the small bowel.[65] If unsuccessful, placement of the patient on the right side and use of agents such as metoclopramide will increase gastric contractions and hopefully move the mercury-tipped catheter into the small bowel. When these combined efforts are unsuccessful, the patient can be brought to fluoroscopy for direct placement of the catheter. A gastroscope can also be used to move the tip of the catheter into the small bowel. We prefer not to feed into the stomach or use bolus feeds. Both are associated with a high incidence of gastric distention and potential aspiration. This is a particular problem in the head-injured patient who usually cannot protect the airway.

Feedings are begun at full strength, usually at rates of 20 to 25 mL/hr. The maximum rate should be 80 to 90 mL/hr. Higher rates seem to be associated with an increased incidence of bowel distention. Most of the diarrhea associated with enteral feeding appears to be related to the protein base and type of carbohydrate substrate used in the formula. Although the osmolarity varies with each formulation, it is not usually the cause of any associated diarrhea. If diarrhea begins with more than two or three watery stools per day, feeding should either be reduced in volume or stopped completely. Another formula can be selected and begun after a minimum 24-hour wait and resolution of the diarrhea. Narcotics administered to stop diarrhea may cause an ileus. If patients have had previous broad-spectrum antibiotic therapy, *Clostridia difficile* toxin screens should be checked.

Long-term enteral therapy may require either percutaneous or operative placement of a jejunostomy combined with a gastrostomy. This will allow for better maintenance, particularly when the patient leaves the ICU. We often combine this procedure at the time of tracheostomy if, in fact, this is deemed necessary for long-term pulmonary care. As indicated, we prefer the enteral to the parenteral route for nutritional support. However, if the gut cannot be utilized because of associated injuries, then we begin parenteral feedings, usually by day 5. Patients who were reasonably healthy prior to their injury can usually withstand the degree of negative nitrogen balance that accumulates over the first several days. It has become increasingly clear that fat, as currently utilized, contributes to inactivation of the immune system. Thus, fat is supplied only as necessary to prevent fatty acid deficiency, and it generally makes up less than 10% of the total caloric requirements.

Caloric requirements for brain-injured patients are usually not excessively high. They ordinarily range between 30 and 35 cal/kg/day. If there are no other associated injuries, the overall needs may be even less. Protein restoration usually requires 1.5 g/kg/day of amino acids.

Other Complications Related to the Head-Injured Patient

Sedation

The head-injured patient will often develop severe and significant agitation. This usually occurs as part of the recovery phase of their injury. On occasion, the agitation may be due to withdrawal from alcohol or other drugs. Pain can also cause significant agitation.

In general, the agitation is usually detrimental to the patient. Indwelling lines can easily be removed and the endotracheal tubes pulled out. Furthermore, both the systemic and brain metabolic rates and oxygen requirements significantly increase.

We prefer to use mild sedation with agents that can be rapidly discontinued. This allows for return to a baseline state so that a complete neurological examination can be performed when required.

We have found that infusions of proprofol or midazolam have both been effective for maintenance of sedation in the brain-injured patient.[66,67] Furthermore, their metabolic properties provide rapid dissipation upon discontinuance and rapid return to baseline for neurological evaluation.[68] Propofol may be somewhat easier to titrate to effect. These agents have minimal effects on ICP except if used in large dosages. Also, they do not directly depress cardiac contractility. Propofol has mild systemic vasodilating effects.

When sedation is undertaken, the end-point of therapy should be clear to the nursing staff. This will allow a more uniform dosing schedule and reliability of recovery time when discontinued. Propofol works well at dosages of 0.03 to 0.06 mg/kg/hr. We generally use midazolam in dosages of 1 to 4 mg/hr. Wakeup occurs within 30 minutes of discontinuation of either agent. We do not recommend the rapid reversal of sedation in patients with known increased ICP with large doses of romazicon for fear of precipitation of further increases in ICP.

Diabetes Insipidus

Diabetes insipidus (DI) usually results because of direct injury to the hypothalamus or nearby structures. Also, inadequate perfusion or hypoxia can cause indirect injury.

Patients develop an increase in urinary output, usually in excess of volumes that are currently being administered. If increased urinary output occurs soon after the initial resuscitation, DI must be differentiated from the diuresis following large volume fluid resuscitation. In addition to large urine volumes, patients with DI will have urine-specific gravity of less than 1.004 and low urine sodium concentrations. Serum sodium will simultaneously increase. Diuresis following fluid resuscitation reveals high urine sodium values and no real change in serum sodium levels.

The high osmolarity associated with hypernatremia can exaggerate water movement from the brain and other cells and lead to dehydration. Steps should be undertaken to correct the problem as soon as apparent. If patients are awake and alert, simple oral intake of fluids is often sufficient to make up the deficit. However, most head-injured patients will not be able to drink and will require IV fluid replacement. Replacement of urine losses at the same rate as urine output will result in a continued increase in both urine volume and fluid requirements. Therefore, we attempt to replace urine at ½ to ¾ of the volume lost. This can be done with a dilute solution of 0.25 saline or 5DW. The use of large volumes of 5DW may lead to hyperglycemia and further problems. With excessive urine volumes, greater than 300 to 400 mL/hr, we use agents such as pitressin or desmopressin acetate (DDAVP®). Pitressin is short-acting, and therefore it should probably be used prior to DDAVP. On occasion, we have seen the latter drug push the patient into syndrome of inappropriate antidiuretic hormone secretion (SIADH). Pitressin can be given in dosages of 5 units intravenously and its effects will last from 4 to 8 hours. DDAVP dosages are 0.5 to 2.0 μg. Its effects will last well beyond 12 and 24 hours.

Syndrome of Inappropriate Antidiuretic Hormone (SIADH)

SIADH can commonly occur following head injury. This results in an excess of water retention, and causes increased cellular and brain swelling.

The diagnosis of SIADH includes hyponatremia, usually less than 130 mEq/L. Urine osmolarity substantially increases while serum osmolarity falls below 280 mOsm/L. The problem is usually self-limited but requires therapy to maintain normal osmolarity. In certain circumstances, fluid can simply be restricted. However, most times these patients still require fluid therapy, which can then be administered as either normal saline or a more concentrated form such as 3% saline. When sodium levels are above 130 mEq/L, 3% saline can be discontinued. When patients are receiving enteral feedings, one to two teaspoons of salt added to the formulation will usually help correct the sodium deficit.

Declaration of Brain Death (See Chapter 18)

Unfortunately, the severity of injury, on occasion, precludes survival, and the patient ultimately becomes brain-dead. This can sometimes be a diagnostic and legal dilemma. Most hospitals have their own stated criteria in order to declare a patient brain-dead. These might include an EEG that is flat on two separate occasions, separated in time by 6 to 24 hours. Others may rely simply on a neurological examination by a qualified individual such as a neurosurgeon or a neurologist.

When possible, we prefer to use the apnea test. This test is carried out when all other portions of the neurological examination show absence of any activity. Provided the patient remains normothermic and has had correction of all electrolytes, the test can be performed. We generally place the patient on 100% oxygen and draw a blood gas, based on the $PaCO_2$ rise of approximately 3 mm Hg/min that will be required for the $PaCO_2$ to reach 60 mm Hg. The patient is then placed on a continuous flow system and observed during this time. If any attempts at breathing occur, the patient is obviously not brain-dead. If there are no breathing attempts, the observation period continues for the duration, consistent with the prediction of $PaCO_2$ in excess of 60 mm Hg. Failure to breathe, despite a $PaCO_2$

of 60 mm Hg, is indicative of brain death. Prior to the tests, it must be clear that the patient has not received any drugs that may interfere with breathing. These include barbiturates, sedatives, and narcotics.

Often because of drug therapy, it is impractical to perform an apnea test. Under these circumstances, a radionuclide scan can help make the determination.[69] Failure to demonstrate blood flow is consistent with brain death. It is a rapid test and precludes waiting for the system to clear various other drugs.

Summary

In conclusion, much new information and data have become available in the treatment of head injury. Clearly, outcomes have continued to improve based on earlier intervention. We appear now to be in a time of transition as our traditional therapies to treat head injury and reduce ICP undergo complete reexamination. Other insights into brain function and an understanding of metabolic pathways will point the way to newer solutions in the future.

References

1. Frankowski RF, Annegers JF, Whitman S: Epidemiology and descriptive studies: Part 1 The descriptive epidemiology of head trauma in the United States. In Eeckerd P, Povlishock JP (eds): Central Nervous System Trauma Status Report, 1985, pp 33–45.
2. Siegel JH, Dunham CM: Trauma, the disease of the 20th Century. In Siegel JH (ed): Trauma Emergency Surgery Critical Care. Churchill Livingston, New York, 1987, pp 1–32.
3. Bullock R, Teasdale G: Head injuries II. Br Med J 300:1576–1579, 1990.
4. Colohan ART, Oyesiku NM: Moderate head injury: An overview. J Neurotrauma 9:S259–S264, 1992.
5. Yamaki T, Murakami N, Iwamoto Y, et al: Pathological study of diffuse axonal injury patients who died shortly after impact. Acta Neurochir 119:153–158, 1992.
6. Shigemori M, Kikuchi T, Ochiai S, et al: Coexisting diffuse axonal injury (DAI) and outcome of severe head injury. Acta Neurochi 55:37–39, 1992.
7. Bommaya AK: Mechanisms of cerebral concussion, contusions and other effects of head injury. In Youmans JR (ed): Neurological Surgery, 2nd ed. WB Saunders Co., Philadelphia, 1982, pp 1877–1895.
8. Zimmerman RA, Bilaniak LT, Gennarelli TA: Computed tomography of shearing injuries of the cerebral white matter. Radiology 127:393–396, 1978.
9. Adams JH, Doyle D, Ford I, et al: Diffuse axonal injury in head injury: Definition, diagnosis and grading. Histopathology 15:49–59, 1989.

10. Adams JH, Graham DI, Murray LS, et al: Diffuse axonal injury due to nonmissile head injury in humans: An analysis of 45 cases. Ann Neurology 12:557–563, 1981.
11. Margiles SS, Thibault LE: A proposed tolerance criterion for diffuse exonal injury in man. J Biomechanics 25(8):917–923, 1992.
12. Graham DI, Clark JC, Adams JH, et al: Diffuse axonal injury caused by assault. J Clin Pathol 45(9):840–841, 1992.
13. Ropper AH, Kennedy SF: Neurological and Neurosurgical Intensive Care. Ashby Publishers Inc., Rockville, MD, 1988.
14. Gennarelli TA: Mechanisms of cerebral, contusion and other effects of head injury. In Youmans JR (ed): Neurolog Surg 3:1953–1963, 1990.
15. Adams JH: Head injury. In Adams JH, Corsellis JAN, Duchen LW (eds): Greenfield's Neuropathology, 4th ed. Edward Arnold, London, 1984, pp 85–124.
16. Adams JH, Gerhan DI, Gennarelli TA: Head injury in man and experimental animals: Neuropathology. Acta Neurochir 32:15–30, 1983.
17. Gade GS, Becker DP, Miller JD, et al: Pathology and pathophysiology of head injury. In Youman's JR (ed): Neurological Surgery, 3rd ed. WB Saunders Co., Philadelphia, 1990, pp 1965–2016.
18. Becker DP, Miller JD, Sweet RC, et al: Head injury management 1977. In Popp AJ, Bourkers, Nelson LR, Kimelverg HK (eds): Neurotrauma Seminars in Neurological Surgery. Raven Press, New York, 1979, pp 313–328.
19. Becker DP, Miller JD, Ward JD, et al: The outcome from severe head injury with early diagnosis is intensive management. J Neurosurg 47:491–502, 1977.
20. Weinman D, Muttucumarub B: Extradural hematoma. Cuilon Med J 14:60–70, 1969.
21. Tsai FY, Teal JS, Hieshima GB: Neuroradiology of Head Trauma. University Park Press, Baltimore, 1984, pp 201–242.
22. Becker DP, Gade GF, Young HF, et al: Diagnosis and treatment of head injury in adults. In Mans JR (ed): Electrical Surgery. WB Saunders Co., Philadelphia, 1990, pp 2051–2053.
23. French BN, Dublin AB: The value of computerized tomography in the management of 1,000 consecutive head injuries. Surg Neurol 7:171–183, 1977.
24. Gallagher TJ: Endotracheal intubation. In Kruse JA (ed): Procedures in Intensive Care. Crit Care Clin 8:665–676, 1992.
25. Giese JL, Stockham RJ, Stanley TH, et al: Etomidate versus thiopental for induction of anesthesia. Anesth Analg 64:871–876, 1985.
26. Heffner JE, Miller KS, Sahn SA: Tracheostomy in the intensive care unit. Part I: Indications, Technique, Management. Chest 90:269–274, 1986.
27. Heffner JE, Sahn SA: The technique of tracheostomy and cricothyrotomy. J Crit Care Illness 2:79, 1987.
28. Fiastro JF, Habib MP, Quan SF: Pressure support compensation for inspiratory work due to endotracheal tubes and demand continuous positive airway pressure. Chest 93:499–505, 1988.

29. Rosner MJ, Daughton S: Cerebral perfusion pressure management in head injury. J of Trauma 30:933–941, 1990.
30. Muizelaar JP, Marmarou A, Young HF, et al: Improving the outcome of severe head injury with the oxygen radical scavenger polyethylene glycol-conjugated superoxide dismutase: A phase II trial. J Neurosurg 78:375–382, 1993.
31. Muzzi DA, Black S, Losasso TJ, et al: Labetalol and esmolol in the control of hypertension after intracranial surgery. Anesth Analg 40:68–71, 1990.
32. Cottrell JE, Tatel K, Ransohoff JR: Intracranial pressure changes induced by sodium nitroprusside inpatients with intracranial mass lesions. Neurosurgery 48:329, 1978.
33. Gunnar W, Jonasson O, Merlotti G, et al: Head injury and hemorrhagic shock: Studies of the blood brain barrier and intracranial pressure after resuscitation with normal saline solution, 3% saline solution and dextran-40. Surgery 103/4:398–407, 1988.
34. Schmoker JD, Zhuang J, Shackford SR: Hypertonic fluid resuscitation improves cerebral oxygen delivery and reduces intracranial pressure after hemorrhagic shock. J Trauma 31:1607–1613, 1991.
35. Zornow MH, Scheller MS, Todd MM, et al: Acute cerebral effects of isotonic crystalloid and colloid solutions following cryogenic brain injury in the rabbit. Anesthesiology 69:180–184, 1988.
36. Zornow MH, Todd MM, Moore S: The acute cerebral effects of changes in plasma osmolality and oncotic pressure. Anesthesiology 67:936–941, 1987.
37. Klatzo I: Neuropathological aspects of cerebral edema. J Neuropathol Exp Neurol 26:1, 1967.
38. Wisner D, Busche F, Sturm J, et al: Traumatic shock and head injury: Effects of fluid resuscitation on the brain. J Surg Res 46:49–59, 1989.
39. Palter MD, Cortes D: Secondary triage of the trauma patient. In Civetta JN, Taylor RW, Kirby RR (eds): Critical Care, 2nd ed. JB Lippincott Co., Philadelphia, 1992, p 617.
40. Chesnut R, Marshall LF: Treatment of abnormal intracranial pressure. Neurosurg Clin North Am 2:267–283, 1991.
41. Muizelaar JP, Marmarou A, Ward JD, et al: Adverse effects of prolonged hyperventilation in patients with severe head injury: A randomized clinical trial. J Neurosurg 75:731–739, 1991.
42. Miller JD, Dearden NM, Piper IR, et al: Control of intracranial pressure in patients with severe head injury. J Neurotrauma 9:S317–S326, 1992.
43. Rosner MJ, Daughton S: Cerebral perfusion pressure management in head injury. J Trauma 933–941, 1990.
44. Bouma GJ, Muizelaar JP: Cerebral blood flow, cerebral blood volume and cerebrovascular reactivity after severe head injury. J Neurotrauma 9:S333–S348, 1992.
45. Brown FD, Johns L, Jafar JJ, et al: Detailed monitoring of the effects of mannitol following experimental head injury. J Neurosurg 50:423, 1979.
46. Muizelaar JP, Wei EP, Knotos HA, et al: Cerebral blood flow is regulated

by changes in blood pressure and in blood viscosity alike. Stroke 17:44, 1986.

47. Shapiro HM: Barbiturates in brain ischemia. Br J Anaesth 57:82–95, 1985.

48. Nordstron CH, Messeter K, Sundbarg G, et al: Cerebral blood flow, vasoreactivity and oxygen consumption during barbiturate therapy in severe traumatic brain lesions. J Neurosurg 68:424–431, 1988.

49. Ward JD, Becker DP, Miller JD, et al: Failure of prophylactic barbiturates in the treatment of severe head injury. J Neurosurg 62:383, 1985.

50. Segal J: Prolonged barbiturate therapy in a patient with closed head injury and jugular venous thrombosis. Neurosurgery 32:468–472, 1993.

51. Feldman Z, Kanter MJ, Robertson CS, et al: Effect of head elevation on intracranial pressure, cerebral perfusion pressure and cerebral blood flow in head-injury patients. J Neurosurg 76:207–211, 1992.

52. Durward QJ, Amacher AL, Del Maestro RF, et al: Cerebral and cardiovascular responses to changes in head elevation in patients with intracranial hypertension. J Neurosurg 59:938–944, 1983.

53. Clifton GL, Christensen ML: Use of moderate hypothermia during elective craniotomy. J Texas Med 88:66–69, 1992.

54. Strachan RD, Whittle IR, Miller JD: Hypothermia and severe head injury. Brain Injury 3:51–55, 1989.

55. Craven DE, Steger KA, Baber TW: Preventing nosocomial pneumonia: State of the are in perspectives for the 1990's. Am J of Med 91:44S–53S, 1991.

56. Borrero E, Bank S, Margolis I, et al: Comparison of antacid and sucralfate in the prevention of gastrointestinal bleeding inpatients who are critically ill. Am J Med 79:62–64, 1985.

57. Atherton ST, White DS: Stomach as a source of bacteria colonizing respiratory tract during artificial ventilation. Lancet 2:948–969, 1978.

58. Powell C, Fabri PJ, Kudsk KA: Risk of infection accompanying the use of single-lumen vs. double-lumen subclavian catheters: A prospective randomized study. JPEN Nutr 12:127–129, 1988.

59. Bonadimani B, Sperti C, Stevanin A, et al: Central venous catheter guidewire replacement according to the Seldinger technique: Usefulness in the management of patients on total parenteral nutrition. JPEN 11: 267–270, 1987.

60. Appel GB, Neu HC: The nephrotoxicity of antimicrobial agents. N Engl J Med 296:663–670, 722–728, 784–787, 1977.

61. Zaloga GP, MacGregor DA: What to consider when choosing enteral or parenteral nutrition. J Crit Illness 5:1180–1200, 1990.

62. Alexander JW: Nutrition and translocation. JPEN 14:170S–174S, 1990.

63. Young B, Ott L, Dentsy R, et al: Relationship between admission hyperglycemia and neurological outcome of severely brain injured patients. Ann Surg 210:466, 1989.

64. Lan AM, Winn HR, Cullen BF, et al: Hyperglycemia and neurological outcome in patients with head injury. J Neurosurg 75:545, 1991.

65. Zaloga GP: Bedside method for placing small bowel feeding tube in critically ill patients: A prospective study. Chest 100:1643–1646, 1991.

66. Farling PA, Johnston JR, Coppel DL: Propofol infusion for sedation of

patients with head injury in intensive care. Anaesthesia 44:222–226, 1989.
67. Chiolero RL, Ravussin PA, Anderes JP, et al: The effects of midazolam reversal by RO 15-1788 on cerebral perfusion pressure in patients with severe head injury. Intensive Care Med 14:196–200, 1988.
68. Ronan KP, Gallagher TJ, George B, et al: Comparison of propofol and midazolam for sedation in intensive care unit patients. Crit Care Med 23:286–293, 1995.
69. Goodman JM, Heck LL, Moore BD: Confirmation of brain death with portable isotope angiography: A review of 204 consecutive cases. Neurosurgery 16:492, 1985.

13

Critical Care Management of Spinal Cord Injuries

Anne F. Boudreaux, MD, T. James Gallagher, MD

Epidemiology

In the United States 10,000 to 11,000 persons yearly suffer traumatic permanent spinal cord injuries (SCI).[1,2] Nearly half become quadriplegic.[3] As with other trauma the majority are males between the ages of 16 and 35 years. Causes include: motor vehicle accidents, stabs, gunshots, industrial accidents, falls, diving injuries, and other sports injuries.[4] Motor vehicle accidents are the leading cause of spinal cord injuries in the United States. Falls, occurring often among the elderly population in their home, rank second.[5] Diving injuries account for 10% of all spinal cord injuries and usually occur in younger patients.[6] Most injuries occur at the level of the cervical spine. Such an injury impacts on every body system as it impairs voluntary motor, sensory, and the autonomic nervous system functions.

Rarely does SCI involve a complete anatomic transection of the

From *Trauma Anesthesia and Critical Care of Neurological Injury,* edited by K. J. Abrams and C. M. Grande. © 1997, Futura Publishing Co., Armonk, NY.

spinal cord. However, 45–65% of all SCI functionally act as a complete spinal cord transection.[7] The trend over the past 20 years reflects a decreasing number of neurological complete injuries.[8] This may represent more informed and careful prehospital care. Generally the spinal cord suffers a contusion or compression secondary to a broken or dislocated vertebrae, disc, or ligamentous encroachment. Those usually follow a component of hyperextension or hyperflexion. Further injury develops when the injured cord undergoes additional biochemical and pathological changes. Postulated mechanisms of these secondary effects include: post-traumatic ischemia, continued direct compression, edema formation, and free radical induced damage. Electrolyte imbalance with intracellular accumulation of calcium and extracellular accumulation of potassium ions, and arachidonate or excitatory amino acids also can induce damage.[9]

Mortality rates following spinal cord injuries have declined dramatically in recent years. This also relates to improved prehospital management and transportation as well as definitive treatment in specialized regional units. Over the past 15 years, admission to a spinal cord injury care system within 24 hours of injury has resulted in a 66% mortality reduction within the first 2 years following injury. Age, level of cord injury, and the presence of preexisting medical problems all contribute to mortality.[10] Older patients with neurologically complete quadriplegia have a particularly poor prognosis with a median cumulative survival time of only 1.8 years.[11] The frequency of complications as well as mortality correlates with a patient's age, premorbid state, the level and severity of the cord lesion, hypotension, and tachypnea.[12]

The leading causes of death following SCI in order of frequency are: pulmonary infections, respiratory failure, heart disease, septicemia, urinary tract complications, pulmonary emboli, and suicide. During a recent 12-year follow-up of SCI patients, a mortality rate of 9.3% was reported.[13] SCI patients are 37 times more likely to die of pneumonia and 82 times more likely to die of septicemia than comparable individuals from the general population. Pneumonia has recently surpassed renal failure and other urological complications as the leading cause of death among SCI patients.

General Management

As with any trauma patient, immediate establishment of the ABCs (airway, breathing, circulation) is mandatory and aids in the maintenance of the critical microcirculation of the spinal cord.

Proper stabilization and immobilization to prevent further damage to the spinal cord is essential. Post-traumatic hypotension is especially damaging to the spinal cord due to loss of spinal cord autoregulation, which makes the cord extremely susceptible to ischemia. Neurological and vertebral assessment should receive emphasis.

In general, following acute injury, the neck and head alignment should not be altered until a well-fitted cervical collar can be applied. Soft collars or the loose-fitting plastic type provide no benefit. In fact, they may add a false sense of security with possibly disastrous consequences. When at all possible, helmets should not be removed in the field. Patients should always be transported on a rigid surface and the neck and head stabilized against lateral movement. All head-injured patients should be considered to have a neck injury until proven otherwise. A brief assessment in the field of neurological function will provide a basis to observe later functional changes.

Airway Management

Airway management of a cervical spinal cord-injured patient usually involves establishment of an airway in a patient whose status has deteriorated. This may rapidly follow the injury or it may later result from pneumonia or some other indirectly related problem.

When a patient requires immediate intubation, the oral method is by far the fastest. Also unlike nasal intubation, it does not require a spontaneously breathing patient.

Oral intubation generally permits placement of a larger-diameter tube. This reduces the overall work of breathing and makes suctioning the tube and, if later necessary, bronchoscopy easier. Nasal tubes have been associated with a higher incidence of maxillary sinusitis and septal necrosis. Because of the more acute bend required, suctioning may be more difficult. As previously described, oral intubation requires that the head be maintained in the current position. A skilled individual such as a neurosurgeon hopefully will be available. Otherwise, the person who helps must be instructed to ensure there is no lateral movement or flexion or extension of the head during the tracheal tube placement. This generally requires a skilled intubationist, preferably an anesthesiologist.

Almost all adult males of normal size can accept a 8.0-mm ID endotracheal tube. In women, a 7.0-mm ID will be satisfactory. The older the patient, the more likely a larger tube will fit as subglottic dilatation occurs with age. Most inexperienced individuals can more easily intubate with a curved-blade laryngoscope. A 4 MacIntosh blade will work for the largest as well as smallest patient.

When nasal intubation is to be performed, the process should proceed slowly and deliberately. Moving ahead rapidly without taking the necessary precautions may lead to epistaxis, aspiration, and failure to actually control the airway. Prior to the intubation the nasal route should be dilated with the use of nasal pharyngeal tubes. This follows local anesthesia with the use of a lidocaine-based gel. The nasal mucosa can be preshrunk with the combination of lidocaine and phenylephrine hydrochloride spray. During progressive dilatation of the nasal pharyngeal airway, sedation can be utilized as previously described.

Almost always, nasal intubation involves a blind attempt. Once the airway has been dilated the tube should be advanced until breath sounds can be clearly heard coming from the tube. On inspiration the tube should be advanced between the vocal chords. Occasionally the patient may buck and cough. This can usually be controlled with a bolus administration of a sedative such as sodium pentothal, which induces sleep without causing hypotension. If the tube is not immediately advanced, the tip may have become entangled on the vallecula. Usually a 90° twist of the tube to the right or the left will redirect it so it can be rapidly passed into place.

Nasal and oral intubation can often be aided with the use of bronchoscopy. The technique may help prevent less head and neck movement during the process. A bronchoscope can be passed through the nasal passages on the mouth and its tip located between the vocal chords. The tracheal tube can then be advanced over the bronchoscope and into the correct position. However, this technique should be used only by those familiar with the bronchoscope and experienced with its use under such conditions. Attempts to do so under emergent situations may result in failure to secure the airway. Likewise, the use of such techniques as a retrograde wire passed through a 14-gauge catheter in the trachea also should not be relied on if the clinician has not previously used the technique under more controlled circumstances.

Awake patients may require some sedation to aid the intubation process. These drugs may alter the patient's sensorium as well as vital signs. Therefore, the patient should be first well oxygenated. This can be best accomplished with a bag and mask. Often an oralpharyngeal or a nasal-pharyngeal airway will effectively help. Oxygenation can usually be confirmed by pulse oximetry. The drugs should be used in small dosages and not cause any other complications by their use. Sodium pentothal in 50-mg increments can produce sedation without causing hypotension, which may be likely in a patient with sympathetic blockade or hypovolemia from hemorrhage. Etomidate has become quite useful as an agent to provide sedation and has minimal vasodilating properties. Dosages are usually 20- to 40-mg increments. Occasionally a benzodiazepine may be helpful. Drugs such as midazolam, 1–2 mg, can be used. Generally there are minimal effects on the cardiovascular system. Narcotics, again in small dosages, such as 1–2 mg of morphine sulphate given intravenously, also provide some degree of sedation. Although sedation is a secondary effect of the drug, the fact that morphine and other narcotic effects can be reversed with naloxone make them desirable under such circumstances.

Muscle relaxants are almost never necessary for intubation under emergency circumstances. However, in some patients it may be difficult to adequately visualize the airway without the aid of a muscle relaxant. We use such agents only after the above-described sedation agents do not help provide satisfactory visualization. In patients with neurological injuries, succinylcholine may cause arrhythmias due to potassium release. This can usually be prevented by low doses of 0.25–0.3 mg/kg. Other choices are nondepolarizers such as rocuronium. However, despite being touted as a short-acting agent, it will last three or four times as long as succinylcholine. This can present potential problems if the airway cannot be easily intubated.

Failure to intubate the patient may require use of the mask and bag again. Consideration should then immediately be given to placement of the cricothyrotomy tube. Problems have developed in the past with cricothyrotomy placement. The technique ordinarily involves cannulation of the trachea with a catheter advanced over a needle. However, the rigid walls of the trachea have on occasion prevented placement of the catheter in the lumen of the trachea although the needle tip itself is already in place. It is advisable to use a small-gauge wire and pass it through the needle once the tracheal lumen has been identified by the air easily aspirated into the barrel of the syringe. Once cricothyrotomy has been safely placed and its position verified, ventilation can commence. Cricothyrotomy kits have their own adaptor that allows attachment to a self-inflating bag. A respiratory rate of 20–30 breaths per minute at a tidal volume that provides chest wall movement will be sufficient. As soon as possible the cricothyrotomy should be converted to a full fledged tracheostomy.

A 14-gauge catheter does not currently seem reasonable as an aid to secure the airway when patients cannot be intubated. The cricothyrotomy kits have all but replaced their utility. Furthermore, the very narrow diameter does not allow ease of ventilation, therefore, CO_2 retention remains a problem.

Since most patients with high spinal cord injuries usually require prolonged intubation that results at some point in tracheostomy, the reader may wonder why tracheostomy should not be performed initially when airway control is a requirement. Tracheostomy is a major operative procedure and should be carried out only under controlled circumstances in the operating room. It should not be considered a method to emergently secure an airway. Attempts to do so in the emergency room can lead to major bleeding, other complications, and possible death of the patient. Furthermore, a tracheostomy incision may interfere with a planned neurosurgical procedure to stabilize the neck early in the post-injury period.

Spinal Shock

Spinal or neurogenic shock may develop immediately or be delayed as long as 60 minutes following a cervical or high thoracic (T6) spinal cord injury. The more cephalad and severe the cord injury, the more profound the neurogenic shock.[14] Manifestations of spinal shock result from insult to the intermediolateral cell column of the cervicothoracic spinal cord, with loss of sympathetic outflow. The imbalance in the autonomic nervous system results from the dissociation of the parasympathetic from the sympathetic nervous system and loss of homeostatic reflexes. Vasomotor instability induces peripheral vasodilation and pooling of the intravascular volume into the capillaries, arterioles, and venules.

The SCI patient in neurogenic shock often has associated bradycardia, increased pulse pressure, and possible conjunctival hemorrhage or priapism. Bradycardia can occasionally progress to heart block with decreased cardiac output or asystole.[15] Bradycardia followed by cardiac arrest occurs in approximately 15% of SCI patients with complete cervical injuries. Spinal shock must be differentiated from other causes of hypotension, such as hemorrhage from associated injuries. Acute alcohol intoxication can also be mistaken for spinal cord shock.

Most define shock as a blood pressure <90 mm Hg or systolic blood pressure decrease of 30% below baseline. In general, these rules apply to the patient in spinal shock. It has been unusual in our experience to see blood pressures <70 mm Hg. Further factors to consider when initiating treatment for reduced blood pressure include loss of consciousness and altered organ profusion manifested by oliguria.

On occasion, if spinal shock has been accompanied by bradycardia, treatment of heart rate alone will increase blood pressure to acceptable levels >90 mm Hg. This can be accomplished with drugs such as atropine in dosages of 1.0 to 2.0 mg. However, most times short-term incremental treatment of heart rate will be insufficient to maintain blood pressure.

Initial therapies to improve blood pressure include volume infusion to meet the demands of the increased vascular capacity secondary to sympathetic stimulation. Typical fluids include a balanced electrolyte solution such as normal saline or Ringer's lactate. Recently, evidence has begun to accumulate with the use of hypertonic saline solutions. This generally involves sodium concentrations between 154 and 450 mEq/L. Hypertonic saline solutions have accomplished the same intravascular expansion with reduced overall volume requirements.[16] Complications of this therapy include hypernatremia if infused at a rapid rate >80 mL/hr or when continuous bolus administration takes place. The use of more than a liter of a hypertonic-containing solution will often result in hyperchloremia and associated metabolic acidosis. This is usually of little consequence but must be differentiated from lactic acidosis due to hypoprofusion. Lactate levels of <2.0 mEq/L confirm that the acidosis is not due to anerobic metabolism and hypoperfusion. Colloid-containing solutions such as 5% albumin can also be used. However, these cost considerably more and should be used sparingly. Again, in comparison to normal saline, the volume requirements will be less. Generally 2 to 4 liters of balanced electrolyte solution will be sufficient to increase intervascular volume and to restore blood pressure.

Vasoactive agents can be used for two reasons: (1) by initiating a degree of vasoconstriction, the overall volume requirements can be decreased; and (2) on occasion, volume expansion alone may not be sufficient to restore blood pressure. Theoretically, alpha adrenergic agents will be adequate to maintain blood pressure. These include phenylephrine hydrochloride and norepinephrine. However, some clinicians fear these agents because of vasoconstriction to vital organs such as the kidney. We have satisfactorily restored blood pressure with dopamine in almost all patients. Although this drug has beta effects within the usual range of 6–15 µg/kg/min, the drug will usually restore blood pressure in the SCI patient. It will also increase heart rate to some degree, which may also aid in further improvement of cardiac output.

Spinal cord injury and hypotension in young patients with previously normal hearts and cardiovascular systems rarely requires more invasive monitoring. However, in older patients or in those with associated injuries, monitoring of either central venous pressure or pulmonary artery pressure may be indicated. In patients suspected of other injuries such as myocardial contusion, the combination of a pulmonary artery pressure catheter and echocardiography may help delineate the extent of any myocardial injury. Patients who have not responded to the previously indicated 2–4 liters of fluid therapy may require increasingly higher dosages of vasoactive drugs to support blood pressure. In such circumstances a pulmonary artery catheter will provide useful information to effectively manage the patient. Long-term therapy in spinal shock may be occasionally required. Drugs such as ephedrine given in 50-mg dosages orally may assist titration of continuous agents such as dopamine or norepinephrine.

Respiratory Complications

The higher the spinal cord lesion, the greater the interference with the abdominal and intercostal muscles as well as the diaphragm, all of which participate in normal respiration.[17] Thoracic injuries and injuries that are higher will interfere with cough mechanisms. Diaphragm innervation occurs at the C4 level. Failure to breathe usually occurs at these higher levels of involvement. Injury at this level will impair normal tidal ventilation. The diaphragm accounts for more than 90% of the tidal volume in C5-level quadriplegic patients. Quadriplegic patients have altered pulmonary function including decreased vital capacity, functional residual capacity, and expiratory reserve volume. Peak inspiratory and expiratory pressures are reduced. Maximum voluntary ventilation decreases to approximately 40% of predicted levels. All of the above alterations in pulmonary function result in complications, including complete respiratory arrest, atelectasis, and pneumonia.

Atelectasis will result from relative hypoventilation.[18] Although patients may be able to maintain tidal volumes, they are ordinarily unable to cough, deep breathe, or sigh. As a result, over time, continued respiration with the usual spontaneous tidal volumes of 4–5 mL/kg will result in micro- and ultimately diffuse atelectasis. Prevention requires close attention to pulmonary care including positioning changes and encouragement of coughing and deep breathing. Other maneuvers include chest physiotherapy and tracheal suctioning to remove secretions when required.

For some patients with hypoventilation, a cuirass-type device has been occasionally prescribed.[19] This is a shell that fits snugly around the thorax. When negative pressure is applied, the chest wall moves out and air enters the lungs. If fitted well, this can act as a negative pressure ventilator and assist during attempts at spontaneous respiration. It can improve overall volumes and to some degree reduce atelectasis.

In almost all patients with spinal cord injury, at some point atelectasis usually becomes severe. Often complete lobar collapse occurs. This almost always requires fiberoptic bronchoscopy through the nasal or oral transtracheal tube. Secretions must be suctioned and removed, particularly if copious in nature. Atelectasis can be a recurrent problem. Positive pressure ventilation with increased levels of PEEP or CPAP can act as a detriment to some degree but is not completely effective. Some restoration of function will return as spinal cord swelling resolves and will result in eventual improvement in these complications.

In our experience few patients with spinal cord injuries escape at least one bout of pneumonia. There are many potential causes for pneumonia. These include retention of secretions, atelectasis, and aspiration of gastric contents at the time of injury or during the course of illness. Spinal cord-injured patients appear to have altered or impaired immune response systems. Failure to continually reposition the patients for removal of secretions may contribute to the development of pneumonia. Some centers feel that a protected suction catheter can be used on multiple occasions in the course of a 24-hour period and is superior to multiple catheters for prevention of pneumonia and tracheal bronchitis. Tracheal toilet is the best preventative measure. There is increasing evidence to suggest that patients who have elevated gastric pH because of H_2 blockers or antacid therapy may have increased colonization in their stomach, particularly with gram-negative bacteria.[20,21] Since up to 80% of intubated patients experience microaspiration, the likelihood of airway colonization increases under such circumstances. Although numerous studies have demonstrated increased airway colonization and even pneumonia, there is no evidence to suggest that the development of such complications increases the already long hospital course or even increases the duration of mechanical ventilation. However, we prefer to maintain the gastric pH as low as possible and use sucralfate to prevent gastritis and potential ulcers.

The most difficult and time-consuming respiratory problem with a quadriplegic patient is an attempt to wean the patient from the mechanical ventilator. In general, patients with cervical cord injuries at the C5 level or higher are particularly difficult and often will never completely wean from mechanical ventilation. We attempt to aid the process in several different ways.

Today almost all patients who require mechanical ventilation and who breathe spontaneously receive some level of pressure support. Pressure support assists the spontaneous ventilation and significantly reduces the work of breathing. However, in addition to its ability to reduce the work of breathing, it also contributes to disuse atrophy of the muscles of respiration. Therefore, during the recovery phase of the patient's illness we will reduce the level of pressure support so that patients begin to incur some work during respiration. This helps to restore tone and hopefully endurance and strength.[22] If the patient continues to improve and we can reduce the required number of mechanical breaths to four or less per minute, we further increase the patient's work and exercise their muscles by short-term discontinuation from mechanical ventilation. This usually involves placement on a T-tube or blow-by at the same FiO_2 for increasing periods of time. This also increases the respiratory work and acts as a form of exercise for the muscles.

As patients are able to tolerate such maneuvers, we will further continue to work their muscles of respiration by using resistance training. This again involves short-term discontinuation of mechanical ventilation. Inserted into the inspiratory limb of the circuit is a 4-cm long tracheal tube at a diameter of 0.5 mm smaller than the current tracheostomy or the tracheal tube. During exercise training a one-way expiratory valve is placed at the airway so that the patient cannot spontaneously breathe from the expiratory side of the system. Patients are then allowed to breathe spontaneously for up to 30 minutes. After each session the patient is rested for 90 minutes with a ventilator rate of 12–14 breaths/min. This is similar to exercise for athletes to increase their overall conditioning level. Once patients are able to tolerate 30 minutes of spontaneous breathing with a resistor in the inspiratory circuit at 1 mm internal diameter smaller than the tracheal or tracheostomy tube in place, they wean almost always successfully from the ventilator. The clinician must remember that with a tracheostomy inner cannula in place, the effective internal diameter is 0.5 mm smaller than the stated size of the tracheostomy tube.

As stated previously, not all patients will completely wean from mechanical ventilation. Those with higher cord injuries or debilitated respiratory muscles due to age and other factors may at the very least require overnight mechanical ventilation. Often they may be able to breathe spontaneously for up to 8–12 hours during the day time. These patients will obviously require a permanent tracheostomy. The ventilators used at home are of a simplified nature usually with a FiO_2 of 0.21 but they do provide for spontaneous breathing coupled with low mechanical rates.[23] However, as a safety factor the rate should not be less than 6 per minute at night, particularly for the out-of-hospital environment.

Patients with injuries at level C4 or above will probably require long-term continued mechanical ventilation. If the phrenic nuclei are in tact, these patients may be candidates for phrenic nerve stimulation. This involves pacers implanted in each phrenic nerve.[24,25] Over 6-8 weeks the phrenic nerves are alternately conditioned so they can tolerate long-term stimulation. With such assistance patients have been weaned from mechanical ventilatory support. In our own practice at least one patient has tolerated up to 2 years of this mode of ventilation. However, its long-term success is somewhat in doubt. In fact, most patients at levels C4 or above generally succumb to a pulmonary infection within 5 years of their injury.

Gastrointestinal Tract

Multiple gastrointestinal tract problems can develop in the quadriplegic.[26] The most usual is that of gastric atony and the ileus following spinal cord injury. Over time GI function returns but it may be delayed as long as 6–8 weeks. Since many of these patients require intubation, they cannot generally tolerate oral feedings. Most patients with an ileus can tolerate duodenal or jejunal feedings. There is some controversy over this aspect and some clinicians may resort to total parenteral nutrition until bowel sounds and gut function return.[27,28] We generally tend to follow this route ourselves over the first 5–7 days. However, parenteral nutrition is clearly associated with a higher incidence of septic complications and not just related to line sepsis. Early utilization of the gut, on the other hand, restores bowel wall function and reduces the likelihood of potential translocation and other problems associated with gut disuse including gut wall atrophy and failure of absorption.

Failure to tolerate enteral feedings will usually be heralded by gastric distention. For that reason we tend to start at low rates of 20–25 mL/hr and increase up to a maximum of 80 mL/hr over 4–7 days. These patients generally cannot be advanced as rapidly as other patients receiving enteral feedings. We see no need to use dilute solutions even when hyperosmotic solutions are used. Diarrhea almost always appears to be related to the particular protein base or glucose fuel in the composition rather than the osmolarity. In fact, the development of diarrhea with more than two stools per day usually requires discontinuation of the current formula until diarrhea has subsided. We then start up with a new formulation in an attempt to find one that the patient can tolerate.

All spinal cord injuries are at risk for duodenal ulcer and perforation. This seems related to the overall severity of their illness plus the use of steroids. Because of the loss of motor tone, the abdominal examination will be notoriously unreliable. However, sudden abdominal distention or other signs of sepsis such as elevated white count, increased immature white cells, or fever should be investigated. In addition to an abdominal and rectal examination, the patient will require upright abdominal and lateral decubitus films to rule out the presence of free air. GI perforation in such patients can have catastrophic consequences.

Patients over the age of 40 years are at risk for the development of acalculous cholecystitis. This complication appears to result from bedrest and the general degree of disability associated with the prolonged course of illness. The older the patient, the more likely that such a problem can occur. Signs and symptoms include right upper quadrant tenderness that will usually be absent in the spinal cord-injured patient. These patients will also have an alteration of liver enzymes, particularly bilirubin and alkaline phosphatase. The diagnosis can be made by ultrasound by localization of a large distended gallbladder with a thickened wall. The diagnosis can also be made by a CT scan. Treatment consists of percutaneous drainage with the tube left in situ.

Pancreatitis may also develop in spinal cord-injured patients.[29]

This is likely to happen if multiple injuries, particularly to the abdomen, have occurred at the time of the accident. Pancreatitis often manifests itself as sepsis with an elevated white blood cell count and a leftward shift as well as hyperpyrexia, tachycardia, and hypotension. Almost all patients with pancreatitis will have an elevated amylase. Diagnosis of pancreatitis can be confirmed by CT analysis.

Urinary Tract

Almost all spinal cord injuries will involve interference of urethral sphincter tone. Such patients will require catheterization of the bladder in order to keep it adequately drained.[30–32] During the initial stages of their illness, continuous catheterization will provide assessment of urinary output and overall fluid balance. However, as the patient's condition stabilizes we remove the indwelling catheter, and catheterization on a regular basis throughout the day is preferred. Although not intuitively so, this methodology results in reduced incidence of urinary tract infections.[33] Patients with spinal cord injury often develop chronic and recurrent urinary tract infections. These can be adequately treated with antibiotics. However, pyelonephritis represents a more severe form of urinary tract infection and may result in permanent damage to the kidneys. Pyelonephritis will present similar to other forms of infection with signs and symptoms as previously described. White cells will be present in the urine and often red cells are also present. Almost all of these infections respond to appropriate antibiotic therapy.

Skin

Many spinal-cord injured patients develop severe and recurring decubiti, particularly in the sacral area. We have seen a number of these lead to significant debilitation with infection and development of systemic signs of sepsis. Often these have required sizable debridement and have resulted in seeding of lung, kidney, and other organs. There are many reports of patient deaths directly attributed to the infected decubitus. These can be best prevented by continued attention to changing the patient's position every 2 hours. Newer hospital beds with pneumatic mattresses that do this on an automatic basis seem to contribute to reduction of such problems. However, patients must still be watched carefully and at the first signs, attempts should be made to reduce pressure in the affected location.

New Therapies and Strategies

Steroids

Over the last 2 to 3 years new pharmacological regimens have appeared that appear to hold promise for improvement of the patient with spinal cord injury. Bracken et al. recently reported on the use of high-dose steroid therapy given within 8 hours of injury.[34] Utilizing methylprednisolone dosages of 30 mg/kg followed by a continuous infusion of 5.4 mg/kg/hr, they demonstrated an overall improvement in sensory functions in incomplete as well as in complete lesions. However, motor function did not improve in those with complete motor injuries.

The effects appear to be directed primarily at the level of the lesion and seem to involve blockade of various mediators released within the first 8 hours such as lipid peroxidases and oxygen radicals. This mode of therapy has now become standardized in most emergency rooms throughout the country. In many areas they are now given in the field.

Although one might suspect an increase in complications in those patients treated with high-dose steroids, the study showed that in fact there was no increase over the placebo group or the third study arm, which received naloxone. The effect of steroids may include perfusion of the microvasculature and reduction of lipid peroxidation. The high doses of the methylprednisolone may improve blood flow to the injured spinal cord and thereby prevent the decline in white matter blood flow, extracellular calcium levels, and evoked potential changes that typically occur following spinal cord injury.[35-37] As the breakdown of the membrane in lipid peroxidation peaks at about 8 hours, treatment begun after that time appears to be ineffective. Today, while all patients with a spinal cord injury receive large-dose methylprednisolone therapy, it should probably be reserved for those with incomplete injury. Patients should expect only possible sensory improvement.

Gangliosides

Another new area of excitement and interest in treatment of spinal cord injury is that of gangliosides. These are complex acidic glycolipids that are components of the cell membrane. Previous animal work has indicated that the gangliosides are able to induce regeneration of neurons.

In a study by Geisler et al., he described 37 patients of an initial 335 who met the criteria for inclusion.[38] All had spinal cord injury with paralysis of a motor group of either the upper or the lower extremity. Ganglioside therapy was started within 72 hours of injury. Compared to placebo there is a statistically significant improvement in motor function. Further analysis identified that the improvement was due to recovery of previously paralyzed rather than already paretic muscle groups.

Animal data would suggest that white matter, when injured, because of its location at the peripheral area of the spinal cord, is not as severely involved as is the more centrally located gray matter. The higher metabolic activity level of gray matter makes it more likely to sustain damaged when traumatized. It requires a higher blood flow and also contains the bodies of the alpha motor neurons. By comparison, gray matter has cell bodies that are at a site distant from that of the injury. The tracts may initially survive the injury and may only be secondarily damaged by ischemia or hypoxia. The authors have contended that only as little as 4–6% of cortical motor neurons need to be regenerated in order to reverse paralysis.[39] It would appear that this may have occurred with the use of gangliosides. Continued work in this area indicates that exciting changes may soon become more readily available for patients with severe paralyzing injuries.

Summary

Acute spinal cord injury results in devastating injuries. Unfortunately, patients cannot expect a full recovery. Almost all patients with cervical spinal cord injury can be expected to develop pulmonary complications requiring mechanical ventilatory support. This usually accounts for their prolonged ICU stay. Likewise, spinal shock usually persists for at least the first week following injury. The need for therapy will be based on the degree of hypotension and organ hypoperfusion. However, careful management while in the ICU can minimize complications that might otherwise prolong the stay or ultimately prove fatal. Furthermore, meticulous care early on can prevent any increase in the level of the lesion. This alone can have profound effects on the patient's ultimate level of recovery.

References

1. Crozier KS, Cheng LL, Graziani V, et al: Spinal cord injury: prognosis for ambulation based on quadriceps recovery. Paraplegia 30:762–767, 1992.

2. Hall ED, Wolf DL: A pharmacological analysis of the pathophysiological mechanisms of posttraumatic spinal cord ischemia. J Neurosurg 64: 951–961, 1986.

3. Castillo RG, Bell J: Cervical spine injury stabilization and management. Postgrad Med Cervical Spine Injury 83:131–138, 1988.

4. Bailes J, Hadley M, Quigley R, et al: Management of athletic injuries of the cervical spine and spinal cord. Neurosurgery 29:491–497, 1991.

5. DeViro M, Rutt R, Black K, et al: Trends in spinal cord injury: Demographics and treatment outcomes between 1973 and 1986. Arch Phys Med Rehabil 73:424–430, 1992.

6. Bailes J, Herman J, Quigley M: Diving injuries of the cervical spine. surg Neurol 34:1558, 1990.

7. Tator CH: Review of experimental spinal cord injury with emphasis on the local and systemic circulatory effects. Neurochirurgie 37:291–302, 1991.

8. DeVivo M, Stover S, Black K: Prognostic factors for 12-year survival after spinal cord injury. Arch Phys Med Rehabil 73:156–162, 1992.

9. Tator C, Fehlings M: Review of the secondary injury theory of acute spinal cord trauma with emphasis on vascular mechanisms. J Neurosurg 75:15–26, 1991.

10. Schmitt J, Midha M, McKenzie N: Medical complications of spinal cord disease. Neurol Clin 9:779–795, 1991.

11. DeVivo M, Kartus P, Rutt R, et al: The influence of age at time of spinal cord injury on rehabilitation outcome. Arch Neurol 47:687–691, 1990.

12. Myllynen P, Kivioja A, Wilppula E: Cervical spinal cord injury: The correlations of initial clinical features and blood gas analyses with early prognosis. Paraplegia 27:19–26, 1989.

13. DeVivo M, Black K, Stover S: Causes of death during the first 12 years after spinal cord injury. Arch Phys Med Rehabil 74:248–254, 1993.

14. Bach-y-Rita P, Illis LS: Spinal shock: possible role of receptor plasticity and non synaptic transmission. Paraplegia 31:82–87, 1993.

15. Gilgoff I, Davidson S, Hohn A: Cardiac pacemaker in high spinal cord injury. Arch Phys Med Rehabil 1991 72:601–603, 1991.

16. Battistella FD, Wisner DN: Combined hemorrhage shock and head injury: Effects of hypertonic (7.5%) resuscitation. J Trauma 31:182–188, 1991.

17. Bergofsky EH: Mechanism for respiratory insufficiency after cervical cord injury. Ann Intern Med 61:435–447, 1964.

18. Fishburn M, Marino R, Ditunno Jr J: Atelectasis and pneumonia in acute spinal cord injury. Arch Phys Med Rehabil 71:197–200, 1990.

19. Bach J, Alba A: Noninvasive options for ventilatory support of the traumatic high level quadriplegic patient. Chest 98:613–619, 1990.

20. Craven DE, Steger DA, Barber TW: Presenting nosocomial pneumonia: State of the art and perspectives for the 1990's. Am J Med 91:44s–53s, 1991.

21. Heyland D, Bradley C, Mandell LA: Effect of acidified enteral feedings on gastric colonization in the critically ill patient. Crit Care Med 20: 1388–1394, 1992.

22. Gross D, Ladd HW, Riley EJ, et al: The effect of training on strength

and endurance of the diaphragm in quadriplegia. Am J Med 68:27–35, 1980.

23. Splaingard M, Frates R, Harrison G, et al: Home positive-pressure ventilation. Chest 84:376–382, 1983.

24. Carter RE, Donovan WH, Halstead L, et al: Comparative study of electrophrenic nerve stimulation and mechanical ventilatory support in traumatic spinal cord injury. Paraplegia 25:86–91, 1987.

25. Bach JR: Alternative methods of ventilatory support for the patient with ventilatory failure due to spinal cord injury. J Am Paraplegia Soc 14: 158–174, 1991.

26. Albert T, Levine M, Balderston R, et al: Gastrointestinal complications in spinal cord injury. Spine 16:S522–S525, 1991.

27. Dietz JM, Bertschy M, Gschaedler R, et al: Reflections on the intensive care of 106 acute cervical spinal cord injury patients in the resuscitation unit of a general traumatology centre. Paraplegia 24:343–349, 1986.

28. Kearns P, Thompson J, Werner P: Nutritional and metabolic response to acute spinal-cord injury. JPEN 16:11–15, 1992.

29. Albuquerque F, Wolf A, Dunham C, et al: Frequency of intra-abdominal injury in cases of blunt trauma to the cervical spinal cord. J Spinal Dis 5:476–480, 1992.

30. Stover S, Lloyd D, Waites K, et al: Neurogenic urinary tract infection. Neurol Clin 9:741–755, 1991.

31. Killorin W, Gray M, Bennett JK, et al: The value of urodynamics and bladder management in predicting upper urinary tract complications in male spinal cord injury patients. Paraplegia 30:437–441, 1992.

32. Beraldo P, Neves E, Alves C, et al: Pyrexia in hospitalized spinal cord injury patients. Paraplegia 31:186–191, 1993.

33. Dewire D, Owens S, Anderson G, et al: A comparison of the urological complications associated with long-term management of quadriplegics with and without chronic indwelling urinary catheters. J Urol 147: 1069–1072, 1992.

34. Bracken M, Shepard M, Collins W, et al: A randomized, controlled trial of methylprednisolone or naloxone in the treatment of acute spinal-cord injury. N Engl J Med 322:1405–1411, 1990.

35. Young W, Flamm E: Effect of high-dose corticosteroid therapy on blood flow, evoked potentials, and extracellular calcium in experimental spinal injury. J Neurosurg 57:667–673, 1982.

36. Anderson D, Means E, Waters T, et al: Microvascular perfusion and metabolism in injured spinal cord after methylprednisolone treatment. J Neurosurg 56:106–113, 1982.

37. Clendenon N, Allen N, Gordon W, et al: Inhibition of Na + -K + -activated ATPase activity following experimental spinal cord trauma. J Neurosurg 49:563–568, 1978.

38. Geisler F, Dorsey F, Coleman W: Recovery of motor function after spinal cord injury A Randomized Placebo-Controlled Trial with GM-1 Ganglioside. N Engl J Med 324:1829–1838, 1991.

39. Nockels R, Young W: Pharmacologic strategies in the treatment of experimental spinal cord injury. J Neurotrauma 9:S211–S217, 1992.

14

Nutritional Care Following Neurotrauma

Andrew B. Leibowitz, MD, John M. Oropello, MD

Introduction

Nutritional support of the critically injured patient can improve nitrogen retention, enhance immune function, potentially modify the response to injury, and may thereby directly effect outcome.

Nutritional support of the patient who has sustained neurological trauma is similar to that given to any critically ill patient. Parenteral nutrition is reserved for patients who cannot meet their caloric requirements from enteral support alone. Neurologically injured patients are more likely to initially require the parenteral route for effective nutritional support due to a high incidence of altered gastrointestinal function. Enteral nutritional support may require special formulations and endoscopic, or even open surgical, placement of feeding tubes into the gastrointestinal tract.

This chapter will review parenteral and enteral nutrition, then

From *Trauma Anesthesia and Critical Care of Neurological Injury,* edited by K. J. Abrams and C. M. Grande. © 1997, Futura Publishing Co., Armonk, NY.

address specific concerns relating to the head and spinal cord-injured patient.

Parenteral Nutrition

Indications

The Association of Parenteral and Enteral Nutrition (ASPEN) has published general guidelines for the institution of parenteral nutrition support.[1] In general, such support should be limited to patients who cannot meet most of their caloric needs enterally and will predictably require intravenous nutritional support for more than 5 days. In metabolically stressed patients, the labile amino acid pool and short-term protein reserves are rapidly catabolized.[2] The absence of nutritional intake for even just a few days may lead toward a state of protein calorie malnutrition. Therefore, the initiation of parenteral or enteral nutritional support should be considered on a daily basis before the patient becomes malnourished.

Formulation

Four major issues need to be considered when writing a parenteral nutrition prescription (Fig. 1): (1) the caloric requirement, (2) the percentage of calories from dextrose versus fat, (3) the protein requirement, and, broadly considered together (4) electrolytes, trace elements, and vitamins.

Caloric Requirement

The number of calories that should be prescribed may be determined in one of three common ways. First, one can estimate that all patients require between 25 and 35 kcal/kg/day. Trauma patients usually fall on the higher end of this spectrum and therefore most often require about 35 kcal/kg/day. Another method is by application of the Harris-Benedict equation, which predicts the resting energy expenditure (REE) based on sex, weight, height, age, and a stress factor (Fig. 2).[3] The third and most accurate method is by application of a metabolic monitor commonly referred to as a "metabolic cart," which directly determines the oxygen consumed and the carbon dioxide produced, and by use of Weir's equation calculates the REE (Fig. 2).[4]

Sample Parenteral Nutrition Formulation

Calculation based on a sample 60-kg patient
Caloric requirement: 30 kcal/kg/day = 1800 kcal

1. CARBOHYDRATE:
60% of caloric requirement from dextrose: 1080 dextrose calories
1 gram dextrose has 3.4 kcal, therefore need 1080 kcal x 3.4 kcal/g
        = 318 g dextrose
D50 contains 500 g dextrose/L, therefore need 318 g x 1 L/50 g
        = 0.618 L of D50

2. FATS:
40% of caloric requirement from fat: 720 lipid calories
1 gram fat has 10.0 kcal, therefore need 720 kcal x 10.0 kcal/g
        = 72 gm fat
Intralipid 20% contains 200 g fat/L, therefore need 72 g x
        1 L/200 g = 0.36 L of intralipid 20%

3. PROTEIN REQUIREMENT: 1.5 g/kg/day = 90 g
Amino acid (aa) solutions usually come as 10%,
containing 100 g amino acid/L and
therefore need 90 g x 1 L/100 g = 0.9 L of aa 10%

4. VOLUME : (618 mL D50) + (360 mL I.L. 20%) +
        (900 mL aa 10%)
Total volume required to deliver this nutrition = 1878 mL/day

Figure 1. Parenteral nutrition prescription. The major issues that need to be considered are: (1) the caloric requirement; (2) the percentage of calories from dextrose vs. fat; (3) the protein requirement; and (4) electrolytes, trace elements, and vitamins.

Resting Energy Expenditure (REE) Calculation

Harris-Benedict Equation[3]

Males: REE = 66.47 + 13.75x(W) + 5.0x(H) - 6.76x(A)

Females: REE = 655.10 + 9.65x(W) + 1.85x(H) - 4.68x(A)

W = weight in kilograms

H = height in centimeters

A = age in years

Weir's Equation[4]

REE = 3.9x(oxygen consumed) + 1.1x(carbon dioxide produced)

Figure 2. The Harris-Benedict equation, which predicts the resting energy expenditure (REE) based on sex, weight, height, age, and a stress factor.

Caloric Distribution

Calories may be given as dextrose, which comes in the form of dextrose 50% (D50), 60% (D60), and 70% (D70), or fat, which comes in the form of lipid emulsions, e.g., intralipid (IL) 10% (IL 10) and 20% (IL 20). In the absence of hypertriglyceridemia, between 30% and 50% of the daily caloric requirements are now routinely administered as fat. Fat is more calorically dense than dextrose. It contains approximately 10 kcal/g, whereas dextrose contains 3.4 kcal/g. Thus, the administration of high caloric parenteral nutrition is possible in a smaller total volume of liquid when a significant percentage of calories come from intravenous fat emulsions.

Protein Requirements

One to 2 g/kg/day of protein in the form of amino acids usually should be administered initially and then adjusted, depending on the results of nitrogen balance studies. Nitrogen balance can be calculated by the following equation:

$$\text{Nitrogen Balance} = (\text{protein intake} \times 6.25) \\ - \text{ urine urea nitrogen excreted} - 2 \text{ g nitrogen}$$

Protein intake is divided by 6.25 to convert it to grams of nitrogen. A 24-hour urine collection is analyzed for urea nitrogen, the major breakdown product of protein. An additional 2 g to 4 g of nitrogen may be lost in the sweat and feces.

Parenterally administered protein is in the form of amino acids that come dissolved in concentrations ranging from approximately 5% to 15%. Intravenous administration of amino acids eliminates the "first-pass" hepatic metabolism of enterally absorbed amino acids and the systemic amino acid profile will much more closely resemble that of the intravenous infusion. The clinical significance of this is unclear but manipulation of this systemic amino acid profile in attempt to influence protein synthesis and patient outcome is the subject of ongoing research.

Protein requirements are influenced in part by energy intake. In general, the ratio of nonprotein calories to grams of nitrogen administered is 150 : 1. For stressed patients with greater protein catabolism and acute phase protein synthesis, a nonprotein calories to grams nitrogen ratio of 100 : 1 is often used in an attempt to achieve positive nitrogen balance.

Failure to achieve positive nitrogen balance is common among critically ill and traumatized patients. Before concluding that it is impossible to achieve positive balance, the patient's nutritional care should be reviewed to determine that there is an adequate caloric and protein prescription, and that there is no hyperglycemia or hypertriglyceridemia.

Electrolytes, Trace Elements, and Vitamins

Sodium and potassium are added to the solution as chloride salts. However, to prevent or treat hyperchloremic metabolic acidosis, bicarbonate, in the form of acetate, may be substituted for the chloride ion. Standard parenteral nutrition formulations usually contain a one-third to one-half normal concentration of sodium chloride (35–70 mEq/L) and approximately 40–70 mEq total of potassium. Phosphorus (10–15 mmol/L), calcium (5 mmol/L), and magnesium (5 mmol/L) are also routinely added to the standard solution. The amounts of electrolytes given vary considerably and are adjusted according to serum levels and the patient's underlying conditions, particularly renal function, and estimated ongoing losses. Trace elements chromium, zinc, manganese, and copper from commercially prepared solutions are added daily as are the recommended daily requirement of multivitamins. Vitamin K is also added one to three times a week.

If necessary, drugs can be added such as the H_2 blockers cimetidine, ranitidine, and famotidine, or insulin, which is commonly added for the treatment of hyperglycemia. Although several other drugs may be soluble in parenteral nutrition, these authors urge against viewing the parenteral nutrition as a drug delivery vehicle. Although drugs may be stable in solution, changes in solution content and temperature may render them less soluble and the bioavailability of drugs administered after prolonged suspension in parenteral nutrition solutions has not been well studied.

Mixing

Dextrose and amino acids are always mixed together prior to administration. Approximately 5 years ago, the addition of fat suspensions to the dextrose and amino acid-containing solutions ("triple mix") became widely accepted and practiced. However, a recent Food and Drug Administration advisory has recommended against this practice because of the remote possibility that precipitation of the mixture may go unrecognized in the presence of the fat suspension. Nonetheless, for adult patients receiving standard prescriptions, this possibility is exceedingly small and triple mix remains widely used, particularly for patients receiving total parenteral nutrition at home.

Monitoring

Monitoring during the first days of parenteral nutrition administration focuses mainly on the physical examination and determination of daily weights to assess volume status. Blood chemistry analyses are performed daily for the evaluation of electrolytes, particularly glucose, potassium, magnesium, and phosphorus (see Table 1 for sample orders).

A 24-hour urine collection for urea nitrogen (baseline nitrogen balance) and a metabolic cart assessment of caloric requirements may be performed within 3 to 4 days after commencing treatment.

Table 1
Sample Orders to Begin TPN Through a Triple-Lumen Central Line

1. Please see the TPN order sheet.
2. TPN to be infused via blue (middle) lumen only and must be infused through a filter.
3. No other solution is to be infused through the blue port.
4. White (proximal) port may be used for blood or other infusion.
5. Brown (distal) port may be used for other infusions, particularly blood.
6. Flush unused lumens with 200 units of heparin in normal saline every 8 hours.
7. Check chemstrips/one-touch glucose checks every 6 hours for 3 days and chart.
8. Weigh patient daily and chart.
9. Strict I's and O's.
10. Chem 6 (Na, K, Cl, HCO_3, BUN, glucose), magnesium, phosphorous, and triglycerides in AM and Chem 6 daily for 3 days.
11. 24-hour urine collection for urine urea nitrogen.
12. Change central line dressing on Monday, Wednesday, and Friday.
13. For any questions please call #45111 or page #1872.

The parenteral formula is adjusted accordingly. At this time, laboratory monitoring may be decreased to every other or every third day. After approximately 10–14 days of parenteral nutrition, an assessment of effectiveness should be made. Generally, this will entail a repeat 24-hour urine to determine nitrogen balance and measurement of serum proteins, particularly albumin. However, albumin may take as long as 3 weeks to rise[5] and some clinicians prefer to measure serum proteins with shorter half-lives, such as thyroxine-binding prealbumin, retinol-binding protein, or serum transferrin. Measurement of these shorter half-life proteins is more expensive and of questionable clinical benefit.

Plasma amino acid profiles have been used to evaluate and follow the response to nutrition but this is an expensive and unproven modality in nutritional assessment. Vitamin levels are also of doubtful value since such deficiencies are rare in the acute care setting and serum vitamin levels may fall during critical illness and not reflect true deficiency at the tissue level.

Complications

Early complications may result from line placement and acute fluid or electrolyte disturbances (Table 2). After 1 to 3 weeks of paren-

Table 2
Complications of Parenteral Nutrition

---

1. Mechanical Complications of Central Line Insertion
Carotid artery puncture
Pneumothorax/hemothorax/chylothorax
Infection/sepsis
Subclavian vein thrombosis
Malignant arrhythmia

2. Fluid and Electrolyte Abnormalities
Hyperglycemia
Hyperlipidemia
Hyperkalemia
Glucosuria
Hyponatremia
Hypernatremia
Hypophosphatemia

3. Other Complications
Liver dysfunction
Elevated liver biochemistries (e.g., AST, ALT, Alk Phos)
Cholestasis
Fatty liver
Acalculous cholecystitis
Ventilator dependence
Overfeeding
High carbohydrate load
Renal dysfunction
Elevation in the blood urea nitrogen level

---

teral nutrition, liver abnormalities may appear.[6,7] This may simply be due to the induction of liver enzymes secondary to refeeding[8] or secondary to cholestasis, fatty liver, or acalculous cholecystitis. Liver biopsies have shown that hepatic steatosis can occur within 2 weeks of parenteral nutrition. The incidence of acalculous cholecystitis (see also Chapter 12) is increasing and is associated with critical illness and parenteral nutrition.[9] It may present as occult sepsis and is very important to consider in any critically ill patient, especially one that has been receiving parenteral nutrition for more than 2 weeks. Of note, neurologically injured patients fed via parenteral nutrition also seem particularly prone toward the development of acalculous cholecystitis.[10]

Miscellaneous Issues

Peripheral Parenteral Nutrition

When most physicians envision parenteral nutrition, they usually think of total parenteral nutrition (TPN), a hypertonic solution administered via a central venous catheter or long-term permanent venous access catheter. Peripheral parenteral nutrition (PPN) is a therapeutic option in particular circumstances. Most commonly it is used either in patients refusing central vascular access or as a bridge until such access can be obtained. PPN can have a maximum osmolarity of 900 mOsms, whereas an average centrally administered formula has an osmolarity of 1,800 mOsms/L.

PPN contains fewer calories per liter and usually consists of dextrose 75 g/L and amino acids 40 g/L. However, the calorically dense fat suspensions are iso-osmolar. Therefore, if a patient is able to tolerate 1,000 kcals from fat per day (500 mL of IL 20%), nearly all of their requirements can be met with the additional administration of 2–3 L of PPN. This requires the ability to tolerate large amounts of intravenous fluid administration and the presence of good peripheral venous access. PPN is usually reserved as a "bridge" between TPN and enteral nutrition, or when central venous access is too difficult to obtain. Aside from avoidance of central venous catheterization, there is no advantage of PPN over TPN.

Access

TPN in the hospitalized patient is best administered through a percutaneously placed central venous catheter. Insertion of permanent access catheters for the administration of TPN when the requirement is on the order of only several weeks will lead to needless expense and operating room time as well as the inevitable removal of catheters during the hospitalization that is fraught with infectious complications that arise from, or contaminate, the catheter.

Percutaneous placement may be via any of the central veins, most commonly the internal jugular and subclavian. Although catheters may be placed at the bedside, they must be inserted under sterile conditions similar to those found in an operating room. They must, then, be maintained in a definitive sterile fashion with a dedicated TPN port. Any fever without a source is presumed to be a line infection until proven otherwise. There must be a low threshold for removal and culture of the central venous catheter. Routine removal and replacement between 7 and 14 days is often recommended but investigation supports the practice of not changing catheters unless there is a suspicion of infection.[11]

Enteral Nutrition

Specialized enteral nutrition should be the mainstay of support for most critically ill patients, including those with neurological injury. Compared with parenteral nutrition, nutrition via the enteral route is associated with less severe and fewer complications, maintains the integrity of the gastrointestinal tract, and is far less costly. For these reasons it should be considered first-line therapy in all patients.

Scientific support for this approach is rapidly accumulating. A recent meta-analysis of eight prospective trials yielding a total of 130 patients for analysis was designed to compare early enteral to parenteral nutrition and found that the enterally patients had significantly lower septic morbidity rates.[12] The exact reasons for such an outcome is unclear but enteral nutrition may help to preserve the normal gut flora, attenuate the injury stress response, and maintain immunocompetence. These effects are in excess of those that are seen with parenteral nutrition administration.

The institution of enteral feeds should not be avoided based on the absence of bowel sounds, which is frequently the case in critically ill patients. Bowel sounds do not necessarily correlate with tolerance to tube feedings, especially if the small bowel is intubated. The rational is that a fully functioning small bowel does not make noises. Bowel sounds emanate primarily from the stomach and large intestine. Many patients with gastric tubes can be enterally fed in the absence of bowel sounds; at least it is worth a trial.

Recent advances in enteral formulations and delivery systems have changed what was previously a relatively small and easy to understand subject into one worthy of textbook-sized treatises. The goal of this short review will be to give the inexperienced practitioner an overview of the methods for intubating the gastrointestinal tract and a means for categorizing and evaluating the growing list of available enteral feeding products.

Access

The gastrointestinal tract may be intubated through one of five ways: (1) nasogastrically or orogastrically, usually with small-bore, soft-tipped feeding tubes, (2) transpyloric fluoroscopically or endoscopically assisted placement of small-bore feeding tubes, (3) via percutaneous endoscopic gastrostomy and/or jejunostomy tubes, (4) open surgical gastrostomy and jejunostomy tubes, (5) laparoscopic placement of gastrostomy and jejunostomy tubes. Tubes inserted through the naso/oropharynx are the most appropriate for short-term access, whereas percutaneous, open surgical, or laparoscopic insertion should be reserved for tubes that will be required for long-term use.

Major complications associated with tubes placed into the naso/oropharynx include misplacement into the tracheobronchial tree or even pleural space, sinusitis, nasal septal erosion, otitis media, esophagitis, and an increased risk of aspiration. Percutaneously inserted tubes have a low complication rate in experienced hands and may be performed at the bedside.[10] In our institution, this is the preferred means for long-term enteral access.

Surgically inserted tubes usually require the administration of general anesthesia and should be reserved for patients with intra-abdominal pathology that contraindicates percutaneous placement.

In patients with large gastric residuals, or in those patients at an extraordinary risk for aspiration, consideration should be given to the placement of a jejunostomy tube along with a gastric tube inserted for drainage of the stomach.[14]

Formulas

Despite the aggressive marketing of several hundred feeding formulas, the similarities between these distinct preparations outnumber their differences. A categorization of their essential, similar properties is what is most important. As with parenteral nutrition, the patient's caloric and protein needs should be thoroughly assessed. Enteral products should then be considered in the following fashion:

Calories

Products contain 1–2 calories per mL. In the absence of high gastric residuals or concern over the fluid intake, calories per mL should rarely be an overriding factor in product selection.

Protein Content

Protein content and quality vary substantially. Formulations range from as low as 35 g/L to as high as 80 g/L of protein. Highly stressed catabolic patients may require as much as 2 g/kg/day of protein and therefore will have their needs more easily met by a formula with a higher protein content. In addition, the kind of protein may vary from completely elemental containing only absorbable amino acids to completely intact protein (polymeric formula). More elemental sources of protein may be of benefit to patients with diarrhea and problems with absorption. In addition, some formulas are now being promoted as having higher concentrations of glutamine, an amino acid that is particularly important for immune function and gastrointestinal mucosal maintenance.[15] It is unclear at present if this has any significant clinical impact.

Osmolarity

Osmolarity ranges from 270 mOsm to as high as 600 mOsm. Hyperosmolar solutions are more likely to cause diarrhea. Solutions with higher osmolarities may be diluted with water when starting enteral feeding to lower the effective osmolarity and thus lessen the likelihood that diarrhea will occur. Alternatively, smaller amounts, on the order of 20–30 mL/hr, may be administered and this infusion increased very slowly.

Caloric Distribution

Caloric distribution between glucose and fat will rarely be a clinically important issue. Formulas containing medium chain triglycerides may be advantageous in that this kind of fat is more easily absorbed. Diabetics with glucose levels that are hard to control should undergo a trial of a formula with a higher fat content and longer glucose polymers. Patients with poor respiratory reserve and carbon dioxide retention may benefit from solutions containing more fat and less sugar, which will result in less carbon dioxide production. In rare instances, the accumulation of excessive carbon dioxide secondary to carbohydrate metabolism may result in respiratory failure. This potential problem is more likely with parenteral nutrition.

Fiber Content

Some products contain fiber, which in some patients may reduce the amount of diarrhea.

Complications

The two major complications associated with enteral feeding are diarrhea[16] and aspiration.[17]

Diarrhea is almost always multifactorial and includes low serum albumin with its associated gastrointestinal tract edema, concomitant antibiotic use, and intolerance of the feeding formula, particularly if the osmolarity is high or the rate of infusion too fast. Infectious causes, particularly pseudomembranous colitis secondary to *Clostridium difficile* toxin, must be excluded. Once an infectious etiology is ruled out, the rate and osmolarity of the feeds should be reduced to as little as 30 mL/hr of an isosmolar or even slightly hypo-osmolar formula. If that does not work, then Kaopectate^R and/or deodorized tincture of opium should be administered via the feeding tube. If diarrhea persists, despite institution of these maneuvers for several days, feeding should be withheld and parenteral nutrition instituted. Diarrhea that persists despite discontinuing oral feeding is secretory in nature and may require further diagnostic investigation.

Aspiration can occur around endotracheal and tracheal tube cuffs. For this reason patients should be fed sitting or with the head of the bed in a 45° head-up position. Residuals are commonly checked every 4 hours and enteral feeding discontinued if the residual is greater than 100 mL. Administration of a promotile agent such as metoclopramide or cisapride might be useful in some circumstances.

Specialized enteral formulas have been devised for use in patients with hepatic, renal, and respiratory failure, and to improve immune function, but there is no evidence that conclusively demonstrates any clinically significant benefits over the standard, less expensive formulas.

Head Trauma

Patients sustaining head trauma are typically hypermetabolic and hypercatabolic. Hypermetabolism refers to the need for more than a usual amount of calories, often 50% to 100% more than baseline. Hypercatabolism refers to the tendency to break down endogenous protein at a greater than normal rate. For example, the average mildly stressed patient may excrete 5 g to 10 g of nitrogen per day in their urine but a hypercatabolic patient often exceeds 20 g of nitrogen excretion in a 24-hour period of time. This response is multifactorial and is probably mediated by sympathetic and autonomic nervous system activation, catecholamine release, stress hormones (e.g., glucagon, cortisol), and cytokine release. As such, it is part of the systemic inflammatory response that occurs after any severe bodily insult. If complications such as systemic hemorrhage, infection, sepsis, or pancreatitis intervene, they will add to the inflammation and hypermetabolism.

After head trauma, resting energy expenditure (REE) may be increased by 50% to 100% above normal and nitrogen excretion often exceeds 20 g/day, which is more than twice normal.[18,19] A previous investigation to determine which factors (determined at the bedside) can be used to estimate the energy expenditure has shown a direct relationship to a combination of the Glasgow Coma Score (GCS), heart rate, and number of days since injury (DSI).[15] That means that the lower the GCS, the higher the heart rate, and the earlier in the patient's course, the higher the REE. However, due to variability in energy expenditure, direct measurement is recommended. Steroid therapy may increase the amount of protein wasting.[20,21]

The primary question is whether early aggressive nutritional support can change outcome and whether this support is best provided by intravenous or enteral routes. There are only a few studies comparing enteral to parenteral nutrition in this group of patients. We have chosen to review the results of the three most often quoted studies that, combined, enrolled only 134 patients. In an initial study of 38 randomized patients, Rapp et al.[22] found a marked effect on the 18-day mortality rate with the prescription of parenteral nutrition. In the 20 patients receiving parenteral nutrition none died, and in the 18 patients receiving enteral nutrition eight died. The authors felt that the parenterally fed group had better nitrogen retention, increased serum albumin, and improved lymphocyte counts. Interestingly, there was no difference in the two groups on day 13, and the parenterally fed group still remained in marked negative nitrogen balance. The choice of an 18-day morbidity is odd and the drastic differences seem suspect. In a follow-up study[23] by the same group reported 4 years later, 51 patients were studied. It was noted that the parenterally fed group received more calories and protein earlier than the enterally fed group. The outcome at 3 months was improved in the parenterally fed group but there was no statistically significant difference at 6 months and 1 year. It was concluded that early outcome was improved with better nutritional support and the increased delivery of enteral nutrition was provided by the improved availability of small-bore feeding tubes and electronic pumps. In a study performed by Hadley et al.,[24] 45 patients were similarly randomized to recieve parenteral or enteral nutrition. No significant differences in outcome, infection, serum albumin, or nitrogen balance were found. Parenterally fed patients received more nitrogen and calories. Again it was noted that patients remained in net negative nitrogen balance and that provision of parenteral nutrition may decrease the degree of nitrogen balance but actually increases the amount of urine urea nitrogen. These authors concluded that parenteral nutrition should be reserved for patients that cannot be fed enterally.

The ability to meet these nutritional requirements via the enteral route has been addressed by Clifton et al.[25] Twenty patients were studied and given an average of 3,500 kcal/day and 188–231 g of protein per day enterally. It was concluded that high caloric and protein feeding may be delivered for a prolonged period of time with few complications.

Given the sparsity of randomized controlled trials, the recent evidence for gut translocation,[26] and the high risk of infection in ventilated patients treated with steroids who would require central venous administration of parenteral nutrition, we recommend early aggressive enteral feedings with a formula that can meet both the caloric and the protein needs of these patients. This will generally be a formula containing at least 1.5 kcal per mL and 60–80 g protein/L administered at a minimum rate of 90 mL/hr for 24 hours or 125 mL/hr for 18 hours. If after 3 or 4 days the patient cannot meet at least 50% of his predicted requirement, we recommend the institution of parenteral nutrition in addition to whatever enteral nutrition the patient can tolerate.

There are several other considerations regarding parenteral nutrition in the head-injured patient.

The standard parenteral nutrition formula is a hyponatremic fluid (0.3 to 0.5 normal saline). If this is not recognized it can contribute to hyponatremia, which in turn may exacerbate cerebral edema. Head-injured patients are prone to hyponatremia either through the syndrome of inappropriate antidiuretic hormone release (SIADH)[27] or a cerebral salt-wasting syndrome. In a patient with a falling serum sodium, the parenteral nutrition formula should be checked and additional sodium added to create a normal saline (0.9%) content.

There is some experimental evidence that hyperglycemia may worsen neurological outcome after brain injury.[28] Clinical studies are needed to confirm these findings. For the time being, it seems prudent to treat serum glucose levels above 200 mg/dL and to maintain serum glucose levels below 250 mg/dL.

Head-injured patients have an increased loss of zinc in the

urine.[29] Although, it is not known yet known if zinc supplementation is of significant benefit, one trial, reported only in abstract form, demonstrated improved levels of the short half-life serum proteins and a more rapid improvement of the GCS score with zinc supplementation.[30]

As stated earlier, it is usually not possible to achieve nitrogen balance in patients following a major injury despite the institution of aggressive, early enteral or parenteral nutrition. In an effort to overcome the brisk nitrogen loss, several anabolic agents are under investigation. They include growth hormone,[31] insulin-like growth factor,[32] and arginine,[33] or glutamine-enriched[34] parenteral nutrition. Although these agents have been shown to promote nitrogen retention, they do not always lead to positive nitrogen balance and it is not known whether they improve outcome in any critically ill patients, including those with head injury. Their use should be considered experimental at this time.

With respect to head-injured patients, it should be noted that one of the proposed mechanisms of secondary neurological injury is via the release of excitatory neurotoxic amino acids, such as glutamine, from damaged neurons.[35] It is theoretically possible that glutamine-enriched feeding, whether enteral or parenteral, may worsen neurological injury. However, this theory has not been subject to human investigation.

Spinal Cord Trauma

The mainstay of spinal cord trauma treatment rests on early stabilization and resuscitation followed by mobilization. The nutritional problems often seen are paralytic ileus, gastrointestinal ulcer formation and resultant bleeding, impaction, and pancreatitis. Other problems that also impact on the nutritional state of the spinal cord-injured patient include denervation atrophy and paralysis, skin and wound breakdown, infection, respiratory failure, atelectasis, pneumonia, neurogenic bladder, and depression. As with the head-injured patient, early nutritional intervention is important to prevent malnutrition.[36,37]

There are some differences in the metabolic response after acute spinal cord injury compared to head injury. The metabolic milieu is marked by severe catabolism that results in a net negative nitrogen balance regardless of nutritional support efforts and is out of proportion to the energy expenditure.[38,39] In a study by Rodriguez et al.,[38]

10 patients with acute spinal cord injury and 20 controls with non-spinal cord injury were matched for time, sex, age, and injury severity score. No spinal cord injury patients established positive nitrogen balance during a 7-week period following the injury despite an average delivery of 2.4 g of protein/kg ideal body weight and 120% of the predicted (via the Harris-Benedict equation) energy expenditure. Metabolic cart determinations in five spinal cord-injured patients showed that caloric intake was 110% greater than the average measured energy expenditures. In contrast, 17 of 20 non-spinal cord-injured patients achieved positive nitrogen balance within 3 weeks of admission. The authors point out that aggressive attempts to achieve positive nitrogen balance will not be effective and may result in overfeeding. A study by Kolpek et al.[39] compared the measured (metabolic cart) versus predicted (Harris-Benedict equation) energy expenditure and urinary nitrogen losses of patients with head trauma (n = 7) to those with spinal cord injury (n = 7). The patients were followed for 18 days after injury. Head trauma patients exhibited a markedly elevated mean measured/predicted energy expenditure ratio (1.5) and mean 24-hour urinary urea nitrogen excretion values (0.18 $\times$ 0.01 g/kg/day). In comparison, spinal cord-injured patients had an equivalent mean 24-hour urinary urea nitrogen loss (0.18 $\times$ 0.04 g/kg/day) but a much lower measured/predicted energy expenditure ratio (0.56). The authors concluded that the elevation in nitrogen loss observed in spinal cord injury was not due to a hypermetabolic state.

Given this severe nitrogen loss, hypoalbuminemia is commonly seen during the early phase of spinal cord injury.[40,41] These authors urge that early aggressive nutritional support is the mainstay in the treatment of this hypoalbuminemia. Several clinical studies have failed to demonstrate the effectiveness of routine albumin supplementation,[42–44] which is particularly expensive.

Hypercalcemia complicates the care of approximately 5% of spinal cord-injured patients.[37,45,46] Mobilization is the most effective means of control. Obviously, while the patient is hypercalcemic, the calcium should be removed from the parenteral nutrition solution. Other suggested means of lowering the serum calcium include the administration of steroids, furosemide, calcitonin, mithramycin, and biphosphanates.[46–48] The long-term effect of calcium homeostasis abnormalities is the development of osteoporosis below the level of injury in the vast majority of patients.[49] There is no widely accepted effective management strategy.

Patients with high spinal cord injuries requiring prolonged mechanical ventilation should receive a gastrostomy or jejunostomy tube as early as possible, preferably at the time of tracheostomy. This will allow easy access to the gastrointestinal tract and avoid the problem of nasogastric tube misplacement and dislodgment as well as the possibility of otitis media and sinusitis.[50]

Future Directions

The general trend in nutritional support has been to develop disease-specific nutritional strategies. This idea is still in its infancy but is best exemplified by a recent study of bone marrow transplant patients who underwent a randomized, double blind, study investigating the utility of glutamine-enriched TPN administration versus standard TPN.[51] The incidence of infection and length of hospital stay was markedly decreased in the group receiving the TPN enriched with glutamine. Similar studies of an arginine and fish oil-enriched enteral feeding product used in the support of perioperative critically ill patients have similarly demonstrated a lower infection rate and shorter length of intensive care unit stay.[52] However, these studies suffer from a variety of methodological flaws and further study will be necessary before these findings are widely accepted and administration of these products becomes routine.

These kinds of specially designed formulations and their rigorous study are the beginning of a new era in the field of nutritional support. The study of these formulas in neurologically traumatized patients has barely begun.

References

1. American Society of Parenteral and Enteral Nutrition Board of Directors: Guidelines for the use of total parenteral nutrition in the hospitalized patient. JPEN 10:441–445, 1986.
2. Elwyn DH: Protein metabolism and requirements in the critically ill patient. Crit Care Clin 3:57–69, 1987.
3. Harris JA, Benedict FG: A biometric study of basal metabolism in man. Carnegie Institute of Washington Publication 279:1–266, 1919.
4. De Weir JB: New methods for calculating metabolic rate with special reference to protein metabolism. J Physiol 109:1–9, 1949.
5. Dowelko JP, Nompleggi DJ: Role of albumin in human physiology and pathophysiology. JPEN 15:207–211, 1991.
6. Touloukian RJ, Downing SE: Cholestasis associated with long-term parenteral hyperalimentation. Arch Surg 106:58–62, 1973.

7. Freund HR: Liver function derangements during total parenteral nutrition. Intensive Crit Care Digest 12:36–39, 1993.
8. MacFadyen BV, Dudrick SJ, Bacquero G, et al: Clinical and biochemical changes in liver function during intravenous hyperalimentation. JPEN 3:438–443, 1979.
9. Messing B, Bories C, Kunstlinger F, et al: Does total parenteral nutrition induce gallbladder sludge formation and lithiasis? Gastroenterology 84:1012–1019, 1983.
10. Murray FE, Stinchcombe SJ, Hawkey CJ: Development of biliary sludge in patients on intensive care unit: Results of a prospective ultrasonographic study. Gut 33:1123–1125, 1992.
11. Cobb DK, High KP, Sawyer RG: A controlled trial of scheduled replacement of central venous and pulmonary artery catheters. N Engl J Med 327:1062–1068, 1992.
12. Moore FA, Feliciano DV, Andrassy RJ, et al: Early enteral feeding, compared with parenteral, reduces postoperative septic complications: The results of a meta-analysis. Ann Surg 216:172–183, 1992.
13. Wolfsen HC, Kozarek RA, Ball TJ, et al: Long-term survival in patients undergoing percutaneous endoscopic gastrostomy and jejunostomy. Am J Gastroenterol 85:1120–1122, 1990.
14. Rombeau JL, Twomey PL, McClean GK, et al: Experience with a new gastrostomy-jejunal feeding tube. Surgery 93:574–578, 1983.
15. Souba W, Austgen T: Interorgan glutamine flow following surgery and infection. JPEN 14:90–93, 1990.
16. Keohane PP, Attrill H, Love M, et al: Relation between osmolality of diet and gastrointestinal side effects in enteral nutrition. Br Med J 288: 678–680, 1984.
17. Olivares L, Segovia A, Revuelta R: Tube feeding and lethal aspiration in neurological patients: A review of 720 autopsy cases. Stroke 5:654–657, 1974.
18. Clifton GL, Robertson CS, Choi SC: Assessment of nutritional requirements of head injured patients. J Neurosurg 64:895–901, 1986.
19. Clifton GL, Robertson CS, Grossman RG, et al: The metabolic response to severe head injury. J Neurosurg 60:687–696, 1984.
20. Robertson CS, Clifton GL, Goodman JS: Steroid administration and nitrogen excretion in the head injured patient. J Neurosurg 63:714–718, 1985.
21. Schiller W, Long C, Blakemore W: Creatinine and nitrogen excretion in seriously ill and injured patients. Surg Gynecol Obstet 149:561–566, 1979.
22. Rapp R, Young B, Twyman D, et al: The favorable effect of early parenteral feeding in survival in head injured patients. J Neurosurg 58: 906–912, 1983.
23. Young B, Ott L, Twyman D, et al: The effect of nutritional support on outcome from severe head injury. J Neurosurg 67:668–676, 1987.
24. Hadley MN, Grahm TW, Harrington T, et al: Nutritional support and neurotrauma: A critical review of early nutrition in forty-five acute head injury patients. Neurosurgery 19:367–373, 1986.

25. Clifton GL, Robertson CS, Contant CF: Enteral hyperalimentation in head injury. J Neurosurg 62:186–193, 1985.
26. Deitch EA: The role of intestinal barrier failure and bacterial translocation in the development of systemic infection and organ failure. Arch Surg 125:403–404, 1990.
27. Lester MC, Nelson PB: Neurological aspects of vasopression release and the syndrome of inappropriate secretion of antidiuretic hormone. Neurosurgery 8:735–740, 1981.
28. Voll CL, Auer RN: The effect of post-ischemic blood glucose levels on ischemic brain damage in the rat. Ann Neurol 24:638–646, 1988.
29. McClain CJ, Twyman D, Ott L, et al: Serum and urine zinc response in head injured patients. J Neurosurg 64:224–230, 1986.
30. Ranseen JD, Schmitt FA, Holt K, et al: Zinc supplementation and early outcome following severe brain injury. J Clin Exp Neuropsychol 12:34A, 1990.
31. Ziegler TR: Use of growth hormone combined with nutritional support in a critical care unit. JPEN 14:574–581, 1990.
32. Guler HP, Zapf J, Foresch ER: Short-term metabolic effects of recombinant human insulin-like growth factor 1 in healthy adults. N Engl J Med 317:137–140, 1987.
33. Daly JM, Reynolds J, Thom A, et al: Immune and metabolic effects of arginine in the surgical patient. Ann Surg 208:512–521, 1988.
34. Stehle P, Zander J, Mertes N, et al: Effect of parenteral glutamine peptide supplements on muscle glutamine loss and nitrogen balance after major surgery. Lancet 1:231–233, 1989.
35. Faden AL, Demediuk P, Panter SS, et al: The role of excitatory amino acids and NMDA receptors in traumatic brain injury. Science 244:798–801, 1989.
36. Kaufman HH, Rowlands BJ, Stein DK, et al: General metabolism in patients with acute paraplegia and quadriplegia. Neurosurgery 16:309–313, 1985.
37. Kearns PJ, Thompson JD, Werner PC, et al: Nutritional and metabolic response to acute spinal-cord injury. JPEN 16:11–15, 1992.
38. Rodriguez DJ, Clevenger FW, Osler TM, et al: Obligatory negative nitrogen balance following spinal cord injury. JPEN 15:319–322, 1991.
39. Kolpek JH, Ott LG, Record KE, et al: Comparison of urinary urea nitrogen excretion and measured energy expenditure in spinal cord injury and nonsteroid-treated severe head trauma patients. JPEN 13:277–280, 1989.
40. Arieff AJ, Pyzik JW, Tigay EL, et al: Some metabolic studies in quadriplegia following SCI. Ill Med J 117:219–223, 1960.
41. Robinson R: Serum protein changes following spinal cord injuries. Proc R Soc Med 47:1109–1113, 1954.
42. Neumann M, Demling RH: Colloid vs. crystalloid: A current perspective. Intensive Care World 9:3–6, 1990.
43. Velanovic V: Crystalloid vs. colloid fluid resuscitation: A meta analysis of mortality. Surgery 105:65–71, 1989.
44. Blackburn GL, Driscoll DF: Time to abandon routine albumin supplementation. Crit Care Med 20:157–158, 1992.

45. Maynard FM, Imai K: Immobilization hypercalcemia in spinal cord injury. Arch Phys Med Rehabil 58:16–24, 1977.
46. Claus-Walker J, Halstead LS, Rodriguez GP, et al: Spinal cord injury hypercalcemia: Therapeutic profile. Arch Phys Med Rehabil 63: 108–115, 1982.
47. Schneider AB, Sherwood LM: Calcium homeostasis and pathogenesis and management of hypercalcemic disorders. Metabolism 23:975–1007, 1974.
48. McCagg CM: Postoperative management and acute rehabilitation of patients with spinal cord injuries. Orthop Clin North Am 17:171–182, 1986.
49. Chantraine A: Actual concept of osteoporosis in paraplegia. Paraplegia 116:51–58, 1978.
50. Green B, Eismont F: Acute spinal cord injury: A systems approach. Cent Nerv Syst Trauma 1:173–195, 1984.
51. Ziegler TR, Young LS, Benfell K, et al: Clinical and metabolic efficacy of glutamine-supplemented parenteral nutrition after bone marrow transplantation: A randomized, double blind, controlled study. Ann Int Med 116:821–828, 1992.
52. Daly JM, Lieberman MD, Goldfine J, et al: Enteral nutrition with supplemental arginine, RNA, and omega-3 fatty acids in patients after operation: immunologic, metabolic, and clinical outcome. Surgery 112: 56–67, 1992.

$$\boxed{15}$$

Therapeutic Advances in Neurotrauma

Gilles A. Orliaguet, MD, Pierre A. Carli, MD

Introduction

Head injury creates not only primary but also secondary insults. The primary insults to the brain usually consist of a diffuse axonal lesion and more localized contusion, and/or hematomas. Apart from some hematomas (e.g., epidural hematoma) that are amenable to surgical intervention, other primary lesions are beyond such treatment. Secondary insults, which are essentially ischemic in nature, are due mainly to hypoxia, hypercarbia, decreased cerebral perfusion pressure (CPP), systemic hypotension, intracranial hypertension, post-traumatic cerebral arterial vasospasm, and transtentorial and cerebellar herniation.

Secondary insults can occur at the scene of the accident and are a major cause of morbidity and mortality.[1-3] Treatment is aimed at preventing and protecting against secondary damage, as well as

From *Trauma Anesthesia and Critical Care of Neurological Injury,* edited by K. J. Abrams and C. M. Grande. © 1997, Futura Publishing Co., Armonk, NY.

providing optimal conditions for tissue repair processes. In fact, it has been suggested that early (prehospital) and aggressive treatment, aimed at preventing and/or treating hypoxia, hypercarbia, and hypotension could decrease mortality and improve neurological outcome after severe head injury.[4] The goals of management to prevent secondary brain damage include: institution of mechanical ventilation, control of any increase in intracranial pressure (ICP), and/or decrease in mean arterial blood pressure (MAP) to maintain sufficient CPP and ensure sufficient O_2 supply to cerebral tissues. The role of the trauma anesthesiologist is of prime importance in this area. After evaluation of the patient and stabilization of life-threatening problems, the trauma anesthesiologist may initiate specific treatment. Recently, new therapeutic interventions have been proposed.

Management of ICP and CPP

In severe head trauma, evidence suggests that CPP should be maintained above 70–80 mm Hg.[5,6] ICP should be reduced and MAP increased to maintain CPP above this threshold, since cerebral autoregulation is impaired following head injury. In order to increase MAP, one can administer fluids (discussed below) or vasopressors. Dopamine with or without phenylephrine is widely used to maintain CPP above 70–80 mm Hg.[5,7]

Alternatively, ICP can be reduced to maintain CPP. High-dose barbiturates have been used to reduce uncontrollable ICP elevation, but the beneficial effects of this treatment have not been documented, and it is possible that only a subset of patients may benefit from this form of therapy.[7] In fact, two controlled studies were not supportive. Ward et al.[8] showed no benefit, while Eisenberg et al.[9] revealed a favorable tendency that did not reach statistical significance. In fact, as has been suggested by Nordström et al.[10] and by Cold et al.[11] there may be a barbiturate reactivity; this so-called "barbiturate reactivity" is observed only in cases with preserved CO_2 reactivity (i.e., in patients with less severe injury). Moreover, a recent experimental study suggested that barbiturate administration is no more effective in reducing ICP than hyperventilation alone, and that the barbiturates reduced cerebral blood flow significantly without providing further relief from increased ICP.[12] Thus, the authors concluded that barbiturate therapy should be utilized cautiously in the treatment of intracranial hypertension that is unresponsive to hyperventilation.

The osmotic diuretic, mannitol, is often administered as treatment for intracranial hypertension, especially in rapidly deteriorating patients, when there is acute loss of pupillary light response.[13] Mannitol has three effects in brain injury: (1) dehydration of the white matter of the normal brain,[14] (2) increased CBF and cardiac output,[15,16] probably by decreasing blood viscosity,[17] and (3) constriction of cerebral vessels.[18] However, the effect of mannitol on outcome has yet to be documented, and a study of mannitol regimens used for several days failed to demonstrated improved prognosis.[19] This study raised the question, as with barbiturate therapy, of whether a small, yet not specifically defined, subset of patients may benefit from mannitol therapy.

Although it is customary to maintain patients with elevated ICP in a head-up position to promote cerebral venous drainage, this may lead to a net reduction in CPP. Recently, Feldman et al.[20] found that although MAP decreased when the head was elevated, ICP also decreased and there was no significant change in CPP or CBF (Fig. 1). As long as MAP exceeds 80 mm Hg, a 30° elevation of the patient's head to treat increased ICP is appropriate.

Hyperventilation, resulting in decreases in $PaCO_2$, CBF, and consequently cerebral blood volume, has been a standard treatment of patients with intracranial hypertension.[21] However, hyperventila-

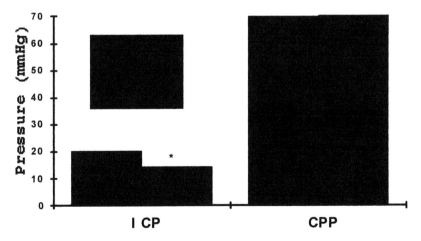

Figure 1. Effect of head elevation on intracranial pressure and cerebral perfusion pressure (CPP) in head trauma patients. *$P = 0.0001$ versus 0° head elevation. Used with permission from Feldman et al.[20]

tion may lead to severe reduction in CBF and development of ischemia.[22] Prophylactic hyperventilation has been reported to retard recovery, and could even be deleterious in head-injured patients with a motor score part of the Glasgow Coma Scale (GCS) of 4 to 5.[23] These studies suggest that, although hyperventilation is a useful tool to control cerebral blood volume and ICP, it should be used judiciously and only as a temporizing measure. Its use is best guided by monitoring of jugular venous bulb oxygen concentration.[24] Without cerebral hemodynamic monitoring, the patient should be moderately ventilated to obtain a $PaCO_2$ of 30–35 mm Hg.

Recent Advances in Fluid Management

The goal of fluid administration in head trauma patients is to maintain cerebral homeostasis, remembering that CBF autoregulation and the blood-brain barrier (BBB) may be altered, resulting in a risk of intracranial hypertension and cerebral edema. Head trauma is often accompanied by hypotension and hypovolemia due to other lesions, and vigorous fluid therapy is mandatory to rapidly restore intravascular volume and to avoid secondary ischemic lesions. In fact, a retrospective analysis of 1,709 patients with blunt head trauma showed that hypovolemic shock increased the mortality rate from 12.8% to 62.1%.[25]

The choice of fluid used for the initial resuscitation of severe head trauma should take into consideration the specific characteristics of the BBB. The BBB is created by the special permeability characteristics of brain capillaries, as well as the choroid plexus. Water-soluble polar compounds are mostly excluded, whereas lipid-soluble compounds easily and rapidly cross the BBB. The endothelial cells of the brain have a unique membranous ultrastructure with "tight junctions," a feature that limits the transfer of macromolecules between adjacent endothelial cells.

They also have highly stereospecific transport systems for sugars, amino acids, and ions. The transcapillary osmolality gradient is a greater driving force for water displacement than the colloid oncotic pressure gradient. Thus, when the BBB is intact, a small reduction in plasma osmolality may result in a greater increase in cerebral water content than a more important reduction in intravascular oncotic pressure.

Several investigators have recently studied the effects of resuscitation with crystalloid or colloid solutions in animal models of head

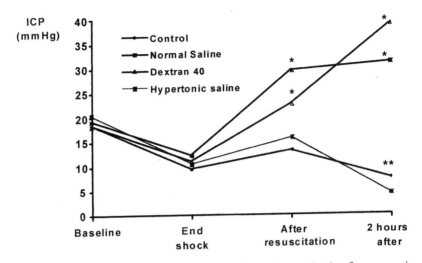

Figure 2. Effect on intracranial pressure (ICP) of resuscitation from experimental hemorrhagic shock with simulated head injury (inflation of an epidural balloon), with normal saline solution, 3% saline solution (hypertonic saline) and dextran-40, *$P < 0.05$ versus control, **$P < 0.05$ versus normal saline and dextran-40. Used with permission from Gunnar et al.[29]

trauma and/or cerebral ischemia associated with hemorrhage.[26–29] Massive administration of both colloids (low molecular dextran, 6% hetastarch, 5% albumin) and crystalloids (saline, Ringer's lactate) increased ICP and cerebral water content, but in the majority of these studies, the increase in ICP was more pronounced and appeared earlier with crystalloids[26–28] (Fig. 2).

The debate over the use of crystalloids versus colloids in patients with cerebral injury and hemorrhagic shock is far from over. In fact, although several studies have reported that a large reduction in cerebral oncotic pressure due to crystalloid infusion contributes to the formation of cerebral edema, most of these studies used Ringer's lactate, which is a hypotonic solution (273 mOsm/L). In contrast, in the studies where isotonic crystalloid solutions were compared with colloids, no significant difference in cerebral water content was found.[29,30] Moreover, recently it has been demonstrated that reduction in cerebral oncotic pressure (with careful maintenance of osmolality) did not increase ICP, and that hypo-osmolality seems more deleterious than hypo-oncosity[27,31] (Fig. 3).

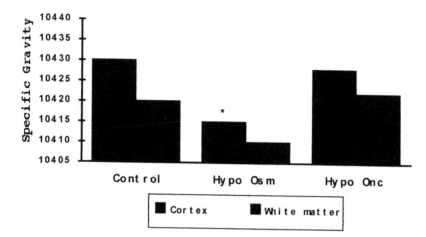

Figure 3. Cortical and white matter specific gravities of the three goups. Utilizing a technique of plasmapheresis to manipulate plasma composition, the authors examined the effects of acute change in either plasma osmolality or colloid pressure on the brain tissue specific gravity of normal rabbits. Animals in which either osmolality (Hypo Osm) or oncotic pressure (Hypo Onc) was decreased by plasma replacement with an appropriate solution were compared to a group of control animals in which both variables were maintened constant. Note: The greater the specific gravity, the lower the water content (i.e., brain tissue with a specific gravity of 1.0430 contains less water than tissue with a specific gravity of 1.0417). *P < 0.01 versus other groups. Used with permission from Zornow et al.[31]

Small Volume Resuscitation

Recently, there has been increased interest in the use of hypertonic saline (HS) solution for fluid administration in severe head trauma patients. In an experimental study on dogs, Prough et al.[32] studied the combined effects of a subdural mass and hemorrhage on regional CBF and treatment with 7.2% NaCl or 0.8% NaCl. In contrast to normal saline, HS lowered ICP and improved both global and regional CBF, despite equal cerebral perfusion pressures in both groups. These results suggest a direct cerebral arteriolar dilatory effect of the hypertonicity. Several authors, using various head injury models with and without hemorrhagic shock, have demonstrated that HS (varying from 1.8% to 7.5%, and from 500 to 2,400 mOsm/L) administration was associated with a lower ICP and lower cerebral water content than administration of isotonic fluids.[32–37] In all of these studies, the decrease of cerebral water content was due to dehydration of the uninjured cortex. Most of the studies have evaluated the effects of acute administration of HS, but few have studied the effects of maintenance of HS therapy for longer periods of time (up to 24 hr).[38,39] Although a sustained effect on the reduction of ICP, improvement of CBF, and cerebral oxygen delivery were reported, there are too few studies to provide definitive conclusions and more work is needed.

Questions about the safety of HS continue to be raised. In particular, Krausz et al.[40] showed that bleeding, in an animal model of uncontrolled hemorrhagic shock, is aggravated by early use of HS. The dangers of hypernatremia after HS administration are often discussed,[38,40,41] but to date no studies, animal or clinical, have reported physiological derangements as a result of HS administration.

Hypertonic saline solutions have already been used clinically, with interesting results in traumatic brain injury. Vassar et al.[42] evaluated the effects of hypertonic (7.5%) saline-dextran or lactated Ringer's solutions in the prehospital resuscitation of severely injured patients. Patients in the HS-dextran group required less fluid administration before hospitalization, had higher blood pressure, and a higher survival rate (32% versus 16%) than those who received lactated Ringer's solution in the subgroup of severely head injured patients. Two other studies, one in children[43] and one in adults,[44] suggest a favorable effect on the reduction of ICP in severe head trauma. Further clinical trials are necessary to confirm not only the acute beneficial effects and the long-term effects of HS, but also to evaluate the impact of a large sodium load on myocardial and renal function in severe head injury with associated systemic hypoperfusion. Once this information becomes available, the exact place for HS in the resuscitation of head trauma patients can be determined.

Clinical studies have demonstrated the degree and duration of post-injury hyperglycemia in severe head trauma patients and its relation to the extent of brain damage. There is a direct relationship between hyperglycemia and poor outcome in head-injured patients.[45,46] In fact, hyperglycemia could contribute to neuronal damage in the setting of focal ischemia and/or hypoxia frequently associated with brain trauma by increasing the production of lactic acid via anerobic metabolism, thereby resulting in cerebral acidosis.[46] Therefore, intravenous administration of glucose in the early post-traumatic period is not recommended. Sometimes, continuous insulin therapy may be required to control hyperglycemia. There may be a relative insulin resistance. However, iatrogenic hypoglycemia resulting from overly aggressive insulin therapy is also undesirable. Thus, careful monitoring of serum glucose concentration is necessary to avoid both hyper- and hypoglycemia, and management should aim to normalize blood glucose gradually over a period of at least 24 hours. Gradual normalization of glucose allows a longer period for osmotic equilibration between cerebral and vascular compartments.

CNS Protection

It has long been believed that the central nervous system (CNS) is irreversibly damaged at the time of the mechanical insult, but studies during the past decade have provided strong support for the concept of secondary ("autodestructive") damage, resulting from more delayed events.[47] These secondary lesions can result from cellular hypoxia, oligemia/ischemia, edema and swelling, and intracranial hypertension, which are manifested over a period of hours to weeks after the initial event. Although the mechanisms underlying delayed tissue injury are poorly understood, they appear to be associated with endogenous neurochemical changes resulting from CNS injury (Fig. 4). Different injury factors, including products of phospholipid hydrolysis (such as polyunsaturated fatty acid, eicosanoids, and free radicals), as well as neuropeptides, monoamines, and changes in cations and amino acids, have been proposed as responsible for this secondary damage. Hypotheses regarding the mechanism of this delayed autodestructive process have provided the theoretical basis for evaluating various pharmacological interventions in CNS trauma.

Steroids

Corticosteroids have been extensively used both in experimental models of neurotrauma and in the clinical setting, based on their theoretical ability to inhibit lipid peroxidation, stabilize lysosomal membranes, and modify production of edema. Very large doses of methylprednisolone have recently been proposed, since such doses are optimal in inhibiting lipid peroxidation.[48] Supporting these experimental results, a recent clinical trial using large intravenous doses of methylprednisolone (30 mg/kg in bolus, followed by 5.4 mg/kg/hr infusion for 23 hr), administered within 8 hours after spinal cord injury, has demonstrated a statistically significant improvement in neurological recovery at 3, 6, and 12 months.[49,50] Despite

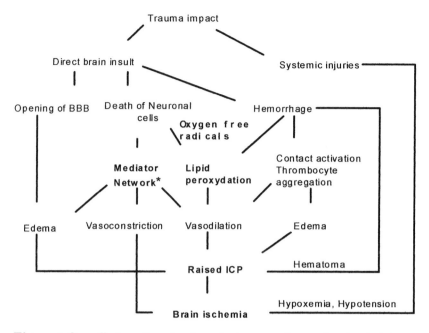

Figure 4. Overall view of mechanism of primary and secondary brain injury.

this beneficial effect of corticosteroids in spinal cord injury, no benefit has been found in traumatic brain injury.[51] On the contrary, some deleterious effects have been reported with corticosteroid administration after CNS trauma, especially septic complications, which may be more frequent and severe.[52,53]

GMM2

There are data to suggest that certain neuroendocrine mechanisms are involved in the regulation of the BBB integrity in normal animals. Nonendocrine fragments and analogs of both adrenocorticotrophic hormone and a-melanocyte-stimulating hormone have been found to reduce BBB permeability.[54,55] An analog of arginine-vasopressin has been found to increase BBB permeability.[56] In a recent study, Goldman et al.[57] investigated the effects of a vasoactive analog of adrenocorticotrophic hormone (GMM2) on time-dependent disturbance in regional cerebral blood flow, permeability-capillary surface area products, and intracranial pressure in a rat model of moderate brain injury. They noted that post-traumatic administration of GMM2 effectively reduced the early hypoperfusion, BBB leakiness, and pathological elevation of ICP.

Lazaroids

Newly developed synthetic 21-aminosteroid compounds (termed "lazaroids"), lacking gluco- and mineralo-corticoid activity, are more potent inhibitors of iron-dependent lipid peroxydation than methyl-prednisolone.[58] In addition, the 21-aminosteroids have recently been shown to have superoxide scavenging properties.[59]

One such 21-aminosteroid, U-74006F (generic name, tirilazad mesylate) has been selected for clinical development for the acute treatment of brain and spinal cord injury, subarachnoid hemorrhage, and stroke. In experimental studies of various head injury models, a beneficial effect of tirizalad has been demonstrated both on the development of brain edema and outcome.[60,61] Tirilazad mesylate also has been investigated for its ability to promote neurological recovery in experimental spinal cord injury. In a model of moderately severe compression injury to the lumbar spinal cord in cats, tirizalad, administered in a random and blinded manner 30 minutes after injury, significantly improved 1 month neurological recovery, to approximately 75% of normal neurological function.[62] Recent experimental studies suggest that tirilazad mesylate retains its effect in improving neurological recovery after spinal cord injury even when it is administered 4 hours after traumatic injury.[63] It has been shown that tirilazad mesylate, administered to healthy volunteers, has no significant effect on global or regional CBF, cerebral metabolic rate of oxygen consumption (CMRO2), or on cerebrovascular carbon dioxide reactivity.[64] Presently, two major clinical trials, one in the United States and Canada, and the other in Europe and Australia, are in progress, to evaluate the effect of tirilazad in head trauma patients, and the results will be available soon.

Glutamate Antagonists

NMDA Receptor Antagonist

Excitatory amino acids (EAAs), modulated by N-methyl-D-aspartate (NMDA) receptors, have been implicated in delayed brain tissue injury after head[65] or spinal trauma.[66] In fact, after brain or spinal trauma, increases in extracellular levels of glutamate and aspartate occur and correlate with injury severity.[65,66] Administered after experimental spinal cord injury, both competitive and noncompetitive NMDA receptor antagonists (MK801, U-50488H, and dextrorphan) have shown a beneficial action on anatomical changes, biochemical variables, and neurological recovery.[67,68] Likewise, comparable beneficial results have been obtained with NMDA receptor antagonists (MK801, U-50488H, and dextrorphan, phencyclidine) in experimental traumatic brain injury.[65,69–72] Although some noncompetitive NMDA receptor antagonists (e.g., phencyclidine and MK801) have potent side effects that limit their usefulness in human beings, other potential therapies (e.g., magnesium and dextrorphan) are considerably safer and may be considered for clinical trials. CGS 19755, a competitive NMDA receptor antagonist that has been shown to be effective in improving outcome after fluid percussion injury and acute subdural hematoma in the rat, has recently been tested in severely head injured patients in a preliminary study.[73] Seventeen severely head-injured patients (Glasgow Coma Score 4-9), requiring supported ventilation and intensive neuromonitoring, were given two doses of CGS 19755 24 hours apart (1–3 mg/kg), and the cerebral hemodynamic and metabolic effects, as well as the effect on outcome were documented. CGS 19755 was well tolerated in all patients, and despite no significant changes in arteriovenous difference in O_2 (AVDO$_2$), mean arterial pressure, and cerebral perfusion pressure, it seems that there was an improvement in outcome as no patient in this series died. These very interesting preliminary results have to be confirmed in larger randomized clinical trials, but the potential impact is exciting.

Non-NMDA Receptor Blockers

Selective blocking of the non-NMDA, AMPA (amino-3-hydroxy-5-methyl-4-isoxazole-propionate), glutamate receptors is a rather new approach in the search for protection against EAA-induced brain damage, and the results are promising.[74] Buchan et al.[75] reported a significant reduction in infarct size following transient (2 hours) middle cerebral artery occlusion, when rats were treated with NBQX, an AMPA-receptor blocker, 90 minutes after occlusion. Also, Nellgard and Wieloch[76] demonstrated that in rats subjected to 30 minutes of global ischemia, NBQX was effective in reducing neuronal damage, whereas MK801 and the competitive NMDA-blocker CGP40116 were not.

Radical Scavengers

Oxygen free radicals are generated, in excess, in ischemic situations and contribute to cell damage. Superoxide dismutase (SOD) is an endogenous scavenger of the superoxide anion, which can act as a precursor for the highly toxic hydroxyl radical, via reactions with H_2O_2 (Fig. 5). Levasseur et al.[77] tested a combination of SOD and ventilation treatment after head injury in rats, and found a markedly reduced mortality in SOD-treated animals. Exogenous SOD penetrates the BBB poorly, and has a very short plasma half-life (5 minutes), but when conjugated to polyethylene glycol (PEG), its half-life is extended and its immunogenicity is limited. Armstead et al.[78] demonstrated that PEG-SOD and PEG-catalase reduced post-ischemic transfer of urea from blood to brain in piglets. The results were taken as evidence for free radical damage of the BBB. In a randomized, double-blind, controlled phase II trial, Muizelaar et al.[79] evaluated the safety and efficacy of PEG-SOD in severely head-injured patients (Glasgow Coma Scale score ≤ 8). At two institutions, 104 patients were randomized to receive either placebo or a single bolus of PEG-SOD (2,000, 5,000 or 10,000 units/kg) 4 hours after head trauma. No complications attributed to the study treatment

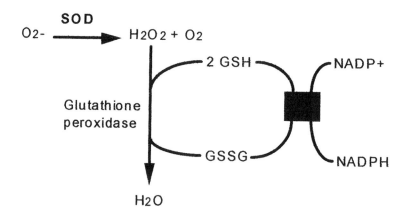

Figure 5. The role of SOD and glutathione peroxidase in removing the superoxide anion and the hydrogen peroxide from human tissues. SOD convert superoxide (O_2-) to hydrogen peroxide (H_2O_2) and oxygen. Glutathione peroxidase uses H_2O_2 to convert reduced glutathione (GSH) to oxidized glutathione (GSSG). Glutathione reductase (GR) reduces GSSG back to GSH at the expense of oxidizing NADPH.

were noted. Average ICP was equal in the four groups, but the percentage of time spent with ICP >20 mm Hg was lower in the 5,000 and 10,000 units/kg groups. Moreover, patients in the 10,000 units/kg group received less mannitol for ICP control than the control group. The 10,000 units/kg group had a statistically significant better neurological outcome at 3 and 6 months than the placebo group (20.0% of patients in a vegetative state and a mortality of 20.8% at 3 and 6 months versus 43.5% and 36.0%, respectively, in the control group). The authors concluded that PEG-SOD was generally well tolerated and appeared promising in improving outcome after head injury. In fact, this very interesting result needs to be confirmed in other studies; and a larger multicenter, phase III trial comparing a higher dose (20,000 units/kg) with placebo and 10,000 units/kg is planned.

Dimethyl sulfoxide (DMSO) is another therapeutic agent possessing free radical scavenger properties,[80] as well as diuretic[81] and cell membrane stabilizing properties.[82] Its effects on the management of brain swelling and increased ICP have been prospectively studied in 10 severely head-injured patients (Glasgow Coma Scale score ≤ 6).[83] The results demonstrate that DMSO rapidly reduces raised ICP, increases CPP, and seems to improve the neurological outcome, without affecting the systemic blood pressure. One patient demonstrated altered responsiveness. It should be noted that this study was fraught with design problems. It was not randomized, there was no control group, and it included only a small number of patients. Again, results must be confirmed in larger, randomized, controlled trials.

Naloxone and Thyrotropin-Releasing Hormone (TRH)

The concept that endogenous opioids play a pathophysiological role in CNS injury was derived from earlier studies on experimental spinal cord injury.[84,85] Initial study showed that naloxone can reverse hypotension, hypoventilation, as well as hypothermia in feline spinal shock.[86] A subsequent study[85] has failed to demonstrate a consistent beneficial effect in the rat spinal cord trauma model.

Among its many effects, TRH antagonizes certain physiological actions of the endogenous opioids without diminishing their analgesic properties, providing a rationale for its use in CNS trauma. Studies with TRH, which has a more potent antagonistic effect than naloxone, yield conflicting results in different species and different spinal cord injury models. A recent experimental study comparing TRH and naloxone, in an experimental spinal cord injury model in rats, found that TRH was effective in improving neurological outcome when given as late as 7 days after trauma, whereas naloxone had no effect.[87]

Gangliosides

Gangliosides are sialic acid-containing glycolipids located in cell membranes, particularly abundant in the CNS, and they appear to play an important role in normal neuronal development and differentiation. GM-1 (an exogenous ganglioside) treatment was reported to enhance 1 year neurological function in humans following spinal cord trauma, even though treatment was not initiated in most patients until 72 hours after injury.[88] The authors concluded that this small study (37 patients) provided evidence that GM-1 enhanced the recovery of neurological function after 1 year, but that a larger study should be conducted before GM-1 could be considered efficacious and safe in treating spinal cord injury. Presently, one major multicenter clinical trial is in progress in the United States, evaluating the effect of GM-1 in spinal cord trauma patients, and the results will be available soon.

Calcium Channels Blockers

Ischemia is a common problem after CNS trauma. In fact, ischemic changes have been noted in more than 90% of patients dying from head injury.[89,90] Intra- and extracellular calcium homeostasis in the brain is disrupted by ischemia and hypoxia. Ionized calcium is thought to enter cells, and trigger catabolic reactions, which affect proteins, phospholipids, and mitochondrial membranes. Vasoconstriction, platelet aggregation, arachidonic acid cascade activation, and uncoupled oxidative phosphorylation in mitochondria are known to occur because of increased intracellular calcium.[91-93]

Treatment with calcium channel blockers has shown promise in incomplete ischemia such as subarachnoid hemorrhage,[94] while results are less convincing in complete cerebral anoxia.[95] There is a rationale for testing calcium antagonists in brain trauma. In fact, multifocal ischemia often develops after head injury, partly caused by traumatic subarachnoid hemorrhage with vasospasm, and, since calcium channel blockers may benefit cerebral ischemia and vaso-spasm, they seem to have potential to improve prognosis following head injury. Two major clinical trials have been conducted evaluating the efficacy of nimodipine in patients with severe head trauma. In the first trial (HIT I), a small but not statistically significant benefit on 6 month outcome from nimodipine was noted.[96] In the second (multicenter European) study (HIT II), which included over 800 severe head trauma patients, nimodipine was administered at a dose of 2 mg/hr, over 7 days.[97] In this study, no significant effect was noted on overall outcome; however, in a subgroup of patients with post-traumatic subarachnoid hemorrhage on the admission CT scan, a statistically significant improvement in outcome in favor of nimodipine was observed. This was most evident in patients below 40 years of age. These results are comparable to those obtained with nicardipine in the treatment of vasospasm following severe head injury.[98] The overall results of the published studies on calcium channel blockers do not support the routine administration of these drugs in head trauma patients, at this time.

Sympathetic Nervous System Modulators

Head injury is followed by prolonged sympathetic hyperactivity, which may indirectly lead to an increase in CBF, cerebral blood volume, and hence, ICP, due to the induced circulatory hyperactivity.[99,100] These circulatory changes and the increase in ICP are attenuated by peripheral α-adrenergic antagonists, such as phentolamine,[101] or by β-blockade[102] in experimental and clinical settings.

Dexmetomidine, a potent and selective agonist of the $\alpha2$-adrenergic receptor, has been shown to possess neuroprotective properties in an animal model of transient global and focal ischemia.[103,104] Previous studies[105,106] conducted in dogs demonstrated that dexmetomidine can decrease cerebral blood flow, presumably by activation of $\alpha2$-adrenergic receptor-mediated vasoconstriction. These findings suggest that the administration of dexmetomidine may decrease ICP by decreasing cerebral blood volume. The effect of increasing doses of dexmetomidine on ICP has been studied in a prospective, randomized, controlled study in rabbits with and without intracranial hypertension.[107] The authors found that, regardless of the presence or absence of raised ICP, dexmetomidine had only minimal effects on ICP in halothane-anesthetized rabbits.

Clonidine, a central $\alpha2$-agonist, has also been shown to reduce elevated peripheral sympathetic activity in patients 3–5 days after head injury, without deleterious cephalic hemodynamic effects.[108] All of the results obtained with sympathetic nervous system modulators remain preliminary and have to be confirmed in the acute phase of human head injury. Finally, the issue of whether a pharmacological reduction in sympathetic activity (or other endocrine modulation) can improve outcome after head trauma needs further investigation.

New Drugs for Anesthesia and Sedation

The absence of any detrimental effects on cerebral perfusion pressure and CBF is one of the most important features of an ideal anesthetic for neurosurgical operations and sedation in the ICU. During the induction of anesthesia and endotracheal intubation, wide swings in blood pressure, hypoxia, hypercarbia, and coughing on the tube should be avoided.

Etomidate

Etomidate has been used as an induction agent (1.5 mg/kg) in a small number of severely head-injured patients[109]; cardiovascular stability was well maintained without an increase in ICP. However, etomidate even as a single dose suppresses the adrenocortical response to stress for up to 6 hours.[110,111] Whether this effect is detrimental is not yet known, but it is probably best not to administer this agent to severely injured patients until its implications are clarified.

Propofol

Propofol has also been used for induction and maintenance of anesthesia in patients undergoing craniotomy.[112] With induction doses of 1.5 mg/kg, followed by a continuous infusion of 100 mg/kg/min, and fentanyl (2 mg/kg before tracheal intubation), propofol significantly decreased cerebrospinal fluid pressure (CSFP) and mean arterial pressure while it maintained CPP above 70 mm Hg. It should be noted that the patients in this study were not head trauma patients, and that all 23 had normal baseline CSFP (11.9 ± 1.4 mm Hg). Moreover, an important assumption in this study was that, in these patients (clinically free of pathology judged likely to obstruct CSF pathways between the intracranial and lumbar CSF spaces), lumbar CSFP reflects ICP in patients with and without intracranial hypertension, as has been shown in a canine experimental study.[113] In fact, the results are somewhat different when the effects of propofol on cerebral hemodynamics and metabolism are investigated in severely brain-injured patients. When administered to severely head-injured patients (Glasgow Coma Scale Score 6–7), previously sedated by 1 mg/hr of phenoperidine, propofol (2 mg/kg IV bolus immediately followed by a 150 mg/kg/min infusion) induced a statistically significant decrease in CPP (from 82 ± 14 to 59 ± 7 mm Hg), a reduction in regional CBF as measured by [133]xenon (from 35 ± 6 to 26 ± 5 mL/100 g/min) and reduced ICP (from 11.3 ± 2.6 to 9.2 ± 2.5 mm Hg), but cerebrovascular resistance and cerebral $AVDO_2$ were unchanged.[114] The authors concluded that propofol reduces ICP in patients with severe brain trauma and ICP ≤ 15 mm Hg, but may decrease CPP because of its effect on MAP. Therefore, propofol should be used with caution in severe head trauma patients because of its potential detrimental effects on CPP. It is possible that by decreasing the dosage to 1–1.5 mg/kg, cerebral hemodynamics would remain more favorable.

Ketamine

Ketamine has been shown to increase ICP and many authors believe that it should not be used in head trauma patients. However, the rise in ICP may be counterbalanced in hypotensive patients by the stability of blood pressure generally obtained with ketamine. Recently, it has been observed that ketamine had a NMDA blocker-like effect.[115,116] Experimentally, Shapira et al.[117] observed that ketamine improved neurological outcome and decreased infarct size in head-injured rats. However, clinical studies on patients with raised ICP are needed before recommending this form of treatment.

Opioids

Opioids are frequently used during anesthesia and sedation in neurosurgical patients.[118,119] However, controversy persists regarding the effects of opioids on ICP.[119–125] Most animal studies report no increase in ICP associated with opioids,[121,122,124] although it has been suggested that increases in CBF may lead to an increase in ICP in the presence of intracranial pathology.[121] Reports in humans vary. Although several investigators have found no increase in ICP after sufentanil[119] or alfentanil,[125] and no increase in CSFP after

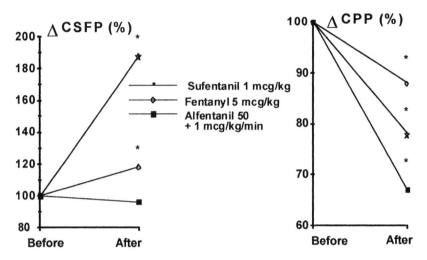

Figure 6. Effects of sufentanil, fentanyl, and alfentanil on cerebrospinal fluid pressure (CSFP) and cerebral perfusion pressure (CPP) in patients with brain tumor. *$P < 0.05$ versus baseline. Used with permission from Marx et al.[120]

sufentanil, alfentanil, and fentanyl,[123] others have reported that sufentanil and alfentanil do increase CSFP in patients with brain tumors[120] (Fig. 6). From et al.[126] have performed a prospective, randomized, and double-blind trial comparing the safety and efficacy of alfentanil, fentanyl, and sufentanil (combined with N_2O) in patients undergoing craniotomy for supratentorial tumor resection. The authors identified only four differences among these three opioids: (1) hypotension before intubation required treatment with ephedrine more frequently in patients receiving alfentanil; (2) respiratory rate and pH were lowest in the sufentanil-treated group (although this did not require naloxone therapy) 30 minutes after entry into the postanesthesia recovery room or in the surgical intensive care unit; (3) there was some suggestion that patients receiving alfentanil were more alert 30 minutes after arrival in the recovery room; and (4) the opioid cost per anesthetic was greatest for alfentanil. Finally, there were no clinically significant differences in the condition of the brain upon dural opening, requirements for isoflurane supplementation, use of either antihypertensives or naloxone, rate at which patients returned to a level of consciousness permitting neurological evaluation, or final patient outcome. These results were obtained during elective craniotomy, and the effects on ICP have not been studied. In fact, in head trauma patients who frequently have abnormal intracranial compliance, altered cerebral autoregulation, and are likely to be sensitive to most factors that may affect ICP, the effect of the potent opioids on ICP should be most apparent and have the greatest clinical significance.

In a recent study, Sperry et al.[127] comparing the effects of fentanyl (3 mg/kg) and sufentanil (0.6 mg/kg) on ICP, and CPP, in a crossover, randomized, double-blind fashion, in nine severe head trauma patients (Glasgow Coma Scale Score: 6 ± 1), found that both drugs significantly increased ICP and decreased CPP, but that there were no significant differences in ICP and CPP effects between the two drugs. Albanese et al.,[128] studying the effects of sufentanil in severe head trauma patients with abnormal intracranial compliance, have found similar results. Sufentanil (1 mg/kg IV over 6 min, followed by a continuous infusion of 0.005 mg/kg/min), administered to 10 head trauma patients with abnormal intracranial compliance (baseline ICP: 17 ± 3 mm Hg), induced a statistically significant increase in ICP of 9 ± 7 mm Hg (+ 53%). This rise peaked at 5 minutes and returned to baseline after 15 minutes. The rise was associated with a significant, persistent decrease in MAP (-24%) and, thus, in CPP (-38%).

Mayberg et al.[129] investigated the effect of two doses of alfentanil (25 or 50 mg/kg) on CBF velocity (measured by transcranial Doppler) and cerebral hemodynamics during isoflurane-N_2O anesthesia in neurosurgical patients. They found no significant change in middle cerebral artery flow velocity and $AVDO_2$, but in the high-dose group there was a statistically (but not clinically) significant increase in ICP (by 2 mm Hg) 4 minutes after injection. Moreover, despite phenylephrine administration (injected if MAP decreased from baseline values), there was an immediate but transient decrease in MAP in the high-dose group, associated with a corresponding decrease in CPP. The authors concluded that despite the absence of clinically significant changes in ICP following these two doses of alfentanil administration, one should be aware that some patients may experience a significant decrease in MAP and perhaps CPP following alfentanil administration.

Remifentanil, a new short-acting opioid, with analgesic and cardiovascular effects similar to those of alfentanil but with a shorter duration of action,[130] has been tested (comparatively with alfentanil) for its effects on cerebral hemodynamics in dogs.[131] The authors observed that the hemodynamic, EEG, and cerebral vascular effects of alfentanil and remifentanil were similar in isoflurane/nitrous oxide anesthetized dogs, but that the recovery from the cardiovascular and cerebral effect of the two opioids occurred sooner with remifentanil than with alfentanil. A possible explanation for the apparent contradictory results observed in these different studies lies with the autoregulatory phenomenon and cerebral compliance. In fact, patients in different studies are not always comparable with respect to their baseline autoregulatory status and ICP, and this may affect the results. Clinically, none of these narcotics appear to pose a problem, but it seems advisable to avoid the association of opioids with a drug shown to increase ICP in order to avoid a sudden increase in ICP and a decrease in MAP and CPP.

Volatile Agents

To further evaluate the impact of anesthetics on the evolution of cerebral injury, Kaieda et al.[132] submitted 33 rabbits to a cryogenic brain lesion, followed by 10 hours of anesthesia at 1 MAC halothane or isoflurane or with an equipotent dose of pentobarbital, and assessed the effects on cerebral hemodynamics and edema formation. Animals given pentobarbital had higher MAP until 3 hours after the lesion had been induced and there were no subsequent intergroup differences in MAP, but ICP increased in all animals without any intergroup differences. Moreover, there were no significant intergroup differences in CPP, lesion volumes, and edema formation in the lesioned hemisphere, but there was statistically less edema on the intact hemisphere in the halothane group. The authors concluded that neither pentobarbital nor isoflurane offer any advantages over halothane with respect to the development of edema after experimental brain injury. In a recent study, performed in hypocapnic neurosurgical patients with supratentorial mass lesions, Muzzi et al.[133] demonstrated that the administration of 1 MAC desflurane resulted in an increase in CSFP, in contrast to 1 MAC isoflurane, which did not produce any increase in CSFP. It should be noted that baseline CSFP was in the normal range in both groups, and that there was no statistically significant decrease in CPP in the two groups. In a more recent study, Ornstein et al.[134] found that desflurane and isoflurane, used at 1, 1.25, and 1.5 MAC, in patients with intracranial mass lesions, were similar in terms of absolute CBF, the response to increasing doses, and the preservation of CO_2 reactivity, but isoflurane induced a more pronounced fall in MAP at MAC 1.5. There is, however, virtually no clinical experience with the use of desflurane in head-injured patients. In another recent prospective, randomized study, Todd et al.[135] compared the effects of propofol-fentanyl, isoflurane-nitrous oxide and fentanyl-nitrous oxide on cerebral hemodynamics, brain swelling score, recovery characteristics, and short-term outcome in neurosurgical patients (undergoing craniotomy for supratentorial mass lesions). They failed to show any clinically significant difference among the three anesthetic regimens (Fig. 7). The authors concluded that, despite their respective cerebrovascular effects, all of the anesthetic regimens used were acceptable in these patients undergoing elective surgery, and that the specific choice of anesthetic agent(s) may not be the most crucial aspect of successful neuroanesthetic practice. Although these results were obtained in patients scheduled for elective craniotomy, they should be able to be extrapolated to stable head trauma patients, without clinical signs of intracranial hypertension. Additional studies are needed in unstable head-injured patients with and without abnormal cerebral compliance before definitively concluding the debate on the cerebrovascular effects of anesthetics.

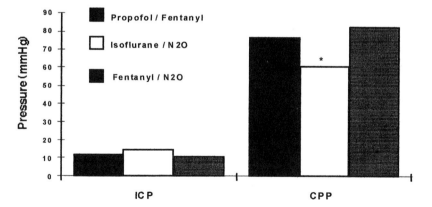

Figure 7. Comparative effect of three anesthetic techniques on intracranial pressure (ICP) and cerebral perfusion pressure (CPP) at the time the first burr hole was drilled in the skull, in neurosurgical patients undergoing elective surgical removal of a supratentorial mass lesion. *$P < 0.05$ versus the two other groups. Used with permission from Todd et al.[135]

Conclusion

The prevention of secondary brain injury is the aim of the emergency management of head trauma patients. The anesthesiologist specialized in trauma care is one of the first specialists to care for these patients. Control of life-threatening problems by simple methods such as mechanical ventilation is the first and probably the most effective step. However, new treatments including anesthetic management have been added to this scheme. Knowledge and familiarity with them is mandatory for the trauma anesthesiologist.

References

1. Shackford SR, Mackersie RC, Davis JW, Wolf PL, Hoyt DB: Epidemiology and pathology of traumatic deaths occurring at a level I trauma center in a regionalized system: The importance of secondary brain injury. J Trauma 29:1392, 1989.
2. Chesnut RM, Marshall LF, Klauber MR, Blunt BA, et al: The role of secondary brain injury in determining outcome from severe head injury. J Trauma 34:216, 1993.
3. Siegel JH, Gens DR, Mamantov T, Geisler FH, et al: Effect of associated injuries and blood volume replacement on death, rehabilitation needs, and disability in blunt traumatic brain injury. Crit Care Med 19:1252, 1991.
4. Baxt WG, Moody P: The impact of advanced prehospital emergency care on the mortality of severely brain-injured patients. J Trauma 27: 365, 1987.
5. Rosner MJ, Daughton S: Cerebral infusion pressure management in head injury. J Trauma 30:933, 1990.
6. Chan KH, Miller JD, Dearden NM, Andrews PJD, Midgley S: The effect of changes in cerebral perfusion pressure upon middle cerebral artery blood flow velocity and jugular bulb venous oxygen saturation after severe brain injury. J Neurosurg 77:55, 1992.
7. Astrup J: Drug therapy in head injury. Curr Opin Anaesth 4:653, 1991.
8. Ward JD, Becker DP, Miller DJ, Choi SC, et al: Failure of prophylactic barbiturate coma in the treatment of severe head injury. J Neurosurg 62:383, 1985.
9. Eisenberg HM, Frankowski RF, Constant CF, Marshall LF, Walker MD: High-dose barbiturate control of elevated intracranial pressure in patients with severe head injury. J Neurosurg 69:15, 1988.
10. Nordström CH, Messeter K, Sundberg G, Schalen W, et al: Cerebral blood flow, vasoreactivity, and oxygen consumption during barbiturate therapy in severe traumatic brain lesions. J Neurosurg 68:424, 1988.
11. Cold G: Measurements of CO_2 reactivity and barbiturate reactivity in patients with severe head injury. Acta Neurochir 98:153, 1989.
12. Louis PT, Goddard-Fineg J, Fishman MA, Griggs JR, et al: Barbiturate and hyperventilation during intracranial hypertension. Crit Care Med 21:1200, 1993.

13. Miller JD: Head injury and brain ischaemia-implications for therapy. Br J Anaesth 57:120, 1985.
14. Hartwell RC, Sutton LN: Mannitol, intracranial pressure, and vasogenic edema. Neurosurgery 32:444, 1993.
15. Mendelow AD, Teasdale GM, Russel T, Flood J, Patterson J, Murray GD: Effect of mannitol on cerebral blood flow and cerebral perfusion pressure in human head injury. J Neurosurg 63:43, 1985.
16. Israel RS, Marx JA, Moore EE, Lowenstein SR: Hemodynamic effect of mannitol in a canine model of concomitant increased intracranial pressure and hemorrhagic shock. Ann Emerg Med 17:560, 1988.
17. Burke AM, Quest DO, Chien S, Cerri C: The effects of mannitol on blood viscosity. J Neurosurg 55:550, 1981.
18. Muizelaar JP, Wei EP, Kontos HA, Becker DP: Mannitol causes compensatory cerebral vasoconstriction and vasodilatation in response to blood viscosity changes. J Neurosurg 59:822, 1983.
19. Smith HP, Kelly DL, McWorther JM, Armstrong D, et al: Comparison of mannitol regimens in patients with severe head injury undergoing intracranial monitoring. J Neurosurg 65:820, 1986.
20. Feldman Z, Kanter MJ, Robertson CS, Contant CF, et al: Effect of head elevation on intracranial pressure, cerebral perfusion pressure, and cerebral blood flow in head-injured patients. J Neurosurg 76:207, 1992.
21. Robertson CS, Contant CF, Gokaslan ZL, Narayan RK, Grossman RG: Cerebral blood flow, arteriovenous oxygen difference, and outcome in head injured patients. J Neurol Neurosurg Psychiatry 55:594, 1992.
22. Cold GE: Does acute hyperventilation provoke cerebral oligaemia in comatose patients after acute head injury? Acta Neurochir Wien 96: 100, 1989.
23. Muizelaar JP, Marmarou A, Ward JD, Kontos HA, et al: Adverse effects of prolonged hyperventilation in patients with severe head injury: A randomized clinical trial. J Neurosurg 75:731, 1991.
24. Mayberg TS, Lam AM: Management of central nervous system trauma. Curr Opin Anaesth 6:764, 1993.
25. Siegel JH, Gens DR, Mamantov T, Geisler FH, Goodarzi S, Mackenzie EJ: Effect of associated injuries and blood volume replacement on death, rehabilitation needs, and disability in blunt traumatic brain injury. Crit Care Med 19:1252, 1991.
26. Poole GV, Prough DS, Johnson JC, Stullken EH, et al: Effects of resuscitation from hemorrhagic shock on cerebral hemodynamics in the presence of an intracranial mass. J Trauma 27:18, 1987.
27. Wisner D, Busche F, Sturm J, Gaab M, Meyer H: Traumatic shock and head injury: Effect of fluid resuscitation on the brain injury. J Surg Res 46:49, 1989.
28. Albricht AL, Latchaw RE, Robinson AG: Intracranial and systemic effects of osmotic and oncotic therapy in experimental cerebral edema. J Neurosurg 60:481, 1984.
29. Gunnar W, Jonasson O, Merlotti G, Stone J, Barret J: Head injury and hemorrhagic shock: Studies of the blood brain barrier and intracranial pressure after resuscitation with normal saline solution, 3% saline solution, and dextran-40. Surgery 103:398, 1988.

30. Shapira Y, Artru AA, Cotev S, Muggia-Sulam M, Freund HR: Brain edema and neurologic status following head trauma in the rat. Anesthesiology 77:79, 1992.
31. Zornow MH, Todd MH, Moore SS: The acute cerebral effects of changes in plasma osmolality and oncotic pressure. Anesthesiology 67:936, 1987.
32. Prough DS, Whitley JM, Taylor CL, Deal DD, Dewitt DS: Regional cerebral blood flow following resuscitation from hemorrhagic shock with hypertonic saline. Anesthesiology 75:319, 1991.
33. Shackford SR, Zhuang S, Schmoker J: Intravenous fluids tonicity: Effect on intracranial pressure and oncotic pressure. J Neurosurg 76:91, 1992.
34. Prough DS, Johnson JC, Poole GV, Stullken EH, Johnston WE, Royster R: Effect on intracranial pressure of resuscitation from hemorrhagic shock with hypertonic saline versus lacted Ringer's solution. Crit Care Med 13:407, 1985.
35. Wisner DH, Schuster L, Quinn C: Hypertonic saline resuscitation of head surgery: Effects on cerebral water content. J Trauma 30:75, 1990.
36. Zornow MH, Scheller MS, Shackford R: Effect of a hypertonic lactated Ringer's solution on intracranial pressure and cerebral water content in a model of traumatic brain injury. J Trauma 29:484, 1989.
37. Walsh JC, Zhuang J, Shackford R: A comparison of hypertonic to isotonic fluid in the resuscitation of brain injury and hemorrhagic shock. J Surg Res 50:284, 1991.
38. Shackford SR, Zhuang S, Schmoker J: Intravenous fluids tonicity: Effect on intracranial pressure, cerebral blood flow and cerebral oxygen delivery in focal brain injury. J Neurosurg 76:91, 1992.
39. Walsh JC, Zhuang J, Shackford SR: A comparison of hypertonic to isotonic fluid in the resuscitation of brain injury and hemorrhagic shock. J Surg Res 50:284, 1991.
40. Krausz MM, Kablan M, Rabinovici R, Klin B, Sherman Y, Gross D: Effect of injured vessel size on bleeding following hypertonic saline infusion in "uncontrolled" hemorrhagic shock in anesthetized rats. Cir Shock 35:9, 1991.
41. Mattar JA: Hypertonic and hyperoncotic solutions in patients [Editorial]. Crit Care Med 17:297, 1989.
42. Vassar MJ, Perry CA, Gannaway WL, Holcroft JW: 7.5% sodium chloride dextran for resuscitation of trauma patients undergoing helicopter transport. Arch Surg 126:1065, 1991.
43. Fisher B, Thomas D, Peterson B: Hypertonic saline lowers raised intracranial pressure in children after head trauma. J Neurosurg Anesthesiol 4:4, 1992.
44. Worthley LI, Copper DJ, Jones N: Treatment of resistant intracranial hypertension with hypertonic saline. J Neurosurg 68:478, 1988.
45. Mouawad E, van Laere E: Troubles de la glycémie chez les traumatisés craniens. Neurochirurgie 19:456, 1973.
46. Lam AM, Winn RH, Cullen BF, Sundling W: Hyperglycemia and neurological outcome in patients with head injury. J Neurosurg 75:545, 1991.

47. Faden AI, Salzman S: Pharmacological strategies in CNS trauma. TiPS 13:29, 1992.
48. Hall ED: Inhibition of lipid peroxydation in CNS trauma. J Neurotrauma 8(Suppl):31, 1991.
49. Bracken MB, Shepard MJ, Collins WF, et al: A randomized controlled trial of methylprednisolone or naloxone in the treatment of acute spinal cord injury. N Engl J Med 322:1405, 1990.
50. Bracken MB, Shepard MJ, Collins WF, et al: Methylprednisolone or naloxone treatment after spinal cord injury: 1-year follow-up data. J Neurosurg 76:23, 1992.
51. Dearden NM, Gibson JS, McDowall DG, Gibson RM, Cameron MM: Effect of high dose dexamethasone on outcome from severe head injury. J Neurosurg 64:81, 1986.
52. Fanconi S, Kloti J, Meuli M, Zaugg H, Zachmann M: Dexamethasone therapy and endogenous cortisol production in severe pediatric head injury. Intens Care Med 14:163, 1988.
53. DeMaria EJ, Reichman W, Kenney PR, Armitage JM, Gann DS: Septic complications of corticosteroid administration after central nervous system trauma. Ann Surg 202:248, 1986.
54. Goldman H, Sandman CA, Kastin A, et al: MSH affects regional perfusion of the brain. Pharmacol Biochem Behav 3:661, 1975.
55. Goldman H, Murphy S: An analog of adrenocorticotrophic-MSH(4-9), ORG-2766, reduces permeability of the blood-brain barrier. Pharmacol Biochem Behav 14:845, 1981.
56. Goldman H, Berman RF, Murphy S: Adrenocorticotrophic-related peptides, kinding and seizure disorders. In Goodwin FK, Sachar EJ, Nerozzi D (eds): Hypothalamic Dysfunction in Neuropsychiatric Disorders. Raven Press, New York, 1987, p 317.
57. Goldman H, Morehead M, Murphy S: Use of adrenocorticotrophic hormone analog to minimize brain injury. Ann Emerg Med 22:1035, 1993.
58. Braughler JM, Chase RL, Neft GL, Yonkers PA, Day JS, et al: A new 21-aminosteroid antioxidant lacking glucocorticoid activity blocks arachidonic acid release and stimulates ACTH secretion from mouse pituitary tumor. J Pharmacol Exp Ther 244:423, 1988.
59. Thomas PD, Mao GD, Rabinovitch A, Poznansky MJ: Inhibition of superoxide generating NADPH oxidase of human neutrophils by lazaroids (21-aminosteroids and 2-methylaminochromans). Biochem Pharmacol 45:241, 1993.
60. Hall ED, Yonkers PA, McCall JM, Braughler JM: Effects of the 21-aminosteroid U-74006F on experimental head injury in mice. J Neurosurg 68:456, 1988.
61. Dimlich RVW, Tornheim PA, Kindel RM, et al: Effects of a 21-aminosteroid (U-74006F) on cerebral metabolites and edema after severe experimental head trauma. Adv Neurol 52:365, 1990.
62. Anderson DK, Braughler JM, Hall ED, et al: Effects of treatment with U-74006F on neurological recovery following experimental spinal cord injury. J Neurosurg 69:562, 1988.
63. Anderson DK, Hall ED, Braughler JM, et al: Effect of delayed administration of U74006F (tirilazad mesylate) on recovery of locomotor func-

tion following experimental spinal cord injury. J Neurotrauma 8:187, 1991.

64. Olsen KS, Videbaek C, Agerlin N, Kroll M, et al: The effect of tirilazad mesylate (UF74006F) on cerebral oxygen consumption, and reactivity of cerebral blood flow to carbon dioxide in healthy volunteers. Anesthesiology 79:666, 1993.

65. Faden AI, Demediuk P, Panter SS, Vink R: The role of excitatory amino acids and NMDA receptors in traumatic brain injury: Science 244:798, 1989.

66. Panter SS, Yum SW, Faden AI: Alterations in extracellular aminoacids after traumatic spinal cord injury. Ann Neurol 27:96, 1990.

67. Faden AI, Ellison JA, Noble LJ: Effects of competitive and non-competitive NMDA receptor antagonists in spinal cord injury. Eur J Pharmacol 175:165, 1990.

68. Gomez-Pinilla F, Tram H, Cotman CW, Nieto-Sampedro M: Neuroprotective effect of MK-801 and U-50488H after contusive spinal cord injury. Exp Neurol 104:118, 1989.

69. Hayes RL, Jenkins LW, Lyeth BG, et al: Pretreatment with phencyclidine, an N-methyl-D-aspartate receptor antagonist, attenuates longterm behavioral deficits in the rat produced by traumatic brain injury. J Neurotrauma 5:287, 1988.

70. McIntosh TK, Vink R, Soares H, Hayes R, Simon R: Effects of the N-methyl-D-aspartate receptor blocker MK-801 on neurologic function after experimental brain injury. J Neurotrauma 6:247, 1989.

71. Shapiro Y, Yadid G, Cotev S, et al: Protective effect of MK801 in experimental brain injury. J Neurotrauma 7:131–139, 1990.

72. McIntosh TK, Vink R, Soares H, et al: Effect of noncompetitive blockade of N-methyl-D-aspartate receptors on the neurochemical sequelae of experimental brain injury. J Neurochem 55:1170, 1990.

73. Stewart L, Bullock R, Jones M, Kotake A, Teasdale GM: The cerebral hemodynamic and metabolic effects of the competitive NMDA antagonist CGS 19755 in humans with severe head injury. 2nd International Neurotrauma Symposium. Glasgow, Abstract 076, 1993.

74. Sheardown MJ, Nielsen E, Hansen AJ, Jacobsen P, Honoe T: 2,3-Dihydroxy-6-nitro-7-sulfamoyl-benzo(F)quinoxaline: A neuroprotectant for cerebral ischemia. Science 247:571, 1990.

75. Buchan M, Xue D, Hung Z-G, Smith KH, Lesiuk H: Delayed AMPA receptor blockade reduces cerebral infraction induced by focal ischemia. Neuroreport 2:471, 1991.

76. Nellgard B, Wieloch T: Postischemic blockade of AMPA but not NMDA receptors mitigates neuronal damage in the rat brain following transient severe cerebral ischemia. J Cereb Blood Flow Metab 1:2, 1992.

77. Levasseur JE, Patterson JL, Ghatak NR, Kontos HA, Choi SC: Combined effect of respirator-induced ventilation and superoxide dismutase in experimental brain injury. J Neurosurg 71:573, 1989.

78. Armstead WM, Mirro R, Thelin OP, Shibata M, et al: Polyethylene glycol conjugated superoxide dismutase and catalase attenuate increased blood-brain barrier permeability after ischemia in piglets. Stroke 23:755, 1992.

79. Muizelaar JP, Marmarou A, Young HF, et al: Improving the outcome of severe head injury with the oxygen radical scavenger PEG-SOD: A phase II trial. J Neurosurg 78:375, 1993.

80. Hammond B, Kontos HA, Hess ML: Oxygen radicals in the adult respiratory distress syndrome, in myocardial ischemia and reperfusion injury, and in cerebral vascular damage. Can J Physiol Pharmacol 63: 173, 1985.

81. Formanek K, Suckert R: Diuretische wirkung von DMSO. DMSO Symposium, Jienna Saladruck. Berlin, West Germany, 1966, p 21.

82. Gorog P, Kovaks W: Effect of dimethyl sulfoxide on various experimental inflammation. Curr Therap Res 10:486, 1968.

83. Kulalt A, Akar M, Baykut L: Dimethyl sulfoxide in the management of patient with brain swelling and increased intracranial pressure after severe closed head injury. Neurochirurgica 33:177, 1990.

84. Faden AL, Molineaux CJ, Rosenberg JG, et al: Endogenous opioids immunoreactivity in rat spinal cord following traumatic injury. Ann Neurol 17:386, 1985.

85. Young W, Flamm ES, Demepoulos HB, et al: Effect of naloxone on postraumatic ischemia in experimental spinal contusion. J Neurosurg 55:209, 1981.

86. Long JB, Martinez-Arizala, Petras JM, Holaday JW: Endogenous opioids in spinal cord injury: A critical evaluation. Cent Nervous Trauma 3:295, 1986.

87. Hashimoto T, Fukida N: Effect of thyrotropin-releasing hormone on the neurologic impairment in rats with spinal cord injury: Treatment starting 24 h and 7 days after injury. Eur J Pharmacol 203:25, 1991.

88. Geisler FH, Dorsey FC, Coleman WP: Recovery of motor function after spinal-cord injury: A randomized, placebo-controlled trial with GM-I ganglioside. N Engl J Med 324:1829, 1991.

89. Graham DI, Adams JH, Doyle D: Ischaemic brain damage in fatal nonmissile head injuries. J Neurosci 39:213, 1978.

90. Graham DI, Ford I, Adams JH, et al: Ischaemic brain damage is still present in fatal non-missile head injury. J Neurol Neurosurg Psychiat 52:346, 1989.

91. Raichle ME: The pathophysiology of brain ischemia. Ann Neurol 13: 2, 1983.

92. Siesjo BK: Cell damage in the brain: A speculative synthesis. J Cereb Blood Flow Metab 1:155, 1981.

93. Choi DW: Calcium-mediated neurotoxicity: Relationship to specific channel types and role in ischemic damage. Trends Neurosci 11:465, 1988.

94. Petruk KC, West M, Mohr G, et al: Nimodipine treatment in poorgrade aneurysm patients: Results of a multicenter double-blind placebo controlled trial. J Neurosurg 68:505, 1988.

95. Bircher NG: Cardiopulmonary-cerebral resuscitation: Brain resuscitation, mediators, glucose and anesthetics. Curr Opin Anaesthesiol 3: 259, 1990.

96. Teasdale G, Bailey I, Bell A, et al: The effect of nimodipine on outcome

after head injury: A prospective randomized controlled trial. Acta Neurochir (Suppl):315, 1990.

97. European Study Group on Nimodipine in Severe Head Injury (HIT II): A multicentre trial on the efficacy of nimodipine on outcome after severe head injury. J Neurosurg 80:797, 1996.

98. Compton JS, Lee T, Jones NR, Waddell G, Teddy PJ: A double blind placebo controlled trial of the calcium entry blocking drug, nicardipin in the treatment of vasospasm following severe head injury. Br J Neurosurg 4:9, 1990.

99. Rosner MJ, Nesome HH, Becker DP, et al: Mechanical brain injury. The sympathoadrenal response. J Neurosurg 61:76, 1984.

100. Millen JE, Clauser FL, Zimmerman M: Physiological effects of controlled concussive brain trauma. J Appl Physiol 49:856, 1980.

101. Clifton GL, Ziegler MG, Grossman RG: Circulating catecholamines and sympathetic activity after head injury. Neurosurgery 8:10, 1981.

102. Robertson C, Clifton GL, Taylor AA, et al: Treatment of hypertension associated with head injury. J Neurosurg 59:455, 1983.

103. Hoffman WE, Kochs E, Werner C, Thomas C, Albrecht RF: Dexmedetomidine improves neurologic outcome from incomplete ischemia in the rat. Anesthesiology 75:328, 1991.

104. Maier C, Steinberg GK, Sun GH, Zhi GT, Maze M: Neuroprotection by the a2-adrenoreceptor agonist dexmedetomidine in a focal model of cerebral ischemia. Anesthesiology 79:306, 1993.

105. Karlsson BR, Forsamn M, Roald OK, Heier MS, Steen PA: Effect of dexmetomidine, a selective and potent $\alpha 2$-agonist, on cerebral blood flow and oxygen consumption during halothane anesthesia in dogs. Anesth Analg 71:125, 1990.

106. Zornow MH, Fleischer JE, Scheller MS, Nakimura K, Drummond JC: Dexmetomidine, an $\alpha 2$-adrenergic agonist, decrease cerebral blood flow in the isoflurane-anesthetized dog. Anesth Analg 70:624, 1990.

107. Zornow MH, Scheller MS, Sheehan PB, Strnat MA, Matsumoto M: Intracranial pressure effects of dexmetomidine in rabbits. Anesth Analg 75:232, 1992.

108. Payen D, Quintin L, Plaisance P, Chiron B, Lhoste F: Head injury: Clonidine decreases plasma catecholamines. Crit Care Med 18:392, 1990.

109. Moss E, Powell D, Gibson RM, et al: Effects of etomidate on intracranial pressure and cerebral perfusion pressure. Br J Anaesth 5:347, 1979.

110. Wagner RL, White PF: Etomidate inhibits adrenocortical function in surgical patients. Anesthesiology 61:647, 1984.

111. Fragen RJ, Shanks CA, Molteni A, et al: Effects of etomidate on hormonal response to surgical stress. Anesthesiology 61:652, 1984.

112. Ravussin P, Guinard P, Ralley F, et al: Effect of propofol on cerebrospinal fluid pressure and cerebral perfusion pressure in patients undergoing craniotomy. Anaesthesia 43:37, 1988.

113. Takizawa H, Gabra-Sanders T, Miller JD: Analysis of changes in intracranial pressure and pressure-volume index at different locations in the craniospinal axis during supratentorial epidural balloon inflation. Neurosurgery 19:1, 1986.

114. Pinaud M, Lelausque A, Fauchoux N, Ménégalli D, Souron R: Effects of propofol on cerebral hemodynamics and metabolism in patients with brain trauma. Anesthesiology 73:404, 1990.
115. Anis NA, Berry SC, Burton NR, Lodge D: The dissociative anaesthetics, ketamine and phencyclidine, selectively reduce excitation of central mammalian neurons by N-methyl-aspartate. Br J Pharmacol 79:565, 1983.
116. Thomson AM, West DC, Lodge D: An N-methylaspartate receptor-mediated synapse in rat cerebral cortex: A site of action of ketamine? Nature 313:479, 1985.
117. Shapira Y, Artru AA, Lam AM: Ketamine decreases cerebral infarct volume and improves neurological outcome following experimental head trauma in rats. J Neurosurg Anesthesiol 4:231, 1992.
118. McKay RD, Varner PD, Henricks PL, Adams ML, Harsh GR: The evaluation of sufentanil-N2O-O2 vs. fentanyl-N2O-O2 anesthesia for craniotomy. Anesth Analg 63:250, 1984.
119. Weinstabl C, Mayer N, Richling B, Czech T, Spiss CK: Effect of sufentanil on intracranial pressure in neurosurgical patients. Anaesthesia 46:837, 1991.
120. Marx W, Shah N, Long C, Arbit E, Galicich J, et al: Sufentanil, alfentanil, and fentanyl: impact on cerebrospinal fluid pressure in patients with brain tumors. J Neurosurg Anesthesiol 1:3, 1989.
121. Milde LN, Milde JH, Gallagher WJ: Effects of sufentanil on cerebral circulation and metabolism in dogs. Anesth Analg 70:138, 1990.
122. Werner C, Hoffman WE, Baughman VL, Albrecht RF, et al: Effects of sufentanil on cerebral blood flow, cerebral blood flow velocity, and metabolism in dogs. Anesth Analg 72:177, 1991.
123. Cuillerier DJ, Mannimen PH, Gelb AW: Alfentanil, sufentanil and fentanyl: effect on cerebral perfusion pressure. Anesth Analg 70:S75, 1990.
124. Bunegin L, Albin MS, Ernst PS, Garcia C: Cerebrovascular responses to sufentanil citrate in primates with and without intracranial hypertension. J Neurosurg Anesthesiol 2:138, 1989.
125. Markowitz BP, Duhaime AC, Sutton L, Schreiner MS, Cohen DE: Effects of alfentanil on intracranial pressure in children undergoing ventriculo-peritoneal shunt revision. Anesthesiology 76:71, 1992.
126. From RP, Warner DS, Todd MM, Sokoll MD: Anesthesia for craniotomy: A double-blind comparison of alfentanil, fentanyl, and sufentanil. Anesthesiology 73:896, 1990.
127. Sperry RJ, Bailey PL, Reichman MV, Peterson JC, Peterson PB, Pace NL: Fentanyl and sufentanil increase intracranial pressure in head trauma patients. Anesthesiology 77:416, 1992.
128. Albanese J, Durbec O, Viviand X, Potie F, Alliez B, Martin C: Sufentanil increases intracranial pressure in patients with head trauma. Anesthesiology 79:493, 1993.
129. Mayberg TS, Lam AM, Eng CC, Laohaprasit V, Winn R: The effect of alfantanil on cerebral blood flow velocity and intracranial pressure during isoflurane-nitrous oxide anesthesia in humans. Anesthesiology 78:288, 1993.

130. Schuster SV, Billota JM, Lutz MK: Analgesic activity of the ultra-short-acting opioid, remifentanil (abstract). FASEB 5:A860, 1991.
131. Hoffman WE, Cunningham F, James MK, Baughman VL, Albrecht RF: Effects of remifentanil, a new short-acting opioid, on cerebral blood flow, brain electrical activity, and intracranial pressure in dogs anesthetized with isoflurane and nitrous oxide. Anesthesiology 79:107, 1993.
132. Kaieda R, Todd MM, Weeks JB, Warner DS: A comparison of the effects of halothane, isoflurane, and pentobarbital anesthesia on intracranial pressure and cerebral edema formation following brain injury in rabbits. Anesthesiology 71:571, 1989.
133. Muzzi DA, Losasso TJ, Dietz NM, Faust RJ, Cucchiara RF, Milde LN: The effect of desflurane and isoflurane on cerebrospinal fluid pressure in humans with supratentorial mass lesions. Anesthesiology 76:720, 1992.
134. Ornstein E, Young WL, Fleischer LH, Ostapkovich N: Desflurane and isoflurane have similar effects on cerebral blood flow in patients with intracranial mass lesions. Anesthesiology 79:498, 1993.
135. Todd MM, Warner DS, Sokoll MD, Maktabi MA, et al: A prospective, comparative trial of three anesthetics for elective supratentorial craniotomy. Anesthesiology 78:1005, 1993.

16

Recent Advances in Central Nervous System Monitoring

Eiichi Inada, MD, Kazuo Okada, MD

Introduction

Monitoring the central nervous system (CNS) represents a real challenge to the anesthesiologist. The major objective of monitoring the CNS is to decrease the mortality and morbidity associated with surgery involving the CNS. Even the most advanced monitoring devices have difficulty in accurately assessing the function of the CNS. The most sophisticated monitors are technically demanding; some are invasive and associated with complications such as infection and bleeding. The ideal monitor should be noninvasive, continuous, have both high sensitivity and specificity, and be user friendly. Although currently available monitoring devices have certain shortcomings and limitations, they may decrease mortality and morbidity.

Numerous monitoring modalities are available to assess the integrity of the CNS. Intracranial pressure (ICP) measurements are popular in patients with head trauma or nontraumatic coma. Cere-

From *Trauma Anesthesia and Critical Care of Neurological Injury,* edited by K. J. Abrams and C. M. Grande. © 1997, Futura Publishing Co., Armonk, NY.

bral perfusion pressure (CPP), the difference between the mean arterial pressure (MAP) and the mean ICP or central venous pressure, is more important than the ICP alone. Cerebral blood flow measurements can be assessed by the transcranial Doppler (TCD) method and are quickly gaining popularity as equipment becomes more readily available. The major determinants of global cerebral circulation are blood flow and perfusion pressure. However, normal flow and pressure does not guarantee normal cerebral circulation and function.

Electrophysiological monitoring, such as electroencephalography (EEG), including computer-assisted EEG and evoked potentials, has been gaining popularity. They can assess the functional integrity of the CNS and may help to localize the sensitivity and specificity of regional abnormalities. In comparison with other monitoring, electrophysiological monitoring is well defined.

The metabolic integrity of the brain can now be determined with SjO_2 and near-infrared spectroscopy (NIRS). Jugular venous oxygen saturation (JvO_2) monitoring provides continuous cerebral oxygenation data. NIRS allows us to assess oxyhemoglobin saturation in the brain as well as the mitochondrial cytochrome-aa3 redox state. This chapter will focus on the use of each of these modalities with respect to the care of the neurologically injured patient.

Intracranial Pressure (ICP)

ICP is one of the major components determining cerebral circulation. Fluid-filled ventricular catheters are the "gold standard" for comparison of ICP monitoring devices. Intraventricular catheters have the advantage of measuring intracranial compliance while allowing removal of cerebrospinal fluid (CSF) in attempt to reduce ICP. Unfortunately, this technique is associated with a high infection rate (of approximately 11%).[1,2]

Other measurement systems such as subarachnoid, subdural, and epidural have been developed to reduce the incidence of infection while maintaining accurate measurements. The Camino ICP system is composed of a no. 4 fiberoptic probe with a transducer at the tip,[3] which can be used for intraventricular, intraparenchymal, or subdural pressure measurements.[4,5] An excellent correlation exists between the intraventricular pressure measured by a standard fluid-filled system and intraventricular pressure measured by the fiberoptic catheter. This strong correlation of pressures is also present in the subdural and intraparenchymal compartments.[6,7] The Camino system has many advantages over fluid-filled catheters. Adjustments for hydrostatic pressure or transducer-level changes based on patient position are unnecessary. It may also provide greater accuracy and less artifact because of the lack of a fluid-filled system, which has a particular resonance frequency and damping factor. Disadvantages include the fact that the device cannot be recalibrated once the catheter has been inserted, and like all fiberoptic catheters, they require careful handling to avoid fiber breakage.[8]

Cerebral Blood Flow

Although ICP is relatively easy to measure, the presence of normal ICP does not necessarily mean that cerebral circulation is normal. Cerebral blood flow (CBF) measurements are a more direct index of cerebral circulation. CBF monitoring reflects global cerebral blood flow and may not demonstrate regional blood flow abnormalities.

Transcranial Doppler (TCD) Monitoring

Recently introduced to clinical practice, TCD has been gaining popularity in the operating room and in the intensive care unit.[9,10] TCD uses Doppler shift to measure blood flow velocity in large arteries such as the middle cerebral arteries. A direction-sensitive probe is placed over the "temporal window" located above the zygomatic arch between the ear and the ocular orbit. Red cell velocity is calculated by measuring the Doppler shift in the reflected sound wave, with mean velocity being calculated from the systolic and diastolic signals. The Gosling pulsatility index (peak systolic velocity–end-diastolic velocity/mean velocity) or Pourcelot resistance index (peak systolic–end-diastolic/peak systolic velocity) are calculated. These values are calculated on the assumption that blood flow velocity in the basal cerebral arteries reflects cortical cerebral blood flow. However, this assumption holds true only when the measured angle of the Doppler probe is nearly constant and when the diameter of the conducting cerebral arteries does not change. The quantitative measurement is difficult to interpret because of dynamic changes in cerebral vessel diameter, linear velocity, and volumetric flow.

It is not known at which point the pulsatile index is increased by increases in distal resistances. Absolute blood flow velocities are affected by many factors such as hematocrit, arterial carbon dioxide pressure ($PaCO_2$), age, and cerebral metabolic rate.[15] Although there are limitations, clinical data are accumulating.

Despite accumulating evidence, the accuracy of TCD remains unclear.[11] Correlations between TCD and other modalities such as EEG, spectral edge frequency parameters, evoked potentials,[12] and electrocorticogram[13] in various clinical settings, as well as in animal models, have been investigated. Significant positive correlation was found between flow velocities measured by TCD and CBF measured by xenon-inhalation technique.[14]

TCD is very sensitive to changes in $PaCO_2$.[16,17] No apparent differences were found in the cerebrovascular reactivity of the middle cerebral artery to CO_2 in healthy children anesthetized with either halothane or isoflurane up to 1 minimum alveolar concentration (MAC).[18] The same authors found that nitrous oxide increased the cerebral blood flow velocity without a change in cerebrovascular resistance index in healthy children.[19]

TCD can be used to evaluate the severity of vasospasm after subarachnoid hemorrhage. Elevation of mean middle cerebral artery (MCA) velocity greater than 120 cm/sec (normal value 35~90 cm/sec)[20] has been used to diagnose vasospasm.[21,22] The degree of MCA velocity parallels the clinical neurological symptoms. Most patients suffering subarachnoid hemorrhage and a rapid rise in MCA velocities subsequently developed a neurological deficit.[23] Thus, TCD may be helpful in identifying patients at risk for cerebral ischemia.

In head-injured patients, TCD can detect cerebral hyperemia as well as ischemia due to vasospasm. Low CBF velocities may be a predictor of early mortality.[26] Bidirectional signals, indicating to and from movement of blood, low systolic spikes without diagnostic signals, and a high pulsatility index indicate brain death.[27]

TCD has been used to detect air embolism during carotid endarterectomy and during weaning from cardiopulmonary bypass.[28,29] Spencer et al. identified air emboli in 38% of patients and formed element emboli in 26% of patients undergoing carotid endarterectomy.[28] Nylor found there was good correlation between stump pressure and MCA mean velocity, as well as a high incidence of air embolism in patients undergoing carotid endarterectomy.[30] Cerebral emboli may often occur during open heart surgery.[31] TCD confirmed that cerebral embolism frequently occurs during aortic cannulation and initiation of bypass.[32] Taylor et al. found that cerebral pressure-flow velocity autoregulation was present during normothermic cardiopulmonary bypass while it became pressure-passive during moderate and profound hypothermic cardiopulmonary bypass.[33]

Xenon Washout

Xenon indicator dilution washout has been the gold standard for evaluation of cerebral blood flow.[34] This is a relatively noninvasive procedure and provides information on regional blood flow. Xenon-133 is injected into either the carotid artery or the jugular vein.[35] The standard technique requires at least 10 minutes to measure CBF. The more recent curve-fitting model reduces the data sampling time by about 75%.[36] Although this measurement can be repeated during surgery, it cannot serve as a continuous monitor of CBF. Furthermore, it measures flow only in the cerebral cortex. Information regarding deeper structures is lacking unless the overlying cortex is infarcted ("look-through phenomenon"). Xenon clearance is not predictive of cerebral ischemia during carotid endarterectomy.[37]

Electrophysiological Monitoring

Evoked Potentials

Sensory evoked potentials (SEPs) are the body's electrophysiological responses to either sensory stimulation or the electrical stimulation of sensory or mixed nerves. SEPs are pathway-specific, while the EEG is a recording of spontaneous electrical activity and is nonspecific. SEPs are commonly elicited by somatosensory, auditory, or visual stimulation.

Somatosensory-Evoked Potential

Somatosensory-evoked potentials (SSEPs) are generated by an electrical stimulus to a peripheral nerve. SSEPs are most often elicited by electrical stimulation of mixed nerves such as the median nerve, the posterior tibial nerve, or peroneal nerve. SSEPs can detect abnormalities in the conduction pathways from peripheral nerves, plexi, nerve roots, the dorsal columns of the spinal cord, the lemniscal pathways to the thalamus, and finally, to the primary sensory cortex. SSEPs have been used to monitor the cerebral cortex as well as to monitor specific neuronal tracts.

SSEPs may be as sensitive as the EEG to decreases in cerebral blood flow. SSEPs were abolished when regional CBF decreased to less than 12 mL/100 g/min while the critical regional CBF associated with EEG changes was 10–18 mL/100 g/min during carotid endarterectomy under isoflurane anesthesia.[38,39] During carotid endarterec-

tomy, SSEP was 100% sensitive and 94% specific for cerebral ischemia, whereas EEG had 92% specificity and 50% sensitivity.[40]
They may be also useful in providing information on prognosis after
cortical tumor resections.[41]

SSEPs arising in the cerebral cortex are sensitive to anesthetic
agents, particularly the volatile anesthetic agents (Fig. 1). Volatile
anesthetics cause a dose-dependent increase in latency and a decrease in amplitude.[42,43] Minimum alveolar concentration (MAC) of
halothane or 0.5 MAC of either enflurane or isoflurane reduced the
amplitude of SSEP more than 50%. Nitrous oxide alone decreases
amplitude with minimal latency changes.[44] Fentanyl and morphine
cause dose-dependent increases in latency of all waves and decreases
in amplitude.

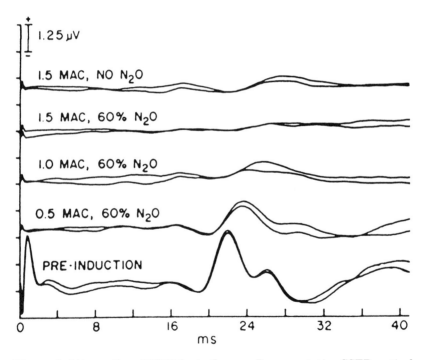

Figure 1. Attenuation of SSEP by isoflurane. Representative SSEP cortical
responses (C3, or C4-FPz) at various MAC levels of isoflurane. From Peterson DO, Drummond JC, Todd MM: Effects of halothane, enflurane, isoflurane and nitrous oxide on somatosensory evoked potentials in humans. Anesthesiology 65:35–40, 1986.

Brain Stem Auditory-Evoked Potentials

Evoked responses may be generated by auditory stimuli. Brain stem auditory-evoked potentials (BAEP) have been used during acoustic neuroma resection and during microvascular decompression[45,46] (Fig. 2). Later peaks will be more affected by cerebral ischemia.[47] BAEPs may have prognostic value after head injury.[48] Although BAEPs are relatively insensitive to anesthetic agents, middle-latency (10–50 ms) auditory-evoked potentials are affected by some anesthetic agents, such as nitrous oxide and inhalation anesthetics.[49–52] Narcotics basically produce minimal to no effect on BAEP recordings. BAEP seems to be resistant to severe hypotension.

Motor-Evoked Potentials

Motor-evoked potentials (MEPs) are usually elicited by direct application of electrical currents or the induction of electrical currents by the application of magnetic fields to the motor system. Transcranial magnetic motor-evoked potentials (tcMMEPs) may be useful to test the continuity of motor pathways from the cortex to the periphery. However, tcMMEPs are very sensitive to nitrous oxide and other inhalation anesthetics.[53,54] Small doses of midazolam and fentanyl produce profound and prolonged attenuation of MEPs. Thiopental and nitrous oxide produce total loss of MEPs. Hypothermia, hypoxia, and hypotension can also alter MEPs.[55] Intraoperative recordability of MEPs can be improved using repetitive stimulation.[56]

Electroencephalogram (EEG)

The traditional EEG (usually 16 channels) is a strip-chart plot of voltage against time. The interpretation of the EEG may require a well-trained technician along with the anesthesiologist, as this is tedious and time-consuming.

The EEG is generated by the pyramidal cells in the granular layer of the cerebral cortex. Slowing of the EEG correlates with a fall in CBF below a threshold value of 18 mL/100 g/min. Cerebral ischemia causes EEG slowing and a decrease in amplitude.[57] The EEG becomes isoelectric as cerebral ischemia worsens and changes within seconds when cerebral ischemia occurs. Hypoxia may initially produce EEG activation, eventually leading to EEG slowing and then electrical silence.

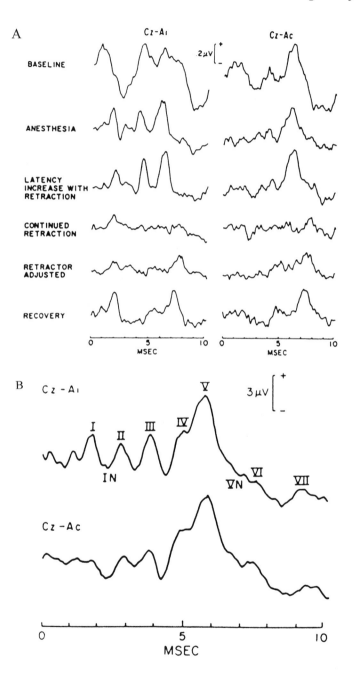

The EEG can be affected by many factors including anesthetic agents. Induction of anesthesia decreases alpha (8–13 Hz) activity and increases beta (>13 Hz) activity. As anesthesia deepens, EEG frequency decreases until theta (4–7 Hz) and delta (0–3 Hz) activity predominate. Further increases in anesthetic depth cause burst suppression. Some ischemic EEG changes are identical to those caused by anesthetics. Isoflurane produces electrical silence at a concentration of 2 MAC. A large dose of thiopental also induces EEG isoelectricity. The EEG is also altered by changes in $PaCO_2$. Hypocapnia causes EEG slowing, while mild hypercapnia increases frequency and severe hypercapnia decreases frequency and amplitude. Hypothermia (<35°C) causes a progressive slowing of EEG activity with the EEG becoming isoelectric at a body temperature of 15–20°C.

Even with these drawbacks, the sensitivity of the EEG in detecting cerebral ischemia ranges from 75% to 100%. Patients at significant risk of intraoperative stroke during carotid endarterectomy can be identified by intraoperative EEG changes.[58] On the other hand, some have reported new postoperative neurological deficits without significant intraoperative EEG changes.[59] EEG is not a direct indicator of cerebral metabolic integrity.[60]

The advent of computer-assisted analysis of the EEG facilitates the interpretation of data by data compression, and can provide results comparable to the conventional EEG interpretation.[61–64]

Spectral Analysis of EEG

Power spectral analysis converts EEG information from the time domain to the frequency domain (Fig. 3). In the compressed spectral array (CSA), the serial power spectra are plotted to provide a time-compressed "mountain and valley" representation of EEG patterns (Fig. 4). Moment-to-moment changes in wave shape may be lost in transformation and subtle changes may become apparent only after

---

Figure 2. Brain stem auditory-evoked potential. **A:** Reversible obiliteration of the brain stem auditor evoked potential with retraction of the eighth cranial nerve. **B:** Normal brain stem auditory-evoked potential. CZ-Ai, vertex to ipsilateral ear, CZ-Ac, vertex to contralateral ear. Peaks in the upper waveform are labeled to show the customary designations. From Grundy BL: Intraoperative monitoring of sensory evoked potentials. Anesthesiology 58:72–87, 1983.

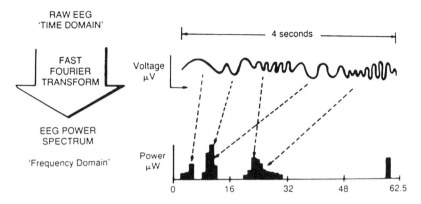

Figure 3. Power spectral analysis. The fast Fourier transform is a mathematical trick that converts a digitized time-varying voltage into a frequency-domain spectrum where the x-axis is frequency in Hz and the y-axis is power in watts. Thus, the slow waves present on the left side of the raw EEG are converted into the low-frequency bars of the spectral histogram, the intermediate frequency waves scattered through the raw EEG are translated in sum to the alpha range bars of the spectrum, and the fast voltage waves become the beta frequency components of the spectrum. There is a spectral signal at 60 Hz, representing the ubiquitous power line interference.

the several epochs (i.e., sampled data of 2–4 seconds in length) of EEG have changed the lines representing power spectra. CSA has proven to be useful during surgery and in the intensive care unit.[65]

Density modulated spectral array (DSA) displays the EEG power spectrum in either shades of gray or different colors, with areas of greatest density or largest dots in the frequencies making the greatest contribution to the EEG (Fig. 5). The sensitivity and specificity of DSA have been evaluated during carotid endarterectomy under general anesthesia.[66] The sensitivity ranged from 59% to 72%, while the specificity ranged from 96% to 99%.

Aperiodic Analysis

This modality analyzes the fast and slow wave components separately, then combines the data for display. Aperiodic analysis does not rely on averaging many waveforms over a given epoch. Aperiodic

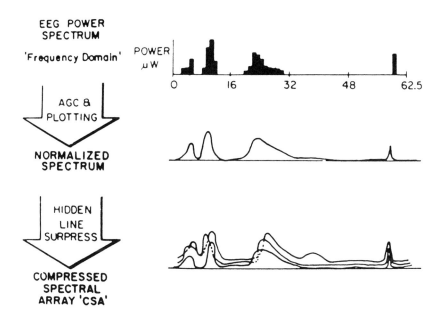

Figure 4. Compressed spectral array (CSA). Once a power spectrum has been formed by the fast Fourier transform (FFT) algorithm, it may be smoothed, its size adjusted for display, and plotted (on paper of screen). A new normalized spectrum is formed with each new epoch of raw EEG. If sequential normalized spectra are plotted adjacent to each other, and the "hidden lines" are identified and not drawn, then the result is a CSA display. Hidden lines are those portions of a spectra which, if spectra were opaque, would not be visible behind prior data. This hidden line suppression reduces visual ambiguity and lends an illusion of a third dimension to the display. A density spectral array replaces the height of the hills with density of dot patterns.

analysis can be useful in detecting intraoperative cerebral ischemia.[67]

Bi-Spectral Analysis of EEG

Bispectral analysis determines both EEG linear (frequency and power) and nonlinear (phase and harmonic) components, and quantitates the interfrequency phase coupling of EEG signals through an examination of the fundamental frequency components and their associated higher-order harmonic relationships. Bispectral analysis

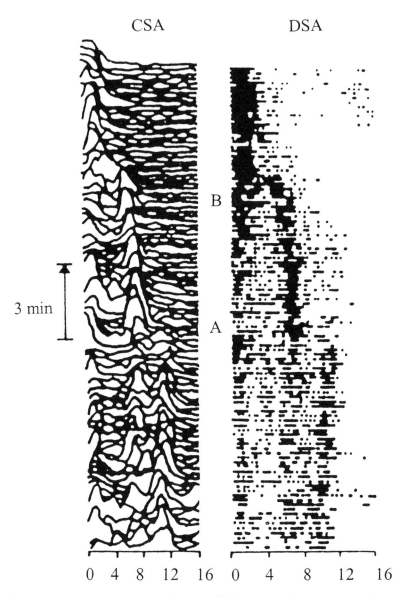

Figure 5. Compressed spectral array (CSA) versus density spectral array (DSA). A comparison of the linear (CSA) and density (DSA) displays of the spectral analysis in a patient during general anesthesia. From Levy WJ, Shapiro AM, Manuchak G, et al: Automated EEG processing for intraoperative monitoring: A comparison of techniques. Anesthesiology 53:223, 1980.

may be used to assess anesthetic depth and to predict hemodynamic responses to endotracheal intubation under opioid-based general anesthesia.[68]

Gas and Metabolic Monitoring

Jugular Venous Oxygen Saturation

Cerebral oxygen balance can be continuously assessed by measuring jugular venous oxygen saturation (SjO_2) with an oximetric catheter placed in the jugular venous bulb (Fig. 6). According to the

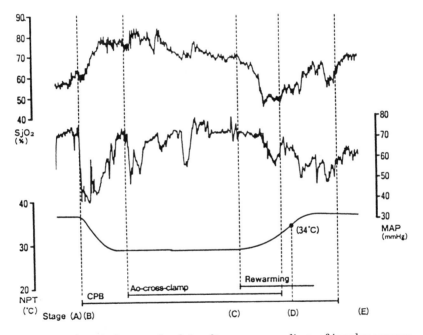

Figure 6. A typical example of simultaneous recordings of jugular venous oxyhemoglobin saturation (SjO_2), mean arterial blood pressure (MAP), and nasopharyngeal temperature (NPT) during cardiopulmonary bypass. Note that SjO_2 increases with cooling and decreases with rewarming. Stage A = within 5 min before initiation of cardiopulmonary bypass (CPB); stage B = within the first minute after initiation of CPB; stage C = during stable hypothermic CPB, 5–10 min before conduction of rewarming; stage D = during rewarming period at 34°C of NPT; stage E = 15 min after CPB. From Nakogima T, Kuro M, Mayashi Y, et al: Anesth Analg 74:630–635, 1992.

Fick principle, the arterio-jugular oxygen content difference ($AJDO_2$) should be equal to the cerebral metabolic rate for oxygen ($CMRO_2$) divided by CBF. If arterial oxygen content remains constant, the ratio of global $CBF/CMRO_2$ is proportional to the SjO_2. $AJDO_2$ above 9 mL O_2/100 mL blood indicates impending global ischemia.[69]

SjO_2 may be useful to manage in patients with raised intracranial pressure head injuries.[70-72] In addition, continuous SjO_2 may be useful during cardiopulmonary bypass.[73,74]

The effectiveness of therapy aimed at reducing ICP can be continuously assessed by SjO_2 monitoring. Hyperventilation is most effective in pediatric patients with cerebral hyperemia.[75] The benefit of barbiturates in providing a favorable outcome exists only when a low $AJDO_2$ returned to normal with therapy.[76] As measured by $AJDO_2$, mannitol is most effective when CBF autoregulation is preserved.[77]

SjO_2 monitoring has the potential for rapid detection and correction of impending global ischemia. Although global cerebral ischemia can be detected, focal cerebral ischemia may be missed by SjO_2. Continuous SjO_2 monitoring provides only relative information about regional cerebral metabolism and CBF.[78] Sampling errors may be increased at low global CBF.[79] The hypoxic threshold to cause cerebral dysfunction and the duration of compromised cerebral oxygen balance have yet to be investigated.

Near-Infrared Spectroscopy

Near-infrared spectroscopy (NIRS) noninvasively measures cerebral hemoglobin and cytochrome-aa3 oxygenation[80,81] (Fig. 7). NIRS is based on the concept that photons in the near-infrared spectrum (650–100 nm) can penetrate human tissue, including the skull and brain tissue, to a depth of several centimeters. Since the signal is not pulse-gated (different from the peripheral pulse oximetry), NIRS can be used under conditions of low flow and circulatory standstill, such as during cardiopulmonary bypass and cardiac arrest. The paradigms of NIRS have been validated in animal models.[82,83] Some individual variability exists for transcranial optical path length and light scattering, which may give rise to errors in quantifying HBO_2%.[84] NIRS measures hemoglobin in the arterial, venous, and capillary circulations; the proportion of those compartments may change at any time although a venous/capillary compartment of 70–80% and an arterial compartment of 20–30% are estimated.[85] In

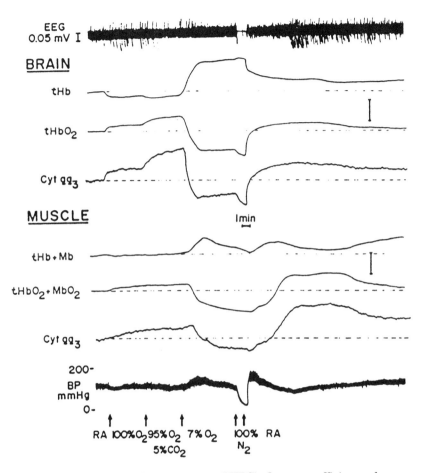

Figure 7. Near-infrared spectroscopy (NIRS). Oxygen sufficiency changes monitored simultaneously in cat's brain (by reflectance) and skeletal muscle (by transillumination of the thigh). EEG = electroencephalogram; tHb = tissue hemoglobin; tHbO$_2$ = tissue oxyhemoglobin; Mb = myoglobin; MbO$_2$ = oxygenated myoglobin; Bp = blood pressure; RA = room air. Adapted with permission from authors and publisher from Piantados CA, Hemstreet JM, VanderVliet FF: Near infrared spectroscopic monitoring of oxygen distribution to intact brain and skeletal muscle tissues. Crit Care Med 14: 698–706, 1986.

spite of these shortcomings, animal and clinical data suggesting the validity of NIRS measurement of cerebral hemoglobin saturation are accumulating. In an animal model, measurement of cytochrome-aa3 was verified by using mitochondrial electron transfer blockers.[86] Mild degrees of hypoxia decrease cytochrome-aa3 oxidation levels in human volunteers.[87] One study showed that isoflurane preserved a favorable redox state during severe hypoxia when compared with sevoflurane.[88] Clinical data are also accumulating in various situations during the intraoperative period and after cardiac arrest.[89–91] McCormick et al. demonstrated that the NIRS measurements were at least as responsive to progressive cerebral hypoxia as EEG.[90,91] Thus, NIRS may be a promising noninvasive monitor of cerebral oxygenation.

Summary

There have been many advances and improvements in monitoring. Although they appear useful in the perioperative period, all monitors have their specific limitations. Sophisticated monitors require special personnel and equipment. The sensitivity and specificity of these monitors should be determined before we regard any of them as the new "gold standard."

References

1. Mayhall CG, Archer NH, Lamb VA, Spadora AC, et al: Ventriculostomy-related infections: A prospective epidemiologic study. N Engl J Med 310: 553–559, 1984.
2. Kanter RK, Weiner LB, Patti AM, Robson LK: Infections complications and duration of intracranial pressure monitoring. Crit Care Med 13: 837–839, 1985.
3. Shellock FG: A fiberoptic transducer-tipped pressure catheter. Med Elec 16:103–106, 1985.
4. Chambers IR, Mendelow AD, Sinar EJ, Mohda P: A clinical evaluation of the Camino subdural screw and ventricular monitoring kits. Neurosurgery 26:421–423, 1990.
5. Yablon JS, Lantner H, McCormack TM, Nair S, et al: Clinical experience with a fiberoptic intracranial pressure monitor. J Clin Monit 91: 171–175, 1993.
6. Cruchflield JS, Narayan RK, Robertson CS, Michael LH: Evaluation of a fiberoptic intracranial pressure monitor. J Nerurosurg 72:482–487, 1990.
7. Gambaredella G, D'Avelia D, Tomasello F: Monitoring of brain tissue pressure with a fiber-optic device. Neurosurgery 31:918–922, 1992.

8. Hollingsworth-Fridlund P, Vos H, Daily EK: Use of fiber-optic pressure transducer for intracranial pressure measurements: A preliminary report. Heart Lung 17:111–120, 1988.
9. Aaslid R, Markwalder T, Nornes H: Noninvasive transcranial Doppler ultrasound recording of flow velocities in basal cerebral arteries. J Neurosurg 57:769–774, 1982.
10. Rahy TN: Cranial Doppler applications in neonatal critical care. Crit Care Clin 8:93–111, 1991.
11. Bishop CCR, Powell S, Rutt D, Brownse NL: Transcranial doppler measurements of middle cerebral artery flow velocity: A validation study. Stroke 17:913–915, 1986.
12. Thiel A, Russ W, Zeiler D, Dapper F, Hempelmann G: Transcranial Doppler sonography and somatosensory evoked potential monitoring in carotid surgery. Eur J Vasc Surg 4:597–602, 1990.
13. Verhaegen MJ, Todd MM, Warner DS: A comparison of cerebral ischemic flow threshold during halothane/N_2O and isoflurane/N_2O anesthesia in rats. Anesthesiology 76:743–754, 1992.
14. Dahl A, Russel D, Nyberg-Hansen R, Rootwelt K: A comparison of regional cerebral blood flow and middle cerebral artery blood flow velocities: Simultaneous measurements in healthy subjects. J Cereb Blood Flow Metab 12:1049–1054, 1992.
15. Caplan LR, Brass LM, DeWitt LD, et al: Transcranial Doppler ultrasound: present status. Neurology 40:696–700, 1990.
16. Pilato MA, Bissonnette B, Lerman J: Transcranial Doppler response of cerebral blood-flow velocity to carbon dioxide in anaesthetized children. Can J Anaesth 38:37–42, 1991.
17. Leon JR, Bissonnette B: Cerebrovascular responses to carbon dioxide in children anaesthetized with halothane and isoflurane. Can J Anaesth 38:817–825, 1991.
18. Leon JE, Bissonnette B: Cerebrovascular responses to carbon dioxide in children anaesthetized with halothane and isoflurane. Can J Anaesth 38:817–825, 1991.
19. Leon JE, Bissonnette B: Transcranial Doppler sonography: nitrous oxide and cerebral blood flow velocity in children. Can J Anaesth 38: 974–979, 1991.
20. Aaslid R, Huber P, Nornes H: Evaluation of cerebrovascular spasm with transcranial Doppler ultrasound. J Neurosurg 60:37–42, 1984.
21. Seiler RW, Grolimund P, Aaslid R, et al: Cerebral vasospasm evaluated by transcranial ultrasound correlated with clinical grade and CT-visualized subarachnoid hemorrhage. J Neurosurg 64:594–600, 1986.
22. Sloan MA, Haley EC Jr., Kassell NF, et al: Sensitivity and specificity of transcranial Doppler ultrasonography in the diagnosis of vasospasm following subarachnoid hemorrhage. Neurology 39:1514–1518, 1989.
23. Grosset DG, Straiton J, Du Trevou M, Bullock R: Prediction of symptomatic vasospasm after subarachnoid hemorrhage by rapidly increasing transcranial Doppler velocity and cerebral blood flow changes. Stroke 23:674–679, 1992.
24. Martin NA, Doberstein C, Zane C, et al: Posttraumatic cerebral arterial

spasm: Transcranial Doppler ultrasound, cerebral blood flow, angiographic foundings. J Neurosurg 77:575–583, 1992.

25. Chan KH, Dearden NM, Miller JD: The significance of posttraumatic increase in cerebral blood flow velocity: A transcranial Doppler ultrasound study. Neurosurgery 30:697–700, 1992.

26. Chan KH, Miller JD, Dearden NM: Intracranial blood flow velocity after head injury: Relationship to severity of injury, time, neurological status and outcome. J Neurol Neurosurg Psychiatry 55:787–791, 1992.

27. Werner C, Kochs E, Rau M, et al: Transcranial Doppler sonography as a supplement in the detection of cerebral circulatory arrest. J Neurosurg Anesthesiol 2:159–165, 1990.

28. Spencer MP, Thomas GI, Nicholis SC, Savage LR: Detection of middle cerebral artery emboli during transcranial Doppler ultrasonography. Stroke 21:415–423, 1990.

29. van Der Linden J, Casimir-Ahn H: When do cerebral emboli appear during open heart operations? A transcranial Doppler study. Ann Thorac Surg 51:237–241, 1991.

30. Nylor AR, Wildsmith JA, McClure J, Jenkins AM, Ruckley CV: Transcranial Doppler monitoring during carotid endarterectomy. Br J Surg 78:1264–1268, 1991.

31. Campbell DE, Raskin SA: Cerebral dysfunction after cardiopulmonary bypass: Aetiology, manifestations and interventions. Perfusion 5: 251–260, 1990.

32. van der Linden, Casimir-Ahn H: When do cerebral emboli appear during open heart operations? A transcranial Doppler study. Ann Thorac Surg 51:237–241, 1991.

33. Taylor RH, Burrows FA, Bissonnette B: Cerebral pressure-flow velocity relationship during hypothermic cardiopulmonary bypass in neonates and infants. Anesth Analg 74:636–642, 1992.

34. Obrist WD, Wilkinson WE: Regional cerebral blood flow measurement in humans by Xenon-133 clearance. Cerebrovasc Brain Metab Rev 2: 283–327, 1990.

35. Young WL, Prohovnik I, Schoroeder T, et al: Intraoperative ^{133}Xe cerebral blood flow measurements by intravenous veusus intracarotid methods. Anesthesiology 73:637–643, 1990.

36. Young WL, Prohovnik I, Ornstein E, Lucas LR, et al: Rapid monitoring of intraoperative cerebral bloodflow using [133]Xe. J Cereb Blood Flow Metab 8:691–696, 1988.

37. Zempella E, Morawetz RB, McDowell HA, et al: The importance of cerebral ischemia during carotid endarterectomy. Neurosurgery 29: 727–730, 1991.

38. Branston NM, Symon L, Crockard HA, Pasztor E: Relationship between the cortical evoked potential and local cortical blood flow following acute middle cerebral artery occlusion in the baboon. Exp Neurol 45:195–208, 1974.

39. Messick JM Jr, Casement B, Sharbrough F, et al: Correlation of regional cerebral blood flow (rCBF) with EEG changes during isoflurane anesthesia for carotid endarterectomy: Critical rCBF. Anesthesiology 66: 344–349, 1987.

40. Lam AM, Manninen PH, Ferguson GG, Nantau W: Monitoring electro-physiologic function during carotid endarterectomy: A comparison of somatosensory evoked potentials and conventional electroencephalogram. Anesthesiology 75:15–21, 1991.
41. Witzmann A, Beran H, Bohm-Jurkovic H, Loffler W: The prognostic value of somatosensory evoked potential monitoring and tumor data in supratentorial tumor removal. J Clin Monit 6:75–84, 1990.
42. Peterson DO, Drummond JC, Todd MM: Effects of halothane, enflurane, isoflurane and nitrous oxide on somatosensory evoked potentials in humans. Anesthesiology 65:35, 1986.
43. McPherson RW, Mahla M, Johnson R, et al: Effects of enflurane, isoflurane, and nitrous oxide on somatosensory evoked potetials during fentanyl anesthesia. Anesthesiology 62:626, 1985.
44. Sloan TB, Koht A: Depression of cortical somatosensory evoked potentials by nitrous oxide. Br J Anaesth 57:328, 1986.
45. Yingling CD, Gardi JN: Intraoperative monitoring of facial and cochlear nerves during acoustic neruroma surgery. Otolaryng Clin N Am 25:413–448, 1992.
46. Woods CC, Spencer DD, Allison T, McCarthy G, et al: Localization of human sensorimotor cortex during surgery by cortical surface recording of somatosensory evoked potentials. J Neurosurg 68:99–111, 1988.
47. Baik NW, Branston NM, Bentivoglio P, Symon I: The effects of experimental brain-stem ischemia on brain-stem auditory evoked potentials in primates. Electroencephalogr Clin Nerurophysiol 75:433–443, 1990.
48. Barelli A, Valente MR, Clemente A, Bozza P, et al: Serial multimodality-evoked potentials in severely head-injured patients: Diagnostic and prognostic implications. Crit Care Med 19:1374–1381, 1991.
49. Jessop J, Griffiths DE, Furness P, Jones JG, et al: Changes in amplitude and latency of the P300 component of the auditory evoked potential with sedative and anaesthetic concentrations of nitrous oxide. Br J Anaesth 67:524–531, 1991.
50. Schender D, Keller I, Schlund M, Klasing S, Madler C: Acoustic evoked potentials of medium latency and intraoperative wakefulness during anesthesia maintenance using propofol, isoflurane and flunitrazepam/fentanyl. Anaesthetist 40:214–221, 1991.
51. Plourde G, Boylan JF: The auditory steady state response during sufentanil anaesthesia. Br J Anaesth 66:683–691, 1991.
52. Madler C, Keller I, Schwender D, Poppel E: Sensory information processing during general anaesthesia: effect of isoflurane on auditory evoked neuronal oscillations. Br J Anaesth 66:81–87, 1991.
53. Stone JL, Ghaly RF, Levy WJ, Karth R, et al: A comparative analysis of enflurane anesthesia on primate motor and somatosensory evoked potentials. Electroencephalogr Clin Neurophysiol 84:180–187, 1992.
54. Firsching R, Heinen LM, Loeschke G: The effects of halothane and nitrous oxide on transcranial magnetic evoked potentials. Anaesthesiol Intensivmed Notfallmed Schmeruztber 26:381–383, 1991.
55. Browning JL, Heizer MI, Baskin DS: Variations in corticomotor and somatosensory evoked potentials: Effects of temperature, halothane an-

esthesia and arterial partial pressure of CO_2. Anesth Analg 74:643–648, 1992.

56. Taniguchi M, Cedzich C, Schramm J: Modification of cortical stimulation for motor evoked potentials under general anesthesia: Technical description. Neurosurgery 32:219–226, 1993.

57. Trojaborg W, Boysen G: Relation between EEG, regional cerebral blood flow and internal carotid artery pressure during carotid endarterectomy. Electroencephalogr Clin Neurophysiol 34:61, 1973.

58. Redekop G, Ferguson G: Correlation of contralateral stenosis and intraoperative electroencephalogram change with risk of stroke during carotid endarterectomy. Neurusurgery 30:191–194, 1992.

59. Kresowik TF, Worsey MJ, Khoury MD, Krain LS, et al: Limitations of electroencephalographic monitoring in the detection of cerebral ischemia accompanying carotid endarterectomy. J Vasc Surg 13:439–443, 1991.

60. Rampil IJ, Litt L, Mayevsky A: Correlated, simultaneous, multiple-wavelength optical monitoring in vivo of localized cerebrocortical NADH and brain microvessel hemoglobin oxygen saturation. J Clin Monit 8: 216–225, 1992.

61. Rampil IJ, Holzer JA, Quest DO, Rosenbaum SH, Correll JW: Prognostic value of computerized EEG analysis during carotid endarterectomy. Anesth Analg 62:533–543, 1983.

62. Russ W, Kling D, Krumholz G, Fraedrich G, Hemplemann G: Experience with a new spectral analyzing system (CSA) during carotid surgery. Anaesthetist 34:85–90, 1985.

63. Baker AB, Roxburgh AJ: Computerized EEG monitoring for carotid endarterectomy. Anaesth Intensive Care 14:32–36, 1986.

64. Tempelhoff R, Modica PA, Grubb RJ, Rich KM, Holtmann B: Selective shunting during carotid endarterectomy based on two-channel computerized electroencephalographic/compressed spectral array analysis. Neurosurgery 24:339–344, 1989.

65. Cant BR, Shaw NA: Electroencephalography and compressed spectral array in severe intracranial disease. Int Anaesthesiol Clin 17:343, 1979.

66. Kearse LA, Martin D, McPeck K, Lopez-Bresnahan M: Computer-derived density spectral array in detection of mild analog electroencephalographic ischemic pattern changes during carotid endarterectomy. J Neurosurg 78:884–890, 1993.

67. Spackman TN, Faust RJ, Cucchiara RF, Sharbrough FW: A comparison of a periodic analysis of the EEG with standard EEG and cerebral blood for detection of ischemia. Anesthesiology 66:229–231, 1986.

68. Kearse LA, Manberg P, deBros F, Chaumon N, Sinai V: Bispectral analysis of electroencephalography during induction of anesthesia may predict hemodynamic responses to laryngoscopy and intubation. Electroencephalogr Clin Neurophysiol 90:194–200, 1994.

69. Opbrist WD, Langfitt TW, Jaggi JL, et al: Cerebral blood flow and metabolism in comatose patients with acute head injury: Relationship to intracranial hypertension. J Neurosurg 61:241–253, 1984.

70. Sutton LN, McLaughlin AC, Dante S, Kotapka M, et al: Cerebral venous oxygen content as a measure of brain energy metabolism with increased

intracranial pressure and hyperventilation. J Neurosurg 73:927–932, 1990.

71. Andrews PJD, Dearden NM, Miller JD: Jugular bulb cannulation: description of a cannulation technique and validation of a new continuous monitor. Br J Anaesth 67:553–558, 1991.

72. Goetting MG, Preston G: Jugular bulb catheterization does not increase intracranial pressure. Intens Care Med 17:195–198, 1991.

73. Nakajima T, Kuro M, Hayashi Y, Kitaguchi K, et al: Clinical evaluation of cerebral oxygen balance during cardiopulmonary byapass: On-line continuous monitoring of jugular venous oxyghemoglobin saturation. Anesth Analg 74:630–635, 1992.

74. Kuwabara M, Nakajima N, Yamamoto F, et al: Continuous monitoring of blood oxygen saturation of internal jugular vein as a useful indicator for selective cerebral perfusion during aortic arch replacement. J Thorac Cardiovasc Surg 103:355–362, 1992.

75. Bruce DA, Raphaely RC, Goldberg AI: Pathophysiology, treatment and outcome following severe head injury in children. Childs Brain 5:174–191, 1979.

76. Sari A. Matayoshi Y, Yonei A, et al: Cerebral arteriovenous oxygen content difference during barbiturate therapy in patients with acute brain damage. Anesth Analg 65:1196–1200, 1986.

77. Muizelaar JP, Lutz HA, Becker DP: Effect of mannitol on ICP and CBF and correlation with pressure autoregulation in severely head-injured patients. J Neurosurg 61:700–706, 1984.

78. Robertson JC, Narayan R, Gokastan Z, et al: Cerebral arteriovenous oxygen difference as an estimate of cerebral blood flow in comatose patients. J Neurosurg 70:222–230, 1989.

79. Robertson CS, Carayan RK, Gokaslan ZL, et al: Cerebral arteriovenous oxygen difference as an estimate of cerebral blood flow in comatose patients. J Neurosurg 70:222–230, 1989.

80. Brazy JE: Cerebral oxygen monitoring with near infrared spectroscopy: Clinical application to neonates. J Clin Monit 7:325–334, 1991.

81. Brown RW: Continuous monitoring of cerebral hemoglobin oxygen saturation. Int Anesth Clin 31:141–158, 1993.

82. McCormick PW, Stewart M, Ray P, Lewis G, et al: Measurement of regional cerebrovascular haemoglobin oxygen saturation in cats using optical spectroscopy. Neurol Res 13:65–70, 1991.

83. Ferrari M, Wilson DA, Hanley DF, Hartmann JF, Rogers MC, et al: Noninvasive determination of hemoglobin saturation in dogs by derivative near-infrared spectroscopy. Am J Physiol 256 (suppl 25):1493–1499, 1989.

84. Kurth CD, Steven JM, Benaron D, Chance B: Near-infrared monitoring of the cerebral circulation. J Clin Monit 9:163–170, 1993.

85. Portnoy H, Chopp M, Branch C: Hydraulic model of myogenic autoregulation and the cerebrovascular bed: the effects of altering systemic arterial pressure. Neurosurgery 13:482–498, 1983.

86. Okada K, Ohsima T, Inada E, et al: Validity of cerebral cytochrome oxidase measurement in vivo by near infrared spectroscopy. Anesthesiology 77:A499, 1992.

87. Hampson NB, Camporesi EM, Stolp BW, et al: Cerebral oxygen avail-ability by NIR spectroscopy during transient hypoxia in humans. J Appl Physiol 69:907–913, 1990.
88. Inada E, Okada K, Ohshima T, et al: Isoflurane is more protective against cerebral hypoxia than is sevoflurane: Near infrared spectro-scopic study. Anesthesiology 79:A394, 1993.
89. Smith DS, Levy W, Maris M, Chance B: Reperfusion hyperoxia in brain after circulatory arrest in humans. Anesthesiology 73:12–19, 1990.
90. McCormick PW, Stewart M, Goetting MG, Dijovny M, et al: Noninvasive cerebral optical spectroscopy for monitoring cerebral oxygen delivery and hemodynamics. Crit Care Med 19:89–97, 1991.
91. McCormick PW, Stewart M, Goetting MG, Balakrishnan G: Regional cerebrovascular oxygen saturation measured by optical spectroscopy in humans. Stroke 22:596–602, 1991.

17

The Role
of the Anesthesiologist
in Rehabilitation

Anthony P. Randazzo III, MD

Introduction

Optimal care of the traumatically injured patient is best provided by a team approach that uses coordinated efforts in all aspects
of the patient's course: from pre-hospital to hospital admission, assessment, therapy, and into the rehabilitative phase. Anesthesiologists are uniquely qualified to provide care throughout this continuum. There is an increasing need for the skills an anesthesiologist
uses that may enhance the overall quality of the care provided. In
particular, these skills lie in the areas of physiological monitoring
and therapeutic interventions typical of the intensive care units, and
in the application of regional anesthesia techniques available for
pain management and rehabilitation.

The impact of trauma on the general well-being of the nation is

From *Trauma Anesthesia and Critical Care of Neurological Injury,* edited by K. J.
Abrams and C. M. Grande. © 1997, Futura Publishing Co., Armonk, NY.

enormous.[1] Well over 50 million injuries occur annually with approximately 100,000 deaths resulting from accidents. Over 400,000 persons have permanently disabling injuries. Additionally, there are over 1 million temporarily disabling injuries. Two million persons annually sustain traumatic brain injury (TBI); of these, over 500,000 have injuries severe enough to warrant hospitalization.[2] Ten thousand individuals annually incur spinal cord injury (SCI).[3] The overall economic toll is staggering with the total lifetime costs of care in excess of 180 billion dollars in 1988.[4] The indirect costs are incalculable in terms of both the loss of income and the long-term care required for the majority of severely injured trauma patients.

In addition to the economic toll, trauma exerts its greatest impact on the patient directly as a result of the physical pain and suffering sustained, as well as the possibility of prolonged and perhaps permanent disability. Rehabilitative efforts are directed at minimizing disability, and in this area anesthesiologists can make a significant contribution to patient care.

The Role of Rehabilitation

Rehabilitation is a process that spans multiple disciplines and physiological applications. For example, one component of rehabilitation is the restoration of proper nutrition, nitrogen balance, and lean body mass. Another is psychological, such as the diagnosis and treatment of post-traumatic stress. Cardiovascular rehabilitation follows myocardial infarction and cardiac surgery. Pulmonary rehabilitation can be as simple as patient positioning and incentive spirometry, or as complex as sophisticated ventilatory management.

The treatment of pain has long been an area of particular interest to anesthesiologists. Beyond the care provided to the patient during the preoperative, intraoperative, and immediate postoperative periods, the importance of understanding pain mechanisms and pain therapy on the rehabilitative process has gained increasing recognition. The objective of any rehabilitation program is to restore the patient to a maximally independent, functional, and pain-free existence, in short, full recovery to their pre-injury state of health. With the great numbers of disabling injuries that occur, this is not always possible. In a 1-year follow-up of 114 severely injured patients, it was revealed that 55% of those surviving had returned to a productive life, which was attributed in large part to the rehabilitation regimens they had undertaken during their hospitalization.[5] Aside from trauma-related deformities such as amputations, blindness, and other injuries that preclude the ability to fully recover, rehabilitation of the trauma patient has become a priority; instituting prompt and aggressive rehabilitative efforts enhances the likelihood of full functional recovery. Also, treatment of spinal cord-injured patients in a comprehensive trauma center that provides early rehabilitation leads to a reduction in medical complications, more appropriate surgical care, and decreased total length of hospitalization, as advances toward recovery are made more efficiently.[6,7]

Patients with central nervous system injury, especially those with traumatic brain injury, present a particular challenge. They may present with associated injuries, such as extremity fractures, dislocations, vascular injuries, etc., that would otherwise be treated with standard therapies (e.g., systemically administered opioids). However, the sedative effects of these medications are undesirable in the setting of an altered sensorium. The pain of associated injuries may impair neurological evaluation and may negatively impact on diagnostic and therapeutic interventions. The application of regional anesthetic techniques should be used in these instances. Anesthesiologists, by virtue of their knowledge of neural anatomy and physiology, coupled with that of applied pharmacology, should be integral members of the team that treats patients during the rehabilitative phase of their injuries. There are several types of injuries and a variety of approaches to their treatment; most will be addressed throughout the remainder of this chapter.

Pathophysiology of Injury

The Effects of Pain

Some of the most common injuries are those involving the extremities with orthopedic, vascular, and neurological injuries presenting individually or, more frequently, in combination. Acute pain is a hallmark of injury, which, in the immediate post-injury phase, is mediated by afferent A delta and C fibers. Segmental reflex responses result in the increase in skeletal muscle tension seen following injury. Other spinal cord components such as wide dynamic range neurons, interneurons, and flexor motor neurons are sensitized and lead to the persistence of tenderness and hyperalgesia seen following injury.[8] The development of chronic pain is a complex process that involves a variety of other nervous system components including the autonomic system, as well as psychological factors.

The response to pain is multifaceted and is modulated by several factors, most notably the patient's particular psyche, the actions of endorphins, and other modifiers. Pain impacts on the rehabilitative process in several ways. First, pain in the affected limb will limit the range of motion and perhaps lead directly to or increase the likelihood of functional impairment. Second, pain results in central sympathetic nervous system activation,[8] leading to increased circulating norepinephrine (from synaptic activity) and epinephrine (from stimulation of the adrenal medulla). These catecholamines have well-documented effects on the cardiovascular system, and continued elevations may be deleterious in certain patients, particularly those with underlying cardiovascular disease.[9] Also, the so-called stress hormones—ACTH, cortisol, glucagon, and ADH—have increased activity and in general promote catabolism, again with the potential for increased activity to be a cause for concern.[10,11] Third, there are alterations in the activity of the kinins, the products of arachidonic acid metabolism—prostaglandins, leukotrienes, and thromboxane—as well as cytokines such as tumor necrosis factor (TNF) and the interleukins. The kinins, interleukins, and prostaglandins are components of the local inflammatory reaction that commences following injury.[12] These and other mediators may have multiple systemic effects predominantly on organ function, regional perfusion, and the development of adult respiratory distress syndrome (ARDS) and multi-organ failure associated with trauma.[13,14] These complications are more frequently seen in the severely injured patient who, in fact, may merit more intensive rehabilitative efforts.

Approaches to Pain Management

The traditional approach to the management of pain had been the administration of parenteral and oral analgesics: narcotics and nonsteroidal anti-inflammatory drugs (NSAIDs). These agents have been supplanted by newer and more physiologically appropriate regimens such as continuous patient-controlled analgesia (PCA) typically administered intravenously, and regional anesthetic techniques. The benefits of these approaches have been well documented: decreased breakthrough pain,[15] increased patient satisfaction,[16] improvements in ventilatory function,[17] and earlier mobilization and ambulation.[18]

With extremity injuries, the benefits of the institution of early rehabilitation cannot be overemphasized because of the implications for improvements in long-term functional outcome. It is essential that care is rendered in an integrated fashion: the appropriate rehabilitation regimen is designed and implemented, and analgesic approaches are then tailored to assist in allowing the patient to maximize their efforts.

It would be ideal to block sensation prior to injury in order to prevent the stress response. To this end, regional anesthetic techniques offer perhaps the most effective interventions. Not only is pain relieved, but the endocrine-metabolic responses to pain are attenuated when compared to systemically administered analgesics.[19-22] However, this relates only to the use of local anesthetics; this attenuation is not seen with narcotics alone given by epidural injection.[23] There may also be a psychological benefit to reduce anxiety relating to the extent of the injury, i.e., a severe (potentially incapacitating) injury will be better tolerated if the patient is pain-free.[24]

In the acute phase of trauma care, the priorities lie in establishing and maintaining physiological integrity: the ABCs of trauma care.[25] Pain management is not often regarded as a priority, but should follow closely once these life-saving maneuvers have been instituted, beginning as early as possible once the patient is stabilized. It is also prudent to consider the approaches to postoperative (or post-admission, if the patient is not brought to the operating room) pain management.

The Role of Regional Anesthesia Techniques

Regional anesthesia has long been used in the acute treatment of trauma. In 1946, Beecher advocated regional (intercostal or paravertebral) blocks for chest wall injuries. He described normalization of pulmonary function and "striking relief."[26] Bion, more recently, used regional anesthetic techniques, including 14 axillary blocks, in 73 patients wounded in combat.[27] He also used isobaric bupivicaine spinal anesthetics in 29 patients with lower extremity injuries (including those in shock) and documented safety and speed of induction, decreased risk of aspiration, and analgesia extending into the postoperative period.[28] Hughes, in 1983, reported a 92% success rate using interscalene blocks to provide analgesia for closed reductions of Colles' fractures in the emergency department.[29] Interscalene blocks have also been successfully performed by non-anesthesiologists in treating orthopedic trauma.[30]

Patients with traumatic brain injury and spinal cord injury resulting in paralysis are of special concern. They are at risk of developing extremity contractures, spastic conditions, pressure ulcers, bowel and bladder dysfunction, and other complications. Of these, spasticity and contractures are often treated by performance of specific nerve blocks. There is also a significant incidence of peripheral nerve injuries (particularly involving the brachial plexus) that often are not diagnosed on initial presentation; these may subsequently lead to functional impairment or spasticity.[31] Early rehabilitative efforts, while medical and neurological status is being stabilized,[32] has been demonstrated to significantly reduce length of hospitalization[33] and lead to functional improvement. The application of regional anesthetic techniques may therefore be of considerable benefit in facilitating the prompt commencement of a rehabilitative regimen.

Regional Anesthesia Approaches and Specific Injuries

Regional anesthesia can be used for almost any operative situation. Its successful application depends on the knowledge of applied neural anatomy, anesthetic pharmacology and physiology, and the complications associated with each.[34] Regional anesthesia is administered by topical application, local infiltration, individual peripheral nerve blocks, plexus blocks, and central neuraxial blockade (subarachnoid or epidural). The successful institution of individual peripheral nerve and plexus blocks may be facilitated by the use of nerve stimulators that can assist in the verification of proper needle location, particularly when these nerves are not superficially situated. Although "single-shot" techniques are effective in the intraoperative and early postoperative phases and may be repeated as indicated (for instance, the use of repeated intercostal blocks for rib fractures), continuous techniques provide analgesia for several days into the recovery phase and facilitate early rehabilitative intervention.

The types of injuries for which regional techniques are particularly well suited have predominantly been extremity injuries. Thoracic injuries, because of the resultant and often significant adverse effects on pulmonary function, are increasingly being managed with regional anesthesia. Orthopedic and vascular trauma comprise the greatest percentage of extremity trauma.[35] Peripheral nerve injury is frequently associated with these and carries the greatest implication in terms of subsequent functional recovery.[36,37] Fractures, dislocations, tendon, muscle, and ligament injuries are typically consequences of blunt trauma, such as falls and motor vehicle accidents involving both pedestrians and passengers. Penetrating trauma, in particular gunshot wounds, also accounts for a percentage of orthopedic trauma.[37] Vascular injuries, with arterial injuries being more significant, are more commonly a result of penetrating trauma from stab and gunshot wounds. They may also appear in conjunction with other injuries, for example, popliteal artery disruption occurring with posterior knee dislocation,[36,38] and brachial artery injury occurring with humeral fracture.[39] Other extremity injuries include amputations and crushing. The development of compartment syndrome is a potentially limb-threatening complication. Some injuries may need to be addressed immediately or subsequently with reimplantation, skin grafting, flap reconstruction, and other surgical techniques. Regional anesthetic techniques should be considered and possibly utilized in all these situations.

Regional anesthetic techniques are also useful in the diagnosis and management of the chronic complications of trauma, for instance, reflex sympathetic dystrophy,[40,41] and phantom limb pain.[42]

Approaches to Extremity Injuries

Upper extremity injuries have the potential for being devastating because of the great potential for subsequent prolonged or permanent disability that may prevent the patient from resuming employment. In perhaps no other situation (other than traumatic brain or spinal cord injury) is rehabilitation as critical to eventual functional outcome than in the setting of an injury to a dominant extremity. Lower extremity injuries impact on subsequent mobility. Even with the development and highly successful use of sophisticated surgical repairs, the rate of functional impairment remains high.[36] This is, in large part, due to associated nerve injuries. However, aside from these considerations, it is usually an objective of postoperative or post-injury care that the patient begin range-of-motion exercises in order to limit the potential for functional disability. For instance, a wrist fracture may require open fixation; postoperatively, the patient may need to do finger flexion-extension exercises to minimize the possibility of scarring of the tendinous sheaths. Continuous passive range-of-motion devices may be used to great benefit. However, pain may limit the patient's ability to maximally comply with therapy.

In the setting of head injury and altered sensorium, the presence of pain resulting from an injured extremity may alter the ability to obtain an accurate neurological evaluation. The treatment of their pain should ideally have minimal effect on their neurological status.

Pain control is obviously a primary concern when considering a regional anesthetic, particularly on a continuous basis; an important secondary concern is the sympathectomy that results in addition to attenuation of somatic impulses. This has implications in terms of extremity blood flow and perfusion.[43-45] A reduction is seen in the incidence and magnitude of vasospasm, as well as improved micro-vascular flow,[46] both of which may directly enhance the integrity of vascular and flap repairs that are used in treating severely injured limbs.[43,44,47,48]

The Upper Extremity

The upper extremity nervous supply is provided by the brachial plexus, which arises from the nerve roots of the fifth through eight cervical segments, and the first thoracic segment (Figs. 1 and 2). Surgery under brachial plexus blockade was first performed by Halsted in 1884, who infiltrated the nerves with cocaine under direct vision following exposure in the neck.[49] Herschel, in 1911, used the first percutaneous approach via the axilla.[50] Today, there are several well-documented and effective approaches to brachial plexus blockade, each with some distinct advantages and disadvantages (Table 1). The plexus may be blocked at various sites as it courses from the neck and joins the subclavian artery and vein beyond the thoracic outlet, and then proceeds into the axilla inferior to the pectoralis minor muscle contained in an investing layer of cervical prevertebral fascia called the axillary sheath.[51] Interscalene, perivascular subclavian (supraclavicular), infraclavicular, infracoracoid, and axillary approaches have all been described. Of these, however, the interscalene and axillary approaches appear to be the most clinically relevant, principally because continuous analgesia is readily achieved. This is accomplished by the percutaneous insertion of a catheter that permits repeated injections or a continuous infusion of local anesthetics. The axillary approach (Fig. 3) has the advantages of easily definable anatomy (identification of the axillary artery at the edge of the pectoralis minor muscle), few associated complications (intravascular injection, direct nerve injury, and hematoma formation), and a high rate of success. DeJong, in a classic article, provided

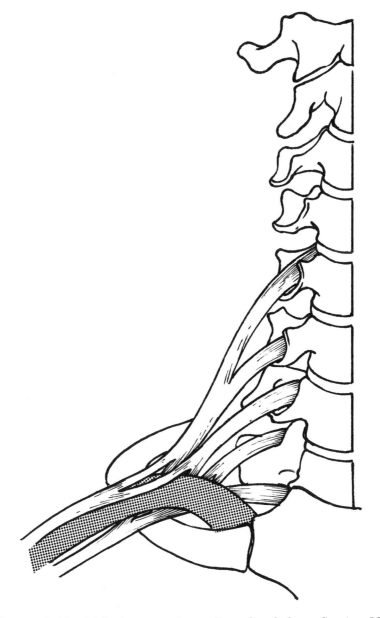

Figure 1. Brachial plexus anatomy. Reproduced from Cousins MJ, Bridenbaugh PO, eds: Neural Blockade in Clinical Anesthesia and Management of Pain, 2nd ed. JB Lippincott Co., Philadelphia, 1988.

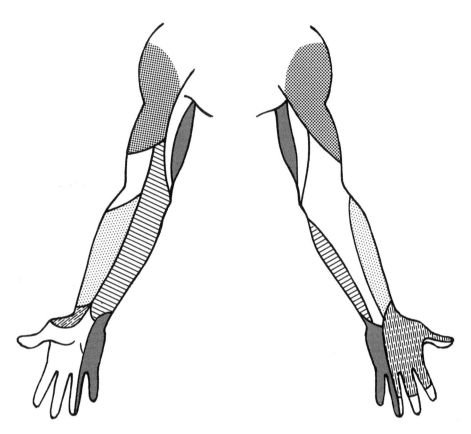

Figure 2. Cutaneous nerve distribution to the upper extremity. Reproduced from Miller RD, ed: Anesthesia, 4th ed. New York, Churchill Livingstone, 1994.

detailed anatomic studies of the axillary approach, and reported a 91.5% success rate in a clinical series of 93 patients.[52] He also noted that a volume of between 40 and 50 mL was necessary to assure adequate infiltration at the level of the cords in the mid-axilla. This is just prior to the division of the plexus into terminal nerves. Infiltration at this level will most reliably result in complete extremity anesthesia. Selander reported on a series of 137 patients; in some cases, analgesia was insufficient in the musculocutaneous and radial distributions. However, a fairly short (47 mm) catheter was used. There

Table 1
Regional Anesthesia Approaches to the Upper Extremity

Methods of Brachial Plexus Blockade
  (Will provide sensory and motor blockade to the entire upper extremity with
    the exception of the area adjacent to the axilla which is supplied by the
    intercostobrachials)
  Interscalene
  Supraclavicular
  Infraclavicular
  Infracoracoid
  Axillary

Individual Nerve Blockade
  (Will provide only sensory blockade to the areas distal to the nerves; typically
    blocked at either the elbow or the wrist)
  Musculocutaneous
  Median
  Radial
  Ulnar
  Digital Nerves (Palmar and Dorsal)

were also several cases of arterial puncture, and the failure rate (no anesthetic effect) was 20%.[53]

Ang et al. placed axillary catheters in 52 patients with a 98% rate; one catheter was left in place for 9 days without sequelae, illustrating the potential for longer-term use.[54] There was one incidence of arterial puncture. The musculocutaneous nerve is sometimes incompletely infiltrated because it departs the axillary sheath at some distance above the axilla.[55] However, if sufficient volume is administered initially (approximately 40 mL), then there is an increased likelihood of obtaining satisfactory blockade of the musculocutaneous nerve. Also, advancing the catheter further cephalad will bring its distal port closer to the takeoff of the musculocutaneous nerve; this was the case in Ang's study, where an 80-mm catheter was inserted. With the use of continuous infusions of local anesthetics, the nerve is also more reliably infiltrated.[56]

Thompson and Rorie performed detailed anatomic, radiographic, and histologic studies in cadavers and volunteers.[51] They demonstrated radiographically the presence of septa that invest individual nerves arising in continuity from the same fascial layer that forms the sheath. These septa are in continuity high in the plexus,

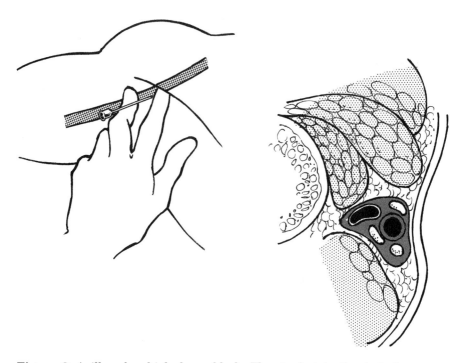

Figure 3. Axillary brachial plexus block. The single injection technique illustrated above can be simply modified for placement of a catheter by using a catheter-through-needle technique. Reproduced from Cousins MJ, Bridenbaugh PO, eds: Neural Blockade in Clinical Anesthesia and Management of Pain, 2nd ed. JB Lippincott Co., Philadelphia, 1988.

but as individual nerves arise, distinct compartments are formed. The factors contributing to a successful block were the diffusion between septa, the extent of proximal spread, and passage between adjacent compartments via interseptal connections.

Winnie in 1970 described the interscalene approach (Fig. 4) to the plexus, and included the use of a continuous catheter technique,[57] which others have also demonstrated to be successful.[58] This study provided radiographic evidence for the presence of an investing perivascular sheath encompassing the plexus and vascular structures. Also demonstrated was the importance of adequate volume administration relating to extent of blockade. The interscalene approach may be somewhat more difficult because of the necessity of identifying the interscalene groove. The use of a nerve stimulator facilitates this process, especially in patients who may not be able to assist (e.g., those under general anesthesia). The interscalene approach is also associated with more significant complications than the axillary approach because of the proximity of several important structures. For example, intravascular injection of local anesthetic into the vertebral artery results in immediate central nervous system toxicity. Phrenic nerve paralysis is an almost universally observed phenomenon; unilateral diaphragmatic palsy has been documented by ultrasonographic studies,[59] and patients with severe underlying pulmonary disease may not tolerate the resultant de-

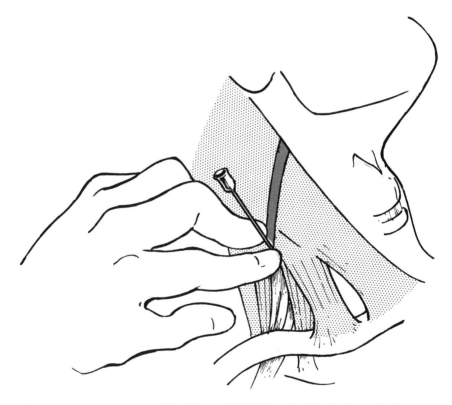

Figure 4. Interscalene brachial plexus block. The single injection technique illustrated above can be simply modified for placement of a catheter by using a catheter-through-needle technique. Reproduced from Cousins, MJ, Bridenbaugh, PO, eds: Neural Blockade in Clinical Anesthesia and Management of Pain, 2nd ed. JB Lippincott Co. 1988.

crease in vital capacity.[60] Subarachnoid and epidural injections have also been seen. Pneumothorax is another complication and is often a reason given to avoid the use of the technique.[52] It is important to note, however, that the plexus lies in a superficial position in the groove, and a probing needle should penetrate no more than 2.5 cm before a paresthesia or nerve stimulator response is elicited. The interscalene approach does require positioning of the arm.[61] With either technique, however, the success rate remains high (greater than 90%) with catheter insertion. Recently, Pham-Dang et al. described a technique of axillary catheter insertion that, utilizing venography and fluoroscopy, had a 100% success rate.[62] Axillary or interscalene catheters may be used for operative anesthesia alone or in combination with a general anesthetic.

Several local anesthetics are available for use singly or in combination; lidocaine 1.5% with epinephrine 1:200,000 or plain bupivicaine 0.5% are certainly effective. For postoperative or nonoperative analgesia, bupivicaine 0.25% by infusion at 6 to 8 mL/hr, following a bolus of 15 to 20 mL, provides excellent results. Catheters can remain in place for several days and should be treated as central venous access lines in terms of local care.

The Lower Extremity

The lower extremities are frequent sites of injury in the traumatized patient. Pedestrian trauma results in fractures of all the long bones and the pelvis, as well as dislocations of all three joints: hip, knee, and ankle. Vascular trauma is also common, due to the superficial course of the femoral artery and its divisions.[63] One of the tenets of rehabilitation is patient mobilization: early ambulation reduces the possibility of complications such as deep venous thrombosis and pulmonary dysfunction. To this end, many fractures are treated operatively, either with internal or external fixation devices. More severe injuries may involve neurovascular injury as well, and some open fractures have extensive soft tissue injury requiring skin grafting and local or free flap reconstruction. These patients may have several procedures within a relatively short period of time (e.g., a week), and in these cases, an epidural catheter can serve to provide intraoperative anesthesia as well as continuous postoperative analgesia. Again, it is essential to maximize the ability of the patient to have pain-free mobility, from passive range-of-motion to ambulation. Although epidural analgesia is the most commonly used technique, there are

Table 2
Regional Anesthesia Approaches to the Lower Extremity

Epidural (will provide bilateral lower extremity sensory and motor blockade)
Lumbar Plexus
Inguinal Paravascular ("3-in-1")
Femoral
Sciatic
Obturator
Popliteal
Lateral Femoral Cutaneous
Saphenous
Tibial
Common Peroneal
Ankle

several alternative approaches. These may be beneficial when there is some concern regarding the complications of epidural analgesia, e.g., hypotension, urinary retention, etc. In patients with unstable cardiovascular status, especially among the elderly, central neuraxial blockade may be undesirable.

Regional anesthesia approaches to the lower extremity are particularly innovative (Table 2) because the nervous supply is not compactly assembled as it is in the upper extremity. The lumbar plexus (Fig. 5) is formed by the ventral rami of the first three lumbar nerves and the major part of the fourth lumbar nerve.[64,65] It passes between the psoas muscle posteriorly and anterior to the quadratus lumborum, and is invested by fascia arising from both muscles. In an effort to avoid the large volumes of local anesthetics necessary to individually block the nerves of the lower extremity (lateral femoral cutaneous, femoral, obturator, and sciatic) (Fig. 6), investigators have sought ways to infiltrate multiple nerves with a single injection. This was demonstrated by Winnie with the infrainguinal, or "3-in-1," block of the femoral nerve[64] (Fig. 7). He noted the necessity of injecting a minimum of 20 mL volume of local anesthetic to achieve satisfactory blockade of the lateral femoral cutaneous, femoral, and obturator nerves. Analgesia will be effectively provided about the hip,[66] and a catheter technique has been demonstrated to successfully provide analgesia both intraoperatively and postoperatively for procedures involving the knee.[67] Radiographic studies demonstrated proximal and distal spread of contrast in the femoral sheath, with analgesia effectively provided in the obturator and lateral femoral

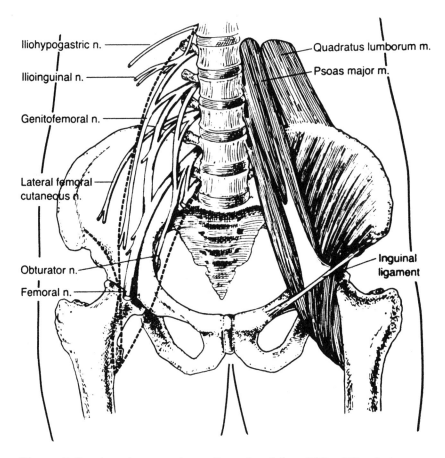

Iliohypogastric n.

Ilioinguinal n.

Genitofemoral n.

Lateral femoral
cutaneous n.

Obturator n.

Femoral n.

Quadratus lumborum m.

Psoas major m.

Inguinal
ligament

Figure 5. Lumbar plexus anatomy. Reproduced from Miller RD, ed: Anesthesia, 4th ed. Churchill Livingstone, New York, 1994.

cutaneous distributions because of proximal spread. The psoas compartment block was described by Chayen et al.[65] Although a single injection was performed, a lumbar plexus catheter may be inserted and has been used to provide analgesia for femur fractures.[68] However, analgesia may not be satisfactory in the desired distribution due the wide spacing of the lumbar nerves.[65]

The lumbar and sacral plexuses are widely separated, without the continuity of fascial sheaths; therefore, the sciatic nerve must be approached separately (Fig. 8). Single injections are most commonly

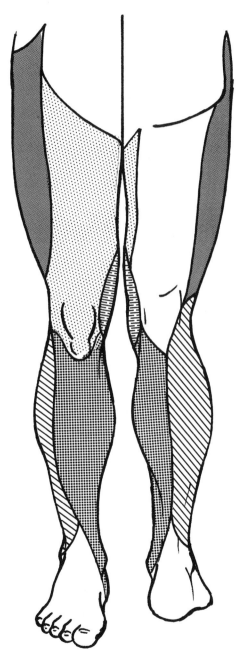

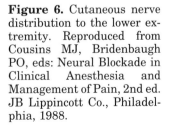

Figure 6. Cutaneous nerve distribution to the lower extremity. Reproduced from Cousins MJ, Bridenbaugh PO, eds: Neural Blockade in Clinical Anesthesia and Management of Pain, 2nd ed. JB Lippincott Co., Philadelphia, 1988.

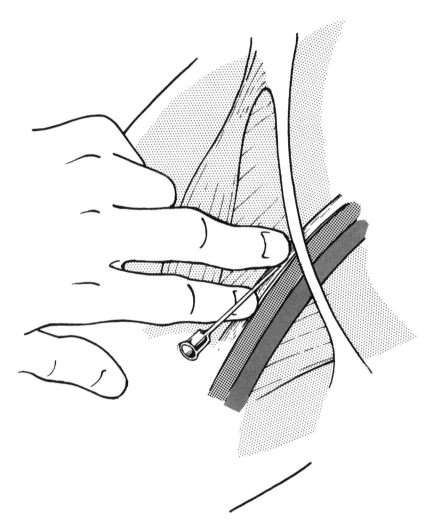

Figure 7. Inguinal paravascular block ("3-in-1"). Reproduced from Cousins MJ, Bridenbaugh PO, eds: Neural Blockade in Clinical Anesthesia and Management of Pain, 2nd ed. JB Lippincott Co., Philadelphia, 1988.

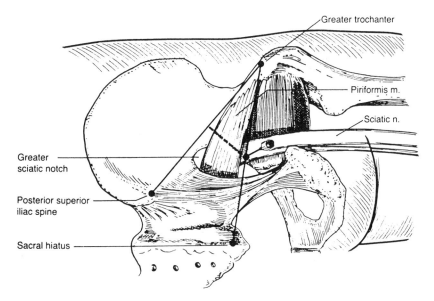

Figure 8. Sciatic nerve block: classical (posterior) approach. Reproduced from Miller RD, ed: Anesthesia, 4th ed. Churchill Livingstone, New York, 1994.

used, but analgesia may also be provided with a catheter placed near the sciatic nerve.[69] Complete analgesia of the lower extremity can be achieved with catheters inserted near the femoral and sciatic nerves. The use of a nerve stimulator-assisted approach is recommended in order to enhance the likelihood of successful catheter placement.

Excellent analgesia for vascular injuries of the lower extremity can be administered with a continuous infusion via an epidural catheter. Although there is scant surgical literature regarding outcome data vis-a-vis anesthetic management of vascular injuries, there is clear improvement in perfusion under regional anesthesia as a result of sympathetic blockade.[44] This may not be of great concern in large vessel injury and repair, but certainly microvascular anastomoses may benefit: (1) a reduction in pain will decrease sympathetically (i.e., alpha-agonist) and humorally (i.e., prostaglandins and thromboxane) mediated vasoconstriction[70]; (2) as a result of sympathectomy, arterial and venous vasodilatation maximizes perfusion.

Whenever a regional anesthetic is used in managing pain associated with an injured extremity, it is imperative that meticulous attention be paid to the affected extremity. Pain is one of the signs of complications such as compartment syndrome and infection, and there have been reports of such diagnoses being masked by regional analgesia,[71] as well as resulting from them.[72]

Approaches to Thoracic Injuries

Thoracic injuries are a common feature of blunt trauma, particularly drivers of motor vehicles involved in collisions. Rib fractures, pulmonary contusions and lacerations, pneumothorax, etc. are frequently observed. Penetrating trauma to the thorax will typically result in a tube thoracostomy being performed and possibly an exploratory thoracotomy. Thoracotomy may also be performed during laparotomy if indicated.

Significant pain is associated with thoracic wounds, and is transmitted by the intercostal nerves supplying the injured area (Fig. 9). This pain has a resultant adverse impact on respiratory function as patients tend to minimize inspirations during tidal breathing and avoid deep inspiratory efforts and coughing.[73] This is particularly true in patients with multiple rib fractures involving the lower segments as these segments have the greatest motion during deep inspirations. Additionally, pulmonary physiotherapy is poorly tolerated. The pulmonary complications are significant: (1) poor inspiratory efforts result in atelectasis and decreased functional residual capacity (FRC), with ventilation/perfusion mismatching leading to hypoxemia; (2) decreased vital capacity; (3) increased dead space to tidal volume ratio results in the need to increase minute ventilation to maintain eucapnia; (4) uncleared secretions can obstruct airways and increase the risk of infectious complications; and (5) possible need for prolonged mechanical ventilatory support.[17,74,75] Patients with underlying pulmonary disease are at markedly higher risk for developing pulmonary complications.[76] Effective rehabilitation then depends on the institution of pulmonary physiotherapy: the use of incentive spirometry and other maneuvers, manual chest physiotherapy, and patient mobilization. Adequate pain management is imperative. Systematically administered (either parenterally or orally) opioid analgesia, at doses sufficient to provide satisfactory analgesia, may produce an undesirable depression of respiratory drive.

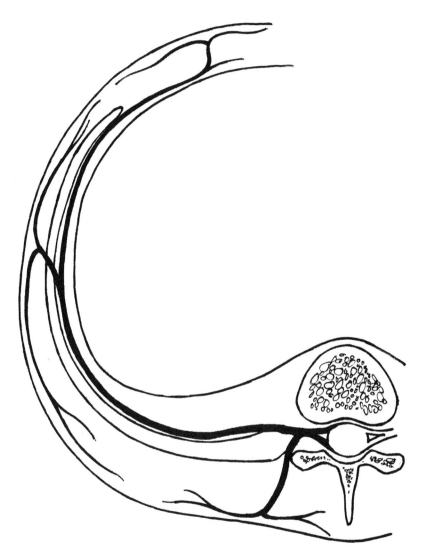

Figure 9. Intercostal nerve anatomy. Reproduced from Raj PP, ed: Practical Management of Pain, 2nd ed. Mosby-Year Book, St. Louis, 1992.

For patients with severe thoracic injuries, especially in conjunction with traumatic brain injury, their use is reasonably avoided.

Regional anesthetic techniques provide a superior approach to pain therapy and have been demonstrated to significantly reduce the need for mechanical ventilation in patients with chest trauma.[77] Improvements in forced expiratory volume at 1 second (FEV_1),[78] increased FRC, and increased vital capacity (VC) are seen as well.[17,79] Obese patients, who are more susceptible to pulmonary complications, or who have received epidural opioids have demonstrated earlier ambulation and improved peak expiratory flows compared to those having received parenteral narcotics.[80] Elderly patients, also at increased risk for pulmonary complications, may benefit as well.[81] The relief of thoracic pain is accomplished by instituting intercostal nerve blockade. This will relieve the somatically transmitted pain and may be achieved by any of three principal approaches: epidural, direct intercostal, or interpleural block. Once successfully implemented, it is possible that other components of thoracic pain (for example, diaphragmatic pain referred to the shoulder) will be "revealed" and other forms of analgesia will be necessary.[82]

Epidural catheters inserted in either the thoracic or lumbar segments provide excellent continuous analgesia. Catheters inserted in the lumbar region tend to require higher infusion rates in order to attain sufficient levels in the desired thoracic region. Previous studies investigated the uses of opioids (e.g., morphine and fentanyl) or local anesthetics. Alone, epidurally administered opioids have been shown to be clinically effective, but are associated with side effects such as respiratory depression, pruritus, nausea and vomiting, and urinary retention.[83,84] Morphine, in particular, given by epidural injection is associated with delayed central respiratory depression due its hydrophilic properties and to rostral spread in the CSF.[85] Local anesthetic solutions (e.g., bupivicaine[86]) were also demonstrated to be clinically effective, but, again, side effects such as hypotension, numbness, urinary retention, and motor blockade were observed.[87-89] More recently, dilute concentrations of local anesthetics (e.g., bupivicaine 0.1% to 0.125%) with opioids added (e.g., fentanyl 10 mcg/mL) have been given by continuous infusions to optimize pain control and minimize side effects.[90] The rate is set to give fentanyl in an initial dose of 1 mcg/kg/min, and is adjusted according to the patient's comfort and clinical condition.

When avoidance of both the physiological and pharmacological side effects of epidural analgesia is desired, intercostal and inter-

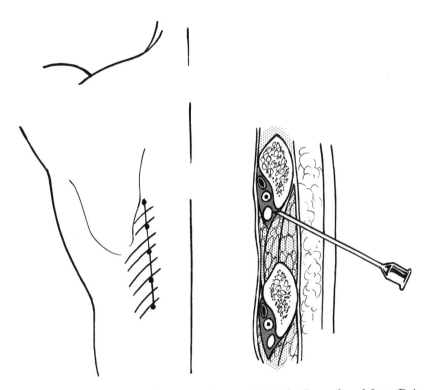

Figure 10. Technique of intercostal nerve blockade. Reproduced from Raj PP, ed: Practical Management of Pain, 2nd ed. Mosby-Year Book, St. Louis, 1992.

pleural catheterization provide excellent analgesia and are attractive alternatives. These techniques should be considered with fractures above the fifth rib because of the effects of epidural blockade on cardiac sympathetic innervation. Intercostal nerve blocks have long been used to provide analgesia for procedures involving the thorax and upper abdomen (Fig. 10). Moore, in 1962, reported on their use in over 4,000 patients.[91] Pneumothorax, often cited as a reason to avoid intercostal nerve block, occurred in less than 1% of these cases. Rib fractures, frequently seen with blunt thoracic trauma, can be treated with individual injections at the corresponding levels (although it may be necessary to block one segment above and one below, as fibers from these segments can contribute to sensation). Injections can be repeated as necessary.[77,92] For multiple rib fractures, continuous intercostal approaches have been described by Crossley[93] and Mowbray et al.[94] Murphy, in cadaveric studies, demonstrated the spread of the injected solution into the paravertebral space, where cephalad and caudad spread occurred.[95] However, the above studies have also indicated the possibility of interpleural spread, and, indeed, some of the catheters had advanced into the interpleural space.[95] One case report has demonstrated the efficacy of continuous intercostal analgesia in a patient with traumatic brain injury and multiple rib fractures where the use of parenteral analgesics was avoided in order to facilitate neurological assessment.[96] This reemphasizes the importance of avoiding agents that may affect mental status in patients with traumatic brain injury, especially in the critical early post-injury period.

Continuous interpleural analgesia has become a focus of several clinical studies since having been described by Reiestad and Stromskag[97] (Fig. 11). They demonstrated excellent analgesia in 78 of 81 patients who had undergone open cholecystectomy, breast, or renal surgery, using bupivicaine 0.5% with epinephrine 1:200,000 given as a 20-mL intermittent bolus. The technique provides unilateral analgesia and has minimal effects on pulmonary function despite the possibility of phrenic nerve blockade, either as it courses along the mediastinal pleura or at its terminal branches in the diaphragm.[98,99] Subsequent studies have validated its effectiveness for the pain of multiple rib fractures.[96,100]

The mechanism of action involves diffusion from the site of catheter placement to the intercostal nerves.[101,102] Murphy described two planes where catheters could be inserted.[103] The first lies deep to the fascia underlying the internal intercostal muscles, and superficial to the parietal pleura. Percutaneous identification of this space relies on the sensing of a "pop" as the needle pierces the fascia of the internal intercostals. The second plane is that between the visceral and the parietal pleura. Identification of this space can be accomplished percutaneously with a loss-of-resistance technique. During thoracotomy, a catheter can easily be inserted into this space under direct guidance by the surgeon. Percutaneous insertion may be associated with pneumothorax and intraparenchymal catheter placement.[104]

The use of interpleural analgesia during thoracic surgery has not been demonstrated to reduce intraoperative anesthetic requirements,[104] and its role in providing post-thoracotomy analgesia has been the subject of several investigations. Earlier studies did not find analgesia to be uniformly satisfactory.[105–108] This was attributed in

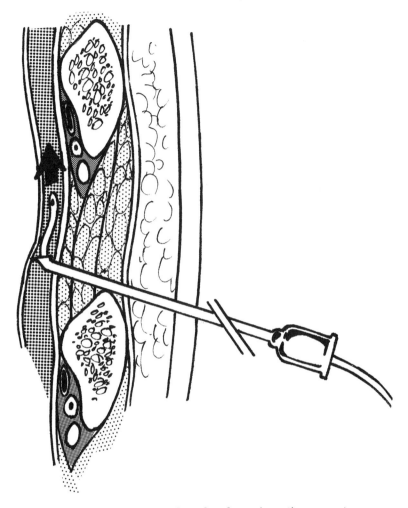

Figure 11. Technique of interpleural catheter insertion: percutaneous approach. Reproduced from Bonica JJ, ed: The Management of Pain, 2nd ed. Lea & Febiger, Philadelphia, 1990.

part to loss of local anesthetic (up to 40% of an instilled bolus) via thoracotomy drainage tubes.[105,106] Also, contused or inflamed lung tissue or pleura may remove local anesthetic due to increased local blood flow. Pooled blood, pleural fluid, or infectious debris may interfere with local anesthetic efficacy. Ferrante et al. noted improved analgesia with a two-catheter technique (one placed paravertebrally and the other laterally).[105] However, significantly higher volumes of local anesthetic must be used, with appropriate concerns regarding serum toxicity. A recent study by Brockmeier et al. compared inter-pleural analgesia to thoracic epidural analgesia in post-thoracotomy patients.[109] In both groups, analgesia was satisfactory, without the need for supplemental opioids. The posterior thoracostomy drainage tube was clamped during and for 15 minutes following the adminis-tration of a 30-mL bolus of bupivicaine with epinephrine 1:200,000; additionally, an infusion rate was titrated upward to provide effec-tive analgesia (from an initial rate of 10 mL/hr to 13 mL/hr). Main-taining the supine position during bolus administration may en-hance local anesthetic infiltration of the intercostal nerves. Other studies have demonstrated satisfactory analgesia with this tech-nique,[98,110,111] and peak serum bupivicaine levels have been shown to be well below the toxic range, especially when epinephrine is added.[110] Interpleural analgesia, therefore, represents an effective option for pain management following chest injury and thoracic sur-gery, and is used at the R Adams Cowley Shock Trauma Center, among the centers nationally with the greatest number of trauma admissions.[34]

Alternatively, the use of continuous paravertebral nerve root analgesia has been described by Matthews and Govenden.[112] With a continuous infusion of local anesthetics via a catheter placed percu-taneously in the paravertebral space (just deep to the transverse processes),[113] they demonstrated analgesia equivalent to that ob-tained with epidurally administered local anesthetics. Again, unilat-eral analgesia and a significant decrease in the incidence of hypoten-sion and urinary retention was seen. This technique has also been successfully used to provide analgesia in children following renal surgery and cholecystectomy.[114]

It is to be emphasized that patients with significant thoracic trauma remain at great risk in the early portions of their hospital course for the development of pulmonary complications, and warrant continuous observation in a critical care unit.

Considerations for Patients with Central Nervous System Trauma

Patients with central nervous system trauma present additional challenges. The long-term objective with these patients, as with all others, is the achievement of maximal functional recovery. Their injuries, however, have a more significant impact on their overall ability to reach this objective. Central nervous system trauma results in impairments which, depending on their extent, can cause functional disability. Impairments are defined as physiological and anatomic derangements, an example of which is paraplegia. Patients who have sustained traumatic brain injury typically have impairments of neurobehavioral and cognitive function,[115] whereas those with spinal cord injury have sensory and motor dysfunction.[116] Disabilities are the resultant impact impairments have on performing certain tasks, for example, climbing stairs. A handicap is a disability that interferes with the ability of the patient to function normally on vocational, educational, and interpersonal levels.[117] The rehabilitative efforts directed at restoring function in these patients are guided by physiatrists, specialists in rehabilitation medicine. However, during the acute care of these patients, two conditions may develop that interfere with their ability to fully participate in the rehabilitation process, namely spasticity and contractures.

Pathophysiology of Spasticity

The definitive pathophysiology of spasticity has not been completely elucidated. It is, however, complex, involving different spinal and supraspinal pathways, and multiple neuronal mechanisms.[118–120] Increased muscle tone and hyperactive reflexes, mediated by loss of upper neuron inhibitory control,[119] are the prominent features. For instance, in patients with spinal cord injuries, intraspinal reflex arcs involving phasic stretch receptors are stimulated. This can be seen in both head and spinal cord-injured patients, and typically develops over the course of several weeks post-injury. The clinical presentation depends on the level of injury: cortical versus brainstem versus spinal cord,[119] and there is a gradient in extent from mild (slight hypertonus – a "catch" when the limb is moved) to severe (a rigid limb). External stimuli, particularly noxious stimuli, can incite the spastic condition. Other features include an anatomic distribution to upper extremity flexors and lower extremity extensors. Spasticity is velocity-sensitive, that is, it increases with the rate of joint movement and occurs primarily in early range-of-motion.[118] In some instances, the spastic condition may be beneficial: lower extremity extensor clonus may actually assist in ambulation, and hypertonus in general may help to maintain muscle mass and bony mineralization in paralyzed extremities.[118] However, it is more often deleterious, interfering with activities of daily living, preventing effective use of a dominant extremity, and interrupting sleep. The evaluation of spasticity includes clinical history and routine physical examination, and is augmented by electrophysiological studies such as electromyography (EMG) studies, as well as other modalities, such as gait analysis. It is of utmost importance to ascertain the muscle and nerve groups involved so as to then address the therapeutic options available.

Therapeutic Approaches to Spasticity

The approaches for the treatment of spasticity can be described in a stepwise fashion as outlined by Merritt[121] (Fig. 12). Initial therapies include simple, conservative, and free-from-side-effect physical modalities such as prevention of noxious stimuli and the use of range-of-motion exercises. The next level utilizes drug therapies such as diazepam and baclofen. Nerve blocks and motor point injections are then performed. Finally, aggressive measures are used: these include surgical procedures such as rhizotomy and myelotomy.

Proper bed positioning and range-of-motion are essential components of spasticity management.[118,120] The topical application of cold for 15 to 20 minutes can reduce phasic stretch reflex responses.[122] Transcutaneous electrical nerve stimulation (TENS) has also been shown to reduce spasticity in spinal cord-injured patients.[123] Other modalities such as serial casting and splinting have been used but are apparently of limited effectiveness.[124]

Oral medications used in the treatment of spasticity include baclofen, diazepam, and dantrolene sodium. Baclofen is an analog of gamma-aminobutyric acid (GABA) and binds at the GABA-B receptor. This inhibits presynaptic calcium influx and suppresses release of excitatory neurotransmitters. Baclofen may be superior in spasticity due to spinal cord pathology.[118,120] Diazepam acts at the GABA-A receptor and increases postsynaptic inhibitory tone.[118,120] Of the benzodiazepines, only diazepam is used for the treatment of spasticity.[125] Dantrolene sodium blocks calcium ion release from the sarcoplasmic reticulum, and decreases the force of muscle contraction, although actual muscle strength may not be clinically affected.[126] It also reduces the activity of phasic stretch receptors and affects fast muscle fibers more selectively than slow ones,[127] and is

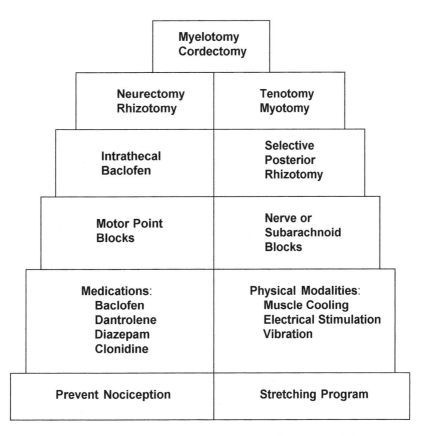

Figure 12. Stepwise approach to the treatment of spasticity. The progression from least to most invasive is ascending. Adapted from Merritt JL: Management of spasticity in spinal cord injury. Mayo Clin Proc 56:614–622, 1981.

the only antispasmodic agent to act at the muscular rather than at the reflex level.[118,120]

Baclofen can also be administered via the intrathecal route. This allows for direct access to the spinal cord, effectively bypassing the blood-brain barrier which limits passage of baclofen into the central nervous system (CNS). After oral administration, serum levels are many times higher than cerebrospinal fluid (CSF) levels; with intrathecal injection, sufficient CSF concentrations are achieved with minimal plasma concentrations and adverse central effects (e.g., symptoms of CNS depression: somnolence, mental status changes, hypotonia, etc.).[128] Initially, doses were administered on an intermittent or trial basis, but chronic administration can now be performed with an indwelling subarachnoid catheter connected to an automated delivery system. Clinical studies by Lazorthes et al.[129] and Parke et al.[130] have demonstrated the safety and efficacy of intrathecal baclofen, and this has become a preferred route of delivery for spasticity secondary to spinal cord injury.

More relevant to anesthesiologists, perhaps, is the use of selected nerve and motor point blocks (so named because they involve blockade of the terminal motor nerve fibers). These are performed most often in cases where drug therapy is inadequate, or their side effects are undesirable or not well tolerated.[131] The use of percutaneous nerve stimulation facilitates the identification of the objective nerves or motor points. Local anesthetics are used primarily for diagnostic purposes[132]; phenol is used for therapeutic blockade of longer duration. In concentrations greater than 5%, phenol infiltration will cause protein denaturation and neurolysis, resulting in block duration of 3 to 6 months or longer. Ideally, predominant motor blockade is achieved. Injection of nerves containing larger numbers of sensory fibers can result in painful paresthesias. Clonus and velocity-dependent tone are most amenable to motor point blockade.[118] Spasticity involving muscles about the hip joint can cause pain and interfere with postural and gait control. Hip flexor spasticity can be treated with psoas muscle motor point blockade. An ultrasound guided technique has been described.[133] Obturator nerve blockade will reduce adductor spasm.[134] The other major nerves of the lower extremity can be blocked as clinically indicated, for example, the tibial nerve in relation to ankle clonus.[132] Finally, there is a case report of intrathecal electrical localization of selected spinal roots for alcohol injection in a patient with severe flexor spasticity of the hips.[135]

Spasticity of the upper extremity typically involves flexor function in the elbow, forearm, and hand. The objective of treatment is to maximize the ability to engage in rehabilitative efforts and to minimize deformity.[136] Treatment of forearm flexor spasticity can unmask intrinsic flexor spasticity in the hand. This may be treated by injection of the ulnar nerve in Guyon's canal in the wrist.[137] The use of motor point injections may be more desirable in the upper extremity in order to avoid injection of phenol into a mixed nerve.[136] Phenol injections of the musculocutaneous nerve can improve elbow range-of-motion for 5 months or more following a single injection.[138]

In some brain-injured patients, blockade of the entire brachial plexus may be desirable, and this can be accomplished by the use of repeated injections via an indwelling catheter.[139] Also, the shoulder girdle may be involved, and this can severely impede arm range-of-motion. Motor point blocks of the pectoralis major muscle may alleviate this condition.[140] The above are merely a few of several clinical applications of straightforward regional anesthetic techniques.

Finally, severely refractive cases of spasticity, typically involving a paretic or contracted limb, may necessitate surgical intervention. Orthopedic procedures such as tenotomy, tendon lengthening, muscle release, and tendon transfers are performed after the neurological condition of the patient has stabilized; this may occur up to 18 months following traumatic brain injury.[140,141] In some selected patients, the use of these procedures can lead to significant functional improvements.[120,141] Release of contractures may be performed in nonfunctional limbs for cosmetic reasons and improved hygiene.[141] Neurosurgical procedures are undertaken as a means of definitively abolishing the spastic condition. Rhizotomy, for example, is the lesioning of spinal nerve roots. A selective rhizotomy involves sectioning of the posterior nerve rootlet, and may use electrical mapping to determine the extent of nerve rootlet involvement in the hypertonic reflex.[118,120] The most severe cases of spasticity may be treated with myelotomy, which is the severing of tracts in the spinal cord. This is reserved for patients who have failed more conservative therapies and who typically have pain in addition to severe spasticity. A recent study demonstrated the effectiveness of this option in 20 such patients.[142]

Pathophysiology of Contracture

A contracture is the lack of full active or passive range-of-motion due to joint, muscle, or soft tissue limitations. Several factors contribute to limited joint movement: pain, paralysis, capsular or periarticular tissue fibrosis, or primary muscle damage. The critical feature of contracture development is the absence of joint mobilization throughout the full allowable range. Contractures can be categorized into three groups: arthrogenic, myogenic, and soft tissue based on where the primary pathological changes occur. Ultimately, however, all tissues about the affected joint will be secondarily involved. The rate of contracture development may be accelerated by concurrent processes such as edema, ischemia, and bleeding. Diabetes mellitus can contribute due to its affects on the microvasculature. Advanced age is also a predisposition because of the relative decrease in muscle fibers and an increase in connective tissue. The ultimate pathology of contracture development is the formation of new collagen, with random arrangements and cross-linkages.[143] The net clinical result is change in joint biomechanics: an increase in joint stiffness (as manifested by an increase in the torque necessary to extend the joint), and a decrease in the stiffness of individual ligaments (making the joint less stable).[119]

Therapeutic Approaches to Contractures

Contractures are treated by active and passive range-of-motion exercises, emphasizing terminal stretching, that is, keeping the joint maximally extended for a sustained period. Patients with neurological trauma may not be able to participate in active exercises; they are then dependent on passive modes of therapy, e.g., nursing or physical therapy staff. Continuous passive motion (CPM) machines have been used for postoperative care of orthopedic patients, particularly those who have undergone total knee arthroplasty.[144–146] Among the advantages of CPM are its ability to provide therapy for long duration (hours or days), decreased analgesic requirements,[145] and earlier mobilization.[144] It is important to emphasize the need to achieve maximal extension in order to minimize the possibility of contracture formation. The benefits of CPM for post-traumatic joint injuries (e.g., intra-articular fractures) has been demonstrated in animal models.[147] Also, there is some evidence to support the addition of neuromuscular stimulation to extensor groups because this may enhance both strength and pain relief.[148] The use of the regional anesthesia approaches described in the preceding sections can be an important therapeutic adjunct for two reasons: (1) pain relief, and (2) muscle relaxation. Both of these may allow the patient to benefit more completely from their rehabilitative interventions.

Contractures due to spasticity are treated primarily by alleviating the underlying spastic condition, as detailed above. Other modalities include serial casting, with progressive extension of the joint, and surgery. Surgery is typically indicated for severe contractures that interfere with positioning in an otherwise bed-bound patient. However, tenotomy and myotomy are performed for the treatment of spastic contractures as well, for instance, in patients with cerebral palsy.

Summary

Trauma often results in severe, incapacitating injuries that require hospitalization, operative repairs, and the need for rehabilitation. Rehabilitation is a process that should commence from the earliest point possible in the patient's post-injury course and continue throughout their hospitalization, as patients may more swiftly and effectively achieve their functional recovery. Any measure that can maximize the ability of the patient to participate in this process should be aggressively used. Regional anesthetic techniques have been demonstrated to provide a superior means of enabling the patient both to tolerate and to fully participate in their rehabilitation. The goal is to progress toward as full a recovery as possible. Those patients who have sustained neurological injuries, particularly those with traumatic brain injury and spinal cord injury, represent a subgroup who may benefit greatly from the application of regional anesthetic techniques applied not only to the treatment of pain, but as therapy for spasticity and contractures. As the acknowledged experts in regional anesthesia, anesthesiologists should become invaluable members of the team caring for the patient during their entire hospital course. Additionally, as physicians responsible for the care of trauma patients in the resuscitation suite, operating room, and intensive care units, anesthesiologists should be aware of injuries that require rehabilitation, as well as the therapeutic regimens used. The use of regional anesthesia techniques applied during the rehabilitative phase is one of several significant areas in which anesthesiologists may contribute outside the arena of the operating room and post-anesthesia care units.

References

1. Jaffin JH, Champion HR, Boulanger BR: Economic considerations. Crit Care Clin 9(4):765–774, 1993.
2. Stachniak J, Layon A: Closed head injury and the treatment of sequelae of motor vehicle accidents. J Clin Anesth 6(5):437–449, 1994.
3. Sonntag VKH, Douglas RA: Management of spinal cord trauma. Neurosurg Clin N Am 1(3):729–750, 1990.
4. Rice DP, MacKenzie ET: Cost of injury in the United States: A report to congress. San Francisco, CA: Institute for Health and Aging, University of California and Injury Prevention Center, The Johns Hopkins University, 1989.
5. Morris JA, Sanchez AA, Bass SM, MacKenzie EJ: Trauma patients return to productivity. J Trauma 31(6):827–834, 1991.

6. Oakes DD, Wilmot CB, Hall KM, Sherck JP: Benefits of early admission to a comprehensive trauma center for patients with spinal cord injury. Arch Phys Med Rehab 71:637–643, 1990.

7. Heineman AW, Yarkony GM, Roth EJ, et al: Functional outcome following spinal cord injury. Arch Neurol 46:1098–1102, 1989.

8. Bonica JJ: Postoperative pain. In Bonica JJ (ed): Management of Pain, 2nd ed. Lea and Febiger, Philadelphia, 1990, pp 461–480.

9. Steen PA, Tiuker JH, Tarhan S: Myocardial infarction after general anesthesia and surgery. JAMA 239:2566–2570, 1979.

10. Wilmore DW: Hormonal responses and their effects on metabolism. Surg Clin North Am 56(5):999–1018, 1976.

11. Kehlet H: The modifying effect of general and regional anesthesia on the endocrine-metabolic response to surgery. Reg Anesth 7(45): S38–S48, 1982.

12. Yates DAH, Smith MA: Orthopaedic Pain after trauma. In Wall PD, Melzack R (eds): Textbook of Pain, 3rd ed. Churchill Livingstone, New York, 1994, pp 409–421.

13. Baker CC, Faist E: Immunologic response. In Moore EE, Mattox KL, Feliciano DV (eds): Trauma, 2nd ed. Appleton and Lange, Norwalk, 1991, pp 881–890.

14. Julien M, Lemoyne B, Denis R, Malo J: Mortality and morbidity related to severe intrapulmonary shunting in multiple trauma patients. J Trauma 27:970–973, 1987.

15. Lanz E, Theiss D, Riess W, Sommer U: Epidural morphine for postoperative analgesia: A double-blind study. Anesth Analg 61:236–240, 1982.

16. Raj PP, Knarr D, Vigdorth E, et al: Comparative study of continuous epidural infusions vs. systemic analgesics for postoperative pain relief. Anesthesiology 63(3A):A238, 1985.

17. MacKersie RC, Shackford SR, Hoyt DB, Karagianes TG: Continuous epidural fentanyl analgesia: ventilatory function improvement with routine use in treatment of blunt chest injury. J Trauma 27(11): 1207–1212, 1987.

18. Pflug AE, Murphy TM, Butler SH, Tucker GT: The effects of postoperative peridural analgesia on pulmonary therapy and pulmonary complications. Anesthesiology 41(1):8–17, 1974.

19. Fellows IW, Woolfson AMJ: Effects of therapeutic intervention on the metabolic responses to injury. Br Med Bull 41(3):287–294, 1985.

20. Engquist A, Brandt MR, Fernandes A, Kehlet H: The blocking effect of epidural analgesia on the adrenocortical and hyperglycemic responses to surgery. Acta Anaesth Scand 21:330–335, 1977.

21. Breslow MJ, Parker SD, Frank SM, et al: Determinants of catecholamine and cortisol responses to lower extremity revascularization. Anesthesiology 79:1202–1209, 1993.

22. Moller IW, Rem J, Brandt MR, Kehlet H: Effect of posttraumatic epidural analgesia on the cortisol and hyperglycaemic response to surgery. Acta Anaesth Scand 26:56–58, 1982.

23. Jorgensen BC, Andersen HB, Engquist A: Influence of epidural morphine on postoperative pain, endocrine-metabolic and renal responses to surgery: A controlled study. Acta Anesth Scand 26:63–68, 1982.

24. Rosenblatt R, Pepitone-Rockwell F, McKillop MJ: Continuous axillary analgesia for traumatic hand injury. Anesthesiology 51:565–566, 1979.
25. Advanced Trauma Life Support: Course for physicians. American College of Surgeons, 1993.
26. Beecher HK: Pain in men wounded in battle. Ann Surg 123(1):96–105, 1946.
27. Bion J: An anaesthetist in a camp for Cambodian refugees. Anaesthesia 38:798–801, 1983.
28. Bion J: Isobaric bupivicaine for spinal anaesthesia in acute war injuries. Anaesthesia 39:554–559, 1984.
29. Hughes TJ, Desgrand DA: Forum: Interscalene block for Colles' fracture. Anaesthesia 38:149–151, 1983.
30. Heffington CA, Thompson RC Jr: The use of interscalene block anesthesia for manipulative reduction of fractures and dislocations of the upper extremities. J Bone Jt Surg 55-A(1):83–86, 1973.
31. Stone L, Keenan MAE: Peripheral nerve injuries in the adult with traumatic brain injury. Clin Orthop 233:136–144, 1988.
32. Bontke CF, Boake C: Traumatic brain injury rehabilitation. Neurosurg Clin North Am 2(2):473–482, 1991.
33. Cope DN, Hall K: Head injury rehabilitation: benefit of early intervention. Arch Phys Med Rehabil 63:433–437, 1982.
34. Desai SM, Bernhard WN, McAlary B: Regional anesthesia: management considerations in the trauma patient. Crit Care Clin 6(1):85–101, 1990.
35. McAndrew W, Johnson KD: Penetrating orthopedic injuries. Surg Clin North Am 71:297, 1991.
36. Flanigan DP, Durham JH: Upper extremity injuries. In Bongard FS, Wilson SE, Perry MO (eds): Vascular Injuries in Surgical Practice. Appleton and Lange, Norwalk, 1991, pp 131–142.
37. Stein JS, Strauss E: Gunshot wounds to the upper extremity. Orthop Clin North Am 26:29–35, 1995.
38. Hsiang YN, White RA: Popliteal and distal injuries. In Bongard FS, Wilson SE, Perry MO (eds): Vascular Injuries in Surgical Practice. Appleton and Lange, Norwalk, 1991, pp 219–229.
39. Thompson PN, Chang BB, Shah DM, et al: Outcome following blunt vascular trauma of the upper extremity. Cardiovasc Surg 1(3):248–250, 1993.
40. Ladd AL, DeHaven KE, Thanik J, et al: Reflex sympathetic imbalance: response to epidural blockade. Am J Sports Med 17(5):660–667, 1989.
41. Wang JK, Johnson KA, Ilstrup DM: Sympathetic blocks for reflex sympathetic dystrophy. Pain 23:13–17, 1985.
42. Melzack R: Phantom limb pain: implications for treatment of pathologic pain. Anesthesiology 35(4):409–419, 1971.
43. McGregor AD, Jones WK, Perlman D: Blood flow in the arm under brachial plexus anaesthesia. J Hand Surg 10-B(1):21–24, 1985.
44. Weber S, Bennett Jones NF: Improvement in blood flow during lower extremity microsurgical free tissue transfer associated with epidural anesthesia. Anesth Analg 67:703–705, 1988.

45. Gross GD, Porter JM: Blood flow in the upper limb during brachial plexus anaesthesia. Anaesthesia 43:323–326, 1988.
46. Berger A, Tizian C, Zenz M: Continuous plexus blockade for improved circulation in microvascular surgery. Ann Plast Surg 14:16–19, 1985.
47. Cousins MJ, Wright CJ: Graft, muscle, skin blood flow after epidural block in vascular surgical procedures. Surg Gyn Obstet 133:59–64, 1971.
48. Bird TM, Strunin L: Anaesthetic considerations for microsurgical repairs of limbs. J Can Anaesth Soc 31(1):51–60, 1984.
49. Halsted J: Halsted Memorial Address. Quoted by R Matas. Johns Hopkins Med J 36:2–27, 1925.
50. Hirschel G: Die anasthesierung des plexus brachialis bei operationen and der oberen extremitaet. Muenchen Med Wschr 58:1555–1556, 1911.
51. Thompson GE, Rorie DK: Functional anatomy of the brachial plexus sheaths. Anesthesiology 59:117–122, 1983.
52. DeJong RH: Axillary block of the brachial plexus. Anesthesiology 22(2): 215–225, 1961.
53. Selander D: Catheter technique in axillary plexus block. Acta Anaesth Scand 21:324–329, 1977.
54. Ang ET, Lassale B, Goldfarb G: Continuous axillary brachial plexus block: A clinical and anatomical study. Anesth Analg 63:690–684, 1984.
55. Raj PP, Montgomery SJ, Nettles D, Jenkins MT: Infraclavicular brachial plexus block: A new approach. Anesth Analg 52(6):897–904, 1973.
56. Sada T, Kobayashi T, Murakami S: Continuous axillary brachial plexus block. J Can Anaesth Soc 30:201–205, 1983.
57. Winnie AP: Interscalene brachial plexus block. Anesth Analg 49(3): 455–466, 1970.
58. Manriquez RG, Palleres V: Continuous brachial plexus block for prolonged sympathectomy and control of pain. Anesth Analg 57:128–130, 1978.
59. Pere P, Pitkanen M, Rosenberg PH, et al: Effect of continuous interscalene brachial plexus block on diaphragm motion and on ventilatory function. Acta Anaesth Scand 36:53–57, 1992.
60. Urmey WF, McDonald M: Hemidiaphragmatic paresis during interscalene brachial plexus block: effects on pulmonary function and chest wall mechanics. Anesth Analg 74:352–357, 1992.
61. Ward ME: The interscalene approach to the brachial plexus. Anaesthesia 29:147–157, 1974.
62. Pham-Dang C, Meunier JF, Poirier P, et al: A new axillary approach for continuous brachial plexus block. A clinical and anatomic study. Anesth Analg 81:686–693, 1995.
63. Leighton TA, Wilson SE, Williams RA: Vascular Injuries of the groin and thigh. In Bongard FS, Wilson SE, Perry MO (eds): Vascular Injuries in Surgical Practice. Appleton and Lange, Norwalk, 1991, pp 207–217.
64. Winnie AP, Ramamurthy S, Durrani Z: The inguinal paravascular

technic of lumbar plexus anesthesia: The "3-in-1 block." Anesth Analg 52(6):989–996, 1973.

65. Chayen D, Nathan H, Chayen M: The psoas compartment block. Anesthesiology 45:95–99, 1976.

66. Howard CB, Mackie IG, Fairclough J, Austin TR: Forum: femoral neck surgery using a local anaesthetic technique. Anaesthesia 38:993–994, 1983.

67. Rosenblatt RM: Continuous femoral anesthesia for lower extremity surgery. Anesth Analg 59:631–632, 1980.

68. Brands E, Callanan VI: Continuous lumbar plexus block analgesia for femoral neck fractures. Anaesth Intens Care 6:256, 1978.

69. Smith BE, Fischer HBJ, Scott PV: Continuous sciatic nerve block. Anaesthesia 39:155–157, 1984.

70. MacDonald DJF: Anaesthesia for microvascular surgery: A physiologic approach. Br J Anaesth 57:904–912, 1985.

71. Strecker WB, Wood MB, Bieber EJ: Compartment syndrome masked by epidural anesthesia for postoperative pain. J Bone Jt Surg 68-A(9): 1447–1448, 1986.

72. Parziale JR, Marino AR, Herndon JH: Diagnostic peripheral nerve block resulting in compartment syndrome. Am J Phys Med Rehab 67(2):82–84, 1988.

73. Staren ED, Cullen ML: Epidural catheter analgesia for the management of postoperative pain. Surg Gyn Obstet 162:389–404, 1986.

74. Georg J, Hornum I, Mellemgaard K: The mechanism of hypoxaemia after laparotomy. Thorax 22:382–386, 1967.

75. Churchill ED, McNeil D: The reduction in vital capacity following operation. Surg Gyn Obstet 44:483–488, 1927.

76. Craig DB: Postoperative recovery of pulmonary function. Anesth Analg 60(1):46–52, 1981.

77. Gibbons J, James O, Quail A: Relief of pain in chest injury. Br J Anaesth 45:1136–1138, 1973.

78. Lomessy A, Magnin C, Viale J, et al: Clinical advantages of fentanyl given epidurally for postoperative analgesia. Anesthesiology 61: 466–469, 1984.

79. Bromage PR, Camporesi EM, Chestnut D: Epidural narcotics for postoperative analgesia. Anesth Analg 59:473–480, 1980.

80. Rawal N, Sjostrand U, Christofferson E, et al: Comparison of intramuscular and epidural morphine for postoperative analgesia in the grossly obese: Influence on postoperative ambulation and pulmonary function. Anesth Analg 63:583–592, 1984.

81. Soliman IE, Safwat AM: Successful management of an elderly patient with multiple trauma. J Trauma 25:806–807, 1985.

82. Benumof JL: Management of postoperative pain. In Anesthesia for Thoracic Surgery, 2nd ed. WB Saunders, Philadelphia, 1995, pp 756–774.

83. Bromage PR, Camporesi EM, Durant PAC, Nielsen CH: nonrespiratory side effects of epidural morphine. Anesth Analg 61(6):490–495, 1982.

84. Renaud B, Brichant JF, Clergue F, et al: Continuous epidural fentanyl:

ventilatory effects and plasma kinetics. Anesthesiology 63(3A):A234, 1985.

85. Bromage PR, Camporesi EM, Durant PAC, Nielsen, CH: Rostral spread of epidural morphine. Anesthesiology 56:431–436, 1982.

86. James EC, Kolberg HL, Iwen GW, Gellatly TA: Epidural analgesia for post-thoracotomy patients. J Thorac Cardiovasc Surg 82:898–903, 1981.

87. Johnston JR, McCaughey W: Epidural morphine: A method of management of multiple fractured ribs. Anaesthesia 35:155–157, 1980.

88. El-Baz NM, Faber LP, Jensik RJ: Continuous epidural infusion of morphine for treatment of pain after thoracic surgery: A new technique. Anesth Analg 63:757–764, 1984.

89. Ross RA, Clarke JE, Armitage EN: Postoperative pain prevention by continuous epidural infusion. Anaesthesia 35:663–668, 1980.

90. Logas WG, El-Baz N, El-Ganzouri A, et al: Continuous thoracic epidural analgesia for postoperative pain relief following thoracotomy: A prospective randomized study. Anesthesiology 67:787–791, 1987.

91. Moore DC, Bridenbaugh LD: Intercostal nerve block in 4333 patients. Anesth Analg 41(1):1–11, 1962.

92. Gibbons J, James O, Quail A: Management of 130 cases of chest injury with respiratory failure. Br J Anaesth 45:1130–1135, 1973.

93. Crossley AWA: Intercostal catheterization: An alternative approach to the paravertebral space? Anasthesia 43:163, 1987.

94. Mowbray A, Wong KKS, Murray JM: Intercostal catheterization. Anaesthesia 42:958–961, 1987.

95. Murphy DF: Continuous intercostal nerve blockade: An anatomical study to elucidate its mode of action. Br J Anaesth 56:627–629, 1984.

96. Graziotti PJ, Smith GB: Multiple rib fractures and head injury: An indication for intercostal catheterization and infusion of local anaesthetics. Anesthesiology 43:964–966, 1984.

97. Reiestad F, Stromskag KE: Interpleural catheter in the management of postoperative pain: A preliminary report. Reg Anaesth 11:89–91, 1986.

98. Seltzer JL, Larijani GE, Goldberg ME, Marr AT: Intrapleural bupivicaine: A kinetic and dynamic evaluation. Anesthesiology 67:798–800, 1987.

99. Gallart L, Gea J, Aguar MC, et al: Effects of interpleural bupivicaine on respiratory muscle strength and pulmonary function. Anesthesiology 83:48–55, 1985.

100. Rocco AG, Reiestad F, Gudman J, McKay W: Intrapleural administration of local anaesthetics for pain relief in patients with multiple rib fractures: preliminary report. Reg Anaesth 12:10–14, 1987.

101. Stromskag KE, Hauge O, Stern PA: Distribution of local anaesthetics injected into the interpleural space, studied by computerized tomography. Acta Anaesth Scand 34:323–326, 1990.

102. Covino BG: Interpleural regional analgesia (editorial). Anesth Analg 67:427–429, 1988.

103. Murphy DF: Interpleural analgesia. Br J Anaesth 71:426–434, 1993.

104. Symreng T, Gomez MN, Johnson B, et al: Intrapleural bupivicaine:

technical considerations and intraoperative use. J Cardiothorac Vasc Anesth 3(2):139–143, 1989.
105. Ferrante FM, Chan VWS, Arthur GR, Rocco AG: Interpleural analgesia after thoracotomy. Anesth Analg 72:105–109, 1991.
106. Rosenberg PH, Scheinin BA, Lepantalo MJA, Lindfors O: Continuous intrapleural infusion of bupivicaine for analgesia after thoracotomy. Anesthesiology 67(5):811–813, 1987.
107. Seltzer JL, Bell SD, Moritz H, Cantillo J: A double-blind comparison of intrapleural bupivicaine and epidural fentanyl for post-thoracotomy pain. Anesthesiology 71(3A):A665, 1989.
108. El-Baz N, Faber LP: Intrapleural infusion of local anesthetic: A word of caution. Anesthesiology 68:809–810, 1988.
109. Brockmeier V, Moen H, Karlsson BR, et al: Interpleural or thoracic epidural analgesia for pain after thoracotomy: A double blind study. Acta Anesth Scand 38:317–321, 1993.
110. Kambam JR, Hammon J, Parris WCV, Lupinetti FM: Intrapleural analgesia for post-thoracotomy pain and blood levels of bupivicaine following intrapleural injection. Can J Anaesth 26(2):106–109, 1989.
111. Mann LJ, Young GR, Williams JK, et al: Intrapleural bupivicaine in the control of post-thoracotomy pain. Ann Thorac Surg 53:449–454, 1992.
112. Matthews PJ, Govenden V: Comparison of continuous paravertebral and erxtradural infusions of bupivicaine for pain relief after thoracotomy. Br J Anaesth 62:204–205, 1989.
113. Govenden V, Matthews P: Percutaneous placement of paravertebral catheters during thoracotomy. Anaesthesia 43:256, 1988.
114. Lonnqvist PA, Olsson GL: Paravertebral versus epidural block in children. Acta Anaesth Scand 38(4):346–349, 1994.
115. Whyte J, Rosenthal M: Rehabilitation of the patient with traumatic brain injury. In DeLisa JA (ed): Rehabilitation Medicine: Principles and Practice, 2nd Ed. JB Lippincott, Philadelphia, 1993, pp 825–860.
116. Staas WE, Formal CS, Gershkoff AM, et al: Rehabilitation of the spinal cord-injured patient. In DeLisa JA (ed): Rehabilitation Medicine: Principles and Practice, 2nd Ed. JB Lippincott, Philadelphia, 1993, pp 886–915.
117. Ditunno JF: Functional assessment measures in CNS trauma. J Neurotrauma 9 (Suppl 1):S301–305, 1992.
118. Little JW, Massagli TL: Movement disorders, including tremors. In DeLisa JA (ed): Rehabilitation Medicine: Principles and Practice, 2nd ed. JB Lippincott, Philadelphia, 1993, pp 666–680.
119. Botte MJ, Nickel VL, Akeson WH: Spasticity and contracture: physiologic aspects of formation. Clin Orthop 233:7–18, 1988.
120. Katz RT: Management of spasticity. Am J Phys Med Rehab 67(3): 108–116, 1988.
121. Merritt JL: Management of spasticity in spinal cord injury. Mayo Clin Proc 56:614–622, 1981.
122. Hartviksen K: Ice therapy in spasticity. Acta Neurol Scand 38 (Suppl 3):79–84, 1962.
123. Bajd T, Eng D, Gregoric M, et al: Electrical stimulation in treating

spasticity from spinal cord injury. Arch Phys Med Rehabil 66:515–517, 1986.

124. Otis JC, Root L, Kroll MA: Measurement of plantar flexor spasticity during treatment with tone-reducing casts. J Pediatr Orthop 5: 682–686, 1985.

125. Greenblatt DJ, Shader RI, Abernethy DR: Drug therapy: current status of benzodiazepines. NEJM 309(7):410–416, 1983.

126. Katrak PH, Cole AMD, Poulos CJ, McCauley JCK: Objective assessment of spasticity, strength, and function with early exhibition of dantrolene sodium after cerbrovascular accident: A randomized double-blind study. Arch Phys Med Rehabil 73:4–9, 1992.

127. Pinder RM, Brogden RN, Speight TM, Avery GS: Dantrolene sodium: A review of its pharmacological properties and therapeutic efficacy in spasticity. Drugs 13:3–23, 1977.

128. Lewis KS, Mueller WM: Intrathecal baclofen for severe spasticity secondary to spinal cord injury. Ann Pharmacother 27:767–773, 1993.

129. Lazorthes, Yves, Sallerin-Caute B, Verdie JC, et al: Chronic intrathecal baclofen administration for control of severe spasticity. J Neurosurg 72:393–402, 1990.

130. Parke B, Penn RD, Savoy SM, Corcos D: Functional outcome after delivery of intrathecal baclofen. Arch Phys Med Rehabil 70:30–32, 1989.

131. Gunduz S, Kalyon TA, Dursun H, et al: Peripheral nerve block with phenol to treat spasticity in spinal cord injured patients. Paraplegia 30:808–811, 1992.

132. Arendzen JH, van Duijn H, Beckmann MKF, et al: Diagnostic blocks of the tibial nerve in spastic hemiparesis. Scand J Rehab Med 24: 75–81, 1992.

133. Koyana H, Murakami K, Suzuki T, Suzuki K: Phenol block for hip flexor muscle spasticity under ultrasonic monitoring. Arch Phys Med Rehabil 1040–1043, 1992.

134. Wassef MR: Interadductor approach to obturator nerve blockade for spastic conditions of adductor thigh muscles. Reg Anesth 18:13–17, 1993.

135. Chabal C, Jacobson L, White J: Electrical localization of spinal roots for the treatment of spasticity by intrathecal alcohol injection. Anesth Analg 68:527–529, 1989.

136. Garland DE, Lilling M, Keenan MA: Percutaneous phenol blocks to motor points of spastic forearm muscles in head-injured patients. Arch Phys Med Rehabil 65:243–245, 1984.

137. Keenan MAE, Todderud EP, Henderson R, Botte M: Management of intrinsic spasticity in the hand with phenol injection or neurectomy of the motor branch of the ulnar nerve. J Hand Surg 12A:734–739, 1987.

138. Keenan MAE, Tomas ES, Stone L, Gersten LM: Percutaneous phenol block of the musculocutaneous nerve to control elbow flexor spasticity. J Hand Surg 15A:340–346, 1990.

139. Keenan MAE: Management of the spastic upper extremity in the neurologically impaired adult. Clin Orthop 233:116–125, 1988.

140. Botte MJ, Keenan MAE: Percutaneous phenol blocks of the pectoralis

major muscle to treat spastic deformities. J Hand Surg 13A:147–149, 1988.
141. Jordan C: Current status of functional lower extremity surgery in adult spastic patients. Clin Orthop 233:102–109, 1988.
142. Putty TK, Shapiro SA: Efficacy of dorsal longitudinal myelotomy in treating spinal spasticity: A review of 20 Cases. J Neurosurg 75: 397–401, 1991.
143. Halar EM, Bell KR: Contracture and other deleterious effects of immobility. In DeLisa JA (ed): Rehabilitation Medicine: Principles and Practice, 2nd ed. JB Lippincott, Philadelphia, 1993, pp 681–699.
144. Ecker ML, Lotke PA: Postoperative care of the total knee patient. Orthop Clin North Am 20(1):55–62, 1989.
145. Colwell CC, Morris BA: The influence of continuous passive motion on the results of total knee arthroplasty. Clin Orthop 276:225–228, 1992.
146. Nadler SF, Malanga GA, Zimmerman JR: Continuous passive motion in the rehabilitation setting. Am J Phys Med Rehab 72(3):162–165, 1993.
147. Namba RS, Kabo JM, Dorey FJ, Meals RA: Continuous passive motion vs. immobilization: the effect on posttraumatic joint stiffness. Clin Orthop 267:218–223, 1991.
148. Haug JY, Wood LT: Efficacy of neuromuscular stimulation of the quadriceps femoris during continuous passive motion following total knee arthroplasty. Arch Phys Med Rehabil 69:423–424, 1988.

Brain Death
and Organ Procurement

W. Andrew Kofke, MD, Joseph Darby, MD, David Powner, MD, Yoo Goo Kang, MD

Brain Death

Definitions

Permanent unconsciousness has been described as follows: "Personality, memory, purpose of action, social interaction and emotional states are gone. What remains is a bodily reminder of a person who once was and might yet have been. Only vegetative functions and reflexes persist. If food is supplied, the gut functions with uncontrolled evacuation; the kidneys make urine and the bladder is incontinent; the heart, lungs, and blood vessels continue to move air and blood, nutrients are distributed in the body and CO_2 and O_2 are exchanged."[1] Permanent unconsciousness is seen in patients in either a persistent vegetative state[2] (also referred to as the apallic

From *Trauma Anesthesia and Critical Care of Neurological Injury,* edited by K. J. Abrams and C. M. Grande. © 1997, Futura Publishing Co., Armonk, NY.

syndrome,[3,4] coma prolonge,[5] neocortical death,[6] and cerebral death[7]) or who are brain dead. The primary difference between the two conditions is that bulbar and some telencephalic functions persist in the vegetative state, but not in brain death. Thus, a patient in a vegetative state may be able to breathe spontaneously and may even have sleep-wake cycles but still exhibits characteristics of permanent unconsciousness.

The concept of brain death represents the extreme end of permanent unconsciousness, as recognized by the *1981 Guidelines for Determination of Death by the President's Commission for the Study of Ethical Problems in Medicine and Biomedical and Behavioral Research.*[8] These guidelines use the Uniform Determination of Death Act definition of death, which states that "(A) An individual with irreversible cessation of circulatory and respiratory functions is dead, and (B) An individual with irreversible cessation of all functions of the entire brain, including the brain stem, is dead." The second part of this statement is commonly referred to as the whole brain death definition of death. The President's Commission guidelines form the basis for current standards used in diagnosing brain death in the United States.

The whole brain death definition of death is the only definition accepted in the United States. However, other definitions for brain death have been adopted elsewhere,[9] which has caused some confusion.[10] Brain stem death refers to the permanent loss of all brain stem functions.[9,11,12] Demonstrating the absence of higher cerebral function is not required and such patients need not have an isoelectric EEG.[11]

Neocortical death[6] refers to necrosis involving variable amounts of the telencephalon but with diffuse destruction of neocortical neurons. Such is the condition of patients in persistent vegetative states. Because the brain stem and some telencephalic structures may be intact, the patient may have sleep-wake cycles and a withdrawal response to pain, but shows no evidence of personality, memory, social interaction, or emotion. Currently, neocortical death is not accepted as a reason for declaring death. However, this has recently been challenged. Fackler and Truog[13] argue that the current operational diagnosis of whole brain death permits continuance of some vegetative functions. They make a persuasive argument that organ removal in any patient diagnosed as irreversibly unconscious should be acceptable.

Table 1
Brain Death Criteria

General Characteristics
- Permit no errors in classifying a living individual as dead.
- Allow as few errors as possible in classifying a dead person as alive.
- Allow determination of brain death to be made without unreasonable delay.
- Adaptable to a variety of clinical situations.
- Explicit and verifiable.

Specific Requirements
- Establish nonremedial brain damage.
- Exclude reversible causes of unconsciousness.
- Demonstrate unresponsiveness and absence of brain stem function by physical examination.
- Verify laboratory studies.
- Re-test over time to confirm unchanging condition.

Used with permission from Beecher HK, ref. 14.

Diagnosis of Brain Death

Definition

A person with irreversible cessation of all functions of the entire brain, including the brain stem, is dead.[8] Conceptually, this definition is straightforward. However, the diagnosis of brain death, in known situations that can imitate brain death, must be cautiously approached. Numerous guidelines for determining brain death have been published.[8,14–29] The criteria used to determine death have the general and specific characteristics outlined in Table 1.[8] No single set of specific diagnostic criteria has been universally accepted or enacted by federal or international legislation.[30] Many authoritative groups have published their own lists of criteria. In general, differences among groups have arisen in regard to time intervals between examinations and the variable importance ascribed to and the choice of confirmatory diagnostic tests.

Patient History

To fulfill the criteria for brain death, without resorting to angiography, an irremediable cause must be established and be sufficient to explain the irreversible cessation of all brain function. The patient's history will provide information (e.g., drug use, anesthetic administration) or medical history (e.g., endocrine abnormalities or severe lung disease) that is needed to properly perform the brain death examination and dictates any tests needed to confirm the diagnosis.

General Considerations

The specific procedures used to certify brain death vary among hospitals and localities. Certification procedures for a specific patient should be based on the "standard of practice" or approved policy in that patient's hospital. Most of the procedures described below have been adapted or quoted from procedures used at the University of Pittsburgh Medical Center[31] and should be regarded only as guidelines:

"The patient must be observed for a reasonable period of time ... after treatment of potentially correctable abnormalities that may contribute to deteriorated brain function, e.g., hypovolemia, hypoxemia, hypotension, hypothermia, hypercapnia or severe electrolyte abnormalities. The exact length of the observation period from the time an experienced observer suspects brain death to the time brain death is finally declared is a matter of clinical judgment. However, when the etiology of the brain injury is due to anoxia or cardiac arrest, the patient should be observed for at least 24 hours before a declaration of brain death is made without a confirmatory test such as an EEG or cerebral blood flow study.

Two separate clinical examinations must demonstrate complete absence of all brain function. At least one of the examining physicians should be experienced in the clinical diagnosis of brain death."[31]

The second examination should be conducted no sooner than 2 hours after the first. If there is any evidence of brain function during either examination, the patient is not considered to fulfill the criteria and cannot be certified as dead. Preferably, the entire certification procedure should be performed with the aid of an institutionally provided checklist.[31,32]

Physical and Laboratory Examination

An important part of the procedure for certification of brain death is physical and laboratory examination, and this must demonstrate absent confounding factors, absent cerebral function, and absent brain stem function.

Absent Confounding Factors

The guidelines of the Presbyterian University Hospital[31] regarding absent confounding factors are as follows:

"Before a clinical diagnosis of brain death can be made, factors which may impair brain function independent of the primary brain injury must be absent:

A. Systolic blood pressure must be above 90 mm Hg with evidence of adequate peripheral tissue perfusion.
B. Core temperature must be at least 32°C.
C. CNS depressants.

When drugs may be implicated by the history or physical examination as a possible etiology of depressed brain function, or in patients with coma of unknown etiology, toxicological screening and/or analysis for specific CNS depressant drugs are indicated.

Drugs known to produce severe CNS depression include tricyclic antidepressants, phenothiazines, lithium, benzodiazepines, methaqualone, glutethimide, barbiturates, and opiates. If, in addition, alcohol has been ingested, the synergistic effect between alcohol and such drugs must be considered and blood alcohol levels determined. Recent general anesthesia, metabolic encephalopathies, hypothermia, and shock may also influence the brain-injured patient's response during evaluation for potential brain death. If neuromuscular blocking agents have been used, absence of the effects of these muscle relaxant drugs must be assured by use of a nerve stimulator, before the examination may proceed. Acceptable levels of CNS depressants will vary depending on severity of injury and certainty of prognosis. Any patients in whom levels of CNS depressants are in the toxic or therapeutic range and/or alcohol levels are greater than or equal to 100 mg% cannot be declared brain dead without a cerebral blood flow study (e.g., cerebral angiogram or technetium cranial radionuclide angiogram) showing absent circulation to the brain. Patients with alcohol levels less than 100 mg% or CNS depressant levels in the sub-therapeutic range may be declared brain dead only when the patient has suffered an obviously lethal brain injury as indicated by clinical examination and supported by CT scanning (e.g., blunt head injury with massive brain swelling and herniation, bihemispheric gunshot wounds, subarachnoid hemorrhage with massive brain swelling and herniation). In patients with an uncertain etiology or prognosis or in whom there is combined presence of multiple sedatives and alcohol, both CNS depressants and alcohol must be absent on blood analysis in order to declare brain death without a cerebral blood flow study showing absent cerebral circulation.

The results of any toxicological studies performed on the patient in relationship to the brain death evaluation must be documented in the comments section of the brain death checklist along with the time at which the sample was obtained."

D. Metabolic disturbances. Uremia, hepatic failure, encephalitis, and electrolyte abnormalities can all cause or contribute to an unconscious state.

E. Anatomic abnormalities should be considered. For example, quadriplegia can give the appearance of unresponsiveness to pain, and facial injuries may depress cranial responses.

Absent Cerebral Function

The diagnosis of brain death in most North American centers requires that absent cerebral function be established. Deep coma (cerebral unreceptivity and unresponsiveness) must be evident.[8] Medical circumstances may require confirmatory studies such as EEG or studies reflecting cerebral blood flow to establish this with absolute certainty.

Patients with pontine infarction who appear comatose occasionally are not comatose but, in fact, are suffering from "locked-in" syndrome.[33] They are conscious and have relatively intact sensation but have lost all motor output except for voluntary vertical eye movements. It is, therefore, essential to exclude this possibility when performing a physical examination.

The entire central nervous system (CNS) has not necessarily ceased to function in brain-dead patients. The spinal cord may function, as may extracranial components of the autonomic nervous system. Thus, the examination strategy is to assess brain function, not spinal cord reflexes. One clinical method for confirming absent brain function in the absence of confounding factors is to observe the patient for a possible motor response to a centrally delivered painful stimulus. This noxious input is applied to a cranial (e.g., trigeminal) rather than a spinal dermatome to avoid provoking spinal cord reflexes. Stereotypical flexor or extensor posturing, purposeful movement, or facial grimacing in response to the noxious stimulus, rules out brain death (Table 2), as does spontaneous movement, shivering, or seizure activity.

Absent Brain Stem Function

Essential to the diagnosis of whole brain death is proof of myelencephalic (brain stem) death. This is established by physical exami-

Table 2
Diagnostic Tests for Establishing Brain Death on Physical Examination*

Response	Technique	Finding Indicating Brain Death	Significance
Pupilliary reaction	Shine bright light in each eye	Completely unreactive pupils in midposition, 4 to 6 mm in diameter	Evidence of sympathetic and parasympathetic denervation of the pupil
Eye movement	Oculocephalic and oculovestibular reflex tests	No spontaneous or elicited movement	Disruption of the centers of eye movement and control of their input and output pathways in the brain stem
Motor response to stimulation	Noxious central stimuli: loud noise, pressure on supraorbital nerves; nasal mucosal stimulation: endotracheal suctioning	Reflexes requiring higher centers are absent; no decerebrate or decorticate posturing; no grimacing	Disruption of the corticospinal, reticulospinal, and vestibulospinal pathways
	Corneal stimulus: touch cornea with tip of a sterile applicator	No blink response bilaterally	Disruption of afferent (cranial nerve V) and efferent (cranial nerve VII) pathways
	Gag response: stimulate posterior pharynx with tongue blade	No gag response or movement of palate	Disruption of afferent and efferent pathways in the medulla (cranial nerves IX and X)
	Suction trachea with catheter	No cough	
Respiratory movement	Observation	No spontaneous ventilatory movement	Disruption of respiratory control centers of medulla
			Disruption of afferent (cranial nerve X) and efferent medullary respiratory pathways
	Apnea testing:** preoxygenate for 20 min; disconnect or decrease ventilator support while patient receives oxygen	No respiratory movement, with $PaCO_2$ >60 mm Hg	Any spontaneous breathing efforts indicate that part of the brain stem is functional
Atropine test	Administer 2 mg atropine IV and observe heart rate response	Heart rate change <5 beats per minute	No vagal efferent activity

Modified from Smith MC, Bleck TP: J Crit Illness 4(11):67–73, 1989.

$PaCO_2$ = Arterial carbon dioxide tension.

* These procedures and techniques can be used to evaluate brain stem function and thus to confirm or exclude a diagnosis of brain death. Any evidence of brain stem function negates the diagnosis of brain death.

** Apnea testing is performed if no other evidence of brain stem function has been noted and there is no spontaneous ventilatory movement.

nation (Table 2) to evaluate the cranial nerves. The following reflexes are tested and medullary function evaluated by the apnea test. The following cranial nerve and brain stem tests must all indicate no function for brain death to be diagnosed:

1. *Pupillary light reflex.* Pupils need not be equal or dilated but must not react to light stimulation. An absent pupillary reflex is nondiagnostic after administration of scopolamine,[35,36] opiates, succinylcholine (with prolonged effect),[37] other neuromuscular blocking agents,[38,39] atropine,[35,36,39] mydriatic eye drops,[40] glutethimide,[36,39,41] monoamine oxidase inhibitors,[42] tricyclic antidepressants,[43] high-dose catecholamines, bretylium overdose,[44] cocaine, or high-dose magnesium, and in the presence of ocular trauma or another relevant eye disease.

2. *Corneal reflexes.* Preexisting seventh cranial nerve dysfunction, facial muscle weakness, neuromuscular blockade, or trigeminal nerve dysfunction can falsely abolish this reflex.

3. *Oculovestibular response.* To assess this response, the patient's head should be at a 30-degree angle and at least 50 mL of ice water injected slowly into each external ear canal, which must be free of cerumen. The patient should be observed for several minutes looking for eye movement, which, if present, indicates brain stem function. Preexisting labyrinthine disease may abolish this reflex, as may neuromuscular blockade, sedatives, anticholinergics, anticonvulsants, and tricyclic antidepressants,[38,43] as well as certain antibiotics and diuretics that are ototoxic. This test is relatively contraindicated if there are inner ear injuries (and possibly a basilar skull fracture).[1]

4. *Oculocephalic (doll's eyes) responses.* To test the reflex, the patient's head is turned rapidly from side to side and through a vertical axis. Any eye movement indicates brain stem function. This test must be used cautiously, because it is contraindicated when there may be cervical spine injury.[1] Neuromuscular blockade and sedatives may abolish the reflex.

5. *Ninth and tenth cranial nerve function.* These nerves are assessed by mechanical stimulation of the oropharynx to elicit a gag reflex or catheter stimulation of the carina to evoke a cough. High quadriplegia, neuromuscular blockade, and heavy sedation may extinguish responses to airway stimulation (no cough or gag in the presence of an intact brain stem).

6. *Atropine test.* If the vagus nerve is actively secreting acetylcholine

at the nicotinic cardiac myoneural junction, atropine will block the receptor and this will accelerate the heart rate. Thus, an increased heart rate after an intravenous atropine (2 mg) challenge indicates an intact vagal nucleus and, therefore, a functioning brain stem.[45,46] This test is not valid with a denervated (transplanted) heart and must be interpreted cautiously in patients who have undergone recent surgery with pharmacological reversal of neuromuscular blockade. The atropine test should be done after other tests have been completed, with the apnea test performed last.

7. *Apnea test.* Apnea in the context of respiratory acidosis is the final condition needed to diagnose absent brain stem function. There are several methods for performing the apnea test.[47-49] Essentially, all require a period when mechanical ventilation is stopped or decreased, with continued administration of oxygen, for a long enough period of time to increase the arterial carbon dioxide tension ($PaCO_2$) above a physiological threshold (e.g., over 60 mm Hg[8]). Starting with a normal $PaCO_2$, 10 minutes of apneic oxygenation will generally suffice to raise the $PaCO_2$ above 60 mm Hg. It is helpful before the test to adjust the ventilator to normalize $PaCO_2$ if hyperventilation was previously used.

Apneic oxygenation can usually be accomplished by keeping the patient on 100% oxygen on a continuous positive airway pressure (CPAP) mode (5 to 10 cm H_2O)[48a,49] or by administering 100% oxygen by cannula or T-piece via the tracheal tube. Adequate oxygenation during the test should be confirmed continuously by pulse oximetry. Some patients, nevertheless, sustain an unacceptable degree of hypoxemia despite these precautions. Such patients may require an occasional manual breath to reverse airway closure, although this may prolong the test of apnea. In situations of recurrent hypoxemia, carbon dioxide may need to be administered or "controlled hypoventilation" may need to be induced in such patients. Finally, patients with chronic hypercapnia or metabolic alkalosis need an increase in $PaCO_2$ (which may exceed 60 mm Hg) sufficient to decrease the arterial pH to less than 7.3.[1] If hypoxic drive is a possible preexisting problem, the inspired oxygen fraction must be decreased to produce an arterial oxygen tension (PaO_2) below 50 mm Hg, after achieving a suitable increase in $PaCO_2$. This is a controversial technique, however, and is seldom done in a clinical setting. Some clinicians may consider

Table 3
Confirmatory Tests

Neuronal Function Studies
- Electroencephalogram
- Evoked Potentials

Blood Flow Studies
- Four-Vessel Angiography
- Radionuclide Angiography
- Stable Xenon CT Cerebral Blood Flow
- Transcranial Doppler

the requisite decrement in arterial oxygen saturation too danger-ous for use in this patient population.

For all of these procedures, a test is positive when careful observa-tion or capnometry reveals no evidence of respiratory effort during 30 seconds of apnea at a $PaCO_2$ above 60 mm Hg (or PaO_2 below 50 mm Hg with hypoxic drive), with an arterial pH under 7.3.[1,8,31] If this test cannot be carried out because of unacceptable or poorly tolerated hypoxemia, a cerebral blood flow study indicating ab-sent brain stem blood flow must be done to certify brain death.[31]

Peripheral nervous system activity and spinal cord reflexes may persist after death.[8,50,51] Striking arm movements can occur in brain-dead patients, with arms flexing quickly to the chest from the patient's side and the shoulders adducting.[51] These move-ments can be precipitated by hypoxia when the patient is taken off the ventilator during apnea testing.

Confirmatory Tests

There are two general categories of confirmatory tests.[30] One depends on neuronal function and the other on blood flow (Table 3).

Neuronal Function Studies

Confirmatory tests of neuronal function useful in diagnosing brain death are currently limited to studies evaluating neuronal elec-trical function.

Electroencephalography. Arising from its inclusion in the Har-vard criteria for the diagnosis of brain death,[14] the isoelectric EEG has become a required component of some brain-death criteria.[39,16] However, its persistent inclusion in brain-death protocols is controversial.[16,17,30] Nevertheless, an isoelectric EEG may be desirable proof when objective documentation is needed to substantiate physical examination findings.[8] Electrocerebral silence verifies absent cortical function, which is assumed to be permanently lacking when there are no confounding factors.[52] In conjunction with the appropriate physical examination findings and lack of confounding factors (see Table 1), an isoelectric EEG supports the diagnosis of brain death. However, it is essential that the EEG recording is done in accordance with strict standards. The important technical details in performing bedside EEG for brain death evaluation have been elaborated by the American Electroencephalographic Society.[53]

An EEG recording from the scalp does not test brain stem function. Moreover, it has been demonstrated that brain stem death can exist despite continued EEG activity[11,17,54,55] but no brain stem blood flow.[11] Thus, the EEG can document loss of cortical functions (in the absence of confounding factors) and, with an appropriate examination demonstrating no brain stem function, can confirm the clinical diagnosis of brain death. Electrocerebral silence in an environment free of artifacts correlates highly with the clinical assessment of brain death,[56] the angiographic absence of intracranial blood flow,[57] and the characteristic pathological changes (total necrosis) of brain death.[58]

Whenever an EEG is obtained to confirm brain death, the physician must be fully aware of conditions that can cause or can contribute to reversible electrocerebral silence, and which could therefore produce a false positive diagnosis of brain death.[52] Such conditions include drug overdose or persistent anesthetic effect (e.g., barbiturates,[59,60] etomidate,[60] propofol[61]), profound hypothermia,[62,63] metabolic encephalopathy,[30,64] encephalitis,[39] hypotension,[65,66] hypoxemia,[67,68] electrolyte and glucose abnormalities,[69,70] or recent cardiac arrest (within 8 hours).[16,54,71] In patients with such confounding problems, electrocerebral silence occasionally has been reversible.[30,71] If confounding factors are possible but are not reversible in a timely fashion, there must be a reliable physical indication of absent intracranial blood flow, such as by four-vessel iodinated contrast angiography.

Evoked potentials. Available sensory evoked potential tests include the visual and somatosensory (median or posterior tibial nerve electrical stimulation) tests, as well as the brain stem auditory evoked response (BAER).[72,73] The BAER is considered the most useful for evaluating brain death.[74]

There have been reports of falsely absent BAERs in patients being evaluated for brain death (the test indicates brain death in a non-brain-dead subject[74,75]), but the presence of any brain stem waves must be considered strong evidence that there is not brain stem death.[74] Therefore, BAER testing is most useful for ruling out brain death. A typical situation would be a patient considered brain dead after recent drug ingestion or anesthetic administration[76] or with facial injuries that prevent appropriate clinical examination. If the BAER examination shows brain stem activity, radionuclide cerebral blood flow testing or four-vessel angiography is not necessary.

Blood Flow Studies

When intracranial blood flow confirmatory tests are indicated, blood flow throughout the brain must be absent for brain death to be diagnosed. Four-vessel iodinated contrast arteriography is considered the "gold standard" of these tests,[8,30] although other, less invasive, tests are also often considered acceptable (e.g., cerebral radionuclide angiography). Because of its high sensitivity and directed distribution to all intracranial vessels, iodinated contrast angiography examines all areas of the brain and may be used confidently, even in the context of CNS depressant therapy, intoxication, or hypothermia. However, its availability may be limited and its complications[77,78] may jeopardize any remaining viable brain tissue or other organs, such as the kidneys.

There is agreement in the literature that radionuclide angiography is an effective, safe bedside procedure for determining absence of cerebral blood flow.[79–82] Goodman and associates[79] concluded that a technically satisfactory single flow study showing arrest of the carotid artery circulation at the base of the skull confirms a carefully established clinical diagnosis of brain death. The primary disadvantages of the technique are that variant blood flow patterns have been observed[83] and that it does not permit good evaluation of vertebral artery flow.[30,82,84] Thus, it seems reasonable to consider radioisotope angiography, like EEG, an excellent adjunct to a careful and complete examination in diagnosing brain death. A test showing no flow, with appropriate corroborating physical examination findings, is highly correlated with brain death.[46,79,81–85]

Stable xenon-enhanced computed tomographic cerebral blood flow has been shown to confirm absent intracranial blood flow in brain-dead patients.[86,87] It is conceptually a promising alternative to iodinated contrast arteriography because it is noninvasive. However, it has not yet been correlated with four-vessel iodinated contrast arteriography in a large series.

Transcranial Doppler ultrasonography (TCD) is a noninvasive bedside technique that allows determination of instantaneous cerebral blood flow velocity. In the event of brain death, TCD usually shows cessation of forward flow and a characteristic oscillating waveform.[88,89] Both false positives and negatives have been reported.[88–90] Thus, TCD is a rapid, safe, and convenient bedside noninvasive technique that can provide some confirmation of a provisional clinical hypothesis, and is most useful when it shows normal blood velocity. However, it is not reliable as the only flow study for confirming brain death.

Certification

Legal Principles

Although most states have patterned their brain death laws after the Uniform Determination of Death Act,[8] the clinical diagnosis of brain death must conform to each state's legislated statute. Therefore, physicians diagnosing brain death must be familiar with the laws and regulations of their locality.

Bernat[91] indicates that even in places that do not have brain death statutes, there are usually judicial decisions favoring brain death. Moreover, physicians can feel secure in diagnosing brain death because such a determination is clearly within the usual standard of clinical practice in the United States.[33]

The diagnosis of brain death is a medical act for which consent is not required, nor should it be requested from the next of kin. However, the family must be informed of the medicolegal consequences of brain death, the certification process involved, and the fact that death has occurred. The time of brain death certification is the time of death for all medical and legal purposes.

Problems and Controversies

Medical Examiner Cases

If the brain-dead patient is liable to be submitted to a legal inquiry (e.g., crime, suicide, accident, occupational disease), the case should be reviewed carefully by the medical examiner before organ donation is considered.[31,92] Permission from the medical examiner is required to remove organs for transplantation.

Uncooperative Family

The decision to certify death in a brain-dead individual is based on medical indications.[93,94] When a patient is brain dead, he or she must be declared dead. Families have opposed disconnecting the ventilator when told that their loved one is brain dead and their permission is sought to discontinue support.[94] To avoid this problem, physicians must present the situation to the family in such a way that there is no choice regarding withdrawal of life support. The family is empathetically informed of the situation, and options for organ retrieval are presented, after which ventilator, pressor, and fluid therapy is withdrawn at the appropriate time. The common-sense precedent for this is the practice of not asking the family whether a relative can be declared dead once his or her heart has stopped beating.

Brain Stem Death

Brain stem death is incompatible with the recovery of human cognition.[9,11,12,17,17a] Darby, Yonas, and Brenner[11] described a patient who had no brain stem function and blood flow but persisting EEG activity. After all appropriate tests were completed, the family was consulted and life support was withdrawn. This seems to be the most appropriate management in such patients, especially in the United States, where these patients cannot be certified dead before the heart stops. In the United Kingdom, documentation of brain stem death is sufficient to certify death.[9,12,17,17a]

Children

In 1987, the Task Force for Determination of Brain Death in Children published separate death certification guidelines for children younger than 5 years.[18] The need for separate guidelines stems from the difficulty in confirming brain death in children because of neural immaturity and plasticity.

Pregnancy

If the potentially brain-dead patient is a woman of childbearing age, a pregnancy test should be done. If it is positive, obstetric consultation should be quickly obtained to ascertain gestational age. What should be done at that point is currently unclear. There have been several reports of prolonged systemic support and successful subsequent cesarean section delivery in pregnant patients.[95–97] However, the gestational threshold (if any) for continuing intensive care is an unusual situation that has not been the subject of extensive public scrutiny and can be expected to be controversial.

Organ Donor Management in the Intensive Care Unit

With the diagnosis of brain death, patient care priorities change and must be refocused on the support of transplantable organs or tissues. The goal of maintaining organs requires a careful balance of priorities so that treatment intended to benefit one organ does not harm another. For example, positive end-expiratory pressure (PEEP) used to improve oxygenation might paradoxically reduce cardiac output and hence oxygen delivery to all organs. Fluid therapy to enhance renal perfusion may injure the lung, or dopamine administered to maintain cardiac output may injure donor splanchnic organs. Such balances require careful attention to many aspects of patient monitoring, the consequences of the patient's primary illness or injury, and the prevention or treatment of physiological changes after brain death.

Many patient care practices that are considered routine extend throughout the patient's admission, regardless of the occurrence of brain death. Turning, skin and wound care, lubrication and protective closure of the eyes, antiseptic management of all catheters, nasogastric suction, bladder drainage, and appropriate laboratory testing for the determination of organ function and for balancing the complex physiological changes underway must be continued until the time of organ removal.[98–100]

Physiological Consequences of the Brain Death Process

Considerable experimental and clinical evidence is now accumulating that donor organs may be harmed during hormonal changes after head injury and during the evolution of brain death.[100a–c] Damage to these organs may cause them to fail in the donor patient and thereby be lost as potential donor organs. Likewise, a higher incidence of early nonimmunologically mediated, so-called primary organ failure in the recipient may result from this injury. Current estimates indicate that 4% to 10% of transplanted hearts, for example, fail in the recipient soon after implantation for unexplained reasons.[101]

Abnormalities in cardiac biopsy specimens from human donors have been reported.[102] These abnormalities are correlated with an increased need for inotropic support and increased mortality among recipients. A myocytolytic lesion has also been reported[103] in the hearts of patients following a variety of intracranial insults, although the relationship of brain death to myocardial performance was not discussed. Serial liver biopsies after brain death in humans showed histologic changes characteristic of central venous congestion in a majority of specimens. Changes consisting of fibrosis, cholangitis, piecemeal necrosis, and fatty metamorphosis were minimal at the time of brain death, but were quite evident days later.[104]

Novitsky and et al.[105] studied hemodynamic events in the baboon after sudden cerebral herniation and brain death caused by abrupt inflation of a subdural balloon. Initial increases in intracranial pressure (ICP) were associated with systemic hypertension, sinus bradycardia, and atrioventricular dissociation. Additional rises in ICP precipitated elevated left atrial pressure, pulmonary capillary wedge pressure, systemic vascular resistance, and further increases in systemic blood pressure. Presumably because of the high systemic vascular resistance, aortic blood flow decreased and pulmonary edema occurred. Supraventricular and ventricular dysrhythmias were also observed during this hypertensive phase. Histologic changes in the heart were noted, and these consisted of disorganization of myocardial fibers and contraction bands.[113]

Novitsky's group hypothesizes that catecholamine release from the injured brain and an accentuated discharge of the sympathetic nervous system may cause severe vasoconstriction and the potential for ischemia and histologic lesions to develop in other organs, especially the heart.[106] They have shown that myocardial lesions are eliminated or reduced by pretreatment with a calcium channel blocker[107] or beta-receptor blocker[105] and after cardiac sympathectomy[108] in a small number of animals. Similar in vivo and in vitro cardiac dysfunction was demonstrated in an ischemic brain death model in pigs[109] and dogs.[110] No data are available confirming such findings or beneficial treatment in patients. Likewise, no data have been obtained in an experimental model concerning other organ injury.

Our observations and the work of others, however, agree with the overall general pattern of hemodynamic change observed during the development of brain death, as described by Novitsky. The patient's cardiovascular system is often stable after acute resuscitation from the primary injury. However, as deterioration in the patient's neurological condition occurs, despite therapeutic measures, a period of remarkable arterial hypertension may ensue that can last for 1 or 2 hours. Often tachycardia and some arrhythmias arise, although these are usually not life-threatening.[111] It has been postulated that cerebral herniation is occurring throughout the hypertensive period, and often brain death can be diagnosed soon thereafter. Neurological function usually continues through the hypertensive period but often erodes toward the end of this time as the patient's blood pressure falls. Following this hypertensive phase, profound hypotension may arise, occasionally precipitously, despite fluid infusion, inotropic support, and even alpha-adrenergic receptor stimulation.[111–115] This hypotension may be caused by loss of sympathetic discharge from the brain, leading to arterial vasodilation and relative hypovolemia.[112,116] Other theories include reduced endogenous catecholamine production[112,116] and the stress-induced release of endorphins, for which treatment with naloxone has been suggested.[118] Although episodic elevations in blood pressure and heart rate may subsequently occur, perhaps brought about by a spinal cord nociceptive reflex,[119] the brain-dead patient often remains hypotensive.

Treatment during the development of brain death may be difficult. Vasoactive drugs that produce general or regional vasoconstriction are best avoided; these include norepinephrine, high-dose dopamine, and digitalis. It has been shown that dopamine infusion (10 mg/kg/min) does not harm donor heart in humans,[101] but dosages exceeding 15 mg/kg/min harmed the liver in a brain-dead dog preparation.[120] Dopamine use may or may not be harmful to the donor pancreas[121,122] or kidney[123] in the human. Iwai and co-workers[124] have reported that a combination of intravenous vasopressin (Pitressin) at 1-2 units/hr and an epinephrine infusion are best able to offset this hypotension and prevent cardiac arrest.

The hypotension may abate in time, and pressor support can often be reduced. However, this cycle of low perfusion followed by resumption of blood pressure, with or without medicinal support, implies that a subsequent reperfusion type of injury may occur.[125] The use of agents to reduce the formation of free radicals or to remove them from susceptible tissues has been proposed.[125,126]

These experimental data and clinical observations suggest options in patient care that must be considered experimental because they remain largely untested and because such treatment would be directed toward donor organ care in a patient who is not yet brain dead. Careful invasive vascular monitoring, titrated beta-adrenergic receptor blockade, intravascular volume expansion or restriction, calcium channel blockers, agents that scavenge or reduce the production of free radicals, and intracellular buffers of acidosis all remain possible future techniques for use in cases of anticipated brain death and organ donation.

Therapy after Brain Death

Once brain death is confirmed, therapy is clearly directed toward preservation and enhancement of donor organs. Previous treatment priorities often will need to be reversed or reconsidered. For example, hyperosmolar therapy for brain edema is no longer appropriate and may be harmful to donor organs during preparation for organ removal. In addition, new physiological changes occur after brain death, which must be anticipated, prevented, or treated.

The primary treatment goal in these cadavers with beating hearts is to maintain optimal intravascular volume and the delivery of oxygen and nutrients to the donor organs. Although the effect is undocumented, significantly reduced total body oxygen consumption is likely to occur because of loss of brain metabolism, flaccidity of the skeletal musculature, and mild hypothermia. This, in general, may benefit other metabolically active tissues and organs, where perfusion remains of critical importance. To accomplish optimal support, appropriate fluid supplementation and monitoring methods should be used, and this should be coordinated with other members of the transplantation team:

1. Some surgeons may prefer the radial artery for arterial line insertion. The sequence in which organs are removed may eliminate monitoring from a femoral arterial line early in surgery when multiple organs are produced.
2. Pulmonary artery catheters may cause endocardial injury and local as well as systemic infection. Their use should therefore be limited to as short a period of time as necessary.[99]
3. Monitoring and the management of arrhythmias should follow routine protocols, but atropine should not be used because it is

ineffective.[127] Therefore, adrenergic chronotropic agents, or transvenous/transcutaneous pacemakers must be used. The response to a sudden cardiac arrest must also be planned in advance by the transplant team. Whether defibrillation or closed chest cardiac massage are to be used is best decided early.

4. The type of fluid to be administered should be coordinated among team members, especially when blood transfusions may be needed. Although some exposure to new antigenic material occurs during transfusion, some surgeons support the transfusion effect, whereby recipient acceptance of the organ is improved after transfusion.[128] Likewise, the need to improve oxygen transport also overrides most concerns about antigenic exposure.

Other more specific treatment challenges and goals that arise are influenced by transplantation needs. These include respiratory failure, poikilothermia, polyuria, hormonal changes, and lactate production.

Respiratory Failure

Aggressive pulmonary care must be continued or increased after brain death. Often patients with head injuries are treated with their heads elevated, which may lead to orthostatic pulmonary changes. Careful posturing and other therapeutic modalities needed to keep the lungs healthy should be instituted without delay. Important issues that need to be coordinated among the transplantation team members include:

1. Endotracheal tube position, which avoids injury to a potential tracheal anastomosis;
2. Inspired oxygen concentration, PEEP, peak airway pressure, or mean intrathoracic pressure, which provide optimal organ oxygenation with minimal lung damage[129]; and
3. Discontinuation of therapeutic hyperventilation, which may precipitate changes in potassium and phosphorous homeostasis or the P50 of hemoglobin.

The success of lung and heart-lung transplantation is inversely correlated with the presence of fungus, large amounts of bacteria, and large numbers of polymorphonuclear cells in tracheal aspirates from donors.[126,129] Likewise, the presence of abnormal bacteria in the oropharynx has been associated with a poor outcome in lung recipients.[126] Techniques to minimize such occurrences including careful suctioning, chest physiotherapy, aerosolization of antibiotics, systemic antibiotics, and pharyngeal decontamination have not been evaluated prospectively.[98]

Poikilothermia

Most patients become poikilothermic after brain death,[114] and may become moderately hypothermic. The degree of hypothermia is usually only modest (mean temperature of 34°C in two series), but temperatures as low as 27°C have been reported.[111,114] Although reduced body temperature does decrease systemic oxygen consumption, more pronounced hypothermia may also produce organ injury.

The potentially harmful effects of hypothermia in these patients include: dysrhythmias,[130] decreased cardiac contractility,[131] reduced glomerular filtration,[132] coagulation defects,[132] vasoconstriction, and changes in P50 of hemoglobin.

Although various protocols for rewarming may be followed, the best plan is to anticipate hypothermia and prevent it by reducing the patient's heat loss or by instituting passive exogenous warming. This can be done easily by heating inspired gases delivered by the ventilator or by applying surface warming devices. Aggressive rewarming should be avoided, as should overwarming, because hyperthermia may increase tissue oxygen consumption and cause tachycardia. There may be topical injury to the trachea if inspired gas is heated above normal body temperatures.[133]

Polyuria

Polyuria is common after brain death[114] and may be multifactorial in origin. Causes include vasopressin deficiency, physiological fluid mobilization, osmotic diuresis, or hypothermia-induced diuresis.[135] Each potential cause must be diagnosed and treated. Careful titration of the patient's intravascular volume with treatment of electrolyte changes, glucose levels, and free water loss is necessary to avoid the harmful consequences of uncontrolled polyuria. Hypovolemia, hyperosmolarity, hypernatremia, hypokalemia, and hypophosphatemia may both separately and collectively be very injurious to donor organs.

The production of vasopressin from the hypothalamus usually ceases after brain death, resulting in diabetes insipidus. However, not all patients demonstrate polyuria,[114] suggesting that some residual nutrient blood flow may persist to this area or that residual vasopressin may be available to the circulation from the hypothalamic-pituitary axis.

The free water deficit can be estimated based on the serum sodium level. Replacement with a dextrose-containing solution can provoke marked hyperglycemia, which may contribute to further fluid and electrolyte changes through osmotic diuretic effects. Persistent hyperglycemia may be related to decreased survival of the transplanted pancreas.[121] Therefore, dilute intravenous saline solutions may be more appropriate, even though they introduce some sodium into a patient who may already be hypernatremic. The volume of fluid required with either method is often very large and difficult to administer. Therefore, treatment of diabetes insipidus usually requires both free water replacement and the administration of vasopressin.

If diabetes insipidus is present, therapy with vasopressin or desmopression is indicated.[134] In this clinical setting, the aqueous preparation of vasopressin may be preferred for subcutaneous or intravenous administration. Either repeated boluses[137] or a constant infusion[138a] is convenient and short-acting. High-dose aqueous vasopressin, however, may produce harmful splanchnic or renal vasoconstriction, and desmopressin has been recommended over vasopressin because it causes less vasoconstriction.[139,140] Urine output should be titrated to ensure a rate approximately 100 mL/hr with any preparation of vasopressin selected.

Other causes of polyuria should also be considered. These include the spontaneous diuresis of excessive fluids accumulated during earlier volume-oriented therapy, prior osmotic diuretic use, and moderate hypothermia.[135] Even if polyuria is present, some authors advocate the use of renal-dose dopamine and add diuretics immediately before kidney removal.

Hormonal Changes and Lactate Production

Several animal and human studies have evaluated other changes in circulating hormones and endocrine gland function.

Novitzky et al.[105] found low levels of triiodothyronine, thyroxine, cortisol, and insulin in their baboon model. Similar changes in circulating thyroid hormone levels have been documented in brain-dead patients,[137–142] although insulin and cortisol levels were low, normal, or increased.[137,140–142] It is suggested that this altered pattern of serum thyroid hormones is most consistent with the "euthyroid sick syndrome" characteristic of many acutely ill patients, rather than true hypothyroidism.[137,141,142] The proposed benefits of hormonal therapy have been reviewed[143] and, although controversial,[140] thyroid hormone administration is not currently recommended.[137-142]

Measurement of pituitary hormones with and without physiological stimulation has produced variable results without consistent evidence of reduced function.[137,144] This suggests that there is some circulation to the hypothalamic-pituitary axis after brain death or that residual hormone stores may be accessible.[137,144]

Interestingly, Novitzky et al.[105] also found modestly elevated serum lactate levels in baboons, a finding also observed in some head-injured and brain-dead patients.[105,140,141] There are insufficient study data to show conclusively that the increased lactate level is caused by a shift from aerobic to anaerobic metabolism, as suggested by Novitzky.[140] Furthermore, any association between the elevated lactate level and any other hormonal change is currently speculative, but the finding is reproducible and although the elevations are only modest, the cause remains unclear.

Organ Procurement from Donors with Brain Death

Organ Procurement

The main goal of organ procurement, as described in the *Organ and Tissue Procurement Manual* of the Pittsburgh Transplant Foundation, is to maintain homeostasis of all organ systems in a potential donor before organs are removed.[145] Specifically, integrity of organs should be maintained by optimal organ perfusion, avoidance of further damage, and removal and preservation of organs with minimal ischemic injury. Care of the donor during organ procurement, therefore, requires a continuation of the intensive care that was provided before brain death and precise surgical procurement procedure.

Preparation for Procurement

Administration and Logistical Considerations

A victim of trauma is normally treated in sophisticated trauma care systems with aggressive medical and surgical resuscitative measures to reverse underlying injury and organ dysfunction. However, if complete and irreversible loss of all brain function occurs despite such treatment, brain death is then declared by the responsible physicians. Administrative and organizational procedures, including obtaining consent for organ donation and identifying the organs and tissues to be procured, are subsequently initiated and a procurement team is deployed. The team usually consists of nurses, anesthesiologists, surgeons, and procurement officers. Experienced members of procurement teams from other institutions frequently participate in this process as well.

Once a decision has been made to proceed with organ procurement, the most important issue is clear communication between the members of the procurement team. A lack of communication at this point can disrupt donor care and compromise organ stability. Therefore, the needs and protocols of the individual procurement teams should be discussed in detail before any organ removal surgery occurs. The host institution that is referring a donor and the visiting procurement teams share the responsibility for evaluation, recovery, preservation of the donor organs, and for the financial aspects involved. In addition, if possible, the logistic arrangements between teams should be expedited so that no time constraints are placed on the host team. Moreover, the host team must be tolerant, because extrarenal organs often have to be flown to distant parts of the country, and some recipient surgery may be quite complex and time-consuming. To facilitate planning, the host team should have information about the donor available to allow a prompt evaluation by the visiting team. In general, donors should not have untreated infection or malignancy other than a primary brain tumor.

During preoperative evaluation of the donor, an anesthesiology care team, led by an experienced anesthesiologist, visits the donor in the ICU to verify the existence and validity of brain death certification, consent from family members, and permission from the coroner, and reviews the donor's medical history, including the cause of brain death and condition of all vital organs (see Table 4). Important medical information includes drug allergies, medications, significant coexisting cardiopulmonary disease, surgical history, and current need for cardiopulmonary support.

Specific test results include the chest x-ray, electrocardiogram (ECG), arterial blood gas tensions, acid-base status, hemoglobin concentration, serum levels of electrolytes, aspartate aminotransferase (GOT), alanine aminotransferase (GPT), amylase, bilirubin, creati-

Table 4
Checklist for Anesthesia for Organ Procurement

1. Consent from family and coroner's permission
2. Donor support guidelines
   • Systolic blood pressure ≥100 mm Hg
   • Central venous pressure ≤12 cm H_2O
   • Urine output ≥100 mL/h
3. Equipment
   • Transport monitor
   • Multiple-channel vital sign monitor
   • Anesthetic gas machine
   • Ventilator
   • Surface warming device and blood warmer
   • Infusion devices
   • Defibrillator
4. Laboratory tests
   • Hemoglobin and hematocrit
   • Arterial blood gas tensions and acid-base state
   • Serum electrolytes, calcium, lactate
   • Blood glucose
5. Medications
   • Packed red blood cells (5 U)
   • Lactated Ringer's solution (12–15 L)
   • Dopamine (400 mg)
   • Heparin (20,000 U)
   • Methylprednisolone (30 mg/kg)
   • Chlorpromazine (250 mg)
   • Mannitol (25%, 100 g)
   • Furosemide (100 mg)

nine, blood urea nitrogen, and glucose. The blood type of the donor is identified to prepare blood products and to match with the blood type of potential recipients.

Generally, donors who are antigen-positive for hepatitis and the acquired immunodeficiency syndrome are excluded from donor candidacy. Serologic markers of these diseases must be identified to ensure the safety of transplant recipients as well as of health care workers.

The transition from the ICU to the operating room is a crucial period. The donor should not be left unmonitored, and management cannot be interrupted. Furthermore, the involvement of several procurement team members may make communication difficult. Generally, the anesthesia care team is responsible for the transport, while the donor is continuously monitored, ventilated, and treated. All necessary life-support equipment must accompany the donor.

Intraoperative Management

Because unique pathophysiological changes occur in the donor with brain death, meticulous medical care is imperative and should be directed by an experienced anesthesiologist in continual communication with the surgical team. In general, donors with brain death should be treated as vigorously as living-related donors,[146] with use of sound medical and ethical judgment.

Equipment and Medications

Equipment and medications necessary for multiple-organ procurement, practical guidelines, and desired laboratory tests are shown in Table 4. A multiple-channel vital sign monitor is essential to keep track of hemodynamic fluctuations associated with the absence of brain stem function, surgical manipulation, and fluid shift. The conventional pressure-cycled ventilator of the anesthetic gas machine is adequate in most cases, but a volume ventilator may be needed for donors requiring high levels of PEEP or airway pressure.

The operating room should be kept warm, and a warming blanket and blood warmer are necessary to prevent hypothermia. Continuous drip infusion devices are needed for titration of potent vasoactive drugs. A laboratory facility in which tests can be done immediately should be available to measure arterial blood gas tensions and acid-base state, hematocrit, hemoglobin, and serum levels of electrolytes, ionized calcium, glucose, and lactate.

A large volume of crystalloids should be prepared, and a colloid solution (e.g., 5% albumin, plasma protein fraction, or hetastarch) may be necessary. Five units of packed red blood cells should be kept on standby, although the quantity requirement depends on the condition of the donor. Coagulation factors and platelets are rarely necessary. Medications other than those listed may be required for procurement of specific organs.

Monitoring

Monitoring of the donor is similar to that of critically ill patients undergoing major surgical procedures. Blood pressure is monitored by an indwelling catheter in the radial artery, allowing abrupt changes in blood pressure to be anticipated. When a radial artery is inaccessible, the brachial artery may be used. The femoral artery is avoided because manipulation or cross-clamping of the aorta is unavoidable. The ECG is monitored, preferably using lead V_5, to detect dysrhythmias or myocardial ischemia, particularly in heart donors. Central venous pressure (CVP) monitoring is essential,[4] and a pulmonary arterial catheter may be used in unstable donors, although it has inherent risks of dysrhythmia and pulmonary injury. Transesophageal two-dimensional echocardiography may be used to assess cardiac contractility in heart donors. Other standard parameters are monitored: urine output is monitored by an indwelling urinary catheter, and body temperature is measured by an oral, rectal, or core blood thermistor. Monitoring of intracranial pressure serves no purpose and is not done. Laboratory variables are monitored hourly or more frequently, as indicated.

Anesthetic Management

It may appear to the uninitiated that anesthetics are unnecessary during organ procurement, since donors without cortical function cannot perceive pain from surgical stimulation. However, donors do respond to surgical stimulation with dramatic hemodynamic changes, such as tachycardia and hypertension, perspiration, and involuntary movement. In a series of human donors, skin incision increased systolic blood pressure by 31 mm Hg, diastolic pressure by 16 mm Hg, and heart rate by 23 beats per minute.[147] This sympathetic response usually occurred within 5 minutes after surgical incision, with maximal response within 5 to 20 minutes. This so-called "mass reflex" is caused by neurogenic vasoconstriction and stimulation of the adrenal medulla by the spinal reflex arc.[148] In addition, abdominal muscle tone may interfere with surgical exposure, and involuntary movement caused by spinal cord reflexes can be erroneously perceived as a sign of life or can cause accidental injury to the donor's organs during a technical procedure.

Anesthetics and neuromuscular blockers are thus given to obliterate the sympathetic response and involuntary movement and to provide satisfactory muscle relaxation. An induction agent is unnecessary because organ donors are normally already intubated and ventilated. Although any available potent inhalation anesthetic can be used to maintain anesthesia, isoflurane is preferred because the degree of myocardial depression is less than with halothane or enflurane. Halothane is avoided because halothane hepatitis may be a concern in the presence of potential hepatic ischemia. Enflurane may increase the blood level of inorganic fluoride, although whether this has an effect on donor kidneys is unknown. In hemodynamically unstable donors, short-acting narcotics such as fentanyl (5–10 μg/kg) are preferred. Muscle relaxants such as vecuronium bromide (0.05 to 0.1 mg/kg) or pancuronium bromide (0.05 to 0.1 mg/kg) are commonly used because of their relatively insignificant hemodynamic effects.

Respiratory Care

Respiratory care during organ procurement includes nasogastric suction, pulmonary toilet, and adjustment of the cuff pressure of the endotracheal or tracheostomy tube to prevent aspiration. Specific goals of ventilatory care are to maintain PaO_2 between 70 and 100 mm Hg, oxygen saturation of arterial hemoglobin (SaO_2) at greater than 95%, and arterial pressure of carbon dioxide ($PaCO_2$) within the range of 35 to 45 mm Hg, and to avoid pulmonary complications.

In hypothermic donors, a mild respiratory alkalosis (pH 7.4 to 7.5) may be preferred to improve tissue perfusion.[149,150] This goal frequently is achieved by ventilating with a tidal volume of 10 to 15 mL/kg, FiO_2 of 30% to 40%, a respiratory rate of fewer than 20 breaths/minute, and a low level of PEEP ($\leq$5 cm H_2O).

When optimal gas exchange is difficult, adjustments are made in tidal volume, respiratory rate, and PEEP to optimize gas exchange. However, an increase in FiO_2 is preferred to an excessive tidal volume and high PEEP because elevated intrathoracic pressure decreases venous return and splanchnic blood flow.

Circulatory Care

Aggressive circulatory care is essential, because hemodynamic instability may damage the heart, making it unacceptable for transplantation,[151] and it may also impair other organs to be procured. Hypotension (systolic blood pressure <80 mm Hg or mean arterial pressure <40 mm Hg) is associated with an increased incidence of acute tubular necrosis and nonfunction of the donor kidneys,[152,153] and poor function of the liver.[154] Many surgeons agree that systolic blood pressure should be maintained between 100 and 120 mm Hg, and CVP at less than 10 cm H_2O with minimal vasopressor support.[155–157]

Management of the circulatory system therefore begins with adjustment of the fluid volume to attain an optimal preload. Volume deficit is usually replaced with a balanced electrolyte solution (e.g., lactated Ringer's) to maintain systolic blood pressure greater than 100 mm Hg and CVP close to 8 mm Hg. A colloid solution such as albumin (5%) or hetastarch may be administered, although crystalloids appear to be as effective as colloids in increasing intravascular volume.[158] Once any fluid deficit is corrected, a hypotonic solution with glucose (e.g., 5% dextrose in 0.45% sodium chloride [NaCl], 1 mL/kg/hr) is administered to replace urine output and insensible loss, guided by CVP and urine output. Fluid loss from excessive urine output (>200 to 250 mL/hr) is replaced by a hypotonic electrolyte solution with supplementation of potassium chloride (KCl, 20 mmol/L). This aggressive volume replacement may decrease the need for vasopressors in many cases,[159] but acute volume expansion may lead to increased myocardial oxygen consumption, congestive heart failure, dysrhythmia, and the need for inotropic support because the compliance of the heart is decreased in most donors.[155] Therefore, CVP should not be permitted to exceed 8 mm Hg in most cases.

The tachycardia that is frequently associated with hypertension should be avoided because it may increase oxygen consumption of the heart, causing secondary pulmonary edema and decreased blood flow to donated organs.[155-157] Tachycardia and hypertension frequently are controlled by general anesthetics, particularly by potent inhalation anesthetics, but in severe cases, a beta-antagonist, such as labetalol hydrochloride or esmolol hydrochloride, or a calcium channel blocker, such as verapamil hydrochloride, is administered.[158a,159] Occasionally, a vasodilator such as hydralazine or sodium nitroprusside may be given to reduce afterload. When bradycardia is a concern, a direct-acting agent such as isoproterenol or epinephrine is used for positive chronotropic effects because donors are unresponsive to centrally acting chronotropic drugs, such as atropine. Supraventricular or ventricular dysrhythmia is treated with conventional antiarrhythmic drugs.

Attempts to increase the afterload with an alpha-adrenergic drug such as phenylephrine hydrochloride, norepinephrine bitartrate, or metaraminol bitartrate may not be desirable in the presence of myocardial depression, and these may decrease splanchnic and coronary blood flow.[159-161] Thus, a low afterload is compensated by increasing the preload. Adequate cardiac output and perfusion pressure are also maintained by adjusting the preload. However, when these goals cannot be met because of preexisting cardiovascular disease or myocardial depression, a vasopressor may indeed be required.

In general, dopamine hydrochloride (2 to 5 μg/kg/min and up to 10 μg/kg/min) is recommended to improve cardiac contractility. Dobutamine hydrochloride (2 to 10 μg/kg/min) and isoproterenol hydrochloride (0.1 to 1 μg/kg/min) are useful when myocardial dysfunction is the cause of hypotension, although these drugs may dilate the peripheral vascular beds, decreasing blood pressure. Doses of all vasopressors should be carefully titrated so as not to compromise blood flow to the organs. Donors without vasopressor support have better renal function and less incidence of acute tubular necrosis.[152]

In general, transfusion of packed red blood cells (1 to 3 units) is necessary to maintain a hematocrit between 25% and 30% or to keep the level of hemoglobin greater than 8 g/dL.[162,163] Blood transfusion may prolong the survival of the kidneys.[162,163]

Circulatory arrest has occurred in 10% of potential donors and in 66% of referred donors.[158,159,164] Treatment is according to conventional circulatory resuscitative measures, except that atropine is ineffective, and no direct intracardiac injection of medication is recommended in heart donors. When circulatory resuscitation is ineffective, organs should be harvested as rapidly as possible to minimize further ischemic damage.

Temperature Regulation

Hypothermia, which is seen in up to 86% of donors,[111,114] plays a major role in hemodynamic instability. To avoid the untoward effects of hypothermia on circulation and metabolism, body temperature is kept warmer than 35°C by increasing the operating room temperature, infusing all fluids through a blood warmer, and using heating lamps, a surface warming device, and a heated humidifier in the inspiratory limb of the ventilation circuit.

Diuresis, Fluid Balance, and Diabetes Inspidus

To maintain adequate diuresis, intravascular volume is replenished as previously described. In addition, urine output is replaced by lactated Ringer's solution or half-normal saline with KCl (20 mmol/L). When urine output is inadequate, fluid is given to maintain CVP close to 8 mm Hg, and dopamine may be given. However, an infusion rate of greater than 10 μg/kg/min should be avoided because the risk of acute tubular necrosis and renal graft failure increases with a higher infusion rate.[152] For persistent oliguria, furosemide (1–2 mg/kg) and mannitol (0.5 g/kg) may be administered.

When diabetes insipidus is present, urine output is replaced by a hypotonic solution (0.45% NaCl with KCl 20 mmol/L), and supplemental antidiuretic hormone is administered to maintain urine output in the range of 100 to 250 mL/min. Vasopressin (0.5 to 1 unit/hr) was used commonly in the past, but desmopressin acetate (DDAVP)[172] is now often used (1–2 μg every 8–12 hr) because of its long duration of action and a low pressor/antidiuretic effect ratio.[165] Hyperglycemia is treated by an infusion of insulin (5 to 10 units).

Acid-Base State and Electrolyte Balance

Metabolic acidosis caused by inadequate tissue perfusion may be compounded by respiratory acidosis. Because of potential myocardial depression, metabolic acidosis is corrected by administration of sodium bicarbonate. When hypernatremia is a concern, tromethamine (tris-[hydroxymethyl]aminomethane, THAM) may be used (0.3 molar THAM [mL] = body weight [kg] × base deficit [mmol/L]) instead of sodium bicarbonate.

Electrolyte imbalance is caused by fluid shift and diabetes insipidus and may result in dysrhythmia and myocardial dysfunction. Common abnormalities are hypernatremia, hypokalemia, hypocalcemia, hypophosphatemia, and hypomagnesemia and should all be corrected.

Coagulopathy

Coagulation abnormalities should be treated conservatively. Replacement of coagulation factors and platelets is rarely necessary during organ procurement, unless massive bleeding is caused by coagulopathy. Antifibrinolytic therapy is not recommended because microvascular thrombi could form.

Other Medications

Although some modifications are expected, depending on the protocol of individual centers, the following medications are frequently administered to organ donors. The donor is given heparin (200 to 300 units/kg) systemically before cannulation of the aorta. Sodium methylprednisolone succinate (1,000 mg) may be given to stabilize cell membranes, to reduce donor lymphocytes, and to decrease the antigenicity of the organ graft. Mannitol (0.25 to 0.5 g/kg) and furosemide (40 mg) may be given to induce diuresis before division of the renal pedicle and to prevent ischemia-induced acute tubular necrosis.[166–168] Alpha-adrenergic receptor blockers such as phenoxybenzamine hydrochloride may be used to promote renal vasodilation and prevent vasospasm.[169] However, these blockers are not recommended in multiple-organ procurement because their effects on other organs are unknown. Prophylactic administration of antibiotics such as broad-spectrum cephalosporins is recommended by some surgeons,[170,171] although efficacy is controversial. Nephrotoxic antibiotics should be avoided.

Termination of Anesthesia

Once cardioplegia is induced, no further supportive care is necessary. Cardiopulmonary support is discontinued, and vital sign monitors and the ventilator are turned off. All intravenous and intra-arterial cannulas may be removed. The organs are swiftly removed in the following sequence: heart, lungs, liver, pancreas, and kidneys. When procurement of other tissues such as the cornea or bone is considered, the procedure is performed without tissue perfusion, because these tissues tolerate ischemia of a longer period without significant injury.

Summary

A diagnosis of brain death represents a tragedy for a patient and his/her family. Up until recently, such patients were supported indefinitely in ICUs, further prolonging the suffering of families. The advent of widely agreed-upon concepts and diagnostic criteria for brain death has resulted in a rational approach that conserves resources and shortens bedside vigils by family.

Out of these evolving issues and procedures has arisen the potential to improve or save the lives of others through transplantation. It thus is essential that intensivists and anesthesiologists are aware of issues in brain death diagnosis and physiology. Clearly, appropriate care of organ donors is an integral and very important component of transplantation.

References

1. Grenvik A: Brain death and permanently lost consciousness. In Shoemaker WC, Thompson WL, Holbrook PR (eds): Textbook of Critical Care. W.B. Saunders, Philadelphia, 1984, pp 968–980.

2. Jennett B, Plum F: The persistent vegetative state: A syndrome in search of a name. Lancet 1:734, 1972.
3. Kretschmer E: Das appalische Syndrom. Z Gesamte Neurol Psychiatr 169:576, 1940.
4. Ingvar DH, et al: Survival after severe cerebral anoxia with destruction of the cerebral cortex: the apallic syndrome. Ann NY Acad Sci 315:184, 1978.
5. Mollaret P, Goulon M: Le coma depasse. Rev Neurol 101:5–15, 1959.
6. Brierly JB, et al: Neocortical death after cardiac arrest. Lancet 2:560, 1976.
7. Korein J: The problem of brain death: development and history. Ann NY Acad Sci 315:19, 1978.
8. Guidelines for the determination of death: Report of the medical consultants on the diagnosis of death to the President's Commission for the Study of Ethical Problems in Medicine and Biomedical and Behavioral Research. JAMA 246:2184–2186, 1981.
9. Pallis C: The declaration of death. Intensive Crit Care Dig 2:21–22, 1983.
10. Youngner SJ, et al: "Brain death" and organ retrieval: A cross-sectional survey of knowledge and concepts among health professionals. JAMA 261:2205–2210, 1989.
11. Darby J, Yonas H, Brenner RP: Brainstem death with persistent EEG activity: evaluation by xenon-enhanced computed tomography. Crit Care Med 15:519–521, 1987.
12. Pallis C: Prognostic significance of a dead brain stem. Br Med J 286:123–124, 1983.
13. Truog RD, Fackler JC: Rethinking brain death. Crit Care Med 20:1705–1713, 1992.
14. Beecher HK: A definition of irreversible coma: Report of the Ad Hoc Committee of the Harvard Medical School to examine the definition of brain death. JAMA 205:337–340, 1968.
15. National Institute of Neurological and Communicative Disorders and Stroke: An appraisal of the criteria of cerebral death: A summary statement; a collaborative study. JAMA 237:982–986, 1977.
16. Powner DJ, Pinkus RL, Grenvik A: Decision-making in brain death and vegetative states: multiple considerations. In Grenvik A, Safar P (eds): Brain Failure and Resuscitation. Churchill Livingstone, Edinburgh, 1981, pp 239–259.
17. Pallis C: The arguments about the EEG. Br Med J 286:284–287, 1983.
17a. Conference of Royal Colleges and Faculties of the United Kingdom: Diagnosis of brain death. Lancet 2:1069–1070, 1976.
18. Task Force for the Determination of Brain Death in Children: Guidelines for the determination of brain death in children. Arch Neurol 44:587–588, 1987.
19. Masland RL: Report of the committee on irreversible coma and brain death. Trans Am Neurol Assoc 103:320–321, 1978.
20. Kaste M, Hillbom M, Palo J: Diagnosis and management of brain death. Br Med J :525–527, 1979.

21. Walker AE: Cerebral death. In Tower DB (ed): The Nervous System, Vol 11. Raven Press, New York, 1975, pp 75–87.
22. Molinari GF: Review of clinical criteria of brain death. Ann NY Acad Sci 315:62–69, 1978.
23. Suter C, Brush J: Clinical problems of brain death and coma in intensive care units. Ann NY Acad Sci 315:398–416, 1978.
24. Hicks RG, Torda TA: The vestibulo-ocular (caloric) reflex in the diagnosis of brain death. Anaesth Intensive Care 7:169–173, 1979.
25. Searle J, Collins C: A brain death protocol. Lancet 1:641–643, 1980.
26. Belsh JM: Brain death: Policy at Middlesex General University Hospital. J Med Soc NJ 82:199–205, 1985.
27. Black PM: Criteria of brain death. Postgrad Med 57:69–74, 1975.
28. Cranford E: Minnesota Medical Association criteria: Brain death. Minn Med 61:561–563, 1978.
29. Harp JR: Criteria for the determination of death. Anesthesiology 40: 391–397, 1974.
30. Powner DJ: The diagnosis of brain death in the adult patient. Intensive Care Med 2:181–189, 1987.
31. Certification of brain death and management of adult brain dead organ donors. Presbyterian University Hospital Policy and Procedure Manual. Presbyterian University Hospital, Pittsburgh, July 5, 1990, p 5108.
32. Kofke WA, Darby JD: Evaluation and certification of brain death. In Grande C, et al (eds): Textbook of Trauma Anesthesia and Critical Care. Mosby, St. Louis, 1993.
33. Bleck TP, Smith MC: Diagnosing brain death and persistent vegetative states. J Crit Illness 4:60–65, 1989.
34. Wetzel RC, et al: Hemodynamic responses in brain dead organ donor patients. Anesth Analg 64:125–128, 1985.
35. Garde JF, et al: Racial mydriatic responses to belladonna premedication. Anesth Analg 57:572, 1978.
36. Black PM: Brain death (2 parts). N Engl J Med 299:338–344, 393–401, 1978.
37. Tyson RN: Simulation of cerebral death by succinylcholine sensitivity. Arch Neurol 30:409–411, 1974.
38. Posner JB: Coma and other states of consciousness: the differential diagnosis of brain death. Ann NY Acad Sci 315:215–227, 1978.
39. Korein J: Brain death. In Cottrell JE, Turndorf H (eds): Anesthesia and Neurosurgery, Mosby-Year Book, St. Louis, 1986, pp 293–351.
40. Finklestein S, Ropper A: The diagnosis of coma: its pitfalls and limitations. Heart Lung 8:1059–1064, 1979.
41. Allen N, Burkholder J, Comiscioni J: Clinical criteria of brain death. Ann NY Acad Sci 315:70–95, 1978.
42. Mallampalli R, Pentel PR, Anderson DC: Nonreactive pupils due to monoamine oxidase inhibitor overdose. Crit Care Med 15:536–537, 1987.
43. Yang KL, Dantzker DR: Reversible brain death: A manifestation of amitriptyline overdose. Chest 99:1037–1038, 1991.

44. Thompson AE, Sussmane JB: Bretylium intoxication resembling clinical brain death. Crit Care Med 17:194–195, 1989.
45. Quaknine GE: Cardiac and metabolic alterations in brain death. Ann NY Acad Sci 315:252–264, 1978.
46. Quaknine GE: Bedside procedures in the diagnosis of brain death. Resuscitation 4:159–177, 1975.
47. Earnest MP, Beresford R, McIntyre HB: Testing for apnea in suspected brain death: methods used by 129 clinicians. Neurology 36:542–544, 1986.
48a. Perel A, Berger M, Cotev S: The use of continuous flow of oxygen and PEEP during apnea in the diagnosis of brain death. Intensive Care Med 9:25–27, 1983.
48. Oboler SK: Brain death and persistent vegetative states. Clin Geriatr Med 2:547–576, 1986.
49. Bruce DL: Blood gas values change slowly in apneic organ donors. Anesthesiology 65:128, 1986.
50. Ropper AH: Unusual spontaneous movements of brain-dead patients. Neurology 34:1089–1092, 1984.
51. Friedman AJ: Sympathetic response and brain death. Arch Neurol 41:15, 1984.
52. Powner DJ: Drug-associated isoelectric EEGs. JAMA 236:1123, 1976.
53. American Electroencephalographic Society. Guidelines in EEG. The Society, Willoughby, 1971.
54. Hughes JR: Limitations of the EEG in coma and brain death. Ann NY Acad Sci 315:121–136, 1978.
55. Younger SJ, Bartlett ET: Human death and high technology: the failure of the whole-brain formulations. Ann Intern Med 99:252–258, 1983.
56. Powner DJ, Fromm GH: The electroencephalogram in the determination of brain death. N Engl J Med 300:502, 1979.
57. Greitz T, et al: Aortocranial and carotid angiography in determination of brain death. Neuroradiology 5:13–19, 1973.
58. Leestma JE, Hughes OR, Diamond JR: Temporal correlates in brain death. Arch Neurol 41:147–152, 1984.
59. Clark DL, Rosner BS: Neurophysiologic effects of general anesthetics. 1. The electroencephalogram and sensory evoked responses in man. Anesthesiology 38:564–582, 1973.
60. Ghoneim MM, Yamada T: Etomidate: A clinical and encephalographic comparison with thiopental. Anesth Analg 56:479–485, 1977.
61. Herregods L, Rolly G, Mortier E, et al: EEG and SEMG monitoring during induction and maintenance of anesthesia with propofol. Int J Clin Monit Comput 6:67–73, 1989.
62. Pearcy WC, Virtue RW: The electroencephalogram in hypothermia with circulatory arrest. Anesthesiology 20:341–347, 1959.
63. Levy WJ: Quantitative analysis of EEG changes during hypothermia. Anesthesiology 60:291–297, 1984.
64. Brenner RP: The electroencephalogram in altered states of consciousness. Neurol Clin 3:615–631, 1985.

65. Dong WK, et al: Profound arterial hypotension in dogs: brain electrical activity and organ integrity. Anesthesiology 58:61–71, 1983.

66. Prior PF: Critical comparison of monitoring EEG, cerebral function (CFM), compressed spectral array (CSA), and evoked response under conditions of reduced cerebral perfusion. In Heuser D, McDowell DG, Hempel V (eds): Controlled Hypotension in Neuroanesthesia. Plenum, New York, 1985, pp 117–132.

67. Kraaier V, Van Huffelen AC, Weineke GH: Quantitative EEG changes due to hypobaric hypoxia in normal subjects. Electroencephalogr Clin Neurophysiol 69:303–312, 1988.

68. Akopyan NS, Baklavadzhyan OG, Karapetyan MA: Effects of acute hypoxia on the EEG and impulse activity of the neurons of various brain structures in rats. Neurosci Behav Physiol 14:405–411, 1981.

69. Young GB, et al: Hypophosphatemia versus brain death. Lancet 1:617, 1982.

70. Aver RN, et al: Hypotension as a complication of hypoglycemia leads to enhanced energy failure but no increase in neuronal necrosis. Stroke 17:442–449, 1986.

71. Tender RL, Sadove M, Becka DR: Electroencephalographic evidence of cortical "death" followed by full recovery: protective action of hypothermia. JAMA 164:1667, 1957.

72. Grundy BL: Monitoring of sensory evoked potentials during neurosurgical operations: methods and applications. Neurosurgery 11:556–575, 1982.

73. Chiappa KH, Ropper AH: Evoked potentials in clinical medicine. N Engl J Med 306:1140–1150, 1205–1211, 1982.

74. Hall JW III, Mackey-Hargadine JR, Kim EE: Auditory brain stem response in determination of brain death. Arch Otolaryngol 111:613–620, 1985.

75. Taylor MJ, Houston BD, Lowry NJ: Recovery of auditory brain stem responses after a severe hypoxia ischemic insult. N Engl J Med 309:1169–1170, 1983.

76. Newton PG, et al: Effects of therapeutic pentobarbital coma on multimodality evoked potentials recorded from severely head-injured patients. Neurosurgery 12:613–619, 1983.

77. Hankq GJ, Warlow CP, Molyneux AJ: Complications of cerebral angiography for patients with mild carotid territory ischaemia being considered for carotid endarterectomy. J Neurol Neurosurg Psychiatry 53:542–548, 1990.

78. Skalpe IO: Complications in cerebral angiography with iohexol (Omnipaque) and meglumine metrizoate (Isopaque cerebral). Neuroradiology 30:69–72, 1988.

79. Goodman JM, Heck LL, Moore BD: Confirmation of brain death with portable isotope angiography: A review of 204 consecutive cases. Neurosurgery 16:492–497, 1985.

80. Schwartz JA, et al: Radionuclide cerebral imaging confirming brain death. JAMA 249:246–247, 1983.

81. Korein J, et al: Radioisotopic bolus technique as a test to detect circula-

tory deficit associated with cerebral death. Circulation 51:924–938, 1975.

82. Korein J, et al: Brain death. I. Angiographic correlation with the radio isotopic bolus technique for evaluation of critical deficit of cerebral blood flow. Ann Neurol 2:195–205, 1977.

83. Brill DR, Schwartz JA, Baxter JA: Variant flow patterns in radionuclide cerebral imaging performed for brain death. Clin Nucl Med 10:346–352, 1985.

84. Tsai SH et al: Cerebral radionuclide angiography: its application in the diagnosis of brain death. JAMA 248:591–592, 1982.

85. Morayati SO, Nagle CE: The determination of death and the changing role of medical imaging. Radiographics 8:967–979, 1988.

86. Darby JM, Yonas H, Gur D, Latchaw RE: Xenon-enhanced computed tomography in brain death. Arch Neurol 44:551–554, 1987.

87. Ashwal S, Schneider S, Thompson J: Xenon computed tomography measuring cerebral blood flow in the determination of brain death in children. Ann Neurol 25:539–546, 1989.

88. Ropper AH, Kehn SM, Wechsler L: Transcranial Doppler in brain death. Neurology 37:1733–1735, 1987.

89. Newell DW, et al: Evaluation of brain death using transcranial Doppler. Neurosurgery 24:509–513, 1989.

90. Velthoven W, Calliauw L: Diagnosis of brain death: transcranial Doppler sonography as an additional method. Acta Neurochir 95:57–60, 1988.

91. Bernat J: Ethics in neurology. In Joynt RJ (ed): Clinical Neurology. Lippincott, Philadelphia, 1988.

92. Nirmel KN, Ropper AH: Brain death. In Kofke WA, Levy J (eds): Postoperative Critical Care Procedures of the Massachusetts General Hospital. Little Brown, Boston, pp 314–319.

93. Black PM: Clinical problems in the use of brain-death standards. Arch Intern Med 143:121–123, 1983.

94. Paris JJ, Reardon FE: Dilemmas in intensive care medicine: an ethical and legal analysis. J Intensive Care Med 1:75–90, 1986.

95. Dillon WP, et al: Life support and maternal brain death during pregnancy. JAMA 248:1089–1091, 1982.

96. Field DR, et al: Maternal brain death during pregnancy: medical and ethical issues. JAMA 260:816–822, 1988.

97. Bernstein IM, et al: Maternal brain death and prolonged fetal survival. Obstet Gynecol 74:434–437, 1989.

98. Darby JM, Stein K, Grenvik A, Stuart SA: Approach to management of the heartbeating "brain dead" organ donor. JAMA 261:2222–2228, 1989.

99. Powner DJ, Jastremski M, Lagler RG: Continuing care of multiorgan donor patients. J Intensive Care Med 4:75–83, 1989.

100. Soifer BE, Gelb AW: The multiple organ donor: identification and management. Ann Intern Med 110:814–823, 1989.

100a. Clifton GL, Ziegler MG, Grossman RG: Circulating catecholamines and sympathetic activity after head injury. Neurosurgery 8:10–13, 1981.

100b. Hamill RW, Woolf PD, McDonald JV, Lee KA, Kelly M: Catecholamines predict outcome in traumatic brain injury. Ann Neurol 21: 438–443, 1987.

100c. Payen D, et al: Head injury: clonidine decreases plasma catecholamines. Crit Care Med 18:392–395, 1990.

101. Trento A, Hardesty RL, Griffith BP: Early function of cardiac homografts: relationship to hemodynamics in the donor and length of ischemic period. Circulation 74:77–79, 1986.

102. Darracott-Cankovic S, et al: Biopsy assessment of myocardial preservation in 160 human donor hearts. Transplant Proc 20:44–48, 1988.

103. Connor RCR: Focal myocytolysis and fuchsinophilic degeneration of the myocardium of patients dying with various brain lesions. Ann NY Acad Sci 156:261–270, 1969.

104. Nagareda T, et al: Clinicopathological study of livers from brain-dead patients treated with a combination of vasopressin and epinephrine. Transplantation 47:792–797, 1989.

105. Novitzky D, et al: Electrocardiographic, hemodynamic and endocrine changes occurring during experimental brain death in the Chacma baboon. J Heart Transplant 4:63–69, 1984.

106. Rose AG, Novitzky D, Copper DKC: Myocardial and pulmonary histopathologic changes. Transplant Proc 20:29–32, 1988.

107. Novitzky D, et al: Prevention of myocardial injury by pretreatment with verapamil hydrochloride prior to experimental brain death. Am J Emerg Med 5:11–18, 1987.

108. Novitzky D, et al: Prevention of myocardial injury during brain death by total cardiac sympathectomy in the Chacma baboon. Ann Thorac Surg 41:520–524, 1986.

109. Novitzky D, et al: Improved cardiac function following hormonal therapy in brain dead pigs: relevance to organ donation. Cryobiology 24: 1–10, 1987.

110. Finkelstein I, Toledo-Pereyre LH, Castellanos J: Physiologic and hormonal changes in experimentally induced brain dead dogs. Transplant Proc 19:4156–4158, 1987.

111. Griepp RB, et al: The cardiac donor. Surg Gynecol Obstet 133:792–798, 1971.

112. Kinoshita Y, et al: Clinical and pathological changes of the heart in brain death maintained with vasopressin and epinephrine. Pathol Res Pract 186:173–179, 1990.

113. Adomian GE, Laks MM, Billingham ME: The incidence and significance of contraction bands in endomyocardial biopsies from normal human hearts. Am Heart J 95:348–351, 1978.

114. Jastremski M, Powner DJ, Snyder JV: Problems in brain death determination. Forensic Sci 11:201–212, 1978.

115. Nygaard CE, Townsend RN, Diamond DL: Organ donor management and organ outcome: A 6-year review from a Level I trauma center. J Trauma 30:728–732, 1990.

116. Emery RW, et al: The cardiac donor: A six-year experience. Ann Thorac Surg 41:356–362, 1986.

117. Feibel JH: Reduced catecholamine excretion at onset of brain death. Lancet I:890–891, 1981.
118. Toledo-Pereyra LH, Castellanos J, Finkelstein I: Improved donor kidney function and hemodynamics following naloxone administration. Transplant Proc 20:733–735, 1988.
119. Wetzel RC, et al: Hemodynamic responses in brain-dead organ donor patients. Anesth Analg 64:125–128, 1985.
120. Okamoto R, et al: Influence of dopamine on the liver assessed by changes in arterial ketone body ratio in brain-dead dogs. Surgery 107: 36–42, 1990.
121. Gores PF, et al: The influence of donor hyperglycemia and other factors on long-term pancreatic allograft survival. Transplant Proc 22: 437–438, 1990.
122. Wright FH, et al: Pancreatic allograft thrombosis: donor and retrieval factors and early postperfusion graft function. Transplant Proc 22: 439–441, 1990.
123. Whelchel JD, et al: The effect of high-dose dopamine in cadaver donor management on delayed graft function and graft survival following renal transplantation. Transplant Proc 18:523–527, 1986.
124. Iwai A, et al: Effects of vasopressin and catecholamines on the maintenance of circulatory stability in brain-dead patients. Transplantation 48:613–617, 1989.
125. Hernandez LA, Granger N: Role of antioxidants in organ preservation and transplantation. Crit Care Med 16:543–549, 1988.
126. Zenati M, et al: Organ procurement for pulmonary transplantation. Ann Thorac Surg 48:882–886, 1989.
127. Ouakanine G, et al: Laboratory criteria of brain death. J Neurosurg 39:429–433, 1973.
128. Opelz G: Current relevance of the transfusion effect in renal transplantation. Transplant Proc 17:1019, 1985.
129. Harjula A, et al: Proper donor selection for heart-lung transplantation. J Thorac Cardiovasc Surg 94:874–880, 1987.
130. Okada M, et al: The J wave in accidental hypothermia. J Electrocardiol 16:23–28, 1983.
131. Okada M: Echocardiographic evaluation of the heart in accidental hypothermia. Keio J Med 31:111–125, 1982.
132. Carden D, et al: Hypothermia. Ann Emerg Med 11:497–503, 1982.
133. Harnett RM, Pruitt JR, Sias FR: A review of the literature concerning resuscitation from hypothermia. II. Selected rewarming protocols. Aviat Space Environ Med 54:487–495, 1983.
134. Hsu T: Diabetes insipidus: current concepts. Comp Ther 10:6–10, 1984.
135. Fitzgerald FT, Jessop C: Accidental hypothermia. Adv Intern Med 27: 128–150, 1982.
136. Muhlberg J, et al: Hemodynamic and metabolic problems in preparation for organ donation. Transplant Proc 18:391–393, 1986.
137. Howlett TA, et al: Anterior and posterior pituitary function in brain-stem-dead donors. Transplantation 47:828–834, 1989.
138a. Levitt MA, Fleischer AS, Meislin HW: Acute post-traumatic diabetes

insipidus: treatment with continuous intravenous vasopressin. J Trauma 24:532–535, 1984.

138. Gifford RRM, et al: Thyroid hormone levels in heart and kidney cadaver donors. J Heart Transplant 5:429–253, 1986.

139. Koller J, et al: Thyroid hormones and their impact on the hemodynamic and metabolic stability of organ donors and on kidney graft function after transplantation. Transplant Proc 22:355–357.

140. Novitzky D, Cooper DKC, Reichart B: Hemodynamic and metabolic responses to hormonal therapy in brain-dead potential organ donors. Transplantation 43:852–854, 1987.

141. Powner DJ, et al: Hormonal changes in brain-dead patients. Crit Care Med 18:702–708, 1990.

142. Robertson KM, Hramiak IM, Gelb AW: Endocrine changes and hemodynamic stability after brain death. Transplant Proc 21:1197–1198, 1989.

143. Debelak L, Pollak R, Reckard C: Arginine vasopressin versus desmopressin for the treatment of diabetes insipidus in the brain dead organ donor. Transplant Proc 22:351–352, 1990.

144. Schrader H, et al: Changes of pituitary hormones in brain death. Acta Neurochir 52:239–248, 1980.

145. Pittsburgh Transplantation Foundation: Organ and Tissue Procurement Manual.

146. Luksza AR: Brain-dead kidney donor: selection, care, and administration. Br Med J 1:1316, 1979.

147. Wetzel RC, Setzer N, Stiff JL et al: Hemodynamic responses in brain dead organ donor patients. Anesth Analg 64:125, 1985.

148. Guyton AC: The autonomic nervous system. In Textbook of Medical Physiology. WB Saunders, Philadelphia, 1981, p 710.

149. Kroncke GM, Nichols RD, Mendenhall JT, et al: Ectothermic philosophy of acid-base balance to prevent fibrillation during hypothermia. Arch Surg 121:303, 1986.

150. Swain JA: Hypothermia and blood pH: A review. Arch Intern Med 148: 1643, 1988.

151. Painvin GA, Frazier OH, Chandler LB, et al: Cardiac transplantation: indications, procurement, operation, and management. Heart Lung 14: 484, 1985.

152. Whelchel JD, Diethelm AG, Phillips MG, et al: The effect of high-dose dopamine in cadaver donor management on delayed graft function and graft survival following renal transplantation. Transplant Proc 18:523, 1986.

153. Wicomb WN, Cooper DKC, Lanza RP, et al: The effects of brain death and 24 hours storage by hypothermic perfusion on donor heart function in the pig. J Thorac Cardiovasc Surg 91:896, 1986.

154. Busuttil RW, Goldstein LI, Danovitch GM, et al: Liver transplantation today. Ann Intern Med 104:377, 1986.

155. Griepp RB, Stinson EB, Clark DA, et al: The cardiac donor. Surg Gynecol Obstet 133:792, 1971.

156. Flanigan WJ, Ardon LF, Brewer TE, et al: Etiology and diagnosis of early post-transplantation oliguria. Am J Surg 132:808, 1976.

157. Toledo-Pereyra LH, Simmons RL, Olson LC, et al: Cadaver kidney transplantation effect of hypotension and donor pretreatment with methylprednisolone and phenoxybenzamine. Minn Med 62:159, 1979.
158. Davidson I, Berglin E, Brynger H: Perioperative fluid regimen, blood and plasma volumes, and colloid changes in living-related donors. Transplant Proc 16:18, 1984.
158a. Slapak M: The immediate care of potential donors for cadaveric organ transplantation. Anaesthesia 33:700, 1978.
159. Kormos RL, Donato W, Hardesty RL, et al: The influence of donor organ stability and ischemia time on subsequent cardiac recipient survival. Transplant Proc 20:980, 1988.
159a. Levinson MM, Copeland JG: The organ donor: physiology, maintenance, and procurement considerations. Contemp Anesth Pract 10:31, 1987.
160. Schneider A, Toledo-Pereyra LH, Seichner WD, et al: Effect of dopamine and pitressin on kidneys procured and harvested for transplantation. Transplantation 36:110, 1982.
161. Hardesty RL, Griffith BP: Multiple cadaveric organ procurement for transplantation with emphasis on the heart. Surg Clin North Am 66: 451, 1986.
162. Frisk B, Berglin E, Brynger H: Positive effect on graft survival of transfusions to the cadaveric kidney donor. Transplantation 32:252, 1981.
163. Jeekel J, Hersche O, Marquet R: Effects of blood transfusions to the donor on kidney grafts survival in man. Transplantation 32:453, 1982.
164. Lucas BA, Vaughn WK, Spees EK, et al: Identification of donor factors predisposing to high discard rates of cadaver kidneys and increased graft loss within one year post transplantation. Transplantation 43: 253–258, 1987.
165. Cowley AW, Monos E, Guyton AS: Interaction of vasopressin and the baroreceptor reflex system in the regulation of arterial blood pressure in the dog. Circ Res 34:505, 1974.
166. Dahlager JL, Bilde T: The integrity of tubular cell function after preservation in Collin's or Sacks' solution. Transplantation 21:365–369, 1976.
167. Rijksen JFWB: Preservation of canine kidneys. The effect of various preservation fluids on renal morphology and function, Thesis, University of Leiden, Netherlands.
168. Schloerb PR, Postel J, Mortiz ED, et al: Hypothermic storage of the canine kidneys for 48 hours in a low chloride solution. Surg Gynecol Obstet 141:545, 1975.
169. Miller CH, Alexander JW, Smith EJ, et al: Salutary effect of phentolamine (Regitine) on renal vasoconstriction in donor kidneys: experimental and clinical studies. Transplantation 17:201, 1974.
170. Abramowicz M: The choice of antimicrobial drugs. Med Lett 24:21, 1982.
171. Abramowicz M: Choice of cephalosporins. Med Lett 25:57, 1983.
172. Richardson DW, Robinson AG: Desmopressin. Ann Intern Med 103: 228, 1985.

Subject Index

Access
  for enteral nutrition, 392–393
  for parenteral nutrition, 391–392
Acid-base state, 528
Administration of fluids, 217–220
  monitoring, 219–220
  volume, 217–219
Adrenocorticotrophic hormone. *See*
      GMM2
Aircraft, fixed-wing, for interhospital
      transport, 52–53
Airway
  in prehospital assessment, 8
  in resuscitation, 74–77
    consciousness, level of, 75–76
    obstruction, 76
Airway control, in intrahospital
      resuscitation, with head injury,
      101–104
Airway management, 121–151
  cervical spine, 138–145
    advanced, 141–145
    basic, 140–141
  closed head injury, 121–138, 346–347
    anesthetic induction agents,
        122–129
      adjunctive therapy, 128–129
      barbiturates, 122–123
      benzodiazepines, 127–128
      etomidate, 123–124
      ketamine, 125
      muscle relaxants, 126–127
      opioids, 125–126
      propofol, 124–125
    patient management, 129–133
      endotracheal intubation,
          emergency, 131–135
      patient profile
        hemodynamically stable
            patient, 135–137
        hemodynamically unstable
            patient, 137–138
      patient management, patient
          profile, 135–138
    epidemiology, 138–139
    failed intubation alternatives,
        144–145

      comtube, 144–145
      cricothyroidotomy, 145
      laryngeal mask airway, 144
    intubation techniques, 141–143
      awake intubation, 142–143
      Bullard laryngoscope, 143
      direct laryngoscopy, 142
      nasotracheal intubation, 143
    physical examination, 139–140
    prehospital, 13–15
    spinal cord injury, 367–370
Altas, fractures of, 318
Ambulance, ground, for interhospital
      transport, 51–52
Amino acid antagonists, excitatory,
      172–173
Anesthesiologists in field, 32–36
Angiography, neurodiagnostic evaluation,
      285–288
Antibiotics, with closed head injury, 355
Antidiuretic hormone, inappropriate,
      syndrome of, 359
Aperiodic analysis, electroencephalogram,
      444–445
Apnea test, brain death and, 507
Arteriography, 247–249
Articulations, spinal cord injury,
      intraoperative mangement,
      312–314
Assessment, initial, for prehospital
      anesthesia, 7–13
  neurological assessment, 9–13
  primary survey, 7–9
    airway, 8
    breathing, 8
    cervical spine, 8
    circulation, 8–9
    disability, 9
    exposure, 9
  resuscitation phase, 9
  scoring, 9–13
Atlanto-occipital dislocations, 316–317
Atropine test, brain death and, 506
Axis
  spondylolisthesis of, traumatic, 320–321
  traumatic spondylolisthesis of, 320–321
Axonal injury, diffuse, 342–344

539

Barbiturates
  brain protection, 168–169
  closed head injury, 122–123
  coma, with closed head injury, 351–352
  intraoperative use of, 299
Benzodiazepines
  closed head injury, 127–128
  intraoperative use of, 301
  in neurodiagnosis, 272
Bi-spectral analysis,
          electroencephalogram,
          445–447
Blood flow studies, brain death, 510–511
Brain coverings, injury to, intraoperative
          anesthesia, 292
Brain death, 499–513
  absent confounding factors, 502–504
  brain stem function, absent, 504–508
  cerebral function, absent, 504–505
  certification, 511
    legal principles, 511
  confirmatory tests, 508–511
    blood flow studies, 510–511
    neuronal function studies, 508–510
      electroencephalography, 508–509
      evoked potentials, 509–510
  controversies, 511–513
  declaration of, 359–360, 499–538
  diagnosis of, 501
  diagnostic imaging and, 257–259
  laboratory examination, 502
  organ procurement, 520–529
  patient history, 501–502
  physical examination, 502
  problems, 511–513
    brain stem death, 512
    children, 512
    medical examiner cases, 511–512
    pregnancy, 512–513
    uncooperative family, 512
Brain stem auditory-evoked potentials,
          441–443
Brain stem death, brain death and, 512
Brain stem function, absent, brain death
          and, 504–508
Breathing, prehospital assessment, 8
Bullard laryngoscope, 143

C_1-C complex, injuries to, 317
Calcium accumulation, intracellular,
          160–161
Calcium channel blockers, 173–174,
          418–419

Caloric distribution
  enteral nutrition formula, 394
  parenteral nutrition formula, 386
Caloric requirement, parenteral nutrition
          formula, 384, 386
Calories, enteral nutrition formula, 393
Cardiovascular changes, during
          interhospital transport, 48–49
Cardiovascular system management,
          closed head injury, 347–350
Central nervous system
  monitoring of, 435–456
    cerebral blood flow, 437–439
      transcranial doppler monitoring,
          437–438
      xenon washout, 439
    electrophysiological, 439–447
      electroencephalogram, 441–447
        aperiodic analysis, 444–445
        bi-spectral analysis of EEG,
          445–447
        spectral analysis of EEG,
          443–446
      evoked potentials, 439–441
        brain stem auditory-evoked
          potentials, 441–443
        motor-evoked potentials, 441
        somatosensory-evoked potential,
          439–440
    gas monitoring, 447
    intracranial pressure, 436–437
    metabolic monitoring, 447
      jugular venous oxygen saturation,
          447–448
      near-infrared spectroscopy,
          448–450
  protection, 412–420
    calcium channels blockers, 418–419
    gangliosides, 418
    glutamate antagonists, 414–415
      NMDA receptor antagonist,
          414–415
      non-NMDA receptor blockers, 415
    GMM2, 413–414
    lazaroids, 414
    naloxone, 417–418
    radical scavengers, 416–417
    steroids, 412–413
    sympathetic nervous system
          modulators, 419–420
    thyrotropin-releasing hormone,
          417–418
  rehabilitation, 482–488
    contracture
      pathophysiology, 487–488
      therapeutic approaches, 488

spasticity
    pathophysiology, 483–484
    therapeutic approaches, 484–487
Cerebral blood flow
    monitoring, 437–439
        transcranial doppler, 437–438
        xenon washout, 439
    nitric oxide, regulation, 162–163
Cerebral function, absent, brain death
        and, 504–505
Cerebral hemodynamics, closed head
        injury, 350–353
Cerebral perfusion pressure, 406–408
Certification, brain death, 511
Cervical fractures, lower, dislocations,
        321–322
Cervical spine
    airway management, 138–145
        advanced, 141–145
        basic, 140–141
        epidemiology, 138–139
        failed intubation alternatives,
            144–145
        intubation techniques, 141–143
            awake intubation, 142–143
            Bullard laryngoscope, 143
            direct laryngoscopy, 142
            nasotracheal intubation, 143
        physical examination, 139–140
    anatomy of, 309–316
    intraoperative management, 315–316
    kinematics, 314–315
    ligaments, 312–314
    penetrating injuries, 322–327
    prehospital assessment of, 8
    stabilization, in intrahospital
            resuscitation, with head injury,
            101–104
    upper, 310–313
Cervical vertebrae, lower, 312–313
Cervicomedullary injury, transaxial, 318
Chest injury
    with head injury, resuscitation, 87–89
    and maxillofacial injury, resuscitation,
        89–90
Children, brain death, 512
Chloral hydrate, in neurodiagnosis, 274
Circulation
    care, 525–527
    prehospital assessment, 8–9
    resuscitation, prehospital, 15–18
Classification, closed head injury, 342
Closed head injury
    airway management, 121–138

anesthetic induction agents, 122–129
    adjunctive therapy, 128–129
    barbiturates, 122–123
    benzodiazepines, 127–128
    etomidate, 123–124
    ketamine, 125
    muscle relaxants, 126–127
    opioids, 125–126
    propofol, 124–125
patient management, 129–133
    endotracheal intubation,
        emergency, 131–135
    patient profile, 135–138
        hemodynamically stable patient,
            135–137
        hemodynamically unstable
            patient, 137–138
anesthetic induction agents, 122–129
    adjunctive therapy, 128–129
critical care, 341–364
    brain death, declaration of, 359–360,
        499–538
    cerebral hemodynamics, 350–353
        barbiturate coma, 351–352
        induced hypothermia, 352–353
        mannitol, 351
        positional changes, 352
    classification, 342
    complications, 357–359
        diabetes insipidus, 358
        selection, 357–358
        syndrome of inappropriate
            antidiuretic hormone, 359
    diffuse axonal injury, 342–344
    etiology, 341
    hematoma space-occupying lesion,
        344–346
        epidural hematoma, 345
        subarachnoid hemorrhage, 345
        subdural hematoma, 344–345
    hyperventilation, 350–353
    incidence, 341
    poor outcome, causes of, 342
    resuscitation, 346–350
        airway, 346–347
        cardiovascular system, 347–350
    sepsis prevention, 353–357
        antibiotics, 355
        nutritional support, 355–377
            glucose homeostasis, 355–356
            tube feeding regimes, 356–357
        pneumonia, 353–354
        septicemia, 354
        urinary tract infection, 354

shear injury, 342–344
types of injuries, 341–346
intraoperative anesthesia, 291–306
anesthetic care, 297–303
emergence, 303
inhalation agents, 297–299
desflurane, 298–299
isoflurance, 297–298
nitrous oxide, 299
intracranial hypertension control,
293–297
fluid replacement, 295–296
steroid administration, 295
intravenous agents, 299–302
barbiturates, 299
benzodiazepines, 301
etomidate, 301
ketamine, 300
muscle relaxants, 301–302
opioids, 299–300
propofol, 300–301
monitoring, 303–304
types of head injuries, 292–293
brain coverings, injury to, 292
epidural hematoma, 293
intracerebral hematoma, 293
missile injuries, 292
subdural hematoma, 293
resuscitation, 85
without herniation syndrome, 85–86
Coagulopathy, 528
Colloid osmotic pressure, changing,
cerebral effects of, 211–212
Colloids, for fluid management, 201
albumin, 201
synthetic, 202
dextrans, 202–203
hetastarch, 202
pentastarch, 202
Combitube, as failed intubation
alternative, 144–145
Communications, prehospital, in
intrahospital resuscitation,
with head injury, 96–98
Complications, of closed head injury,
357–359
diabetes insipidus, 358
selection, 357–358
syndrome of inappropriate antidiuretic
hormone, 359
Computed tomography, 243, 270–276
head injury, 243–246
pediatric patient, 273–276
spinal cord injury, 246–247

Confirmatory tests, brain death, 508–511
blood flow studies, 510–511
neuronal function studies, 508–510
electroencephalography, 508–509
evoked potentials, 509–510
Contrast agents, 232–234
intrathecal, 233–234
intravenous, 232–233
Corneal reflexes, brain death and, 506
Coverings, of brain, injury to,
intraoperative anesthesia, 292
Cricothyroidotomy, as failed intubation
alternative, 145
Critical care, during interhospital
transport, 60–61
Crystalloid solutions, fluid management,
191, 197–200
hypertonic, 198–200
hypotonic, 197
isotonic, 191, 197

Death, brain, declaration of, 359–360,
499–538
Desflurane, intraoperative use of, 298–299
Detection, untreated life-threatening
injuries, before interhospital
transport, 55
Dextrans, 202–203
Diabetes insipidus, with closed head
injury, 358
Diagnostic imaging, 227–268
acute neurotrauma, 234–251
arteriography, 247–249
computed tomography, 243
head injury, 243–246
spinal cord injury, 246–247
digital subtraction angiography,
249–250
plain film radiography, 234–242
head injury, 234–235
spinal cord injury, 235–243
ultrasound, 250–251
brain death, 257–259
contrast media, 232–234
intrathecal agents, 233–234
intravenous agents, 232–233
intraoperative, 251–252
nonacute neurotrauma, 252–257
head injury, 252, 253
magnetic resonance imaging,
254–257
myelography, 253–254
spinal cord injury, 252
radiological diagnosis, 228–232

Diazepam, in neurodiagnosis, 272
Diffuse axonal injury, 342–344
Digital subtraction angiography, 249–250
Disability, prehospital assessment, 9
Distribution, of infused fluids, 194–197
Diuresis, fluid balance, and diabetes inspidus, 527–528
Documentation, prehospital anesthesia, 36–39
Doll's eyes. *See* Oculocephalic response
Dopamine, extraneuronal, 159–160

EEG. *See* Elecroencephalogram
Electroencephalogram
  brain death and, 508–509
  in CNS monitoring, 441–447
    aperiodic analysis, 444–445
    bi-spectral analysis of EEG, 445–447
    spectral analysis of EEG, 443–446
Electrolytes
  balance, 528
  parenteral nutrition formula, 387–388
Electrophysiological CNS monitoring, 439–447
  electroencephalogram, 441–447
    aperiodic analysis, 444–445
    bi-spectral analysis of EEG, 445–447
    spectral analysis of EEG, 443–446
  evoked potentials, 439–441
    brain stem auditory-evoked potentials, 441–443
    motor-evoked potentials, 441
    somatosensory-evoked potential, 439–440
Endotracheal intubation, emergency, 131–135
Enteral nutrition, 392–395
  access, 392–393
  complications, 394–395
  formulas, 393–394
    caloric distribution, 394
    calories, 393
    fiber content, 394
    osmolarity, 394
    protein content, 393–394
Enzymatic quenching, of free radicals, 177–178
Epidural hematoma
  with closed hed injury, 345
  intraoperative anesthesia, 293
Etomidate, 420
  brain protection, 169–170
  closed head injury, 123–124
  intraoperative use of, 301

Europe, system of interhospital transport in, 62–64
Evoked potentials
  brain death, 509–510
  electrophysiological CNS monitoring, 439–441
    brain stem auditory-evoked potentials, 441–443
    motor-evoked potentials, 441
    somatosensory-evoked potential, 439–440
Excitatory amino acids, 156–158
  antagonists, 172–173
Exposure, prehospital assessment, 9
Extremity injuries, rehabilitation, 463–476
  lower extremity, 470–476
  upper extremity, 464–470
Extrication, of patient, prehospital anesthesia, 18–22

Failed intubation alternatives, combitube, 144–145
Family, uncooperative, brain death, 512
Fiber content, enteral nutrition formula, 394
Fixed-wing aircraft, for interhospital transport, 52–53
Flail chest, ventilation, in resuscitation, 78–79
Fluid management, 189–226
  administration, 217–220
    monitoring, 219–220
    volume, 217–219
  advances in, 408–412
  colloidal solutions, 201
    albumin, 201
  crystalloid solutions, 191, 197–200
    hypertonic solutions, 198–200
    hypotonic solutions, 197
    isotonic solutions, 191, 197
  distribution, infused fluids, 194–197
  in head-injured patient, 203–216
    colloid osmotic pressure, changing, cerebral effects of, 211–212
    hemodilution, cerebral effects of, 207–211
    hemorrhage, resuscitation
      bi cerebral effects of, 215–216
      cerebral effects, 212–215
    infusion, cerebral effects of, 204–209
    isovolemic hemodilution, cerebral effects of, 207, 209
    osmolality, changing, cerebral effects of, 211–212

physiological principles, 190–197
plasma, 201–202
small volume resuscitation, 410–412
solutions, for intravenous
administration, 197
synthetic colloids, 202
dextrans, 202–203
hetastarch, 202
pentastarch, 202
Fluid replacement, intraoperative,
295–296
Formulation
enteral nutrition, 393–394
caloric distribution, 394
calories, 393
fiber content, 394
osmolarity, 394
protein content, 393–394
parenteral nutrition, 384–388
caloric distribution, 386
caloric requirement, 384, 386
electrolytes, 387–388
mixing, 388
protein requirements, 386–387
trace elements, and vitamins,
387–388
vitamins, 387–388
Free radical
chain reaction, neuronal cell, 162
enzymatic quenching of, 177–178
formation, 161–162
excessive, 161
scavengers, 175–177

GABA. See Gamma-aminobuyric acid
Gamma-aminobutyric acid, 157–159
Gangliosides, 378–379, 418
Gas monitoring, central nervous system,
447
Gastrointestinal tract
changes, during interhospital transport,
50
with spinal cord injury, 375–377
Glucose homeostasis, with closed head
injury, 355–356
Glutamate antagonists, 414–415
NMDA receptor antagonist, 414–415
non-NMDA receptor blockers, 415
GMM2, 413–414
Goals, prehospital anesthesia, 3–7
Ground ambulance, for interhospital
transport, 51–52

Hangman's fracture. See Spondylolishesis
of axis

Head injury. See also Closed head injury
with chest injury, resuscitation, 87–89
closed, 350–357
airway management, 121–138
anesthetic induction agents,
122–129
adjunctive therapy, 128–129
barbiturates, 122–123
benzodiazepines, 127–128
etomidate, 123–124
ketamine, 125
muscle relaxants, 126–127
opioids, 125–126
propofol, 124–125
patient management, 129–133
endotracheal intubation,
emergency, 131–135
patient profile, 135–138
hemodynamically stable
patient, 135–137
hemodynamically unstable
patient, 137–138
barbiturate coma, 351–352
brain death, declaration of, 359–360,
499–538
cerebral hemodynamics, 350–353
classification, 342
complications, 357–359
diabetes insipidus, 358
selection, 357–358
syndrome of inappropriate
antidiuretic hormone, 359
critical care management, 341–364
diffuse axonal injury, 342–344
hematoma space-occupying lesion,
344–346
epidural hematoma, 345
subarachnoid hemorrhage, 345
subdural hematoma, 344–345
incidence, 341
induced hypothermia, 352–353
intraoperative anesthesia, 291–306
anesthetic care, 297–303
emergence, 303
inhalation agents, 297–299
desflurane, 298–299
isoflurance, 297–298
nitrous oxide, 299
intracranial hypertension control,
293–297
fluid replacement, 295–296
steroid administration, 295
intravenous agents, 299–302
barbiturates, 299

benzodiazepines, 301
etomidate, 301
ketamine, 300
muscle relaxants, 301–302
opioids, 299–300
propofol, 300–301
monitoring, 303–304
types of head injuries, 292–293
brain coverings, injury to, 292
epidural hematoma, 293
intracerebral hematoma, 293
missile injuries, 292
subdural hematoma, 293
mannitol, 351
poor outcome, causes of, 342
positional changes, 352
resuscitation, 85, 346–350
airway, 346–347
cardiovascular system, 347–350
without herniation syndrome,
85–86
sepsis prevention, 353–357
antibiotics, 355
glucose homeostasis, 355–356
nutritional support, 355–377
pneumonia, 353–354
septicemia, 354
tube feeding regimes, 356–357
urinary tract infection, 354
types of injuries, 341–346
computed tomography, 243–246
diagnostic imaging, 252, 253
fluid management, 203–216
hemodilution, cerebral effects of,
207–211
hemorrhage
and resuscitation, cerebral effects,
212–216
resuscitation and, cerebral effects
of, 212, 213
infusion, cerebral effects of, 204–209
isovolemic hemodilution, cerebral
effects of, 207, 209
osmolality, changing, cerebral effects
of, 211–212
intrahospital resuscitation, 95–120
airway control, 101–104
assessment, initial, 99–109
cervical spine stabilization, 101–104
hemodynamic management, 105–109
intensive care unit, transfer to, 117
intracranial pressure, control of, 116
monitoring, in resuscitation room,
115–116

operating room, transfer to, 117
other injuries, evaluation of, 112–115
prehospital communications, 96–98
prioritization of care, 109–112
secondary injury, prevention of,
99–101
secondary survey, 109–115
trauma team, set-up of, 98–100
ventilatory management, 104–105
nonacute neurotrauma, 252–253
nutritional care after, 395–398
plain film radiography, 234–235
types of, intraoperative anesthesia,
292–293
brain coverings, injury to, 292
epidural hematoma, 293
intracerebral hematoma, 293
missile injuries, 292
subdural hematoma, 293
Helmet removal, 23, 24–25
Hematoma
epidural, 345
intraoperative anesthesia, 293
intracerebral, intraoperative anesthesia,
293
space-occupying lesion, 344–346
subarachnoid hemorrhage, 345
subdural, 344–345
intraoperative anesthesia, 293
Hemodilution
cerebral effects of, 207–211. *See also*
Fluid managemen
isovolemic, cerebral effects of, 207, 209
Hemodynamic management, in
intrahospital resuscitation,
with head injury, 105–109
Hemodynamic stabilization, before
interhospital transport, 56–58
Hemodynamic support, in resuscitation,
79–85
abdominal bleeding, 81–82
cardiac tamponade, 83–84
extremity bleeding, 82–83
intrathoracic bleeding, 80–81
myocardial injury, 84–85
retroperitoneal bleeding, 82
Hemodynamically stable patient, closed
head injury, 135–137
Hemodynamically unstable patient, closed
head injury, 137–138
Hemorrhage, resuscitation and, cerebral
effects, 212–216
Herniation syndrome, resuscitation, 86
Hetastarch, 202

History, of patient, resuscitation and, 72–73
Hormonal changes and lactate production, 519–520
Hypertension, intracranial, 26–27
intraoperative control, 293–297
Hypothermia, 165–167
induced, with closed head injury, 352–353
mechanisms of protection, 165–166
outcome studies, 166–167

ICP. *See* Inracranial pressure
Imaging, diagnostic, 227–268
acute neurotrauma, 234–251
arteriography, 247–249
computed tomography, 243
head injury, 243–246
spinal cord injury, 246–247
digital subtraction angiography, 249–250
plain film radiography, 234–242
head injury, 234–235
spinal cord injury, 235–243
ultrasound, 250–251
brain death, 257–259
contrast media, 232–234
intrathecal agents, 233–234
intravenous agents, 232–233
intraoperative, 251–252
nonacute neurotrauma, 252–257
head injury, 252, 253
magnetic resonance imaging, 254–257
myelography, 253–254
spinal cord injury, 252
radiological diagnosis, 228–232
Immobilization, of patient, prehospital, 18–22
Inappropriate antidiuretic hormone, syndrome of, 359
Incidence, closed head injury, 341
Induced hypothermia, with closed head injury, 352–353
Infusion, fluid, cerebral effects, 204–209
Inhalation agents, intraoperative, 297–299
desflurane, 298–299
isoflurance, 297–298
nitrous oxide, 299
Initial assessment, for prehospital anesthesia, 7–13
Initial resuscitation, 69–93
Intensive care unit, transfer to, after intrahospital resuscitation, with head injury, 117

Interhospital transport, 47–67
critical care, during transport, 60–61
evaluation, pretransport, 54
neurological assessment, 54
vital function assessment, 54
indications for, 47–48
life-threatening injuries, untreated, detection of, 55
modes of, 51–54
aircraft, fixed-wing, 52–53
ambulance, ground, 51–52
rotocraft, 53–54
monitoring, during transport, 59–60
pathophysiology, 48–51
cardiovascular changes, 48–49
gastrointestinal changes, 50
metabolic changes, 50
movement, physiological changes secondary to, 50–51
respiratory changes, 49–50
thermoregulation, 50
stabilization, pretransport, 55–59
hemodynamic stabilization, 56–58
intracranial pressure, increased, treatment of, 58–59
respiratory status stabilization, 55–57
system organization, 61–63
in Europe, 62–64
in United States, 61–62
Intracellular calcium accumulation, 160–161
Intracerebral hematoma, intraoperative anesthesia, 293
Intracranial hypertension, 26–27
intraoperative control, 293–297
fluid replacement, 295–296
steroid administration, 295
Intracranial pressure, 406–408
increased, treatment of, before interhospital transport, 58–59
in intrahospital resuscitation, with head injury, 116
monitoring, 436–437
Intrahospital resuscitation, head injury, 95–120
airway control, 101–104
assessment, initial, 99–109
cervical spine stabilization, 101–104
hemodynamic management, 105–109
intensive care unit, transfer to, 117
intracranial pressure, control of, 116
monitoring, in resuscitation room, 115–116
operating room, transfer to, 117

other injuries, evaluation of, 112–115
prehospital communications, 96–98
prioritization of care, 109–112
secondary injury, prevention of, 99–101
secondary survey, 109–115
trauma team, set-up of, 98–99
ventilatory management, 104–105
Intraoperative diagnostic imaging, 251–252
Intraoperative management, 523–529
  closed head injury, 291–306
    anesthetic care, 297–303
    emergence, 303
    inhalation agents, 297–299
      desflurane, 298–299
      isoflurance, 297–298
      nitrous oxide, 299
    intracranial hypertension control, 293–297
      fluid replacement, 295–296
      steroid administration, 295
    intravenous agents, 299–302
      barbiturates, 299
      benzodiazepines, 301
      etomidate, 301
      ketamine, 300
      muscle relaxants, 301–302
      opioids, 299–300
      propofol, 300–301
    monitoring, 303–304
    types of head injuries, 292–293
      brain coverings, injury to, 292
      epidural hematoma, 293
      intracerebral hematoma, 293
      missile injuries, 292
      subdural hematoma, 293
  spinal cord injury, 307–340
    anesthetic management, 330–333
    articulations, 310, 312–314
    cervical spine, 315–316
      anatomy, 309–316
      upper, 310–313
    cervical vertebrae, lower, 312, 313
    epidemiology, spinal cord injury, 308–309
    injuries, mechanisms of, 316–322
      altas, fractures of, 318
      atlanto-occipital dislocations, 316–317
      axis, traumatic spondylolisthesis of, 320–321
      C$_1$-C complex, injuries to, 317
      lower cervical fractures, dislocations, 321–322

odontoid fractures, 318–320
penetrating injuries, cervical spine, 322–327
transaxial cervicomedullary injury, 318
kinematics, cervical spine, 314–315
ligaments, cervical spine, 310, 312–314
pathophysiology, 322–327
resuscitative modalities, 327–330
stability, cervical spine, 315–316
Intrathecal contrast agents, 233–234
Intravenous agents, 232–233, 299–302
  barbiturates, 299
  benzodiazepines, 301
  etomidate, 301
  ketamine, 300
  muscle relaxants, 301–302
  opioids, 299–300
  propofol, 300–301
Intravenous solutions, fluid management, 197
Intubation, 141–143
  awake, 142–143
  Bullard laryngoscope, 143
  direct laryngoscopy, 142
  failed, alternatives, 144–145
    combitube, 144–145
    cricothyroidotomy, 145
    laryngeal mask airway, 144
Ischemic neuronal damage, 153–156
Isoflurane, 171, 297–298
Isovolemic hemodilution, cerebral effects of, 207, 209

Ketamine, 421
  closed head injury, 125
  intraoperative use of, 300
  in neurodiagnosis, 274
Kinematics, cervical spine, 314–315

Laryngeal mask airway, as failed intubation alternative, 144
Laryngoscope, Bullard, 143
Laryngoscopy, direct, 142
Lazaroids, 414
Legal principles, certification, of brain death, 511
Life-threatening injuries, untreated, detection of, before interhospital transport, 55
Ligaments, cervical spine, 310, 312–314
Lipid antioxidants, 175–177
LMA. See Laryngeal mask airway
Lorazepam, in neurodiagnosis, 272

Magnetic resonance imaging, 276–285
  anesthetic techniques, 279–284
  critically ill patient, 284–285
  head injury, 254–257
  monitoring, 278–280
  nonacute neurotrauma, 254–257
Mannitol
  with closed head injury, 351
  prehospital, 26–27
Maxillofacial injury, and chest injury,
    resuscitation, 89–90
Mechanisms, spinal cord injuries,
    316–322
  altas, fractures of, 318
  atlanto-occipital dislocations, 316–317
  axis, traumatic spondylolisthesis of,
    320–321
  C_1-C complex, injuries to, 317
  lower cervical fractures, dislocations,
    321–322
  odontoid fractures, 318–320
  penetrating injuries, cervical spine,
    322–327
  transaxial cervicomedullary injury, 318
Medical examiner cases, brain death,
    511–512
Metabolic changes, during interhospital
    transport, 50
Metabolic monitoring, central nervous
    system, 447
  jugular venous oxygen saturation,
    447–448
  near-infrared spectroscopy, 448–450
Methohexital, in neurodiagnosis, 274
Midazolam, in neurodiagnosis, 272, 274
Missile injuries, intraoperative anesthesia,
    292
Mixing, parenteral nutrition formula, 388
Monitoring, 523–524
  of central nervous system, 435–456
  during interhospital transport, 59–60
  in intrahospital resuscitation, with head
    injury, 115–116
  prehospital, 29–31
Morphine sulfate, in neurodiagnosis, 272
Motor-evoked potentials,
    electrophysiological CNS
    monitoring, 441
Movement, physiological changes
    secondary to, 50–51
Muscle relaxants
  closed head injury, 126–127
  intraoperative use of, 301–302
Myelography, 253–254
  head injury, 253–254

N-methyl-D-aspartate. See NMDA
Naloxone, 417–418
Nasotracheal intubation, 143
Neurodiagnostic evaluation, anesthesia,
    269–289
  angiography, 285–288
  computed tomography, 270–276
    pediatric patient, 273–276
    traumatized patient, 270–273
  future developments, 287–288
  magnetic resonance imaging, 276–285
    anesthetic techniques, 279–284
    critically ill patient, 284–285
    monitoring, 278–280
  role of, 269–270
Neurological assessment
  before interhospital transport, 54
  prehospital, 9–13
Neurological trauma, prehospital
    anesthetic management, 1–45
  anesthesia, induction of, 27–29
  anesthesiologists, in field, 32–36
  assignment, 35–37
  documentation, 36–39
  goals of, 3–7
  initial assessment, 7–13
    neurological assessment, 9–13
    primary survey, 7–9
      airway, 8
      breathing, 8
      cervical spine, 8
      circulation, 8–9
      disability, 9
      exposure, 9
    resuscitation phase, 9
    scoring, 9–13
  monitoring, prehospital, 29–31
  neurological injury, signs of, 4–7
  patient transportation, 31–32
  personnel, 32–36
  primary injury, vs. secondary injury, 1–3
  procedures, 13–27
    airway management, 13–15
    circulatory resuscitation, 15–18
    exposure, 23–25
    extrication, 18–22
    helmet removal, 23–25
    immobilization, 18–22
    intracranial hypertension, 26–27
    mannitol, 26–27
    spinal cord injury, 23–26
  quality assurance, 36–39
  triage, 35–37
  vehicles, 33–35

Neuronal cell pathophysiology
  brain protection, pharmacological,
      165–178
    anesthetic agents, 167–171
      barbiturates, 168–169
      etomidate, 169–170
      isoflurane, 171
      propofol, 170–171
    calcium channel blockers, 173–174
    excitatory amino acid antagonists,
        172–173
    free radicals
      enzymatic quenching of, 177–178
      scavengers, 175–177
    hypothermia, 165–167
      mechanisms of protection,
          165–166
      outcome studies with hypothermia,
          166–167
    nitric oxide synthase manipulation,
        174–175
  free radicals
    chain reaction, 162
    formation, 161–162
      excessive, 161
  intracellular calcium accumulation,
      160–161
  ischemic neuronal damage, 153–156
  lipid antioxidants, 175–177
  neurotransmitter release, 156–160
    dopamine, extraneuronal, 159–160
    excitatory amino acids, 156–158
    gamma-aminobutyric acid, 157–159
  nitric oxide, 162–164
    neurotransmitter release, modulation
        of, 163–164
    regulation of cerebral blood flow by,
        162–163
  reperfusion, 161–162
    cerebrovascular instability, 161
Neuronal function studies, brain death,
    508–510
  evoked potentials, 509–510
Neuronal injury, after trauma,
    pathophysiology of, 164–165
Neurotransmitter release, 156–160
  dopamine, extraneuronal, 159–160
Ninth cranial nerve function, brain death
    and, 506
Nitric oxide, 162–164
  intraoperative use of, 299
  neurotransmitter release, modulation
      of, 163–164
  regulation of cerebral blood flow by,
      162–163
  synthase manipulation, 174–175

NMDA receptor antagonist, 414–415
NO. See Niric oxide
Nutritional care, after neurotrauma,
    383–403
  closed head injury, 355–377
  enteral nutrition, 392–395
    access, 392–393
    complications, 394–395
    formulas, 393–394
      caloric distribution, 394
      calories, 393
      fiber content, 394
      osmolarity, 394
      protein content, 393–394
  head trauma, 395–398
  parenteral nutrition, 384–392
    access, 391–392
    complications, 389–390
    formulation, 384–388
      caloric distribution, 386
      caloric requirement, 384, 386
      electrolytes, 387–388
      mixing, 388
      protein requirements, 386–387
      trace elements, and vitamins,
          387–388
      vitamins, 387–388
    indications, 384
    monitoring, 388–389
    peripheral, 391
  spinal cord trauma, 398–400

Oculocephalic responses, brain death
    and, 506
Oculovestibular response, brain death
    and, 506
Odontoid fractures, 318–320
Operating room, transfer to, after
    intrahospital resuscitation,
    with head injury, 117
Opioids, 421–424
  closed head injury, 125–126
  intraoperative use of, 299–300
  in neurodiagnosis, 272
Organ donor management, in intensive
    care unit, 513–520
Organ procurement, 520
  from donors with brain death, 520–529
Osmolality, changing, cerebral effects of,
    211–212
Outlying areas, transport of patient from,
    90–91

Pain
  effects of, 459–460
  management of, 460–461
Parenteral nutrition, 384–392
  access, 391–392
  complications, 389–390
  formulation, 384–388
    caloric distribution, 386
    caloric requirement, 384, 386
    electrolytes, 387–388
    mixing, 388
    protein requirements, 386–387
    trace elements, and vitamins,
        387–388
    vitamins, 387–388
  indications, 384
  monitoring, 388–389
  peripheral, 391
Patient history, resuscitation and, 72–73
Patient transportation, prehospital, 31–32
Pediatric patient, computed tomography,
    273–276
Penetrating injuries, cervical spine,
    322–327
Pentastarch, 202
Pentobarbital, in neurodiagnosis, 274
Perioperative management, 69–93
Peripheral parenteral nutrition, 391
Personnel, for prehospital anesthesia,
    32–36
Physical examination, brain death, 502
Physiology
  brain death process, 513–516
  fluid resuscitation, 190–197
Plain film radiography, 234–242
  head injury, 234–235
  spinal cord injury, 235–243
Plasma, fluid management, 201–202
Pneumonia, with closed head injury,
    353–354
Pneumothorax, tension, in resuscitation,
    78
Poikilothermia, 518
Polyuria, 518–519
Positional changes, with closed head
    injury, 352
Pregnancy, brain death, 512–513
Prehospital airway management, 13–15
Prehospital anesthetic management, 1–45
  anesthesia, induction of, 27–29
  anesthesiologists, in field, 32–36
  assignment, 35–36
  documentation, 36–39
  goals of, 3–7

initial assessment, 7–13
  neurological assessment, 9–13
  primary survey, 7–9
    airway, 8
    breathing, 8
    cervical spine, 8
    circulation, 8–9
    disability, 9
    exposure, 9
  resuscitation phase, 9
  scoring, 9–13
monitoring, prehospital, 29–31
neurological injury, signs of, 4–7
patient transportation, 31–32
personnel, 32–36
primary injury, vs. secondary injury, 1–3
procedures, 13–27
  airway management, 13–15
  circulatory resuscitation, 15–18
  exposure, 23–25
  extrication, 18–22
  helmet removal, 23–25
  immobilization, 18–22
  intracranial hypertension, 26–27
  mannitol, 26–27
  spinal cord injury, 23–26
quality assurance, 36–39
triage, 35–37
vehicles, 33–35
Prehospital communications, in
        intrahospital resuscitation,
        with head injury, 96–98
Preparation for procurement, 520–523
Primary neurological injury, vs. secondary
        injury, prehospital anesthesia,
        1–3
Priorities, in resuscitation, 86–87
Prioritization of care, in intrahospital
        resuscitation, with head injury,
        109–112
Propofol, 420–421
  brain protection, 170–171
  closed head injury, 124–125
  intraoperative use of, 300–301
  in neurodiagnosis, 272, 274
Protein
  content, enteral nutrition formula,
        393–394
  requirements, parenteral nutrition
        formula, 386–387
Pupillary light reflex, brain death and,
        506

Quality assurance, prehospital, 36–39

Radical scavengers, 416–417
Radiological diagnosis, 228–232
Rehabilitation, 457–497
    central nervous system trauma, 482–488
        contracture
            pathophysiology, 487–488
            therapeutic approaches, 488
        spasticity
            pathophysiology, 483–484
            therapeutic approaches, 484–487
    extremity injuries, 463–476
        lower extremity, 470–476
        upper extremity, 464–470
    injury, pathophysiology of, 459–462
        pain
            effects of, 459–460
            management, 460–461
            regional anesthesia techniques, role
                of, 461–462
        regional anesthesia approaches, specific
            injuries, 462–463
        role of, 458–459
    thoracic injuries, approaches to,
        476–482
Reperfusion, 161–162
    cerebrovascular instability, 161
Respiratory changes, during interhospital
    transport, 49–50
Respiratory complications, with spinal
    cord injury, 372–375
Respiratory failure, 517–518
Respiratory status stabilization, before
    interhospital transport, 55–57
Resuscitation, 85–86, 90–91
    airway, 74–77
        consciousness, level of, 75–76
        obstruction, 76
    anesthetic management, 90–91
    cervical spine injury, 327–330
    chest
        head, combined, 87–89
        maxillofacial and, injury, 89–90
    circulatory, prehospital, 15–18
    closed head injury, 85, 346–350
        airway, 346–347
        cardiovascular system, 347–350
        without herniation syndrome, 85–86
    epidemiology, 69–72
    head, chest injuries, combined, 87–89
    hemodynamic support, 79–85
        abdominal bleeding, 81–82
        cardiac tamponade, 83–84
        extremity bleeding, 82–83
        intrathoracic bleeding, 80–81

        myocardial injury, 84–85
        retroperitoneal bleeding, 82
    herniation syndrome, 86
    immediate concerns, 74–91
    initial, 69–93
    intrahospital, head injury, 95–120
        airway control, 101–104
        assessment, initial, 99–109
        cervical spine stabilization, 101–104
        hemodynamic management, 105–109
        intensive care unit, transfer to, 117
        intracranial pressure, control of, 116
        monitoring, in resuscitation room,
            115–116
        operating room, transfer to, 117
        other injuries, evaluation of, 112–115
        prehospital communications, 96–98
        prioritization of care, 109–112
        secondary injury, prevention of,
            99–101
        secondary survey, 109–115
        trauma team, set-up of, 98–100
        ventilatory management, 104–105
    management, immediate, 72–91
    maxillofacial, and chest, injury, 89–90
    neurogenic hypotension, 85
    patient history, 72–73
    priorities, 86–87
    recognition, 72–73
    tension pneumothorax, 78
    tracheal disruption, 76–77
    ventilation, 77–78
    transport, to outlying areas, 90–91
    ventilation
        flail chest, 78–79
        open pneumothorax, 78
        pulmonary contusion, 78–79
Rotocraft, for interhospital transport,
    53–54

Scoring, neurological, prehospital, 9–13
Sepsis prevention, closed head injury,
    353–357
    antibiotics, 355
    glucose homeostasis, 355–356
    nutritional support, 355–377
    pneumonia, 353–354
    septicemia, 354
    tube feeding regimes, 356–357
    urinary tract infection, 354
Septicemia, with closed head injury, 354
SIADH. See Syndrome of inappropriae
    anidiureic hormone
Signs, of neurological injury, 4–7

Skin, spinal cord injury and, 377
Small volume resuscitation, 410–412
Somatosensory-evoked potential,
          electrophysiological CNS
          monitoring, 439–440
Spectral analysis, electroencephalogram,
          443–446
Spinal cord injury, 365–381
    airway management, 367–370
    computed tomography, 246–247
    diagnostic imaging, 252
    epidemiology, 308–309, 365–366
    gastrointestinal tract, 375–377
    general management, 366–377
    intraoperative management, 307–340
       anesthetic management, 330–333
       articulations, 310, 312–314
       cervical spine, 315–316
          anatomy, 309–316
          upper, 310–313
       cervical vertebrae, lower, 312, 313
       epidemiology, spinal cord injury,
          308–309
       injuries, mechanisms of, 316–322
          altas, fractures of, 318
          atlanto-occipital dislocations,
             316–317
          axis, traumatic spondylolisthesis of,
             320–321
          C_1-C complex, injuries to, 317
          lower cervical fractures,
             dislocations, 321–322
          odontoid fractures, 318–320
          penetrating injuries, cervical spine,
             322–327
          transaxial cervicomedullary injury,
             318
       kinematics, cervical spine, 314–315
       ligaments, cervical spine, 310,
          312–314
       pathophysiology, 322–327
       resuscitative modalities, 327–330
       stability, cervical spine, 315–316
    new therapies, 378–379
       gangliosides, 378–379
       steroids, 378
    nutritional care after, 398–400
    plain film radiography, 235–243
    prehospital anesthesia, 23–26
    respiratory complications, 372–375
    skin, 377
    spinal shock, 370–372
    urinary tract, 377
Spinal shock, with spinal cord injury,
          370–372

Spondylolisthesis of axis, 320–321
    traumatic, 320–321
Stability, cervical spine, 315–316
Stabilization
    cervical spine, in intrahospital
          resuscitation, with head injury,
          101–104
    before interhospital transport, 55–59
Steroid administration, intraoperative, 295
Steroids, 378, 412–413
Subarachnoid hemorrhage, with closed
          hed injury, 345
Subdural hematoma, 344–345
    with closed hed injury, 344–345
    intraoperative anesthesia, 293
Sympathetic nervous system modulators,
          419–420
Syndrome of inappropriate antidiuretic
          hormone, 359
Synthetic colloids, fluid management, 202
    dextrans, 202–203
    hetastarch, 202
    pentastarch, 202
System of interhospital transport,
          organization of, 61–63

TCD monitoring. See Transcranial doppler
          monioring
Temperature regulation, 527
Tension pneumothorax, in resuscitation,
          78
Tenth cranial nerve function, brain death
          and, 506
Termination of anesthesia, 529
Thermoregulation, during interhospital
          transport, 50
Thoracic injuries, rehabilitation, 476–482
Thyrotropin-releasing hormone, 417–418
Tracheal disruption, resuscitation and,
          76–77
    ventilation, 77–78
Transaxial cervicomedullary injury, 318
Transcranial doppler monitoring, cerebral
          blood flow, 437–438
Transport
    interhospital, 47–67
       critical care, during transport, 60–61
       evaluation, pretransport, 54
          neurological assessment, 54
          vital function assessment, 54
       indications for, 47–48
       life-threatening injuries, untreated,
          detection of, 55
       modes of, 51–54

aircraft, fixed-wing, 52–53
ambulance, ground, 51–52
rotocraft, 53–54
monitoring, during transport, 59–60
pathophysiology, 48–51
cardiovascular changes, 48–49
gastrointestinal changes, 50
metabolic changes, 50
movement, physiological changes
secondary to, 50–51
respiratory changes, 49–50
thermoregulation, 50
stabilization, pretransport, 55–59
hemodynamic stabilization, 56–58
intracranial pressure, increased,
treatment of, 58–59
respiratory status stabilization,
55–57
system organization, 61–63
in Europe, 62–64
in United States, 61–62
from outlying areas, 90–91
prehospital, 31–32
Trauma team, set-up of, in intrahospital
resuscitation, 98–100
TRH. See Thyroropin-releasing hormone
Triage, prehospital, 35–37

Tube feeding regimes, with closed head
injury, 356–357

Ultrasound, 250–251
United States, system of interhospital
transport in, 61–62
Untreated life-threatening injuries,
detection of, before
interhospital transport, 55
Urinary tract
closed head injury and, 354
spinal cord injury and, 377

Vehicles, usage of, prehospital, 33–35
Ventilation
flail chest, in resuscitation, 78–79
in intrahospital resuscitation, with head
injury, 104–105
in resuscitation
open pneumothorax, 78
pulmonary contusion, 78–79
Vital function assessment, before
interhospital transport, 54
Volatile agents, 424–425

Xenon washout, cerebral blood flow, 439